Heart Disease in Primary Care

Heart Disease in Primary Care

EDITOR
Michael L. Hess, M.D.
Chairman
Division of Cardiopulmonary Labs and Research
Professor of Internal Medicine
Division of Cardiology
Virginia Commonwealth University
Medical College of Virginia
Richmond, Virginia

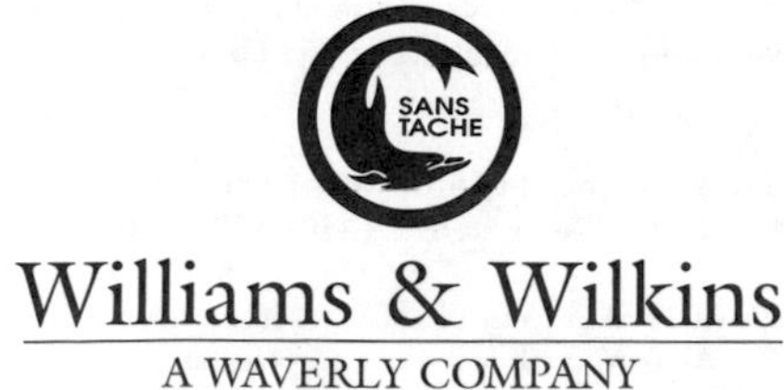

Williams & Wilkins
A WAVERLY COMPANY
BALTIMORE • PHILADELPHIA • LONDON • PARIS • BANGKOK
BUENOS AIRES • HONG KONG • MUNICH • SYDNEY • TOKYO • WROCLAW

Editor: Timothy Hiscock
Managing Editor: Leah Ann Kiehne Hayes
Marketing Manager: Daniell Griffin
Production Editor: June Choe

351 West Camden Street
Baltimore, Maryland 21201-2436 USA

Rose Tree Corporate Center
1400 North Providence Road
Building II, Suite 5025
Media, Pennsylvania 19063-2043 USA

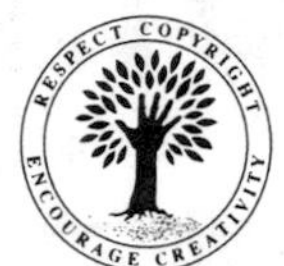

Printed in the United States of America

Library of Congress Cataloging-in-Publication Data

Heart disease in primary care / editor, Michael L. Hess ; associate editor, Andrea Hastillo.
p. cm.
Includes bibliographical references and index.
ISBN 0-683-03988-1
1. Cardiovascular system—Diseases. 2. Primary care (Medicine) I. Hess, Michael L. II. Hastillo, Andrea.
[DNLM: 1. Heart Diseases—diagnosis. 2. Heart Diseases-therapy. 3. Vascular Diseases—diagnosis. 4. Vascular Diseases—therapy. 5. Primary Health Care—methods. WG 210 H4347 1999]
RC667.H433 1999
616.1—dc21
DNLM/DLC
for Library of Congress
98-3520
CIP

To purchase additional copies of this book, call our customer service department at **(800) 638-0672** or fax orders to **(800) 447-8438.** For other book services, including chapter reprints and large quantity sales, ask for the Special Sales department.

Canadian customers should call **(800) 665-1148,** or fax **(800) 665-0103.** For all other calls originating outside of the United States, please call **(410) 528-4223** or fax us at **(410) 528-8550.**

Visit Williams & Wilkins on the Internet: **http://www.wwilkins.com** or contact our customer service department at **custserv@wwilkins.com.** Williams & Wilkins customer service representatives are available from 8:30 am to 6:00 pm, EST, Monday through Friday, for telephone access.

99 00 01 02 03
1 2 3 4 5 6 7 8 9 10

This book is dedicated to the spirit of Sir William Osler and the great tall timbers of Medicine that followed. It was Osler who recognized the importance of the combination of teaching, patient care and knowledge. Teaching, not only at the bedside and in the lecture hall, but in the written word. A man who sat down and wrote in long hand the first comprehensive textbook of Medicine truly deserves the title of the Father of American Medicine. To the late Dr. Jack Myers who demanded excellence and intellectual discipline, which combined with his fiery personality, created a legend in his time. To Jim Leonard who has taught generations of physicians the skills and art of cardiac physical diagnosis. To Douglas Chamberlain once the Senior Registrar in Cardiology at St. Bartholomew's and now recently retired president of the British Cardiac Society—undoubtedly—the best bedside physical diagnostician I have ever met. To F. Norman Briggs, Ph.D., a physiologist supreme, who introduced me to the cardiac cell and a career in the intellectual pursuit of the mysteries of the beating heart. And finally to Dr. Bob and Bill W. who suggested the steps to take that are so necessary to be able to work with a clear and bright mind and offered me the tools to accomplish this task. It is to the legacy of these men that this book is dedicated so that our patients can and will receive better high quality medical care.

Preface

History will record many fundamental changes in American society during the last decade of the twentieth century. One of the most important changes is a restructuring of our model for the delivery of medical care and the placing of the primary care team at the center of this model. Whether it be a health maintenance organization, a large multidisciplinary group, a corporate entity, a solo or group practice, the primary care physicians and their team have been asked to see more patients and assume more responsibility. In the world of adult medicine, cardiovascular-related disease still is the leading cause of morbidity and mortality in the western world. Sixty percent of all patients seen by the primary care physicians will have cardiovascular disease contributing to their clinical problems. Finally, compounding this problem for the primary care team is a knowledge base of cardiovascular medicine that exceeds all other medical disciplines.

With this background Dr. Hess and his co-authors have written a textbook of Cardiovascular Medicine for the primary care physician, nurse, and nurse practitioner. This is not another encyclopedia of Cardiovascular Medicine but rather an organized presentation of the problem as presented, with a brief discussion of pathophysiology, recommendations for appropriate diagnostic modalities, and finally therapeutic recommendations.

A great deal of emphasis is placed on clinical pharmacology and cost effectiveness of diagnostic and therapeutic tools: problems that the primary care team must face on a daily basis. It is hoped that this book will become a well-worn addition in the many offices, nursing stations, and examining rooms where you, the primary care provider will be fighting your battles.

MICHAEL L. HESS

Acknowledgments

This book was dedicated to a bunch of "Grumpy Old Men," but the real credit belongs to two outstanding women. A heart felt thank you to Leah Hayes—my managing editor at Williams & Wilkins—Leah—you have the patience of Job—putting up with this writer for a year while he tried to complete the book in the middle of the chaos and turmoil of Academic Medicine.

To Dr. Andrea Hastillo—friend and colleague—who designed the intent and flow based on her superb course in Cardiovascular Medicine at the Medical College of Virginia. She then turned around and wrote four chapters in her usual, excellent style. Again Andrea, thank you for your help. A heart felt thank you to my fellow authors who are really my friends and colleagues in the Cardiology division at Virginia Commonwealth University. They all work with a large number of primary care physicians and nurses. They know the problems, know what has to be learned, and are excellent teachers. A special thanks to Bill Moskowitz in Pediatric Cardiology for his input and knowledge, in Pediatrics and Adolescent Cardiology, to Yves Janin, Senior Fellow in Cardiology in our program for his hidden talent in writing the English language—his chapters probably would have been masterpieces if written in French and to my friend and colleague Dave Propert at Eastern Virginia School of Medicine for his life long dedication to teaching the History and Physical Exam. Finally, a special thank you to Carol Gaithwright and Sylvia Converse for their excellent typing, editing, and communication skills. Thank you, Sylvia, for your dry, keen sense of humor that helps to keep me sane.

From the bottom of my heart—Thank you one and all.

MICHAEL L. HESS, M.D.

Acknowledgments

Contributors

James A. Arrowood, M.D., F.A.C.C.
Assistant Professor of Internal Medicine
Division of Cardiology
Director, A.D. Williams Cardiology Clinic
Virginia Commonwealth University
Medical College of Virginia
Richmond, Virginia

Henry F. Clemo, M.D., Ph.D.
Assistant Professor of Internal Medicine and Physiology
Division of Cardiology
Virginia Commonwealth University
Medical College of Virginia
Richmond, Virginia

Jeffery B. Dattilo, M.D.
Vascular Research Fellow and
Resident in General Surgery
Virginia Commonwealth University
Medical College of Virginia
Richmond, Virginia

Kenneth A. Ellenbogen, M.D., F.A.C.C.
Associate Professor of Internal Medicine
Division of Cardiology
Director, Electrophysiology and Pacing
Virginia Commonwealth University
Medical College of Virginia
McGuire Veterans Affairs Medical Center
Richmond, Virginia

R. Paul Fairman, M.D., F.A.C.P., F.C.C.P.
Professor of Internal Medicine
Division of Pulmonary and Critical Care Medicine
Virginia Commonwealth University
Medical College of Virginia
Richmond, Virginia

David Gilligan, M.D.
Assistant Professor of Internal Medicine
Division of Cardiology
Virginia Commonwealth University
Medical College of Virginia
Richmond, Virginia

Andrea Hastillo, M.D., F.A.C.C.
Associate Professor of Internal Medicine
Division of Cardiology
Virginia Commonwealth University
Medical College of Virginia
Richmond, Virginia

Michael L. Hess, M.D., F.A.C.C.
Professor and Chairman
Division of Cardiology
Cardiopulmonary Labs and Research
Virginia Commonwealth University
Medical College of Virginia
Richmond, Virginia

Yves Janin, M.D.
Medical Resident in Internal Medicine
Division of Cardiology
Virginia Commonwealth University
Medical College of Virginia
Richmond, Virginia

Raymond G. Makhoul, M.D., F.A.C.C.
Associate Professor of Surgery
Chairman, Division of Vascular Surgery
Virginia Commonwealth University
Medical College of Virginia
Richmond, Virginia

Johnny Moore, Rh.P.
Registered Pharmacist
Richmond, Virginia

Carlos A. Morillo, M.D.
Professor of Internal Medicine
Universidad Industrial de Santander
Director, Department of Cardiology and Cardiovascular Sciences
Fundacion Cardiovascular del Oriente Colombiano
Bucaramanga, Santander, Colombia

William B. Moskowitz, M.D., F.A.C.C.
Associate Professor of Pediatrics
Division of Cardiology
Director, Pediatric Cardiac Catheterization Laboratory
Director, Pediatric Heart and Heart Lung Transplantation Program
Children's Medical Center
Virginia Commonwealth University
Medical College of Virginia
Richmond, Virginia

Walter H.J. Paulsen, M.D., F.A.C.C.
Associate Professor of Internal Medicine
Division of Cardiology
Virginia Commonwealth University
Medical College of Virginia
Richmond, Virginia

David B. Propert, M.D., F.A.C.C., F.A.C.P.
Professor of Internal Medicine
Eastern Virginia Medical School
Norfolk, Virginia
Chief, Medical Service
Veterans Affairs Medical Center
Hampton, Virginia

David W. Richardson, M.D., F.A.C.C.
Professor of Internal Medicine, Emeritus
Division of Cardiology
Virginia Commonwealth University
Medical College of Virginia
Richmond, Virginia

Elizabeth B. Ripley, M.D.
Assistant Professor of Internal Medicine
Division of Nephrology
Virginia Commonwealth University
Medical College of Virginia
Richmond, Virginia

Dominic A. Sica, M.D.
Professor of Internal Medicine and Pharmacology
Chairman, Clinical Pharmacology and Hypertension
Virginia Commonwealth University
Medical College of Virginia
Richmond, Virginia

Richard K. Shepard, M.D.
Assistant Professor of Internal Medicine
Division of Cardiology
Virginia Commonwealth University
Medical College of Virginia
Richmond, Virginia

David M. Tolman, M.D., F.A.C.C.
Assistant Professor of Internal Medicine
Division of Cardiology
Medical Director, Heart Failure and Transplant
Virginia Commonwealth University
Medical College of Virginia
Richmond, Virginia

Mark A. Wood, M.D., F.A.C.C.
Associate Professor of Internal Medicine
Division of Cardiology
Virginia Commonwealth University
Medical College of Virginia
Richmond, Virginia

Contents

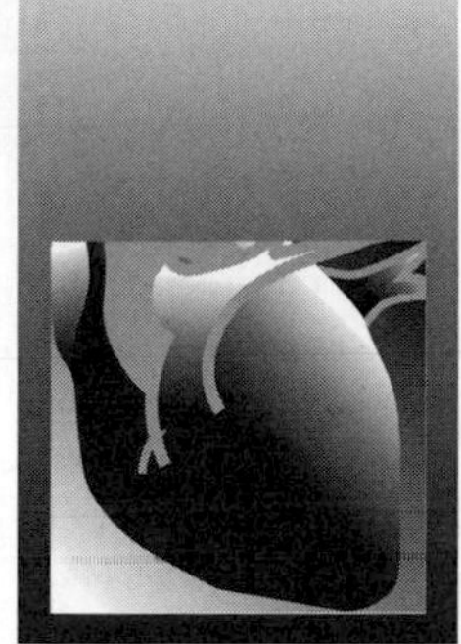

CHAPTER 1

History and Physical Examination

David B. Propert

PREFACE TO CHAPTER 1

This chapter may be the most important chapter in the entire book. Dr. Propert has been a student of bedside diagnosis for more years than he cares to remember. In this chapter he develops a framework and a mindset of the history based on logic and the modern concepts of specificity and sensitivity.

He takes the reader from the symptoms that the patient presents with and then logically leads to a differential diagnosis. He then describes a step-by-step method of physical diagnoses, incorporating the physical findings into the development of an hypothesis. Thus, this chapter is distinctly different from all the chapters that follow, for it is based on the *art* of medicine and is buttressed by the *science* of medicine.

This chapter is essential for all members of the primary care team who evaluate patients with suspected cardiovascular disease. From an economic point of view, Dr. Propert delivers a resounding "no" to the question, "Should all patients with a murmur be referred for echocardiography?" He clearly points out that the examining physician can arrive at a clear and firm diagnosis by using the mind, hand, ears, and stethoscope.

Michael L. Hess, MD, Editor

DIAGNOSTIC PROCESS

When a patient presents with a **problem,** the health provider immediately begins to develop multiple **hypotheses** as to the cause of the problem. In addition, one **ranks** the hypotheses on the basis of highest to lowest probability. This process begins with the initial problem presented by the patient. The diagnostic process (Fig. 1.1) is the method whereby one strengthens or weakens (rules in or rules out) a particular hypothesis until the probability reaches a level at which intervention, or no intervention, is indicated or required.

For example, if a patient presents with chest pain, the physician immediately begins to consider a cardiac or pulmonary problem. Depending on additional information, one may be more specific and consider cardiac pain due to coronary disease or pericarditis. If the patient is a 60-year-old man, the **probability** of coronary disease is high; if the patient is a 13-year-old girl, pericarditis is a more likely diagnosis. Therefore, the probability of a particular diagnosis depends on the age of the patient, character of the pain, and risk factors that are already known or are elicited.

INQUIRY STRATEGY

The **inquiry strategy** includes the history, physical examination, and laboratory testing (blood tests, electrocardiography [ECG], and such imaging methods as radiography and echocardiography). Therapeutic interventions can also be part of the inquiry strategy: for example, does the patient respond to therapy directed at a specific diagnosis? For the diagnostic process to be efficient, timely, accurate, low risk, and low cost, each question to the patient should be directed at a specific hypothesis, and the response (results) should either support or dispute a particular diagnosis.

The inquiry strategy is an iterative process, constantly recycling and revising the ranking and probability level of the different hypotheses. The order in which the physician performs particular parts of the inquiry depends on four factors:

1. Rank of the hypothesis
2. Risk of testing to the patient
3. Cost of testing (monetary value)
4. Risk of diagnosis, that is, possible emergency intervention

For example, if the health care provider suspects an acute myocardial infarction, an ECG should be done immediately because urgent intervention is indicated and is effective in improving outcomes.

A focused history and physical examination are the first parts of the inquiry strategy; when focused on the leading hypotheses, they are effective, quick, and inexpensive and can be done while waiting for the results of

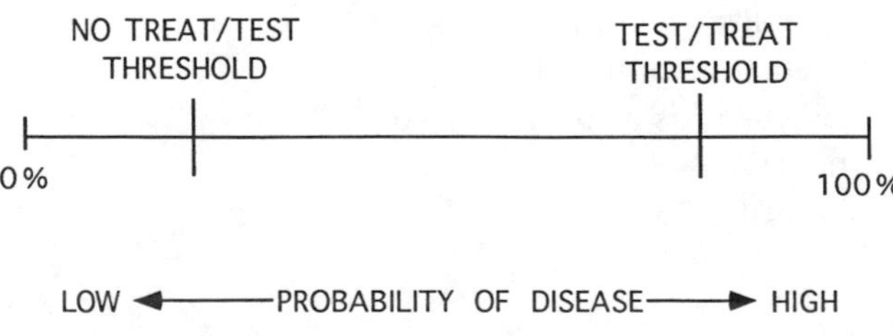

FIGURE 1.1.
Diagram of the clinical problem-solving process.

other tests. A complete history and physical examination should be done for each patient presenting with cardiac distress, which may reveal other problems requiring diagnosis.

Test/Treat Threshold

The diagnostic decision is the most complex decision physicians must make. Associated with that crucial decision is the question of testing for a suspected diagnosis.

Pauker and Kassirer developed the concept of *threshold* (Fig. 1.2) in deciding whether to continue testing or whether to treat or not treat. They define two thresholds of probability for a diagnosis:

1. No test/treat threshold
2. Test/treat threshold

When the probability exceeds the test/treat threshold, the clinician begins treatment, with no further testing. When probability is low enough, treatment is not necessary and no further testing for that diagnosis is needed. One should continually keep these thresholds in mind as a part of the inquiry strategy so that unnecessary testing is not done for patients with either high or low probability of disease.

The limits of these thresholds depends on many factors, including the risk of the abnormality, risk of testing, and risk of therapy. At the test/treat threshold, the probability at which one treats depends on the risk of disease versus withholding treatment and the risk of treatment. For example, in the case of cancer, the health provider should require a probability of 100% through means of a tissue diagnosis before initiating most treatments (surgery, chemotherapy, radiation).

The no test/treat threshold probability depends on

- Risk of disease
- Risks and costs of testing
- Accuracy of the tests (sensitivity and specificity)

For example, in a 25-year-old woman with atypical chest pain, the physician would require a higher probability that the pain may be cardiac before doing an exercise stress test (consider the test cost and risk of disease) than he or she would for a 60-year-old hypertensive man who smokes cigarettes and has a chest pain syndrome (consider the risk of disease). In a 70-year-old patient with typical angina and an unstable pattern, stress testing adds little to the probability that the patient has coronary artery disease and adds some significant risk (consider the risk of testing). Thus, one may initiate treatment without further testing or proceed with a higher-risk procedure (coronary angiography)

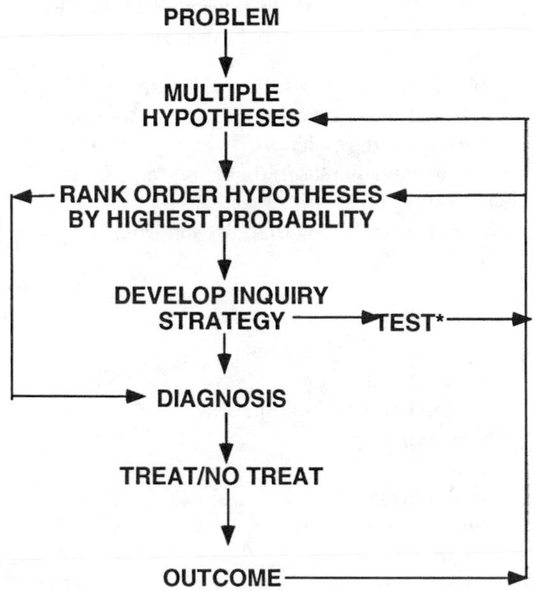

FIGURE 1.2.
Thresholds of testing, diagnosis, and treatment of diseases. *Tests include history, physical examination, blood tests, imaging, and assessment of pulmonary and cardiac function.

that will help determine the need for surgical intervention.

In the problem-solving process, once a threshold is crossed, the hypothesis is either eliminated (no treat) or becomes the diagnosis (treat), wherein therapy is initiated. This thought process results in an outcome that, in itself, becomes part of the **inquiry strategy** and should either support the diagnosis or raise a question that it was not correct and lead to continuation of the problem-solving process.

Patient History

The **history** is the first part of any inquiry strategy and, in many patients with cardiac problems, may give the diagnosis. As with any test, the information obtained from the historical information will have **sensitivity and specificity** for a particular hypothesis. For example, dyspnea is a very sensitive symptom of congestive heart failure that has low specificity.

Information about a patient's past or concurrent conditions may point to causes of the present problem. The clinician should seek information, as outlined in Table 1.1.

The pathology of many diseases affects the heart or vascular system. The presence or absence of these diseases should be sought (Table 1.2) because the disease

TABLE 1.1. Useful Information from History

The physician should ask the patient about
- Military service (rejection for military service?)
- Blood pressure results
- Insurance examinations (rejection for insurance?)
- High rating on insurance
- Previous electrocardiography (abnormal?)
- Childhood illnesses
  - Arthritis
  - Diphtheria
  - Long periods of bed rest
  - Sore throats
- Enlarged heart on radiography
- Medications for
  - Fluids
  - Blood pressure
  - Blood thinning
  - Heart
  - Cholesterol
- Obesity
- Murmurs (as child or adult)

may suggest the cause of the symptom complex. Frequently, the past or accompanying condition occurred many years previously and does not require treatment. In some cases, however, the current cause itself requires treatment: for example, in mitral valve regurgitation that produces heart failure as a result of rheumatic fever. The rheumatic fever episode may have occurred 10 years to 20 years previously and should not be treated, whereas mitral regurgitation due to endocarditis requires active and extensive antibiotic therapy, as well as treatment of the heart failure and possible valve surgery.

Risk Factors

The probability that a diagnosed condition is the cause of the patient's problem is determined, in many cases, by the risk factors for the condition, which can be obtained from the initial history. These factors are well-documented for coronary heart disease but may also be helpful in congenital or genetic diseases, such as the long Q-T syndrome or Wolff-Parkinson-White syndrome. Table 1.3 lists many of the risk factors that have been identified for the most common cardiac conditions.

Symptoms

In general, the symptoms of cardiovascular disease are due to the **altered pathophysiology** directly or to **compensatory mechanisms** for the altered physiology. In congestive heart failure, for example, weakness and fatigue are due to the impaired cardiac output, whereas dyspnea and edema result as compensatory mechanisms that attempt to maintain cardiac output. Treating the symptoms often impairs the body's ability to compensate.

The key (but not specific) symptoms that direct one to the cardiovascular system are the following:

- Chest pain
- Dyspnea
- Edema
- Palpitations
- Dizziness and syncope
- Claudication (extremities)

TABLE 1.2. Some Possible Causes of Heart Disease

Physician should ask patients if they currently experience or have experienced any of the following:
- Alcohol abuse
- Anemia
- Ankylosing spondylitis
- Arteriovenous fistula
- Atherosclerosis (other vascular disease present)
- Cancer and cancer therapy (adriamycin)
- Carcinoid
- Cocaine use
- Congenital-prenatal history of drugs or rubella
- Dental treatment (endocarditis)
- Familial diseases (Wolff-Parkinson-White syndrome, hypertrophic cardiomyopathy, Marfan's syndrome)
- Hemochromatosis
- Hypertension
- Hyperthyroidism
- Hypothyroidism
- Infections (pneumonia, sepsis)
- Muscular dystrophy
- Pulmonary disease
- Pulmonary embolism
- Radiation therapy to chest
- Renal insufficiency (uremia)
- Rheumatic fever
- Rheumatoid arthritis
- Sarcoidosis
- Syphilis
- Trauma

Cardiovascular Risk Factors **TABLE 1.3.**

Risk Factor	Possible Cardiac Condition
Age	CAD
Sex	CAD
Race	HTN
Smoking	CAD
Hypertension	CAD, CHF, ARR
Hypercholesterolemia	CAD, CVD, PVD
Diabetes	CAD
Obesity	CAD, HTN
Diuretics	CAD, ARR
Inactivity	CAD, HTN
Stress	CAD
Alcohol	HTN, CHF
Cocaine abuse	CAD
Personality type	CAD
Kidney disease	HTN
Family history of	
Early death due to CAD (< 60 years)	CAD
Hypertension	HTN
Childhood cyanosis, failure to grow and develop	CHD
Sudden death	CHF, HCM, ARR, CAD
Wolff-Parkinson-White syndrome	ARR
Abnormal electrocardiogram	CAD, CHF

ARR, arrhythmias; CAD, coronary artery disease; CHD, congenital heart disease; CHF, congestive heart failure; CVD, cerebral vascular disease; HCM, hypertrophic cardiomyopathy; HTN, hypertension; PVD, peripheral vascular disease.

Fatigue, weakness, cold extremities, and sweating may be manifestations of cardiovascular disease and frequently accompany the key symptoms but are usually not presenting symptoms. Such associated symptoms should be sought because the pattern of symptoms is helpful in strengthening a diagnosis. For example, the acute crushing chest pain of myocardial infarction is commonly associated with sweating (diaphoresis), shortness of breath, and anxiety.

Chest Pain

Chest pain is the prime symptom related to **ischemic heart disease** caused by inadequate blood supply to the myocardium. Disease of almost any structure in the chest and upper abdomen may produce pain that, in many cases, may mimic and must be distinguished from cardiac pain (see Chapter 7 for an in-depth discussion). **Patterns** of the pain, radiation, and quality are all relevant, but the symptom of chest pain may be one of the most difficult to sort out. Table 1.4 lists many of the noncardiovascular causes of chest pain.

Pain arising from the heart is usually the result of ischemia of the myocardium (cardiac pain), inflammation of the pericardium (pericardial pain), or dissection of the aorta. In general, pain arising from the heart and aorta is deep pain that is not well-localized (diffuse). This is true of any visceral pain (from the esophagus, stomach, and gall bladder to the colon), but a patient's **inability to specify the location of pain** is helpful in distinguishing deep, diffuse pain from chest-wall pain (pleuritic, musculoskeletal), which is usually localized to a fairly circumscribed area.

Pericardial pain is retrosternal but may occur to the right and left of the sternum and in the epigastrium (see Chapter 12 for an in-depth discussion). Pain may radiate to the neck and shoulder but rarely radiates to the arms. Involvement of the diaphragm can produce pain radiating to the trapezius ridge or top of the shoulder. The pain is deep; is not easily localized; and is described as *fullness, pressure,* and *aching* and as *sharp,* a *tightness,* and *constricting.* The quality of the pain is not as relevant to diagnosis as other patterns and is intermittent over hours and days, waxing and waning. Pericardial pain is

TABLE 1.4. Noncardiovascular Causes of Chest Pain

Body area	Causes
Esophagus	Esophagitis Esophageal spasm Acute esophageal obstruction
Trachea and bronchi	Tracheitis and bronchitis
Pleural cavity	Pleurisy Pneumonia Pulmonary infarction
Chest wall	Myositis Interstitial neuritis (e.g., herpes zoster) Chondritis Arthritis Rib fracture Trauma Muscle spasm
Stomach or Duodenum	Peptic ulcer disease Gastritis
Gall bladder	Cholecystitis Biliary colic
Liver and pancreas	Hepatitis Pancreatitis Acute hepatic congestion
Colon	Splenic flexure syndrome Obstruction Irritable bowel syndrome
Spleen	Infarction
Spine	Ruptured cervical disc Radiculitis

usually worse when the patient is lying flat and is relieved by sitting or leaning forward. Swallowing food may aggravate the pain. This pain frequently has a "pleuritic" character in that it is aggravated by body movement, breathing, and coughing. Respiration is frequently shallow, giving the patient a sensation of shortness of breath. The pain is usually not as severe as the cardiac pain of a myocardial infarction but may be so severe as to be associated with diaphoresis or vagal symptoms of nausea, hypotension, and bradycardia. Characteristics that are most specific for pericardial pain are the "pleuritic" nature, radiation to the trapezius ridge, and relief by sitting up or leaning forward.

Cardiac pain due to ischemia is caused when oxygen demand exceeds oxygen supply in the myocardium. The rapidity with which this excessive demand occurs determines the pattern of the pain syndrome. Sudden occlusion of supply due to an intracoronary clot results in prolonged and unrelenting pain. Obstruction to oxygen flow caused by coronary artery spasm also produces pain similar to that seen with an intracoronary clot; also like the pain caused by an intracoronary clot, this pain is not related to activities that increase demand (Prinzmetal's or variant angina). A transient increase in oxygen demand when the supply is fixed, as in the case of atherosclerotic coronary disease, produces the classic symptom complex of angina pectoris. Activities that increase oxygen demand may precipitate angina; this pain is relieved by ceasing or slowing the activities that produce the increased oxygen demand. The major determinants of oxygen demand are contractility, heart rate, and wall tension (which is related to arterial pressure). Table 1.5 lists factors that affect oxygen demand and supply and that should be considered in the evaluation of possible cardiac pain and its syndromes.

Cardiac pain is described as a *squeezing, constricting, tight, heavy, choking, burning, aching,* and *pressure-like* pain. Patients use such terms as "an elephant sitting on my chest" or "a tight band around my chest" to describe the pain. When asked to localize the pain with one finger, the patient uses the whole hand in a circular, up and down, or lateral movement over the precordium. If unable to verbally describe the pain, the patient may use a clenched fist over the sternum to illustrate the symptom (Levine's sign).

The pain is typically located in the lower retrosternal area but may also occur in the upper sternum. It is more often to the left of the sternum (precordium) than the right. Many patients can localize the pain to the epigastrium. **Radiation of cardiac pain** has some typical patterns:

- Pain radiating to the base of the neck and jaw typically originates on the patient's left side but may also originate on the right side or both sides simultaneously.
- Pain also radiates to the left shoulder region (in the distribution of the pectorals) and down the inner aspect of the arm and forearm as far as the fingers (ulnar side, fourth and fifth fingers). Similar radiation may occur on the right side or both sides.
- Pain radiation often stops at the elbow. Pain may radiate to the back, but this suggests the diagnosis of aortic dissection.
- Pain begins or is localized in one of the areas of radiation, such as the jaw or elbow.

Cardiac pain develops and disappears gradually. Sudden onset of chest pain (occurring, for example,

Factors and Possible Causes that Affect the Oxygen Supply and Demand of the Myocardium **TABLE 1.5.**

Decreased Oxygen Supply

Factors	Possible Causes
Coronary artery narrowing	Clot Atherosclerotic plaque Plaque rupture Spasm
Decreased oxygen in blood	Anemia Hypoxia Carbon monoxide (smoking)
Shortened diastolic filling time	Tachycardia
Decreased coronary perfusion pressure	Hypotension Aortic stenosis Aortic regurgitation Elevated ventricular diastolic pressure (e.g., congestive heart failure, diastolic dysfunction)

Increased Oxygen Demand

Factors	Possible Causes
Increased contractility	Exercise Emotion (e.g., anger, anxiety, fear) Postprandial state
Increased heart rate	Exercise Emotion Arrhythmias Postprandial state
Increased myocardial-wall tension	Hypertension Aortic stenosis Pulmonary hypertension Ventricular dilatation—congestive heart failure, volume overloads, such as mitral and aortic regurgitation Cold ambient temperature (elevates blood pressure)

with the speed of a snap of a finger) is rarely cardiac in origin. The duration is finite: approximately 3 to 5 minutes for angina pectoris and longer for variant angina, unstable angina, or myocardial infarction. Shooting, fleeting pains, lasting less than a minute, are not likely to be cardiac in origin. In **classic angina pectoris,** the pain builds, precipitated by some activity that increases oxygen demand (such as exercise and emotion), reaches its peak, and gradually subsides when demand decreases or nitroglycerin is taken. The pain build-up occurs over 1 to 2 minutes, with subsidence of similar duration. Persistence in the activity prolongs the pain or increases its severity. Although a "walk through" phenomenon may occur, whereby the pain dissipates with continued activity, most persons must stop what they are doing to obtain relief. The persistence of activity without relief of pain is less likely to be angina. When factors such as cold weather or having just eaten a meal add to oxygen demand that is already increased by a particular activity, the probability that the pain is caused by cardiac angina increases.

The pain of **variant angina** and **unstable angina** has the quality and radiation of classic angina pectoris but is frequently more severe, is prolonged (lasting longer than 5 minutes), and is often not associated with precipitating factors, occurring at rest or during sleep. The pain of an **acute myocardial infarction** is prolonged and severe (lasting 30 minutes or more) and, like angina, is not associated with precipitating factors. Accompanying breathlessness, diaphoresis, nausea, and anxiety with a sense of doom are common. Shortness of breath is also common in patients with angina. Acute myocardial infarction is often preceded by days or weeks with less severe or shorter periods of pain or by a pattern of increasingly severe episodes of angina along with pain at rest or at night (preinfarction angina, unstable angina). In contrast, **classic anginal pain** is *stable* over periods of weeks and *only gradually increases* in severity. A *rapid progression* in frequency or severity or change in precipitating factors strongly suggests **unstable angina** and requires urgent intervention.

The pain of **dissection of the aorta** is similar to cardiac pain; originates in the retrosternum; and may radiate to the neck, back, and abdomen (see Chapter 17 for an in-depth discussion). Its quality is similar to that of cardiac pain and may be indistinguishable from cardiac pain. Accompanying symptoms of diaphoresis, dyspnea, and anxiety are common. Acute "massive" pulmonary embolism producing acute pulmonary hypertension leads to cardiac pain that is also indistinguishable from the ischemic pain of myocardial infarction (see Chapter 13 for an in-depth discussion.)

In recording a patient's history of chest pain, it is critical to elicit the following:

- Character of the pain
- Location and radiation of the pain
- Precipitating factors
- Relieving factors
- Duration
- Associated symptoms

The aforementioned factors assist in distinguishing among several causes of the pain. The most valuable information in diagnosing or hypothesizing coronary artery disease as the cause of chest pain before an exercise stress test is the character of chest pain: typical angina, atypical angina, noncardiac chest pain, or no chest pain.

In patients with known coronary disease who have angina, have had a myocardial infarction, or have undergone coronary bypass surgery or percutaneous transluminal coronary angioplasty, evaluation of chest pain should include a comparison of the current pain with previous pain of angina or myocardial infarction before angioplasty or bypass surgery. Patients who undergo percutaneous transluminal coronary angioplasty experience pain when the balloon is inflated; this provides another comparison with which to evaluate new onset of pain. Patients can distinguish these types of pain, which helps the clinician diagnose noncardiac chest pain or exclude cardiac pain.

Dyspnea

Shortness of breath is the major symptom of heart failure and is frequently the patient's presenting symptom (see Chapter 19 for an in-depth discussion). Dyspnea is a sensitive symptom but is very nonspecific; possible causes include pulmonary, neuromuscular, and psychogenic disorders or anemia and deconditioning. The shortness of breath in heart failure occurs in several patterns but initially occurs as dyspnea on exertion.

Patients who have **shortness of breath** at rest or when assuming a certain position but not on exertion are extremely unlikely to have **cardiac dyspnea.** Although the stimulus that is experienced as dyspnea is not completely understood, the cardiac pathophysiology associated with dyspnea is related to elevated pulmonary venous pressure (and subsequently pulmonary edema), usually due to elevated left ventricular diastolic pressure caused by impaired systolic or diastolic function. An exception to this is mitral stenosis, in which the elevated pulmonary venous pressure is secondary to the obstruction to mitral valve flow and elevated left atrial pressure. In early heart failure, the left ventricular diastolic pressure is normal at rest but increases with exertion and increased venous return; this increased pressure causes lung congestion and allows the patient to sense dyspnea. With rest and a decrease in venous return, the pressures decrease and the symptom is relieved. As failure progresses, the increased venous return that occurs when the patient assumes a supine position may increase left ventricular diastolic pressure and cause shortness of breath (orthopnea); when this occurs, patients must elevate the upper body to be comfortable. If, after questioning, a patient informs the physician that he or she uses more than one pillow while sleeping, orthopnea is not necessarily indicated unless the patient further explains that breathing is eased with the use of more than one pillow. At night, patients sometimes have peripheral edema that has accumulated during the day; this fluid is resorbed rapidly into the vascular system from the areas no longer dependent. This fluid absorption causes an increase in venous return, elevating the left ventricular diastolic pressure and producing paroxysmal nocturnal dyspnea. If patients describe waking from sleep and sensing dyspnea, it is important to ask about what they do to relieve the shortness of breath. Patients with paroxysmal nocturnal dyspnea *must* sit to obtain relief. They often get out of bed and walk to a cooler area. Patients who change position and go back to sleep are not likely to have heart failure as a cause of their nocturnal dyspnea. Sitting up to breathe is not, in itself, diagnostic of paroxysmal nocturnal dyspnea because patients with lung disease and asthma may also sit up for the me-

TABLE 1.6. Causes of Palpitations and Suggestive Symptoms

Cause	Symptoms
Premature beats	Skipped beats Thumps in chest Fullness in neck Heart jumps Flip-flopping
Regular tachycardia: atrial tachycardia, flutter, ventricular tachycardia	Heart racing Heart beating fast Heart pounding
Irregular tachycardia: atrial fibrillation	Heart racing Heart fluttering
Increased sympathetic stimulation: sinus tachycardia of anxiety	Heart pounding (not very fast)

chanical advantage afforded. To strengthen a diagnosis of paroxysmal nocturnal dyspnea, orthopnea must accompany the nocturnal dyspnea.

Trepopnea is shortness of breath present when the patient lies on one side; when due to heart failure, this condition is usually associated with marked cardiomegaly. Pleural effusion may also produce this symptom.

Cough may be a symptom of heart failure with pulmonary congestion. Cough that occurs when the patient is lying down may indicate orthopnea but is not diagnostic. With advanced heart failure, patients may become dyspneic at rest, aggravated by any exertion; orthopnea is also likely. Some patients initially present with extensive edema. It is critical to investigate for the symptom complex of dyspnea on exertion, paroxysmal nocturnal dyspnea, and orthopnea; this complex indicates that the patient initially had left ventricular failure and now has biventricular failure. If there were no previous symptoms of left-sided failure, the hypothesis is that of "pure" right heart failure; the cause of the latter may be quite different.

Edema

Edema is another key symptom of heart failure; however, it is rarely the first symptom in left ventricular failure and is almost always preceded by dyspnea. "Pure" right-sided heart failure is an exception. **Salt and water retention,** a compensatory mechanism for a failing heart, increases venous return to maintain stroke volume. The patient may not notice mild edema or notice only that his or her shoes are tighter. In early stages of heart failure, fluid accumulates during the day and returns to the vascular system at night. This pattern also correlates with decreased urination during the day and new onset of nocturia. Retention of at least 5 pounds of fluid occurs before edema is seen; in very large or obese persons, however, 10 or more pounds may be retained before edema is observed. The edema of heart failure is position-dependent and is typically seen in the feet, ankles, and lower legs. Edema is not a sensitive symptom or sign of heart failure, nor is it specific.

Other causes of lower-extremity edema include venous disease, lymphatic obstruction, and mechanical factors, such as prolonged sitting and standing. Hypoalbuminemia and salt and water retention from renal disease may be indistinguishable from retention due to heart failure. Because the edema of heart failure is dependent, a patient put to bed with heart failure may have edema shift to the sacral area or posterior aspects of the legs and thighs. Careful measurement of weight in the morning (after voiding and before breakfast) is the best way to quantify diuresis and is something that the patient can do at home.

Palpitations

Palpitations are commonly encountered by the primary care physician. Simply stated, palpitations are an awareness of the heart beat. They usually are associated with a change from "normal." Palpitations are *not* synonymous with an arrhythmia, and many patients will have marked arrhythmias without any symptoms. This information may be helpful in evaluating patients who have premature beats on examination that they are not aware of, suggesting that the palpitations have been occurring over a length of time.

The threshold for the awareness of the heart beat

varies and may be lower in the presence of anxiety. It is beneficial to **characterize the nature of the palpitations** to distinguish tachyarrhythmias from premature beats and from the increased forceful contractions associated with sympathetic stimulation (Table 1.6). Dr. Proctor Harvey popularized a technique to help the patient express the feeling of the palpitations, especially to distinguish a regular from an irregular tachycardia. He suggested that the physician tap rapidly on the patient's chest with a finger and an open hand. A regular, rhythmic tap simulates such conditions as atrial tachycardia and flutter; a very irregular tap simulates atrial fibrillation. The physician can also mimic premature beats, which may be sensed as thumping in the chest and a "flopping" sensation, occasionally accompanied by a sensation of fullness in the neck. Asking patients if they take their pulse can yield diagnostic information. How fast was it? Did it feel as if there were skipped beats? The palpitation associated with sudden increase in adrenergic stimuli (e.g., sympathetic symptoms of hypoglycemia) is felt as a pounding that is not very fast. The physician should elicit the nature of the onset of palpitations, precipitating factors, time of day of onset, and the suddenness of onset and offset if that has been noted. Dizziness and presyncope (blurring or graying of vision) may accompany the onset of any tachyarrhythmia and is useful information to obtain.

Dizziness and Syncope

A decrease in cerebral blood flow results in a loss of consciousness (see Chapter 16 for an in-depth discussion). A transient decrease or a less severe reduction may give a feeling of unsteadiness, weakness of the legs, and dizziness that is often associated with presyncope. Loss of consciousness resulting from cardiac distress must be distinguished from loss of consciousness caused by such neurologic conditions as epilepsy. In the case of true syncope, several potential causes relate to the cardiovascular system. Orthostatic hypotension occurs when the blood pressure decreases in the sitting position or, more frequently, in the standing position. This form of hypotension develops when there has been loss of intravascular volume as a result of hemorrhage or dehydration; it can also occur with loss of sympathetic reflexes (primary orthostatic hypotension).

PHYSICAL EXAMINATION

After obtaining appropriate information from the history, the physician has a resulting set of hypotheses of the most probable cause of the patients' symptoms or problem and can then investigate each in the order of probability. The physical examination, the second part of the inquiry strategy, should be focused to **uphold or nullify a specific hypothesis.** For example, if congestive heart failure is the most probable diagnosis, then one would specifically look for findings that would support the diagnosis, such as rales (crackles) in the lungs, an S_3 gallop, venous distention, and peripheral edema. The presence of all of these strengthens the diagnosis to a probability approaching 100%, allowing the health care provider to intervene appropriately.

Pulses and Pulsations

Arterial

The arterial pulses are examined to

- Determine rate and rhythm
- Assess local peripheral flow, absent or present, bilaterally equal or not
- Evaluate cardiac function

With normal or low diastolic pressures, the fullness of the pulse is related to the pulse pressure (pressure difference between systole and diastole), which from moment to moment is related to the stroke volume.

Bounding pulses (wide pulse pressure) occur with increased stroke volume in high-output states such as anemia, hyperthyroidism, exercise, and atrioventricular fistula as well as aortic regurgitation. A patient with increased diastolic pressure, such as that found in essential hypertension, or a stiff (noncompliant) arterial system has increased pulse pressure. Thus, the finding of full pulses with wide pulse pressure indicates different treatment, depending on the patient's blood pressure and age.

Thready pulses (narrow pulse pressure) of a low stroke volume occur in the low-output states of cardiogenic shock or shock due to decreased preload, such as that found in hemorrhage or dehydration. In the evaluation of hypotension or shock, the presence of bounding pulses (usually with warm extremities) supports the presence of a normal or high cardiac output and directs diagnosis toward decreased blood pressure caused by decreased arterial resistance, a condition typical of early septic shock or secondary to vasodilating drugs.

Other functional information obtained from palpation of the pulses (especially the carotid) include a narrow and slowly increasing pulse (pulsus parvus and pulsus tardus, respectively), occurrence with valvular aortic stenosis, and usually moderate severity. Double-beating pulse (two impulses with each beat) occurs in severe aortic regurgitation and hypertrophic cardiomyopathy with obstruction. In low cardiac output due to heart failure, the pulse may have a double component, but a narrow pulse pressure distinguishes it from aortic regurgitation and hypertrophic cardiomyopathy with obstruction.

Alternating pulse (pulsus alternans) (Fig. 1.3A), in which every other beat is weaker (narrower pulse pressure), indicates left ventricular dysfunction. Alternating pulse may occur transiently after a premature ventricular beat and is a clue to poor left ventricular function.

Paradoxical pulse (pulsus paradoxicus) (Fig. 1.3B and 1.3C) is defined as an exaggerated inspiratory decrease in blood pressure. Normally, the inspiratory decrease in blood pressure is less that 10 mm Hg. A decrease greater than 10 mm Hg during the patient's quiet respiration is considered abnormal. Decrease in blood pressure is measured by gradually decreasing the pressure in the cuff until Korotkoff sounds (indicating systolic pressure) are heard to appear during expiration and disappear during inspiration. The blood pressure at that point is noted. The pressure is decreased further until the sounds are heard throughout the respiratory cycle. This marks the second point of blood pressure measurement; the difference between the first and second measurements should be less than 10 mm Hg.

The causes of the wide variation in intrathoracic pressure include obstructive and restrictive pulmonary disease. Pulse pressure does not vary significantly during the respiratory cycle; thus, one cannot usually palpate the respiratory variation (Fig. 1.3B). Other causes of variation in the intrathoracic pressure are pericardial tamponade and, to a lesser degree, pericardial constriction. These differ from pulmonary disease in that stroke volume markedly decreases; thus, the pulse pressure (volume) during inspiration causes the decrease in systolic pressure (Fig. 1.3C). Because the pulse narrows, the reduction in systolic pressure becomes palpable as a diminished or absent pulse during inspiration.

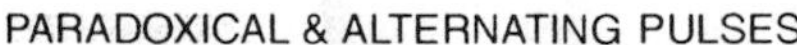

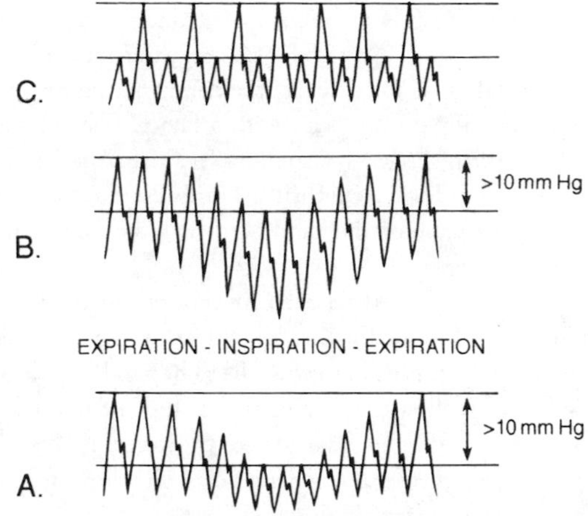

FIGURE 1.3.
Diagram of the arterial pulse and blood pressure variations. **A.,** Alternating pulse. See text for discussion. **B.,** Paradoxical pulse in pericardial tamponade. **C.,** Paradoxical pulse occurring in pulmonary disease.

Precordial

The precordium should be examined from the patient's right side by use of the right hand. This part of the physical examination is used to find evidence of cardiac enlargement and hypertrophy, as well as to palpate for taps or shocks arising from loud heart sounds and thrills (palpable vibrations associated with murmurs). Movements of the heart are very-low-frequency vibrations and are best felt as pulsations with the fingers or whole hand. The point of maximal impulse is produced by the movement of the apical portion of the heart toward the chest wall during the isovolumic contraction. Upon ejection, the impulse moves away from the chest wall. In the supine position, the point of maximal impulse is usually in the fourth intercostal space at or medial to the midclavicular line. Left ventricular dilatation and hypertrophy move the point of maximal impulse leftward and downward. When hypertrophy is caused by aortic stenosis and hypertension, the impulse is sustained, in part because of a prolonged isovolumic contraction period. When the dilatation and hypertrophy are results of volume overload (aortic and mitral regurgitation), the point of maximal impulse is quick or normal. The normal point of maximal impulse is usually contained in an area less than 1 inch in diameter. With dilatation, the point becomes larger and more diffuse. Hypertrophy of the right ventricle produces an enlargement along the left parasternal area in the region of the third to fifth intercostal spaces (a hand placed here feels "lifted," and the lift is sometimes visible). A parasternal enlargement can also occur with severe mitral regurgitation. With right ventricular hypertrophy, the lift coincides with the point of maximal impulse. The right ventricular lift with mitral regurgitation occurs after the point of maximal impulse, giving a rocking motion to the two pulsations.

Two impulses (a double pulsation) may occur at the apex with each beat produced, either by early ventricular filling (early diastole, after S_2) or at the time of the atrial contraction (presystolic, before S_1). These double pulsations correspond to the timing of S_3 and S_4. If double pulsations are felt, the physician should carefully listen for these extra heart sounds.

The last precordial vibrations for which the physician should palpate are taps or shocks, which represent heart sounds of high intensity (loudness) and thrills (vibrations associated with high-energy murmurs). Taps are best felt with the palm of the hand and can be simulated by tapping the palm with a finger. The palm at the base of the fingers is also more sensitive than the tips of the fingers for feeling thrills. Thrills are simulated by placing the palm of the hand over the larynx and humming.

The timing of the thrills or shocks can be determined by palpating the carotid with the left hand while palpating the precordium with the right hand. Taps arising from S_2 follow the peak of the carotid and those due to S_1 precede the carotid upstroke. Systolic thrills occur during the carotid pulse, whereas diastolic thrills follow the peak of the carotid upstroke.

Venous

The pulsations of the jugular vein give information about the function of the right heart.

The **height of the venous pulse** indicates right atrial pressure. Normally, the jugular vein is collapsed in the erect position and distended when lying flat. With decreased intravascular volume, such as that occurring with hemorrhage and dehydration, the right atrial pressure is low and the veins collapse in the supine position with absent pulsations. Veins become distended with pressures exceeding 7 cm H_2O (about 5 mm Hg) in the right atrium. It is important to quantify the pressure rather than just noting distention because the health care provider can monitor the changes in pressure by measuring the distention over a length of time.

Although distention is often measured by describing the angle at which a patient's body lies from supine, this variable is of little importance and lacks accuracy. Certainly, a distended jugular vein in a patient lying 30° from horizontal indicates elevated venous pressure. To quantify the pressure, the patient should be elevated in bed until the venous pulsations can be observed. The internal jugular pulsations should be noted (located anterior to the sternocleidomastoid muscle) and distinguished from the carotid by palpation of the opposite carotid pulse. When the top of the pulsating column is found, measurement from the top of the column vertically to the sternal angle (angle of Louis) is made. Because the sternal angle is approximately 5 cm from the mid-to-right atrium in both the supine position and erect sitting position, the venous pressure can be estimated by adding the measured vertical distance to 5 cm. Thus, if the top of the pulsations in the jugular vein are 9 cm above the angle, then the venous pressure is 12 cm of H_2O, regardless of the angle at which the patient is sitting.

Veins become distended with either high-right atrial pressure or obstruction of the superior vena cava. It is therefore important to search for venous pulsations because their absence with distention indicates obstruction. Another feature useful for distinguishing between vena cava obstruction and increased right atrial pressure is the partial collapse of the venous pressure with inspiration. This collapse does not occur with obstruction. An unusual finding is an inspiratory increase in venous pressure within constrictive pericarditis, right heart failure, and restrictive heart disease. Elevation of the venous pressure during gentle pressing on an enlarged liver supports the presence of a congested liver secondary to heart failure (hepatojugular reflux). The physician should ask that the patient not strain (Valsalva) during the maneuver because doing so mimics reflux. An enlarged liver without jugular venous distention indicates that heart failure is probably not the cause of hepatomegaly.

The venous pulse usually has two visible components, both measurable on phlebography: the A wave (presystolic) and the V wave (late systolic) (Fig. 1.4). In the presence of tricuspid regurgitation, the V wave becomes prominent and is best observed by noting its collapse (negative wave, Y descent), which occurs just after the carotid pulse. Because the most common cause of tricuspid regurgitation is right ventricular failure, the neck vein also becomes distended.

The relationship of the A and V waves is helpful in the evaluation of certain cardiac rhythms. When there is atrioventricular dissociation (as in ventricular tachycardia and complete atrioventricular block), the atria sometimes contracts if the tricuspid valve is closed and produces a large A wave (canon A wave). Thus, the venous pulse varies in ventricular tachycardia, with periodic large A waves; in supraventricular tachycardias, the relationship of the A and V waves is consistent.

Patient's Physical Appearance

The **patient's general appearance** is important in detecting heart conditions. Hyperlipidemia, the presence of **clubbing** (seen in congenital heart disease with right to left shunts), and **cyanosis** are all helpful signs that may alter the probability of the hypothesis being considered. When cyanosis is present, the physician must distinguish peripheral cyanosis caused by poor peripheral flow (whether local, caused by arterial obstruction, or general, caused by shock) from central cyanosis caused by low oxygen saturation. For example, low blood pressure in a patient who has very **pink and warm**

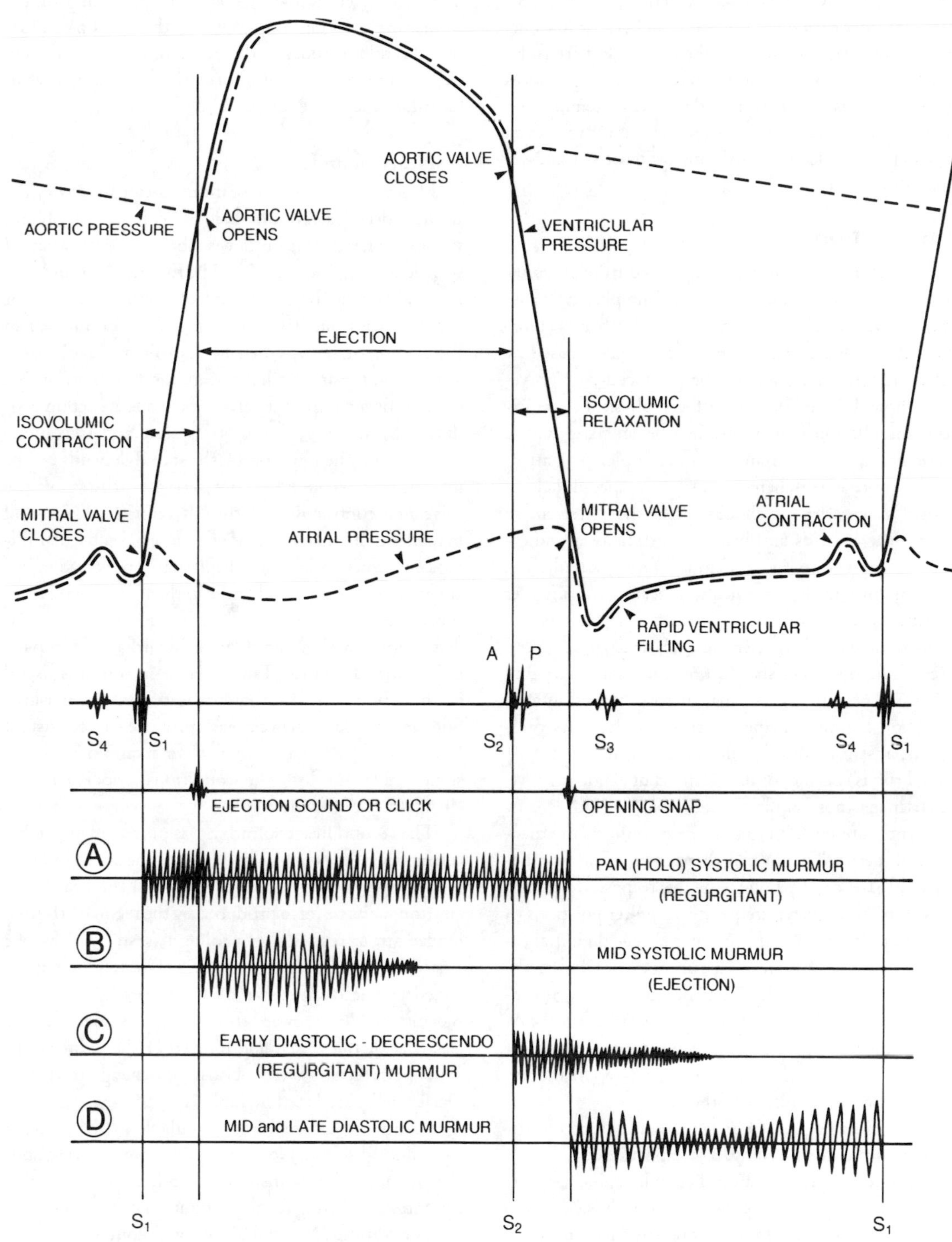

FIGURE 1.4.
Diagram of the cardiac cycle with pressures, heart sounds, and the timing of common murmurs.

extremities is probably caused by peripheral arterial dilatation rather than low cardiac output because low output usually results in low peripheral flow and arteriolar constriction. Poor venous return also produces cyanosis; this is usually seen in the lower extremities but can occur in the face and neck (with superior vena caval obstruction) or locally (with any acute or chronic venous obstruction).

Auscultation

Diagnostic information can be obtained from auscultation of both vessels and the heart. The physician auscultates over vessels primarily to listen for **bruits** (murmurs in vessels). These murmurs are usually caused by obstructed flow but can also be produced by high velocity flow. Like other parts of the physical examination, auscultation is most useful when focused with a particular hypothesis in mind. For example, in a patient with a transient ischemic attack, the possibility of carotid atherosclerosis should direct the physician to palpate the carotids and listen for bruits as an indication of obstruction due to plaque. During auscultation of a patient with leg claudication, hearing a bruit over the femoral artery would strengthen the hypothesis that the patient has atherosclerotic disease of the femoral artery. The physician should know the sensitivity and specificity of a particular auscultatory finding in each condition before drawing conclusions about its presence or absence. For example, a three-component pericardial rub is specific for pericarditis but is not sensitive. Its absence is not helpful for diagnosis (it is often only transiently present), but its presence confirms the diagnosis of pericarditis. When there is significant probability that the chest pain may be due to pericarditis, the physician should listen frequently and alter positions of the patient if pericardial friction is absent on initial examination. The absence of a rub does not lessen the probability of pericarditis, but detection of a rub increases the probability of pericarditis toward 100%. As with all methods of physical examination, the value of auscultation is greatest when it is part of an inquiry strategy for a particular hypothesis.

Another principle of efficient auscultation is to **listen specifically** for a finding. It is important to listen for heart sounds (see next section) before listening for murmurs because identification of heart sounds is critical to diagnosing murmurs. In addition, information in the heart sounds, such as loudness and splitting, helps to diagnose the significance of murmurs (e.g., extra heart sounds may be the only physical finding supporting heart failure).

Interpretation of heart sounds and murmurs requires complete knowledge and understanding of the cardiac cycle (Figure 1.4), as well as the relation of heart sounds and murmurs to the different phases of the cycle. The most important information for the analysis of murmurs and heart sounds is their timing.

Heart Sounds

Heart sounds (brief vibrations) are produced by the sudden deceleration of flow of columns of blood within the heart; this produces vibrations that, when of sufficient energy, are audible. The **first heart sound** (S_1) is associated with the closure of the atrioventricular valves (mitral and tricuspid), primarily mitral. When the column of blood (the end-diastolic volume) that is accelerated toward the left atrium (and right atrium) is checked by a competent valve, vibrations are set up producing S_1 at the beginning of systole and isovolumic contraction. The loudness of the sound depends on the integrity of isovolumic contraction, stiffness of the valve, and contractility of the left ventricle. The sound may vary in intensity, with differences in ventricular filling times, such as in atrial fibrillation. The sound intensity may also vary with changes in the P-R interval measured on ECG, such as occurs in atrioventricular dissociation with ventricular tachycardia or complete atrioventricular block. This variance in sound is useful in the evaluation of tachycardias of unknown cause. Supraventricular tachycardias produce a consistent loudness of S_1 because the P-R interval remains constant. Table 1.7 lists the conditions associated with changes in the loudness of S_1.

The **second heart sound** (S_2) is produced by the deceleration of the column of blood in the aorta and pulmonary artery as it moves back toward the heart after ejection with the force produced by the recoil of the distended great vessels. This column is stopped by the closed aortic and pulmonic valves. The loudness is affected by the competence of the valves and the force moving the blood toward the heart and is related to the elasticity of the vessels and fullness of the pulmonic or systemic arterial systems. Causes of change in the intensity of S_2 are listed in Table 1.8.

Additional information is available in the form of the splitting of S_2. Normally, S_2 becomes two sounds (i.e., it splits) during inspiration and one sound during expiration. Splitting during expiration occurs in pathologic conditions. Normally, the aortic component of S_2 occurs first and pulmonic valve closure follows. During inspiration, because of the increased compliance associated with increased pulmonary vascular volume, the sound on the pulmonic side occurs later, producing splitting. Splitting during expiration can be associated

TABLE 1.7. Changes in Intensity of the First Heart Sound (S_1)[2]

Increased Intensity (loud S_1)	Decreased Intensity (faint or absent (S_1)	Variable Intensity
Stiff and thickened mitral valve—mitral stenosis	Absent isovolumic contraction: significant mitral regurgitation, acute aortic regurgitation with premature closure of mitral valve and high left ventricular end-diastolic pressure with low aortic diastolic pressure, immobile valve in fibrotic/calcific mitral stenosis	Atrial fibrillation, multifocal atrial tachycardia
Increased contractility of left ventricle (exercise, pregnancy, hyperthyroidism)	Poor contractility Left ventricular failure, acute myocardial infarction, heart failure, dilated cardiomyopathy	Atrioventricular dissociation, complete atrioventricular block, ventricular tachycardia
Short PR interval	Prolonged PR interval	

[2]Increased tissue, air, or fat between the heart and the chest wall decreases the loudness of S_1, children, young adults, or lower-than-average-weight adults have increased intensity of S_1.

with persistent or further splitting during inspiration and is termed "fixed splitting." It is caused by conditions on the right side of the circulation. Two sounds on expiration that become one sound with inspiration indicate an abnormality on the left side of the heart or in the circulation (in this situation, the aortic component is later than the pulmonic component). This is called "paradoxical splitting." Table 1.9 lists the causes of the abnormalities of splitting of S_2. Proper identification of S_1 and S_2 is critical in identifying extra heart sounds and murmurs.

The **extra heart sounds,** S_3 and S_4, are associated with filling of the heart during early diastolic filling (rapid ventricular filling phase of diastole) and during the filling associated with atrial contraction, respectively. They are produced when the vibrations associated with the column of blood moving during that phase suddenly decelerate. In the adult, these vibrations are normally of such low intensity that they are inaudible. The intensity increases with stiffness of the ventricles or dilated "full" ventricles with congestive heart failure. The S_4 (atrial gallop or presystolic gallop) occurs with decreased compliance of the ventricles, as in hypertrophy, fibrosis, and aging. It is never a normal sound but rather a physical sign compatible with diastolic dysfunction. Atrial contraction and a normal opening of the mitral valve are required; thus, S_4 is not heard in atrial fibrillation or mitral stenosis.

TABLE 1.8. Changes in Intensity of the Second Heart Sound (S_2)

Increased Intensity (Loud S_2)	Decreased Intensity (Faint of Absent S_2)
Decreased compliance of arterial system Systemic or pulmonic hypertension	Decreased arterial blood pressure Decreased mobility of aortic valve or immobile aortic valve—calcific aortic stenosis
Stiff arterial system, as in aging or arteriosclerosis	Incompetent aortic valve—significant aortic regurgitation

The S_3 (ventricular gallop, protodiastolic gallop) may be heard in a normal heart. In children and young adults, S_3 may be audible because of the thin chest wall. With the increased cardiac output of pregnancy and higher velocity of early diastolic flow, S_3 may also be heard and is considered "normal." In any other circumstance, the presence of S_3 is considered abnormal and a diagnostic sign of ventricular systolic dysfunction (failure).

Both S_3 and S_4 can occur with disease of the right or left heart. A right ventricular S_3 or S_4 is heard best

TABLE 1.9. Changes in the Splitting of the Second Heart Sound

Fixed Splitting (Inspiratory and Expiratory Splitting)	Paradoxical Splitting (Expiratory Splitting, single on inspiration)
Delay in activation of right ventricle	Delay in activation of left ventricle
Complete right bundle-branch block	Complete left bundle-branch block
	Right ventricular pacing
Prolonged ejection of right ventricle	Prolonged ejection of left ventricle
Acute pulmonary hypertension	Acute systemic hypertension
Right ventricular failure	Severe left ventricular failure
Pulmonic stenosis	Severe aortic stenosis
	Myocardial infarction
	Transient angina
Increased pulmonary artery compliance	
Atrial septal defect	
Idiopathic dilatation of pulmonary artery	

along the left sternal border at the third or fourth intercostal space. The left ventricular S_3 is heard at the point of maximal impulse. Because they are both low-frequency sounds, the bell portion of the stethoscope must be used. Increasing ventricular filling increases the intensity of the sounds; thus, the patient should be examined in the supine position and turned to the left to bring the heart closer to the chest wall. Mild exercise or elevating the legs may also increase venous return and elicit these filling sounds.

Other extra heart sounds are associated with valve motion:

- Opening snap of mitral stenosis
- Ejection click of pulmonic stenosis or aortic stenosis, especially congenital aortic stenosis
- Midsystolic clicks of mitral valve prolapse

Each of the aforementioned is associated with sudden stopping of the motion of a valve and thus the column of blood accompanying that motion during opening (aortic, pulmonic, or mitral stenosis) or the checking of the prolapsing valve in mitral valve prolapse. The timing depends on the valve involved. In aortic stenosis, the clicks are in early ejection immediately after S_1; for mitral stenosis, the clicks are in early diastole after S_2. Clicks are of shorter duration and higher frequency than S_3 or S_4 and therefore can be heard through the diaphragm. The timing of the midsystolic click of mitral valve prolapse can be altered by bedside maneuvers or day-to-day variation in cardiac filling and chamber size, as outlined in Figure 1.5. Table 1.10 lists the differential diagnosis of extra heart sounds associated with S_1 and S_2.

Murmurs and Bruits

General Principles Distinct from heart sounds that are caused by vibrations due to the deceleration of blood movement within the heart and circulation, **murmurs** are produced by the vibrations that occur when normally smooth (or laminar) flow within the heart or vessels becomes turbulent. When these vibrations arise within the heart, they are called murmurs. When they arise in the peripheral circulation, they are commonly called bruits. When the energy is high enough, the vibrations can be felt as a thrill.

Heart murmurs are produced when turbulence occurs with blood flow in the normal direction, such as during ejection across the aortic or pulmonic valves or during ventricular filling with flow across the atrioventricular valves. The increased velocity in these circumstances may be produced by a marked increase in velocity of flow within normal valves or obstruction to flow, as in stenosis. In the case of aortic and pulmonic flow, ejection into a dilated aorta or pulmonary artery may also produce turbulence and a murmur. In the case of murmurs occurring during normal flow, the physician must determine whether the murmur is organic (caused by valvular disease) or functional (caused by increased flow). In severe aortic regurgitation, for example, the stroke volume may be more than twice normal because part of the stroke volume regurgitates into the left ventricle during diastole (regurgitant volume). Therefore, a systolic ejection murmur may be produced by the increased velocity of flow during ejection without aortic stenosis. A similar situation may occur with increased mitral diastolic flow with mitral regurgitation and ventricular septal defect, producing a rumbling diastolic

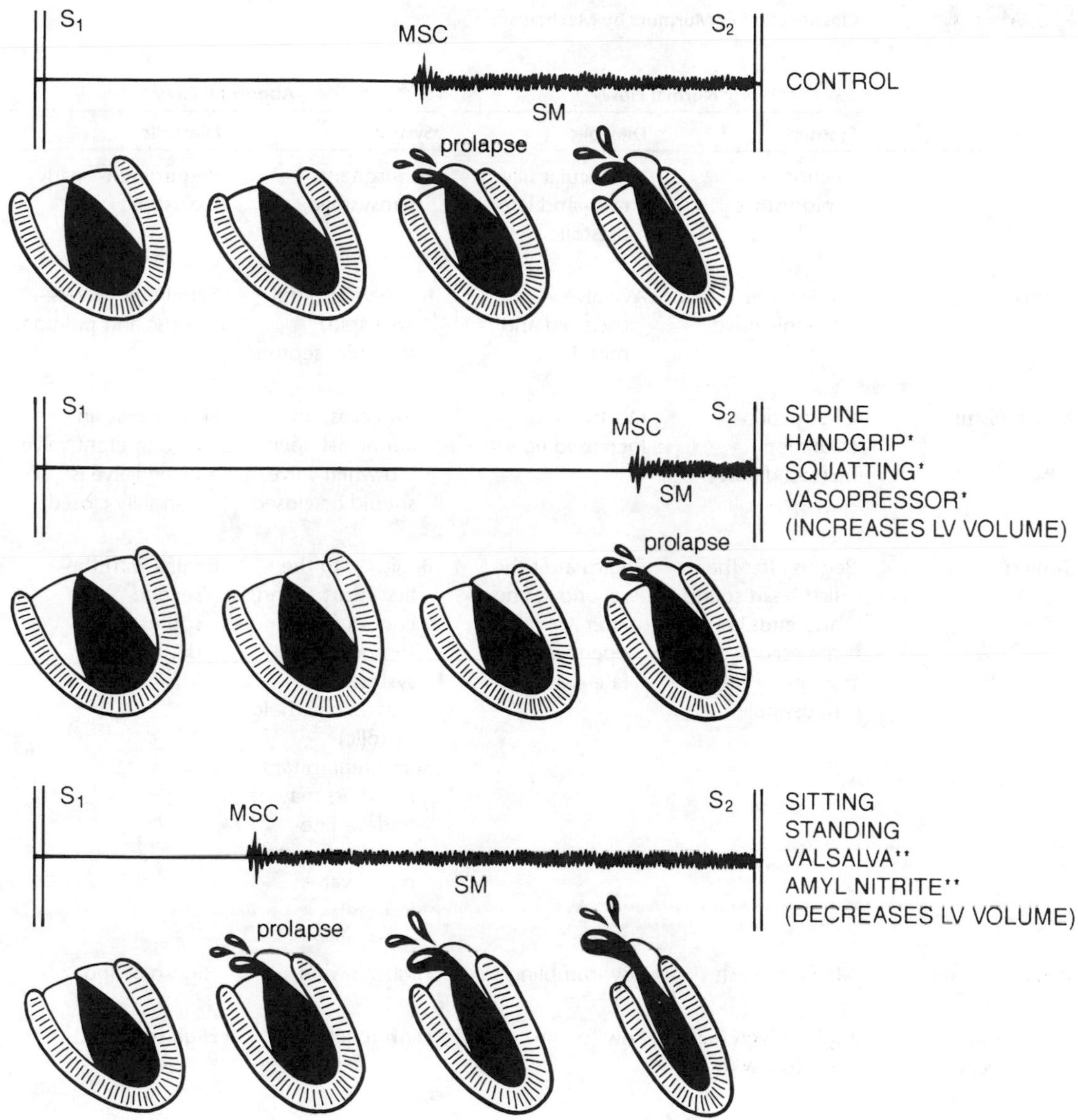

FIGURE 1.5.

Effects of position and maneuvers on mitral valve prolapse. *LV,* left ventricle; *MSC,* midsystolic click. *Murmur intensity increases; **murmur intensity decreases.

Differential Diagnosis of Extra Heart Sounds **TABLE 1.10.**

Extra Sounds at the Time of the First Heart Sound (S_1)	Extra Sounds at the Time of the Second Heart Sound (S_2)
Split S_1	Widely split S_2
S_4, then S_1	S_2, then S_3
S_1—Ejection sound	S_2—Pericardial knock
S_1—Ejection click	S_2—Opening snap
S_1—Early midsystolic click of mitral valve prolapse	S_2—Late midsystolic Click
	S_2—Summation gallop (S_3, S_4)

TABLE 1.11. Classification of Murmurs by Mechanism

	Normal Flow		Abnormal Flow	
Variable	**Systolic**	**Diastolic**	**Systolic**	**Diastolic**
	Ejection—midsystolic	Ventricular filling—mid- and late-diastolic	Regurgitant—pansystolic	Regurgitant—early diastolic
Source	Aortic valve Pulmonic valve	AV valves—tricuspid and mitral	AV valves (mitral-tricuspid) Ventricular septum	Semilunar valves—aortic and pulmonic
Mechanisms	Obstruction Dilatation Increased flow	Obstruction Increased flow	Flow across an abnormal opening when valve should be closed	Flow across an incompetent valve when valve is normally closed
Timing	Begins after the first heart sound and ends before the second sound—midsystolic	Begins after the second sound after AV valves open—mid- to late-diastolic	Begins with the first heart sound, continues throughout systole—pansystolic (holosystolic) Some regurgitant murmurs may be mid- or late-systolic in certain mitral valve lesions[b]	Begins with the second sound—early diastolic
Pitch	Medium-harsh	Low-rumbling	High-blowing	High-blowing
Pressure in chambers[a]	High to high (left) High to low (right)	Low to low	High to low	High to low
Location	Base Second and third intercostal spaces Right or left sternal border	Apex (mitral stenosis) Lower sternal border (tricuspid stenosis)	Apex—mitral valve Lower sternal border—tricuspid and ventricular septal defect	Base Second intercostal space Left and right sternal border
Radiation[c]	Neck and subclavicular areas	Very localized	Axilla, sternum, occasionally back	Left sternal border Third and fourth intercostal spaces

AV, atrioventricular.

[a]Indicates pressure in the chambers on the two sides of the orifice (valve) producing the murmur.

[b]Pansystolic murmurs by definition are regurgitant and thus indicate mitral or tricuspid regurgitation or ventricular septal defect. Not all mitral or tricuspid regurgitations produce pansystolic murmurs (e.g., mitral valve prolapse)

[c]Radiation is determined by the direction of flow of blood producing the murmur (chamber into which the turbulent blood flows).

TABLE 1.12. Effect of Hemodynamic Changes on the Loudness of Murmurs[a]

Change	Normal Response: Systolic	Normal Response: Left-Sided Diastolic	Abnormal Response: Systolic	Abnormal Response: Left-Sided Diastolic
Increased blood pressure	Decreases	No change	Increases	Increases
Decreased cardiac output	Decreases	Decreases	No change	No change
Decreased blood pressure	Increases	No change	Decreases	Decreases
Increased cardiac output	Increases	Increases	No change	No change

[a]Maneuvers that change blood pressure may later change cardiac output; thus, the net effect is not always clear. Complex maneuvers such as squatting and the Valsalva maneuver have variable effects but are useful in the "dynamic" conditions of hypertrophic cardiomyopathy with obstruction and mitral valve prolapse. The changes reflect the responses to left-sided lesions. The effects on right-sided lesions may be different, but, in general, increased flow (cardiac output) increases the intensity of stenotic murmurs.

murmur similar to that present in mitral stenosis. These murmurs must be distinguished from the murmurs heard in stenotic lesions. Associated heart sounds, evaluation of the pulses, and cardiac size are all helpful in this analysis. The characteristics of murmurs produced during normal direction of flow and abnormal direction of flow are noted in Table 1.11. Normal and abnormal effects of hemodynamic changes on the loudness of murmurs are listed in Table 1.12.

Vibrations produced by turbulence have many frequencies and thus sound like static. Occasionally, a particular frequency produces a musical-type murmur. These are associated with flail valve leaflets that vibrate at a particular frequency.

Murmurs vary in frequency depending on the velocity of flow; this, in turn, is determined by the driving force of the blood flow. For example, the driving force in regurgitation across the aortic valve is the pressure in the aorta during diastole, whereas the driving force in mitral regurgitation is the systolic pressure in the left ventricle. In general, the lower the gradient and the driving pressure, the lower the frequency (pitch) of the murmur. Flow across the stenotic mitral valve has a low-pressure driving force. Turbulence produces a low-pitch rumbling murmur heard best with the bell of the stethoscope. The murmur of acute regurgitation, conversely, has a high driving force and thus a high frequency; it is best heard with the diaphragm of the stethoscope. In the case of flow in the abnormal direction (Table 1.11), turbulence is due to a high velocity of flow produced when an incompetent valve produces regurgitation or a ventricular septal defect. These murmurs are always abnormal because they indicate the presence of structural heart disease. Murmurs resulting from abnormal directional flow occur as soon as the valves are closed and there is a gradient across the valve (aortic valve to left ventricle, pulmonic valve to right ventricle, left ventricle to left atrium, right ventricle to right atrium) or between the left ventricle and right ventricle chambers (ventricular septal defect). Because this gradient exists at the closure of the valves and the onset of increasing pressure in the ventricles during systole, the murmurs start with S_1, proceed to and beyond S_2, and are pansystolic (holosystolic). A pansystolic murmur is abnormal and is caused by mitral or tricuspid regurgitation or a ventricular septal defect. Mitral regurgitation may begin later in systole when due to mitral valve prolapse. Such murmurs may begin after a midsystolic click associated with the prolapse but may occur without a click. These murmurs are dynamic; the time of onset changes with different hemodynamic states or bedside maneuvers. Figure 1.5 illustrates the timing of murmurs of mitral valve prolapse. Mitral regurgitation murmurs usually go through systole, but in severe acute regurgitation with a noncompliant left atrium, the left atrial pressure rapidly increases during systole (large V wave) and the gradient from the left ventricle to left atrium decreases. The flow therefore decreases during late systole and the murmur may only be heard in early systole.

Murmurs in the Normal Heart In normal hearts, murmurs may be produced during ejection by turbulence across the aortic or pulmonic valve. These are considered innocent murmurs, not associated with heart disease; they are common in children. One characteristic of an innocent murmur is variation in the murmur from day to day over time. This is typical of ejection murmurs, with the peak velocity of flow normally in the first third of ejection. These murmurs peak early in systole (but begin after S_1) and usually end before the last third of systole. They are sensitive to positional change: They are best heard when the patient is lying down and usually diminish or disappear when the patient sits or stands or during the Valsalva maneuver. Because systolic murmurs are the most common murmurs (and the easiest to hear), the differential diagnosis is among innocent, functional (high velocity and flow states), or organic (stenosis or regurgitation) conditions. In clinical decision making, the presence of systolic murmurs is important. For example, if one considers endocarditis as a possible cause of a febrile illness, the presence of a new murmur is sought. A new regurgitant murmur is more specific (indicating mitral regurgitation, tricuspid regurgitation, aortic or pulmonic regurgitation) than an ejection murmur, which could be stenotic (unusual due to endocarditis) or functional (due to high flow associated with fever). Diastolic murmurs are almost always associated with organic disease.

Differential Diagnosis The most important feature in determining the cause of a murmur is the **timing of the murmur:** systolic or diastolic, ejection, or regurgitant. Careful observation into whether the murmur starts with or after S_1 or with or after S_2 and the duration in the cycle (early systolic, late systolic) are important features in the differential diagnosis.

Location of the murmur and its pattern of radiation are also helpful but may mislead. Aortic stenosis may radiate to the apex of the heart and be loudest in that location, mimicking mitral regurgitation, but the timing should distinguish the two murmurs.

The **pitch and shape** are also helpful for the diagnosis. The shape is determined by the characteristics of the flow producing the murmur. Because the gradient between the aorta and left ventricle in diastole decreases during diastole as the diastolic pressure decreases, the flow decreases; thus, murmurs of aortic regurgitation arc decrescendo. In mitral stenosis, increased flow occurs at the time of atrial contraction; thus, this murmur increases in the presystolic period when the patient is in sinus rhythm (presystolic accentuation), illustrated by murmur D in Figure 1.4.

In fixed lesions (either stenosis or regurgitation), the **loudness** of murmurs can be altered by changing the velocity of flow. The **velocity** in normal flow direction is related to the cardiac output, whereas in fixed regurgitation murmurs, the flow is altered by changing the driving pressure producing the regurgitation. The loudness of murmurs (grade) depends on the velocity of flow; in stenotic murmurs, the velocity is due to the degree of stenosis and flow. Higher-degree stenosis produces louder murmurs when cardiac output is normal. In heart failure, because flow may be decreased, the murmur may become less pronounced; thus, the physician may be misled as to the severity of the stenosis. In the case of regurgitant murmurs, the size of the leak (hole) affects the loudness in the opposite-direction flow. The smaller leak is associated with the louder murmurs, whereas large leaks may not produce as much turbulence and thus are diminished. The more faint the murmur, the greater the likelihood that severe regurgitation is occurring. Loudness is also affected by the thickness of the chest wall, intervening lung, and obesity.

Mitral valve prolapse produces a midsystolic click or clicks, mitral regurgitation murmurs, or both. The timing of the click or the beginning of the murmur varies and depends on the degree of redundancy of the mitral valve apparatus (length of chordae, thickening of the valve leaflets, papillary muscle function, and the integrity of atrioventricular annulus) and the left ventricular chamber at the beginning of systole. The murmur of mitral valve prolapse may vary from day to day and can be late systolic to pansystolic depending on hemodynamic changes, which affect the chamber size and timing (Fig. 1.5).

Hypertrophic obstructive cardiomyopathy is also a dynamic process in which outflow is obstructed by the hypertrophic septum and systolic anterior motion of the anterior leaflet of the mitral valve into the outflow tract of the left ventricle. The mechanism is illustrated in Figure 1.6 (see Chapter 15 for an in-depth discussion). Hemodynamic maneuvers described in the next section will help the reader distinguish this lesion from valvular aortic stenosis. Effects of hemodynamic changes for common systolic and diastolic murmurs are presented in Table 1.13.

Specific Lesions Basic features of common valvular lesions are the following (see Chapter 9 for an in-depth discussion):

Aortic stenosis Ejection; crescendo-decrescendo; harsh; base of heart (right second intercostal space); radiation to left side of sternum, neck, and apex; ejection sound in congenital conditions; disappearance of ejection sound and S_2 with calcification.

Pulmonic stenosis Ejection; late peaking crescendo-

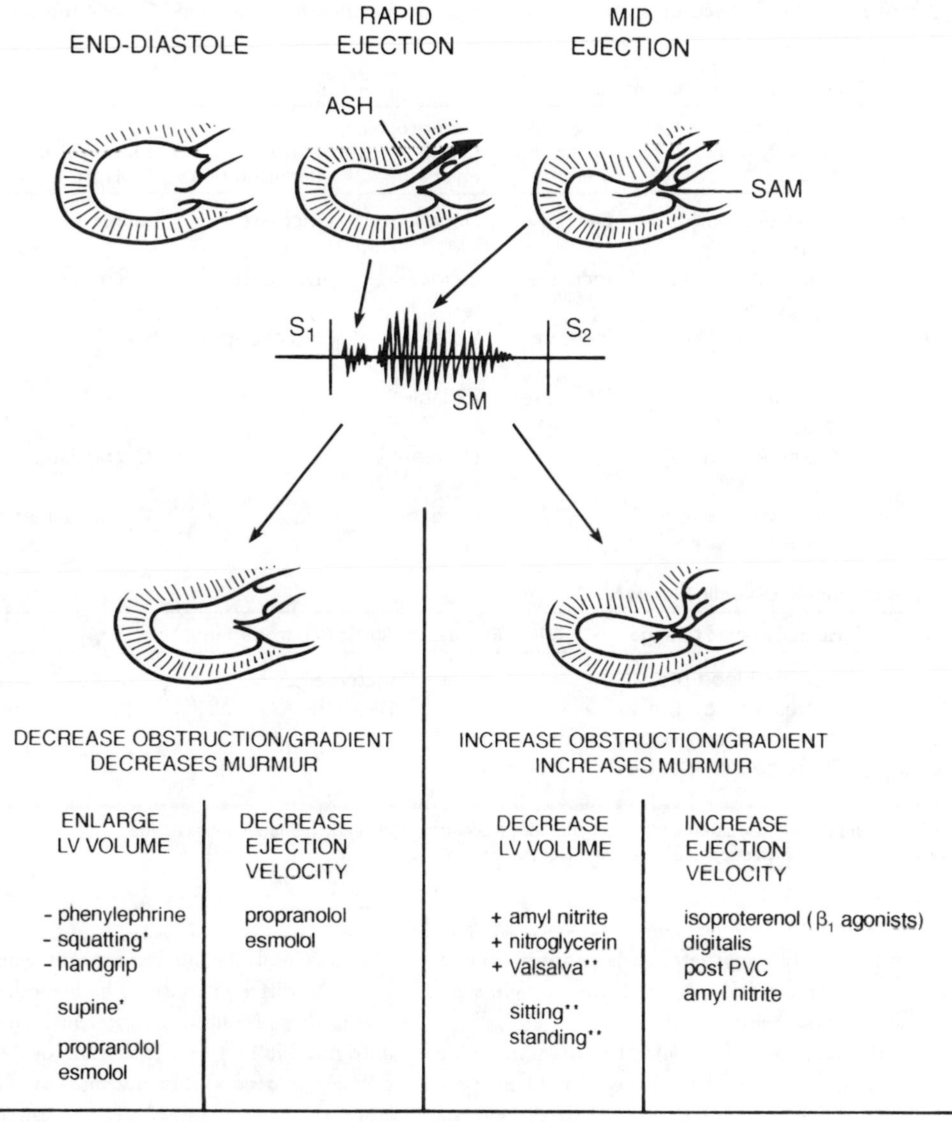

FIGURE 1.6.

Changes in murmur loudness in hypertrophic obstructive cardiomyopathy. *ASH,* asymetric septal hypertrophy; *LV,* left ventricle; *PVC,* premature ventricular contraction; *SAM,* systolic anterior motion. *Increases venous return; **decreases venous return; −increases blood pressure and decreases ejection velocity; +decreases blood pressure and increases ejection velocity.

decrescendo; harsh; base of heart (left second intercostal space); radiation to left infraclavicular area; ejection sound present; delayed pulmonic component of S_2.

Hypertrophic obstructive cardiomyopathy See Figure 1.6.

Innocent Ejection; peaks early; short, medium-pitch blowing; base of heart (right side more often than left side); little radiation; may be vibratory (buzzing); varies over time and with position; rarely loud.

Mitral regurgitation Pansystolic; flat; medium- to high-pitched blowing; apex; radiation to axilla and back; S_1 decreased or absent with severe regurgitation; diastolic rumble and S_3 may be present with severe regurgitation.

Tricuspid regurgitation Pansystolic; medium- to high-pitched blowing; lower left sternal border; increased intensity with inspiration (see Figure 1.5).

Ventricular septal defect Pansystolic; harsh;

TABLE 1.13. Effects of Hemodynamic Changes on the Intensity of Common Systolic and Diastolic Murmurs

Effects on Common Systolic Murmurs

Flow	Hemodynamic Change	Aortic Stenosis	Hypertrophic Cardio-myopathy	Mitral Regurgitation	Mitral Valve Prolapse	Ventricular Septal Defect
Decrease	Increase blood pressure	Decrease	Decrease	Increase	Increase	Increase
Increase	Decrease blood pressure	Increase	Increase	Decrease	Decrease	Decrease
Increase	Increase cardiac output	Increase	Variable[a]	No change	Variable[b]	No change
Decrease	Decrease cardiac output	Decrease	Variable[a]	No change	Variable[b]	No change
	Increase chamber size		Decrease		Occurs later	
	Decrease chamber size		Increase		Occurs earlier	

Effects on Common Diastolic Murmurs

Flow	Hemodynamic Change	Mitral Stenosis	Aortic Regurgitation
–	Increase blood pressure	–	Increase
–	Decrease blood pressure	–	Decrease
Increase	Increase cardiac output	Increase	–
Decrease	Decrease cariac output	Decrease	–

[a]Effects depend on the associated changes in chamber size and velocity of ejection, which depend on the maneuver used to produce the hemodynamic change.

medium-pitched blowing; left sternal border; fourth, fifth, and sixth intercostal space; radiation to right sternal border; thrill common.

Mitral stenosis Mid- and late-diastolic with presystolic accentuation; low-pitched rumbling; preceded by opening snap; apex; very localized; loud S_1. With calcification, S_1 and opening snap diminish and may disappear.

Aortic regurgitation Early diastolic begins with S_2; decrescendo; high-pitched blowing; base (second right intercostal space) radiates to left sternal border (third and fourth intercostal space); best heard with patient sitting and leaning forward with forced expiration; severe regurgitation may have loud ejection murmur without stenosis.

Pulmonic regurgitation If associated with pulmonary hypertension, similar to aortic regurgitation.

BEDSIDE MANEUVERS Because changing the velocity of flow alters the loudness of murmurs, one can use maneuvers easily done at the beside or in the office to change murmur intensity or timing and help distinguish the different causes. The hemodynamic changes that can be produced by different maneuvers are outlined in Table 1.14. (see Table 1.12 for the effects on the different murmurs). The murmurs of mitral valve prolapse and hypertrophic obstructive cardiomyopathy are dynamic in intensity; the timing, in the case of mitral valve prolapse, may vary from examination to examination under different hemodynamic states. These changes can be reproduced in the office setting. Figure 1.6 illustrates the effect of the maneuvers or changes in hemodynamic state on the loudness of the murmur in hypertrophic obstructive cardiomyopathy.

Maneuvers such as the **Valsalva maneuver** produce more complex changes: not only does cardiac output decrease, but with decreased venous return the size of the left ventricular chamber size decreases, blood pressure falls, and the velocity of ejection increases (secondary to reflex sympathetic stimulation, which increases contractility). The net effect is to increase the systolic anterior motion of the mitral valve, which is the major cause of

TABLE 1.14. Effect of Maneuvers on Hemodynamics

	Hemodynamic Effects				
Position or Maneuver	**Venous Return**	**Cardiac Output**	**Aortic Pressure**	**Ventricular Volume**	**Velocity of Ejection**
Recumbency (leg-raising)	Increase	Increase	Increase[a] No Change[a]	Increase	Decrease[a] No Change
Sitting to standing	Decrease	Decrease	Decrease No change	Decrease	Increase
Squatting	Increase (transient)	Increase (transient)	Increase	Increase	Increase
Valsalva maneuver (straining)	Decrease	Decrease	Decrease	Decrease	Decrease
Handgrip[b]	–	–	Increase	Increase[a]	Decrease
Vasopressor (phenylephrine)	–	Decrease[a]	Increase	Increase	Decrease
Vasodilator (amylnitrate)	Increase	Increase	Decrease	Decrease	Increase

[a]Minor changes.
[b]Not well studied.

TABLE 1.15. Examples of Specific Physical Findings Useful in the Inquiry Strategy

Hypothesis	**Findings**	**Sensitivity[a]**	**Specificity[a]**
Pericarditis	Pericardial rub	Low	Very high
Endocarditis	New murmur		
	Ejection murmur	High	Low
	Regurgitant murmur	Low	High
Congestive heart failure			
Systolic dysfunction	S_3	Moderate	High
Diastolic dysfunction	S_4	Moderate	Moderate
Angina	New S_4 during pain	Low	Moderate
Valvular disease	Regurgitant murmur	High	High
	Ejection murmur	High	Moderate to Low

[a]Sensitivity and specificity are author's estimates.

obstruction in hypertrophic obstructive cardiomyopathy. The murmur then intensifies. This process is distinct from valvular aortic stenosis, in which decreasing cardiac output decreases flow across the aortic valve and thereby causes the murmur to diminish in intensity. Shock or other low-output states would produce the same result. In contrast, increasing the aortic pressure (handgrip) decreases aortic flow (sudden increase in afterload), increases left ventricular chamber size, and decreases the velocity of ejection, thus reducing the intensity of the murmur. This is similar to increasing blood pressure in valvular atrial stenosis and therefore is not helpful in distinguishing these two lesions. Conversely, raising left ventricular systolic pressure (when systemic blood pressure is elevated) increases the driving pressure for flow across an incompetent mitral valve and increases the velocity of regurgitant flow and the loudness of the murmur; this helps distinguish atrial stenosis and hypertrophic obstructive cardiomyopathy from mitral regurgitation.

Changes in venous return alter the chamber size of the left ventricle, as do acute changes in blood pressure. In the case of mitral valve prolapse, the major effect is on the time of onset of the regurgitant murmur and time of the associated clicks. Depending on where the prolapse occurs in the cycle, the result could be complete disappearance of the murmur. With maneuvers that move the murmur later, the prolapse will occur late. In early prolapse, a maneuver that would cause increasing prolapse (e.g., the Valsalva maneuver) might then produce a pansystolic murmur as the prolapse occurs with the onset of contraction. Figure 1.5 illustrates these concepts and the effect of different maneuvers in mitral valve prolapse.

To evaluate the cause and significance of a murmur, routine examination should be performed with the patient in the **supine position;** it should also include auscultation in the **sitting and squatting positions** (the changes that occur in these positions are outlined in Table 1.14). The use of a sustained handgrip (the patient squeezes a partially inflated blood pressure cuff to about 50 mm Hg and maintains it for 15 to 30 seconds while the health care provider listens continually) or the Valsalva maneuver (patient blows on his or her thumb without letting air out and sustains this for at least 15 seconds to 20 seconds) should be considered, especially when one suspects hypertrophic obstructive cardiomyopathy or mitral valve prolapse. Murmurs that depend on the normal forward flow of blood will increase in intensity with increased flow and decrease with decrease in flow. Patients should be examined in the supine position to assure maximum flow because these murmurs may diminish in intensity in the sitting and standing position to an inaudible level.

SUMMARY

As with any historical information or laboratory test, a finding is most valuable when it is used to evaluate a specific hypothesis. Table 1.15 illustrates some hypotheses, the findings that are helpful in strengthening or weakening the hypotheses, and the sensitivity and specificity of these findings. The history and physical examination of a patient suspected of having heart disease must be approached with specific hypotheses in mind. The cost of these tests is low, but the potential usefulness is high.

KEY POINTS

History

- Patient presents with a **problem;** the examiner develops a **hypothesis** and initiates the **inquiry strategy** (history, physical examination, laboratory studies).
- Focused history and physical examination on the hypothesis. Arrive at a threshold for a treat/test or test/treat.
- Remember that symptoms, like any test, include specificity and sensitivity. Do not forget history and other conditions, risk factors and then the specific symptoms.
- Symptoms that rapidly point to a cardiovascular hypothesis (problem) that can carry significant mortality and morbidity: **Chest pain** (coronary artery disease, aortic stenosis, hypertrophic cardiomyopathy), **dyspnea** at rest or with exertion, **orthopnea, paroxysmal nocturnal dyspnea** (e.g., congestive heart failure and chronic obstructive pulmonary disease), **edema** (e.g., cardiac, renal, hepatic, and venous disease), **palpitations, dizziness and syncope.**

Physical examination

- Guided by a complete and thorough history.
- General: patient appears "well" or "unwell" and has signs of
  Xanthomas
  Clubbing
  Cyanosis
  Edema
- Arterial pulses: present or absent, full or weak.
  Narrow and slow increase = arterial stenosis
  Double = aortic insufficiency, hypertrophic cardiomyopathy with obstruction, congestive heart failure
  Paradoxical pulse = pericardial disease
- Precordial pulses:
  Point of maximal impulse present or displaced = left ventricular volume or pressure overload
  Right ventricular lift = pulmonary hypertension
  Double pulsations = S_3 and S_4 gallops
- Venous pulsations:
  Right heart function (venous distention with right atrial pressure > 5 mm Hg)
  Hepatojugular reflux with congestive heart failure
  Prominent jugular V wave (indicates tricuspid regurgitation)
  Auscultate: Arch of the aorta, abdominal aorta, and peripheral arterial system
- S_1: Tricuspid and mitral closure
  S_2: Aortic and pulmonic closure with physiologic splitting (nonclosure of S_2, think atrial septal defect)
- Loud S_1 = mitral stenosis, increased contractility
  Soft S_1 = mitral regurgitation, aortic insufficiency, congestive heart failure
  Variable S_1 = atrial fibrillation, atrioventricular dissociation
- Extra sounds:
  S_3 = congestive heart failure
  S_4 = hypertension, aortic stenosis
  Ejection clicks = mitral valve prolapse, aortic stenosis

Common Murmurs

- Systolic ejection murmur at the left sternal border: innocent in children and adolescents and occurs in high-output states, such as pregnancy, anemia, and exercise.
- Harsh, systolic murmurs at the base with radiation to the neck:
  Second right intercostal space = aortic stenosis
  Second left intercostal space = pulmonic stenosis
- Harsh systolic murmur at the left sternal border that increases with the Valsalva maneuver = hypertrophic cardiomyopathy with obstruction
- Apical pansystolic murmur to the axilla = mitral regurgitation
- Left lower sternal border that increases with inspiration = tricuspid regurgitation
- Harsh, left sternal border radiation to the right = ventricular septal defect
- Apical diastolic rumble with a loud S_1 = mitral stenosis
- Early diastolic murmur at the left sternal border:
  Blowing, best heard in the sitting position = aortic regurgitation
  If pulmonary hypertension is present, could be pulmonic regurgitation

SUGGESTED READINGS

Abrams J. Essentials of cardiac physical diagnosis. Philadelphia: Lea & Febiger, 1987.

Abrams J. Synopsis of cardiac physical diagnosis. Philadelphia: Williams & Wilkins, 1989

Benditt DG, Sakaguchi S, Scultz JJ, et al. Syncope. Cardiol Rev 1993;1:146–156.

Constant J. Bedside cardiology. 4th ed. New York: Little, Brown, 1993.

Council of Clinical Cardiology. Examination of the heart. Parts 1–4. New York: American Heart Association; 1991.

Gillespie DJ, Staats BA. Unexplained dyspnea. Mayo Clin Proc 1994;69:657–663

Grewe K, Crawford MH, O'Rourke RA. Differentiation of cardiac murmurs by dynamic auscultation. Curr Probl Cardiol 1988;13:669–721.

Kassirer JP, Kopelmanm RI. Learning clinical reasoning. Baltimore: Williams & Wilkins, 1991.

Leon DF, Shaver JA, eds. Physiologic principles of heart sounds and murmurs. Monograph # 46. New York: American Heart Association; 1975.

Lewis RP. Cardiac examination pearls. Cardiol Rev. 1996;4: 34–46.

Manning HL, Schwartzstein RM. Pathophysiology of dyspnea. N Engl J Med 1995;333:1547–1553.

Miller AJ. Diagnosis of chest pain. New York: Raven Press; 1988.

Pauker SG, Kassirer JP. Decision analysis. N Engl J Med 1987;316:P250–258.

Ronan JA Jr. What comprises an adequate initial evaluation of the patient with a heart murmur? ACC Current Journal Review. 1996 Jan/Feb; 76–80.

Ross RT. Syncope. In: Major problems in neurology. Philadelphia: W.B. Saunders; 1996.

Schneiderman H. Bedside diagnosis: an annotated bibliography of recent literature on interviewing and physical examination. Philadelphia: American College of Physicians; 1988.

Shaver JA. Cardiac auscultation: a cost-effective diagnostic skill. Curr Probl Cardiol 1995;20:443–530.

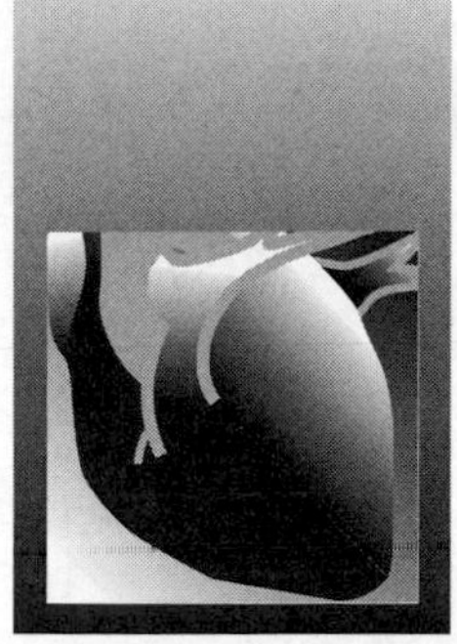

CHAPTER 2

Electrocardiography

Andrea Hastillo

BACKGROUND

The electrocardiogram (ECG) is an intricate component of the examination of any patient suspected of having cardioventricular disease. This common diagnostic tool is available in the offices of all primary care teams; in most cases, interpretation of the ECG is not difficult when approached by using "steps." The fundamental approach to the ECG begins with an analysis of rate, rhythm, and axis. This chapter focuses on atrioventricular (AV) conduction abnormalities, atrial and ventricular hypertrophy, bundle-branch blocks, coronary and pericardial disease, and potassium and calcium abnormalities. Treatment of cardiac arrhythmias is discussed in Chapter 3.

ATRIOVENTRICULAR CONDUCTION ABNORMALITIES

Atrioventricular conduction abnormalities are often caused by natural disease and medication (Table 2.1). In adults, prolongation of the P-R interval for more than the normal 0.20 seconds is called first-degree AV block and may be present in more than 1% of the healthy population.

The well-conditioned individual may, in fact, even develop type I second-degree AV block. Both type I and type II, the two common forms of second-degree AV block, are characterized by relatively regular P-to-P intervals and intermittent failure of the P wave to be followed by a QRS complex. These characteristic intervals are caused by a block in the conduction system that prevents the atrial electrical impulse from producing ventricular depolarization. Although it was previously believed that type I second-degree AV block was due to blockage *within* the AV node and that type II second-degree AV block was due to blockage *below* the AV node, an electrophysiologic study is necessary to determine the true location of the conduction block.

Type I Second-Degree Atrioventricular Block

In type I second-degree AV block, which includes the Wenckebach phenomenon, the P-R interval lengthens as the R-R interval shortens and a P wave is eventually not followed by a QRS interval (Fig. 2.1). Although the P-R interval progressively lengthens, the decremental increase in the P-R interval lessens, thus explaining the

TABLE 2.1. Common Causes of First-Degree Atrioventricular Block

Normal variant
Conditioning
High vagal tone
Medication
Digitalis
β-blockers
Certain calcium-channel blockers (e.g., verapamil, diltiazem)
Certain antiarrhythmic agents (e.g., amiodarone)

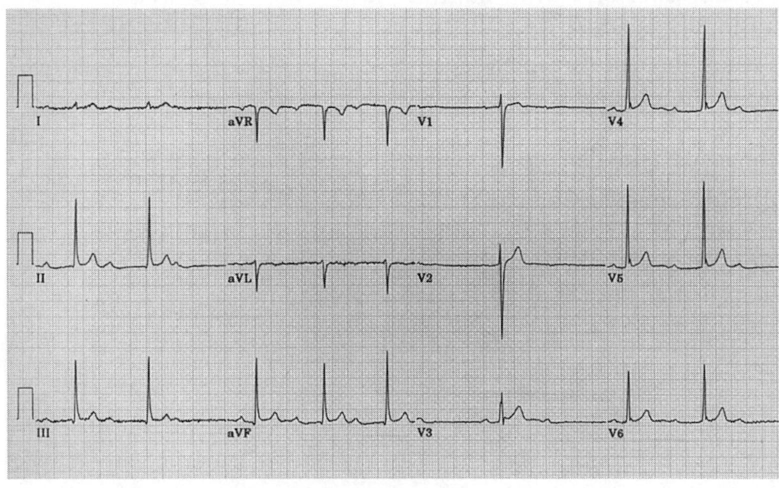

FIGURE 2.1.
Type I second-degree atrioventricular block. The QRS complex is narrow.

TABLE 2.2. Second-Degree Atrioventricular Block

Type	Cause	Conduction Abnormality
Type I	High vagal tone Acute inferior infarction Medications: Digitalis β-blockers	Usually nonprogressive
Type II	Destruction Acute anteroseptal infarction	Usually progressive

shortening R-R intervals. After the single nonconducted P wave, AV conduction resumes. The pause between the last conducted and the next conducted QRS complex is less than twice the shortest R-R interval. This cyclic conduction and subsequent failure to conduct may occur frequently and result in readily perceptible "group beating" on rhythm strips. Unless the patient has preexisting intraventricular conduction delay, the duration of the QRS complex is usually normal. Many variations of type I second-degree AV block with Wenckebach phenomenon exist.

Type II Second-Degree Atrioventricular Block

Type II second-degree AV block demonstrates a fixed P-R interval (two P waves must successively conduct to determine the "fixed" P-R interval) with sudden failure of a P wave to be followed by a QRS complex. The QRS complex is often prolonged. Type II second-degree AV block is often a harbinger of complete heart block with an unstable escape rhythm, especially when it develops during an acute anterior myocardial infarction (Table 2.2).

High-Grade Second-Degree Atrioventricular Block

A third form of second-degree AV block is termed high-grade. In this instance, two or more successive P waves do not conduct. The diagnosis of high-grade second-degree AV block also requires that the atrial rate be reasonably slow (<135 beats/min) to avoid physiologic AV block. The latter might result in successive nonconducted P waves.

Third-Degree Atrioventricular Block

Third-degree AV block results when conduction from the atrium to the ventricle is completely blocked. This mechanism must be distinguished from another form of AV dissociation in which atrial control of the ventricular depolarization is usurped by a more rapidly depolarizing junctional or ventricular focus. Third-degree AV block may be congenital. If so, it is usually accompanied by a junctional escape rhythm; this rhythm, whose rate may vary in response to sympathetic activity, is usually well tolerated. More often, however, third-degree AV block is caused by medications or diseases of varying severity (Table 2.3). Third-degree AV block is diagnosed by the presence of more P waves than QRS complexes (if sinus mechanism is present), a variable P-R interval, and a relatively fixed atrial rate (Fig. 2.2A and 2.2B). The QRS complex may be due to a ventricular

TABLE 2.3. Causes of Third-Degree Atrioventricular Block

- Congenital
- High vagal tone
  - Vomiting
  - Myocardial infarction
  - Myocardial ischemia
- Conduction system interruption—anatomical
  - Myocardial infarction
  - Iatrogenic: surgical, thermal
  - Endocarditis
  - Calcification or fibrosis
- Inflammatory
  - Post-surgery
  - Endocarditis
  - Lyme disease
- Medication
  - Digitalis
  - β-blockers
  - Certain calcium-channel blockers
  - Certain antiarrhythmic agents

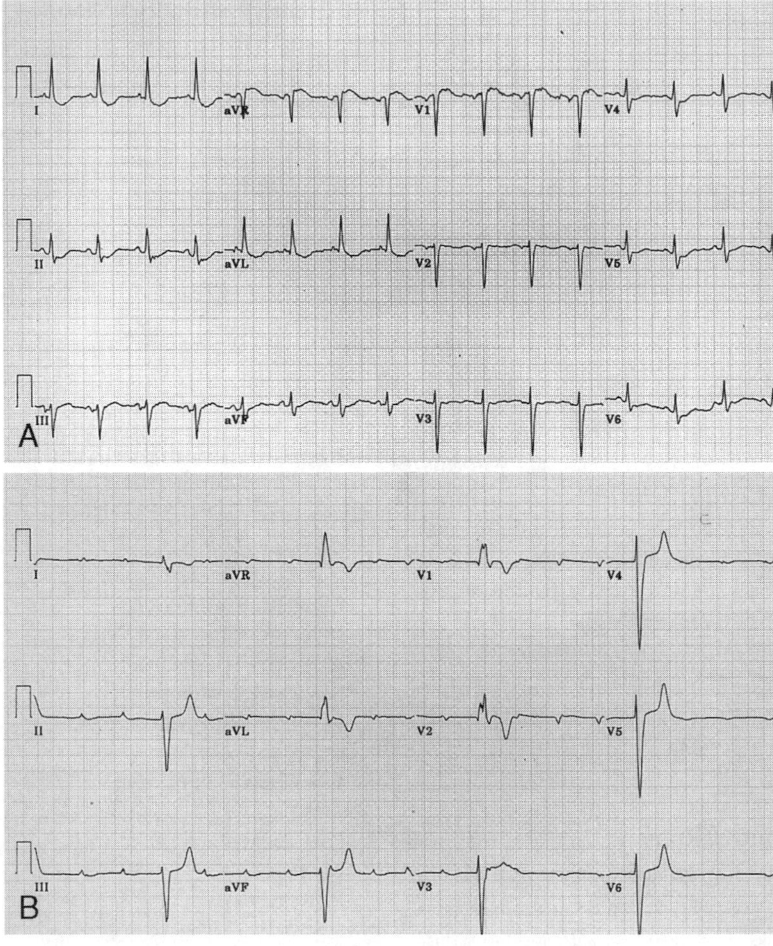

FIGURE 2.2.

A. Normal sinus rhythm with a normal P-R interval and normal QRS duration. **B.** Two days later, sinus tachycardia is present but there is no relationship between the P waves and the QRS complexes. The QRS is wide and clearly different from that noted in part A. The ventricular escape rate is 28 beat/min.

(Fig. 2.2B) or junctional (Fig. 2.3; see also Fig. 2.17B) escape focus at a rate of 60 beats/min or less. In atrial fibrillation complicated by complete heart block, the fibrillatory waves are seen; unlike the typical irregularly irregular QRS rhythm, however, the QRS complex is regular and occurs at a rate of 60 beats/min or less. When atrial fibrillation is the native rhythm but the ventricular rate is regular and exceeds 60 beats/min, the clinician must consider increased automaticity as the mechanism for the regularization. Increased automaticity may be due to the development of ventricular or junctional tachycardia and may occur with ischemia, certain drugs (e.g., isoproterenol), or myocardial inflammation.

VENTRICULAR HYPERTROPHY

Right Ventricular Hypertrophy

Right ventricular hypertrophy may be due to

- Congenital heart disease
- Acquired valvular disease, such as mitral stenosis
- Pulmonary hypertension
- Chronic lung disease, specifically emphysema

As ventricular mass increases, it generates more electrical amplitude in a rightward and anterior direction. If this increase is great enough, it may lead to a frontal axis shift to the right and a gain in anterior forces. A variety of ECG

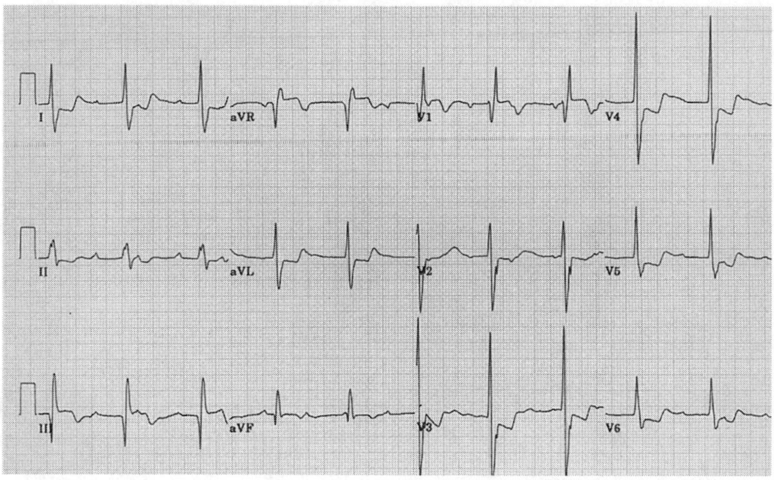

FIGURE 2.3.

Sinus tachycardia is present in a patient with a preexisting right bundle-branch block. There are more P waves than QRS complexes and no fixed P-R interval. The junctional rate is slightly faster than the usual escape rate of 60 beats/min or less.

changes may occur (Table 2.4). The increase in anterior forces may lead to a dominance of right-sided precordial forces. Right ventricular hypertrophy may be indicated if the height of the R wave in lead V1 is greater than or equal to the depth of the S wave in lead V1 (the R/S ratio). More pronounced right ventricular hypertrophy is characterized by prominent S waves in the left lateral leads and by right axis deviation (Fig. 2.4). A right ventricular strain pattern may develop in right ventricular hypertrophy as a result of systolic pressure overload. This is seen in early precordial and inferior leads. The ST-T segment will be depressed, although the ST segment will be in a convex upward shape (an inverted T wave). An incomplete right bundle-branch block pattern may be present in right ventricular hypertrophy associated with atrial septal defect or mitral stenosis. A less impressive ECG pattern may be associated with right ventricular hypertrophy caused by emphysema or chronic obstructive pulmonary disease. Normally, the R/S ratio increases from leads V1 to V6, reaching 1 or more by lead V4. In this form of right ventricular hypertrophy, the precordial R-wave progression proceeds slowly and the R/S ratio may not become 1. Right axis deviation accompanies this abnormal precordial R-wave progression (Figs. 2.5 and 2.6). Low voltage may also be present, defined as the following:

- Total QRS amplitude in leads 1, 2, and 3 $\leq$ 5 mm
  or
- Average amplitude in limb leads $<$ 5 mm
  and
- Average amplitude in precordial leads $<$ 10 mm

TABLE 2.4. Diagnosis of Right Ventricular Hypertrophy

R/S $\geq$ 1.0 in lead V1
Right axis deviation
Incomplete right bundle-branch block pattern
Poor precordial R-wave progression
Low voltage
P-wave pulmonale
S/R $>$ 1.0 in leads 1, 2, 3, in children

Left Ventricular Hypertrophy

Left ventricular hypertrophy is most commonly caused by systemic hypertension. It also occurs in valvular lesions, especially aortic stenosis and mitral and aortic insufficiency; certain congenital lesions; and other disease states. The increased muscle mass increases the normal QRS voltage in the usual leftward and posterior direction and lengthens the duration of depolarization to, at most, the upper limits of normal. The amplitude of the QRS voltage generated is important to the diagnosis of left ventricular hypertrophy but varies depending on the patient's age. Many schemata are available to diagnose left ventricular hypertrophy using an ECG. Although good specificity may be achieved, sensitivity is poor. Two commonly used criteria are the following:

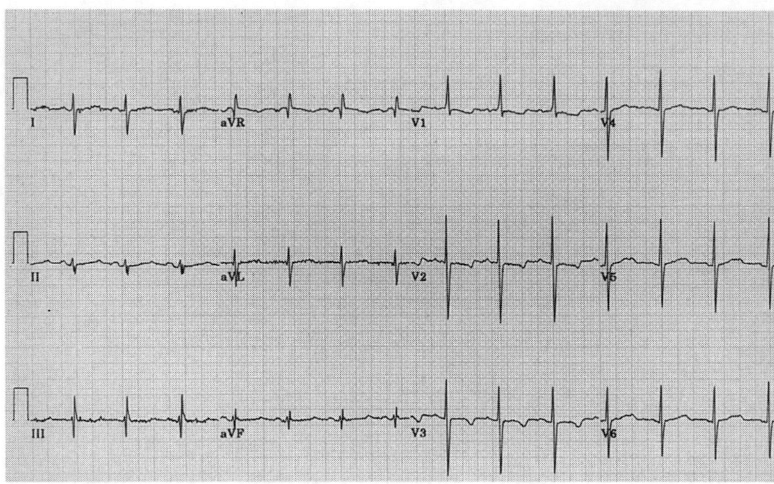

FIGURE 2.4.
Right ventricular hypertrophy.

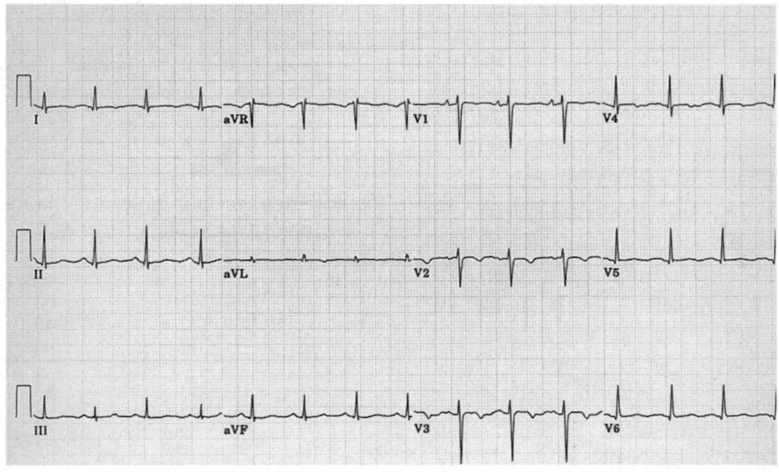

FIGURE 2.5.
Young woman with primary pulmonary hypertension.

Sokolow and Lyon:
S wave in lead V1 plus R wave in V5 or V6 (whichever is taller) ≥35 mm

Romhilt and Estes:

1. R or S in limb lead: ≥20 mm 3 points
   S in V1, V2, or V3 ≥25 mm 3 points
   R in V4, V5, or V6 ≥25 mm 3 points
2. Typical "strain" ST-T (without digitalis) 3 points
   Typical "strain" ST-T (with digitalis) 1 point
3. Left axis deviation: −15° or more 2 points
4. QRS interval: ≥0.09 seconds 1 point
5. Intrinsicoid delay in leads V5 and V6: ≥0.04 seconds 1 point
6. Negative terminal P in lead V1 ≥ 0.04 3 points

Total: score of 5 = left ventricular hypertrophy; score of 4 = probable left ventricular hypertrophy.

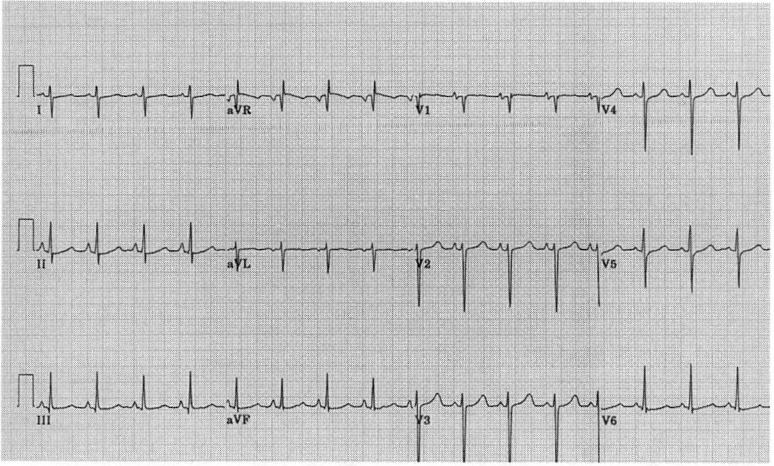

FIGURE 2.6.
Same patient as in Figure 2.5 Her pulmonary pressures have increased over 3 years and the electrocardiogram now shows right-axis deviation and right atrial enlargement.

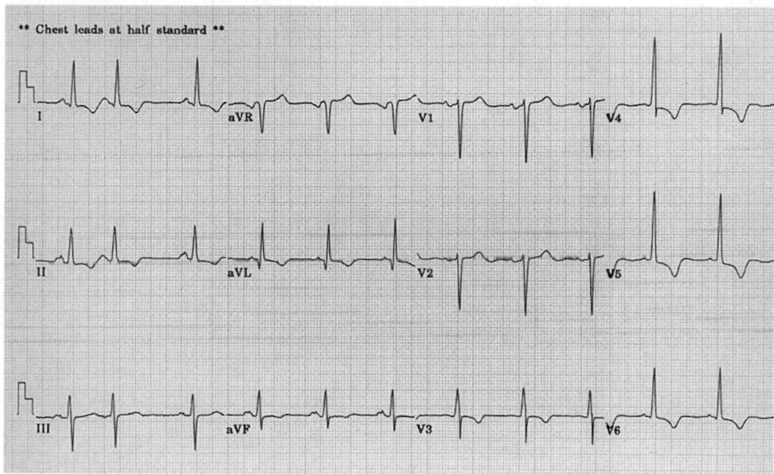

FIGURE 2.7.
The chest leads were obtained at half-standard in this 49-year-old hypertensive man who has left ventricular hypertrophy and marked increase in QRS voltage.

The "strain" pattern seen in left ventricular hypertrophy occurs in various nonprecordial leads, depending on the frontal axis. This ST-segment depression is often seen in leads V5 and V6 as a convex ST-segment depressed into an inverted T wave (Fig. 2.7). Reciprocal concave ST-segment elevation occurs in the early precordial leads and is confusing in patients in whom an acute ischemic pain syndrome is suspected. The "strain" pattern is common in patients with systolic pressure overload; in the pure diastolic overload syndromes (such as those occurring with aortic or mitral insufficiency), the ST-T wave abnormalities may be absent.

ATRIAL HYPERTROPHY

Left atrial hypertrophy is a misnomer because the ECG abnormalities reflect intra-atrial conduction abnormalities, not an increase in atrial mass or a shift in axis.

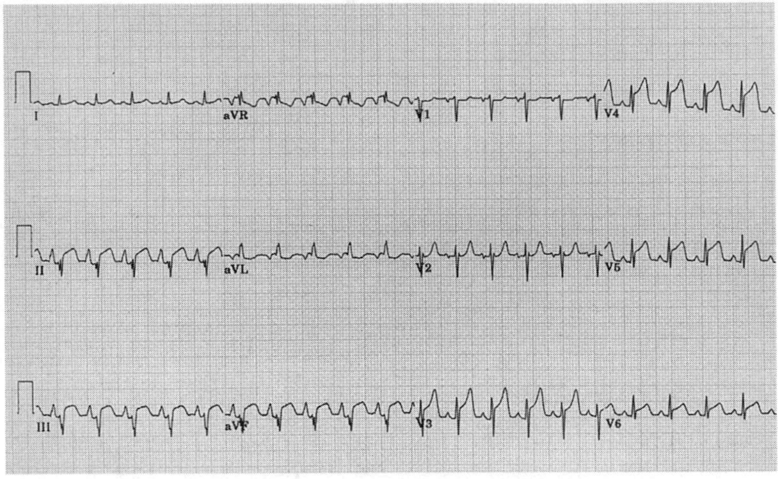

FIGURE 2.8.
Middle-aged man with lung cancer. The P waves are at least 3 mm in height in inferior leads. The ST-segment elevations reflect pericardial involvement from the tumor.

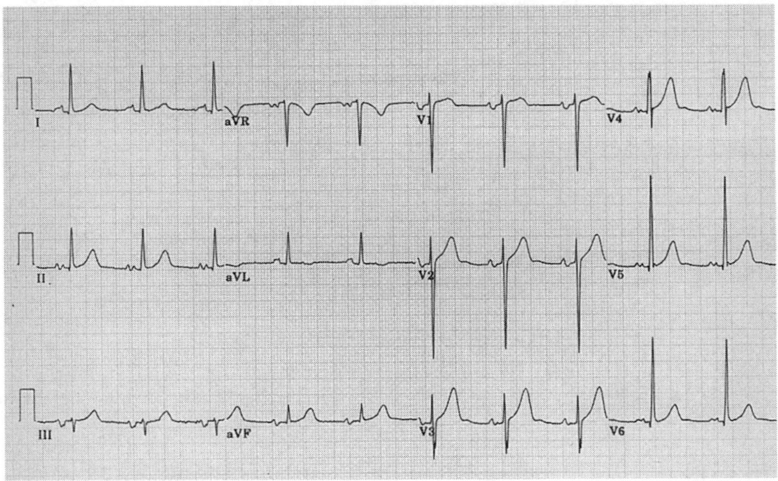

FIGURE 2.9.
Both criteria for left atrial enlargement are present.

Thus, a better term is intra-atrial conduction abnormality or atrial abnormality.

Right Atrial Hypertrophy

Right atrial hypertrophy may lead to a prominent P wave in lead V1 and is often caused by congenital heart disease. P-wave pulmonale, often seen in adults with primary pulmonary hypertension or pulmonary parenchymal disease, is due to a shift in the P-wave vector to a more inferior axis that results in a tall P wave ($\geq$2.5 mm) in the inferior leads (Fig. 2.8). The P-wave duration remains normal at 0.11 seconds or less.

Left Atrial Hypertrophy

Left atrial hypertrophy represents slowed intra-atrial conduction. Fibrosis of the left atrium, as might be seen with rheumatic mitral valve disease, prolongs the dura-

Bundle-Branch Block TABLE 2.5.

Variable	Right Bundle-Branch Block	Left Bundle-Branch Block
QRS duration	0.12 seconds	0.12 seconds
Initial QRS complex	Unaltered: Q wave in leads I and V6; R wave in leads V1, and 2	Altered: No Q wave in leads I, and V6
QRS delay	Results in triphasic wave in leads I, V1, and V6 (Large S wave in leads I, and V6; "rabbit ears" in lead V1)	Results in monophasic R wave in leads I, and V6
Intrinsicoid delay	Lead V1 > 0.02 seconds	Lead V6 > 0.04 seconds
Secondary T wave changes	T-wave inversion in lead V1	T-wave inversion in leads I, and V6
Ability to diagnose Q-wave myocardial infarction	Not usually difficult	More difficult, but sometimes possible

tion of the P wave and explains the second deflection noted in P-wave mitrale, best seen in leads 3 and aVF (Fig. 2.9). The first deflection represents right atrial depolarization, and the latter deflection represents the slowed left atrial depolarization. The duration of the P wave exceeds 0.11 seconds. Specific to the diagnosis of left atrial hypertrophy is the presence of 0.04 seconds between the two peaks of the P wave. Left atrial hypertrophy may also be diagnosed by certain criteria noted in lead V1 (Fig. 2.7). The P wave in lead V1 should be biphasic; the initial deflection is positive and is followed by a negative deflection whose area is at least 0.04 mm-sec. This is determined by multiplying the duration (in seconds) of the negative deflection by the negative depth (in mm). This is the left atrial hypertrophy criterion used in the Romhilt and Estes criteria for left ventricular hypertrophy.

INTRAVENTRICULAR CONDUCTION ABNORMALITIES

Bundle-Branch Block

Right Bundle-Branch Block

Right bundle-branch block is characterized by a QRS duration of 0.12 seconds or more (Table 2.5). The initial portion of the QRS complex is normal in direction and time, but later conduction is shifted rightward and anteriorly. This shift gives the QRS a large S wave in leads I and V6 and the second S wave in leads V1 and V2 (the second "rabbit ear"; Fig. 2.10). The QRS complex is usually 0.12 seconds. Drug effect or conditions that further slow conduction may lead to a longer duration. In typical right bundle-branch block, the T wave may invert in leads V1 to V3. In otherwise uncomplicated right bundle-branch block, T waves are normally upright in leads V4 to V6. Therefore, symmetrical T-wave inversion in the face of a right bundle-branch block in leads V1 to V3 do not necessarily indicate myocardial ischemia; however, similar T-wave inversion in leads V4 to V6 or ST-segment depression is abnormal (Fig. 2.3). Myocardial infarction can be diagnosed according to the presence of right bundle-branch block. Loss of the first "rabbit ear" (R wave) in leads V1 to V3 should alert the physician to the possibility of a septal myocardial infarction (Fig. 2.11).

Left Bundle-Branch Block

Unlike right bundle-branch block (Table 2.5), left bundle-branch block usually precludes diagnosis of myocardial infarction. The QRS duration is 0.12 seconds or slightly more in uncomplicated left bundle-branch block; early depolarization is abnormally directed toward the left (thus, no Q wave should be seen in leads I, aVL, and V6; Fig. 2.12). The QRS complex shifts more to the left and more posteriorly. Therefore, R-wave progression in the precordial leads may be delayed and the R waves in leads V1 to V3 may be small. Finally, T-wave inversion in leads I, aVL, and the left precordial leads, especially V6, is anticipated. The presence of a Q wave in leads I, aVL, and V6 is not anticipated in left bundle-branch block and should alert the clinician to the possibility of concomitant anteroseptal myocardial infarction. Significant ST-segment changes may be interpretable in the presence of a left bundle-branch block if sequential ECGs show changing ST segments (Fig.

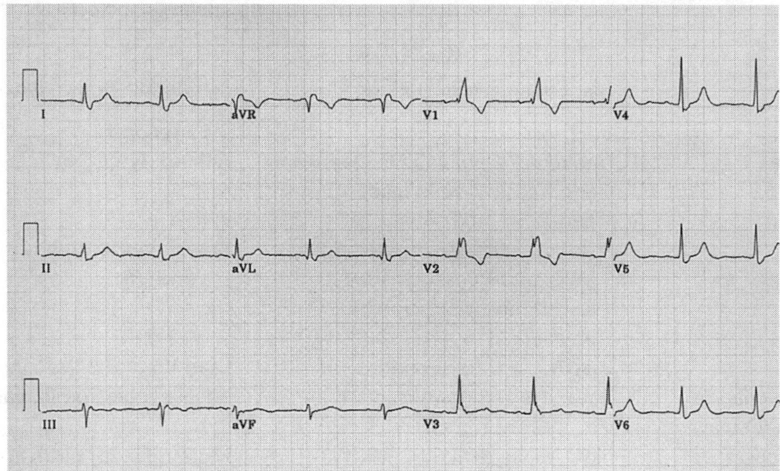

FIGURE 2.10.
Right bundle-branch block.

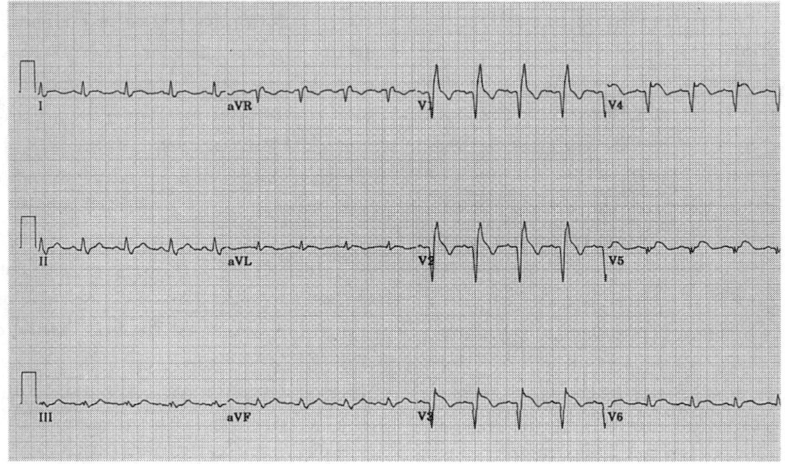

FIGURE 2.11.
Middle-aged man with extensive coronary artery disease and anterior-wall aneurysm. The initial R wave in V1–V5 is missing because of infarction.

2.13). This might occur with infarction or ischemia. A left bundle-branch block complicated by left axis deviation implies the presence of more severe conduction disease, worse myocardial function, and decreased survival rate than if left axis deviation were absent.

Hemiblock

The left bundle branch divides into two fascicles: The longer and thinner left anterior or left superior fascicle has a single blood supply, and the stouter left posterior or inferior fascicle has a dual blood supply. This dual blood supply partly explains why the incidence of left posterior hemiblock is uncommon relative to left anterior hemiblock.

A block in conduction down either of these fascicles leads to a shift in the frontal plane axis and tends to increase limb lead voltage. The block of the anterior fascicle shifts the frontal axis leftward to at least −45° (Table 2.6). A block in the posterior fascicle shifts the frontal axis right to at least 120°. In pure fascicular block, the QRS complex should not be abnormally prolonged. Fascicular block also tends to increase limb lead voltage. Variation in the initial QRS deflections depends on which fascicle is affected.

Left anterior hemiblock is the diagnosis if leads II,

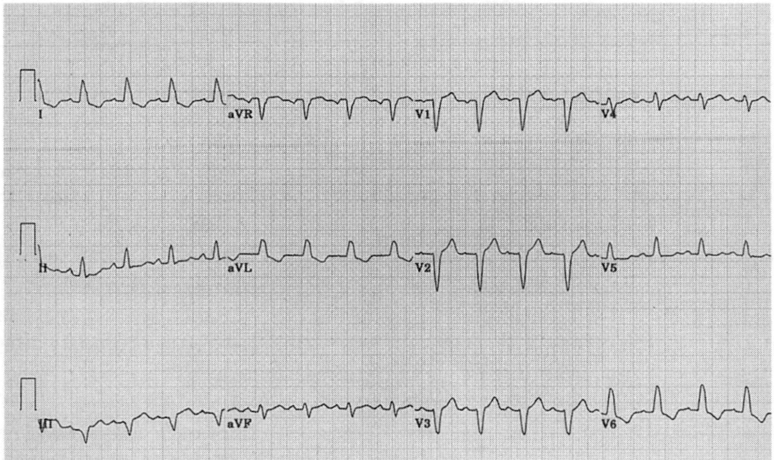

FIGURE 2.12.
Left bundle-branch block.

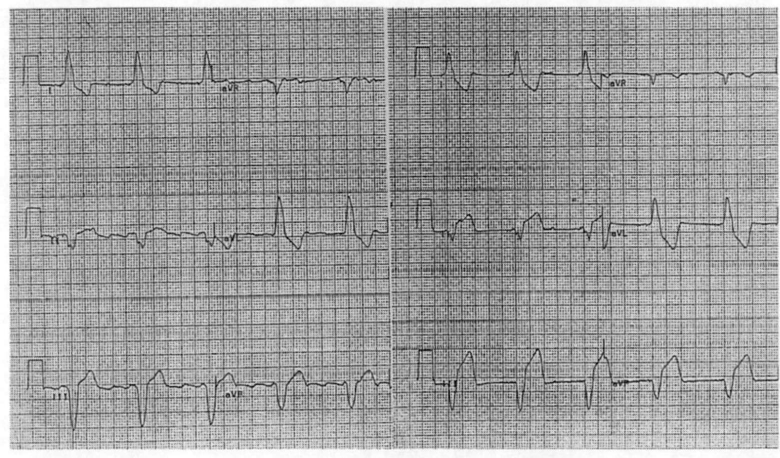

FIGURE 2.13.
Elderly man with permanent ventricular pacemaker and left bundle-branch pattern. The electrocardiogram was obtained on 2 consecutive days: the first after successful right coronary artery angioplasty and the second soon after thrombosis developed in the right coronary artery. Note that the ST-segment elevations in leads II, III, and aVF are more marked on the second day, a finding compatible with a current of injury involving the inferior wall.

III, and aVF display a small R wave followed by a large S wave (Fig. 2.14). Left posterior hemiblock is the diagnosis if the opposite is seen: Tiny Q waves followed by a large R wave must be present in leads II, III, and aVF. Intrinsicoid delay is prolonged in both hemiblocks. Left posterior hemiblock is difficult to diagnose if right ventricular hypertrophy is present because the latter condition alone may shift the frontal axis rightward. However, left posterior hemiblock is usually diagnosed in association with a right bundle-branch block. The physician must determine the frontal axis during the first half of the QRS complex because the right bundle-branch block subsequently slows depolarization; this alone may shift the axis rightward.

Although isolated left anterior hemiblock may be found in persons with normal hearts, the incidence of future right bundle-branch block may be increased in these individuals. In contrast, left posterior hemiblock usually occurs concomitantly with right bundle-branch block and is usually associated with extensive coronary artery disease. Unfortunately, hemiblocks may both mimic and mask myocardial infarction and ventricular

TABLE 2.6. The Hemiblocks

Variable	Left Anterior Hemiblock	Right Inferior Hemiblock
Frontal axis	Usually −60°	Usually +120°
Leads II, III, and aVF	Small R wave, large S wave Small Q wave in leads I and aVL	Small Q wave, large R wave Small R wave in leads I and aVL
Usual QRS duration	≤ 0.10 seconds	≤ 0.10 seconds
Intrinsicoid delay	Lead aVL > 0.045 seconds	Lead aVF > 0.045 seconds
Etiology	Normal variant Aortic valve calcification Cardiomyopathy Ischemic heart disease Transient with hyperkalemia, trauma	Usually seen in presence of right bundle-branch block and associated with extensive coronary artery disease
Other		Cannot be diagnosed in presence of right ventricular hypertrophy

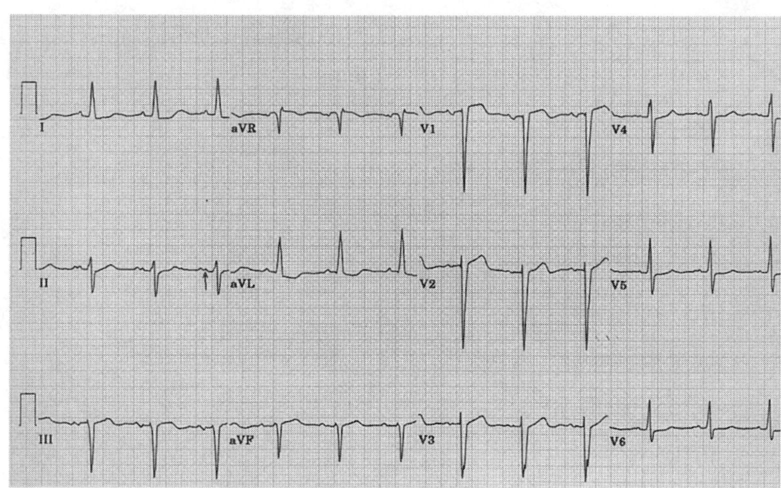

FIGURE 2.14.
Left atrial enlargement, left ventricular hypertrophy, and left anterior hemiblock.

hypertrophy. This may result from (*a*) the changes in initial depolarization and (*b*) a shift of voltage caused by unopposed depolarization or axis shifts that result from the alterations in depolarization sequences.

Atherosclerotic Heart Disease

Atherosclerotic heart disease alters the ECG by three mechanisms: Myocardial ischemia, myocardial injury, and myocardial infarction. Myocardial ischemia is characterized by the development of symmetrical T-wave inversions (Figs. 2.15 and 2.16), which resolve as the ischemia resolves. With prolonged ischemia, ST-segment elevation may occur over the ischemic areas (Fig. 2.17A and 17B). This ST-segment elevation is termed a "current of injury" but, like the ischemic T-wave inversion, may resolve as the ischemia resolves.

The next stage of ischemia is myocardial infarction or necrosis: ischemia has persisted long enough to induce irreversible myocardial changes. Myocardial tissue necroses and may result in the development of Q waves (Fig. 2.17C). Any Q wave lasting 0.03 seconds or longer should be considered suspicious. Q waves develop because necrosed myocardium fails to generate electrical forces. When the electrode reflecting the electrical force generated by this now necrosed area is placed over the infarcted tissue, the R wave is not generated and the unopposed depolarizing areas of the ventricle cause a negative deflection.

Changes in the T wave, ST segment, and QRS complex may occur rapidly, over hours to days. One of the early signs in the evolution of infarction is development of tall "hyperacute" T waves over the affected myocardium (Fig. 2.18). ST segments then begin to elevate, demonstrating the characteristic upward convexity (Fig. 2.19). ST-segment elevation is relatively transient, and the segment may return to baseline within hours to days. As the ST segment elevates, T-wave inversion begins and may continue to invert as the ST segment returns toward baseline. Q waves or decreasing R-wave voltage over necrosed areas may develop within hours to days of infarction. T-wave inversion may last for weeks. Persistent ST-segment elevation suggests aneurysm formation. Pericarditis associated with Q-wave myocardial infarction may also lead to diffuse ST-segment elevations. Because chest pain is so protean and because ST-segment elevation may occur in early

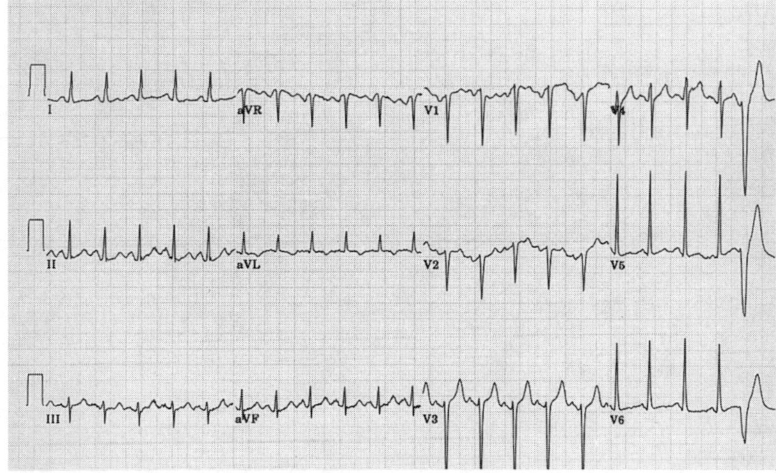

FIGURE 2.15.
Elderly woman examined in the emergency department after having chest pain 2 hours earlier.

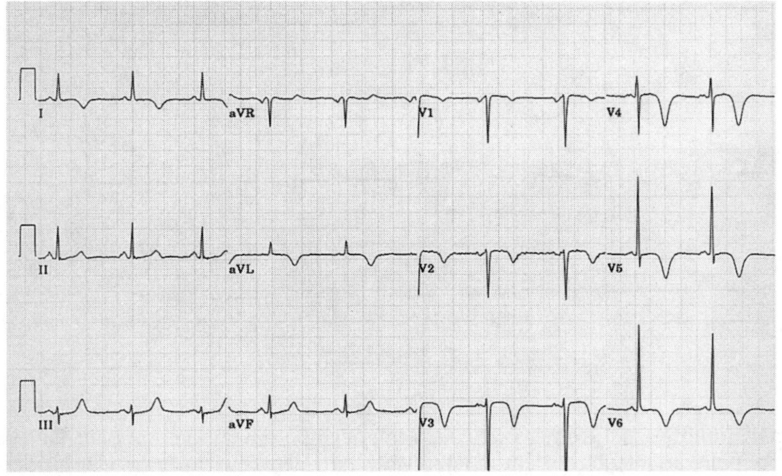

FIGURE 2.16.
The same patient shown in Figure 2.15 while having chest pain the following day.

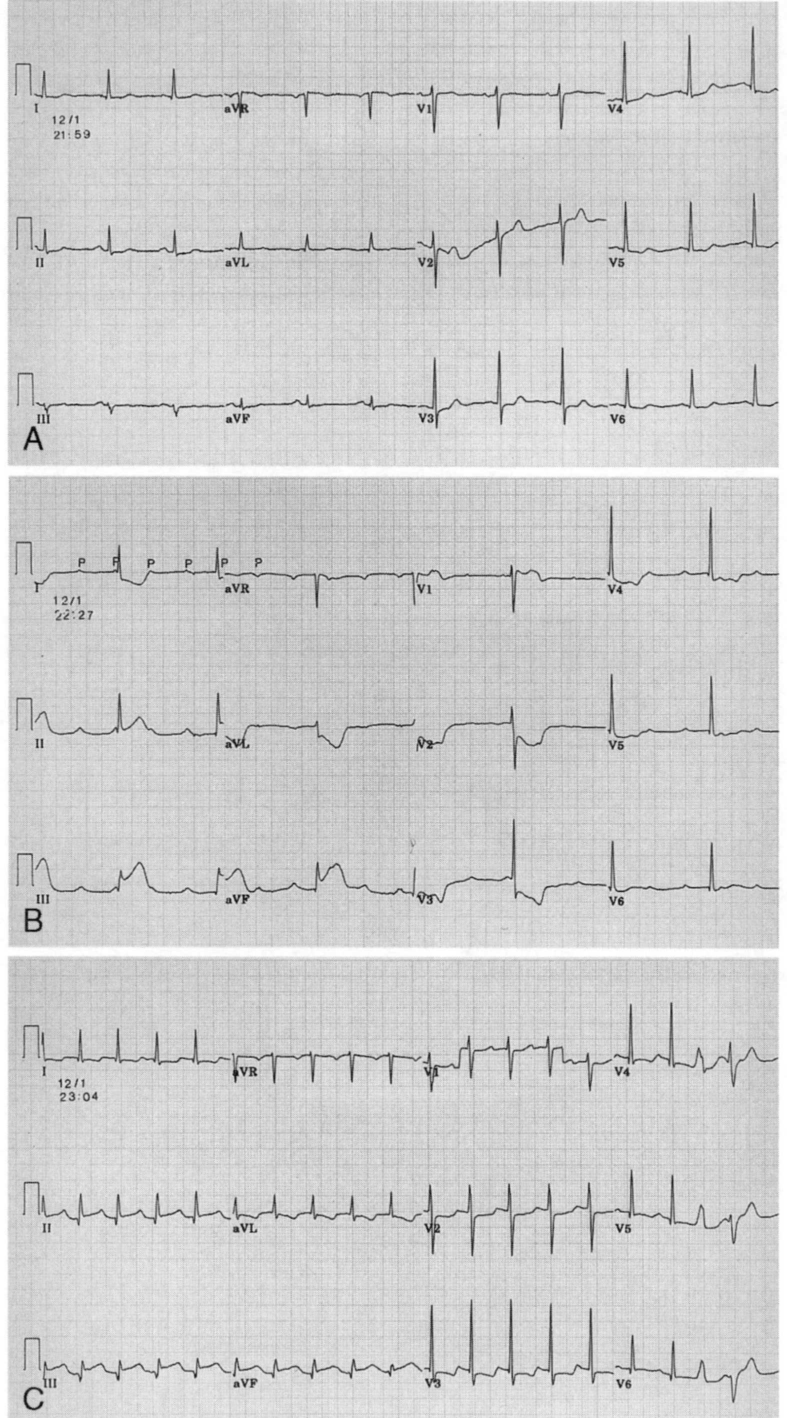

FIGURE 2.17.

A. A 65-year-old man admitted to the emergency department with new-onset chest pain. **B.** Twenty-eight minutes later, with more pain, an inferior current of injury and third-degree atrioventricular block develops with a junctional escape rhythm at a rate of 46 beats/min. **C.** 37 minutes later, atrioventricular conduction is restored. The ST-segment elevations are less prominent, and new Q waves (but not lasting 0.03 seconds) have developed. These Q waves are important because they are new.

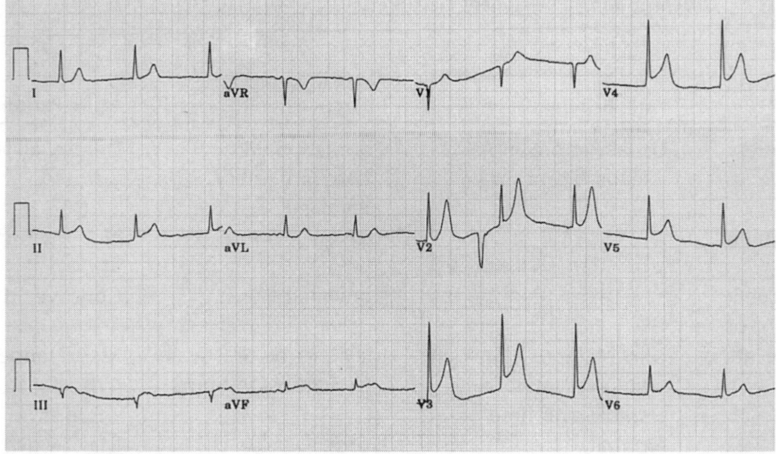

FIGURE 2.18.
Although the baseline is moving, the peaked T wave in lead V2 without significant ST-segment elevation is characteristic of the hyperacute T wave seen in early transmural ischemia. The next stage is development of ST-segment elevation (Figure 2.19).

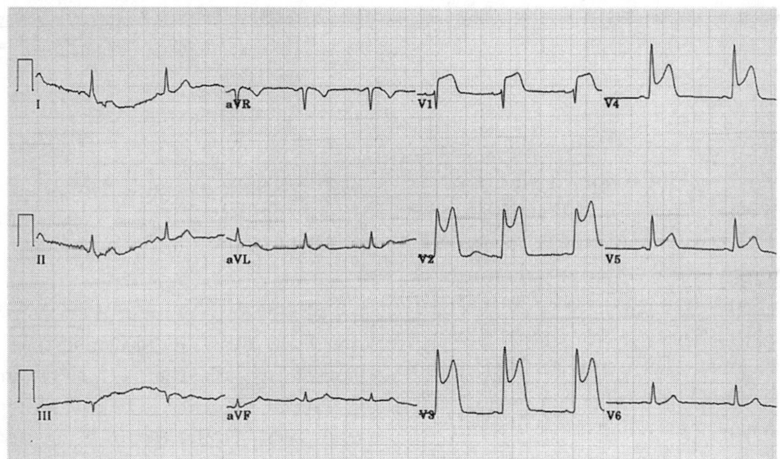

FIGURE 2.19.
Same patient shown in Figure 2.18. He has impressive ST-segment elevation 22 minutes later.

repolarization as well as in acute myocardial infarction and acute pericarditis, certain associated ECG features might be helpful in reaching a diagnosis (Table 2.7). In about 15% of patients, the Q wave, although considered permanent, disappears within a few years after infarction.

Reciprocal changes may develop in acute infarction when ST-segment elevation occurs over the necrosing myocardium. Areas of myocardium that are absolutely opposite the involved myocardium should demonstrate opposite ST-segment changes; for example, if a current of injury is present in the infarcting area, the reciprocal changes are ST-segment depressions in the opposite areas.

Leads II, III, and aVF reflect the inferior wall. Acute inferior infarction with ST-segment elevation results in reciprocal changes in the opposite leads I, aVL, and, at times, anterior leads. An anterior infarction may cause ST-segment elevation in certain anterior leads. Reciprocal changes are thus expected in leads II, III, and aVF. Other opposing lead placements, over the posterior wall, are not routine. Such is

TABLE 2.7. **Differentiating ST-Segment Elevations**

Variable	Early Repolarization	Acute Myocardial Infarction	Acute Pericarditis
ST-segment location	Usually in precordial leads except for V6	Correlation with coronary artery involved	Diffuse, all leads except aVR, and V1
Height of ST-segment elevation		May be > 5 mm	Not > 5 mm
Shape of ST-segment		Convex upward	Concave upward
Changes in height of ST-segment elevation	May be more prominent at lower rates; fairly stable over time	May change drastically in minutes to hours	May change over days, usually not minutes to hours
PR segment	Normal	Normal	May be depressed
QT interval	Normal	Often long	Normal
Q wave	Fails to develop	Develops	Rarely develops
Reciprocal changes between lead I and lead III		Often present	ST-segment elevated in both lead I and lead III

the problem in lateral-wall infarction, in which the ST-segment elevation is expected in leads I and aVL. The routine 12-lead ECG may show only reciprocal ST-segment depression in lead V1. Reciprocal changes of true posterior-wall involvement are seen in leads V1 and V2.

Subendocardial myocardial ischemia may result in ST-segment depression (Figs. 2.20A and 2.20B). Myocardial infarction may not result in the development of Q waves. Loss of myocardium, which generates QRS voltage, sometimes leads only to a decrease in R-wave voltage over the infarcted myocardium. The infarcted area may not be seen on the surface ECG because of its anatomic location.

Electrocardiographic Leads

The 12-lead ECG can "look" at certain areas of the heart. Generally accepted anatomic correlations with the ECG leads are the following:

Anteroseptal area	V1–V4
Anterolateral	V1–V6
Lateral	I, aVL
Inferior	II, III, aVF
Inferolateral	II, III, aVF, V5, V6
Inferoapical	II, III, aVF, V4, V5
Inferoposterior	II, III, avF, V1, V2
Posterior	V1, V2

With the exception of the posterior wall, electrodes over these areas should demonstrate the T-wave inversion of ischemia, the ST-T elevation of injury, or the Q wave of infarction. The true posterior wall is not directly seen because electrodes are not normally placed on the posterior chest. The physician therefore infers involvement of the posterior wall by determining whether reciprocal changes are present in leads V1 and V2. Posterior injury should cause ST-segment depression in leads V1 and V2 and infarction should cause a gain in R-wave voltage in leads V1 and V2 (Fig. 2.21). In the presence of a posterior myocardial infarction, the R wave should be greater than or equal to the S wave (therefore, the R/S ratio is ≥ 1). True posterior-wall infarctions are usually accompanied by an inferior- or lateral-wall infarction, which may help in the diagnosis.

Because of collateral circulation and coronary artery bypass grafting, interpretation of the ECG may not reliably indicate which coronary vessel is responsible for the infarction. Infarction of the right ventricle

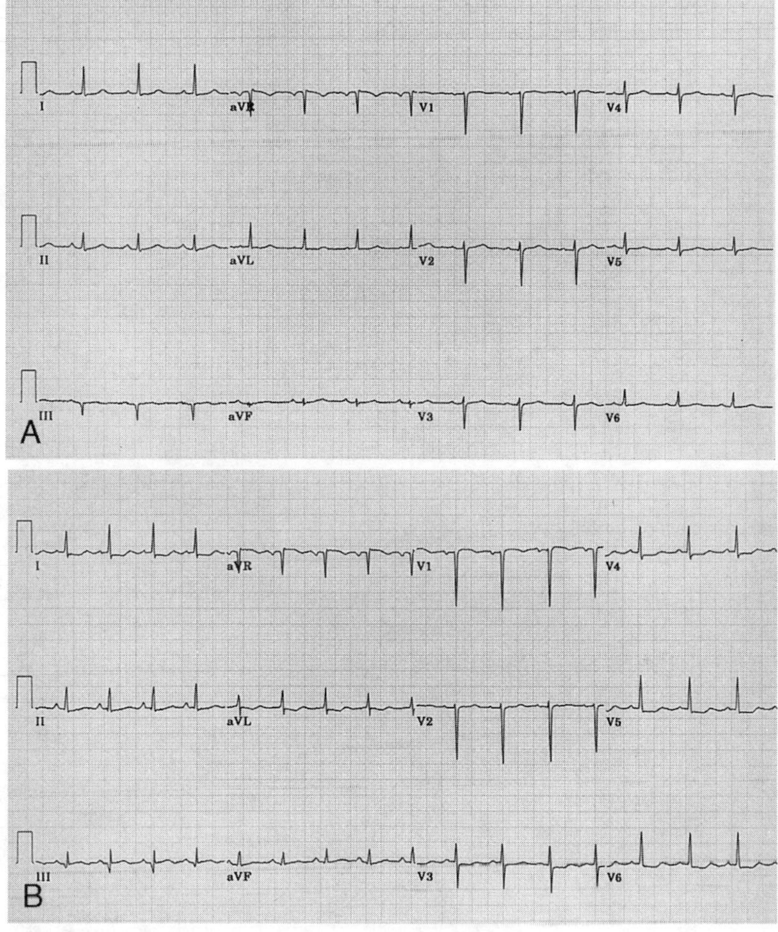

FIGURE 2.20.

A. Baseline electrocardiogram (ECG) of a 45-year-old woman. She had had chest pain before presentation; in the emergency department, however, this ECG was obtained in a pain-free state. **B.** ECG with chest pain. Note planar ST-segment depression in leads I, aVL, and V3 to V6. The ST-segment depression in lead V5 is greater than 1 mm and is diagnostic of subendocardial ischemia. Cardiac catheterization revealed 70% stenoses of both the ostial left main and proximal left anterior descending coronary arteries.

may be as deadly as infarction of the left ventricle. It may be associated with medically recalcitrant heart block and cardiogenic shock. During an acute inferior infarction, right ventricular involvement should be suspected. This is strongly suggested by ST-segment elevation of at least 1 mm in V3R or V4R (Figs. 2.22A and 2.22B).

Atrial infarction, which is usually limited to inferior-wall infarction, is suspected when P-R depression occurs. Atrial arrhythmias commonly develop when the atrium infarcts. P-R depression may also occur in acute pericarditis.

Pericardial Disease

Acute pericarditis may lead to diffuse ST-segment elevation in all leads except aVR and V1. The P-R segment may be depressed. Because both acute myocardial infarction and acute pericarditis may be associated with ST-segment elevations and chest pain, differentiating the two diseases is sometimes difficult. In addition, early repolarization is associated with ST-segment elevation; the latter, however, is normally not seen in all leads and may be resolved by increasing the heart rate (unlike the ST-segment elevations of acute myocardial

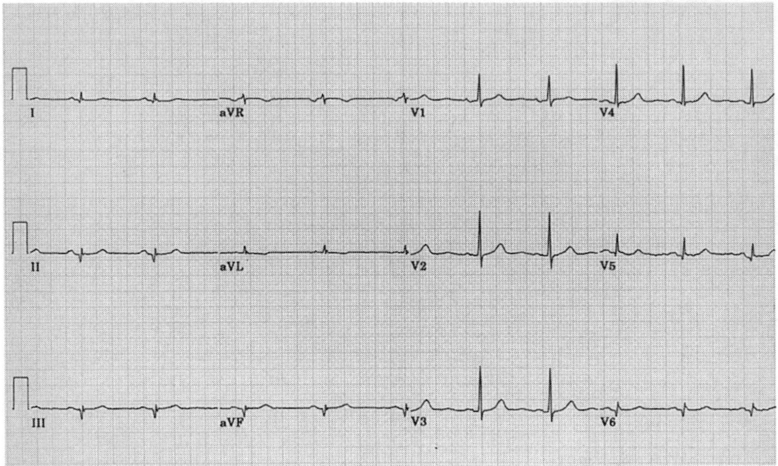

FIGURE 2.21.
Inferior and posterior myocardial infarction.

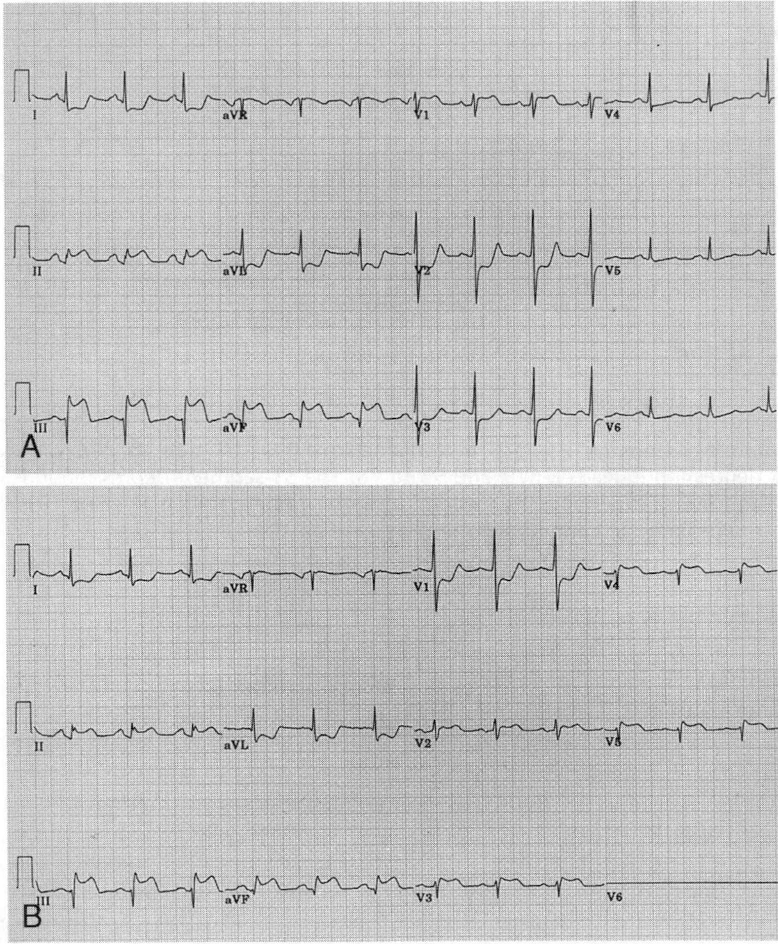

FIGURE 2.22.
A. Elderly woman in the midst of myocardial infarction involving the inferior and posterior regions after failed angioplasty. **B.** These are right-sided leads; thus, V1 equals V2, V2 equals V1, and V3 to V5 are placed on the right chest. Note the 2-mm ST-segment elevation in leads V3R and V4R. This patient also had right ventricular infarction. Emergency cardiac surgery was successful.

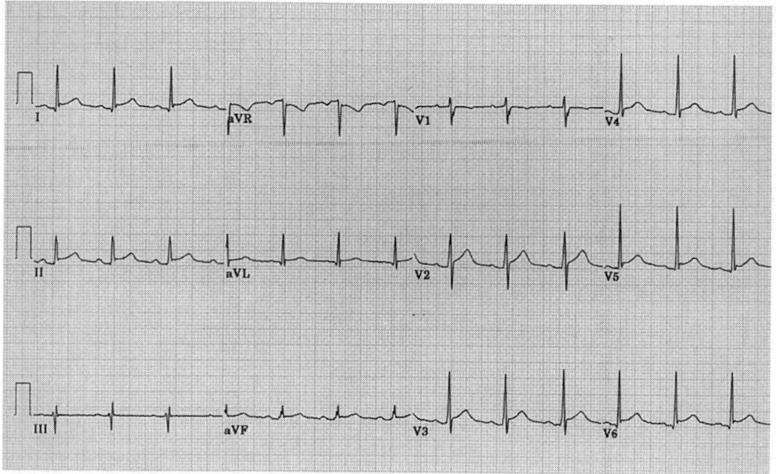

FIGURE 2.23.
ST-segment elevations should traditionally be present in all leads except aVR and V1. In this patient, lead III is spared.

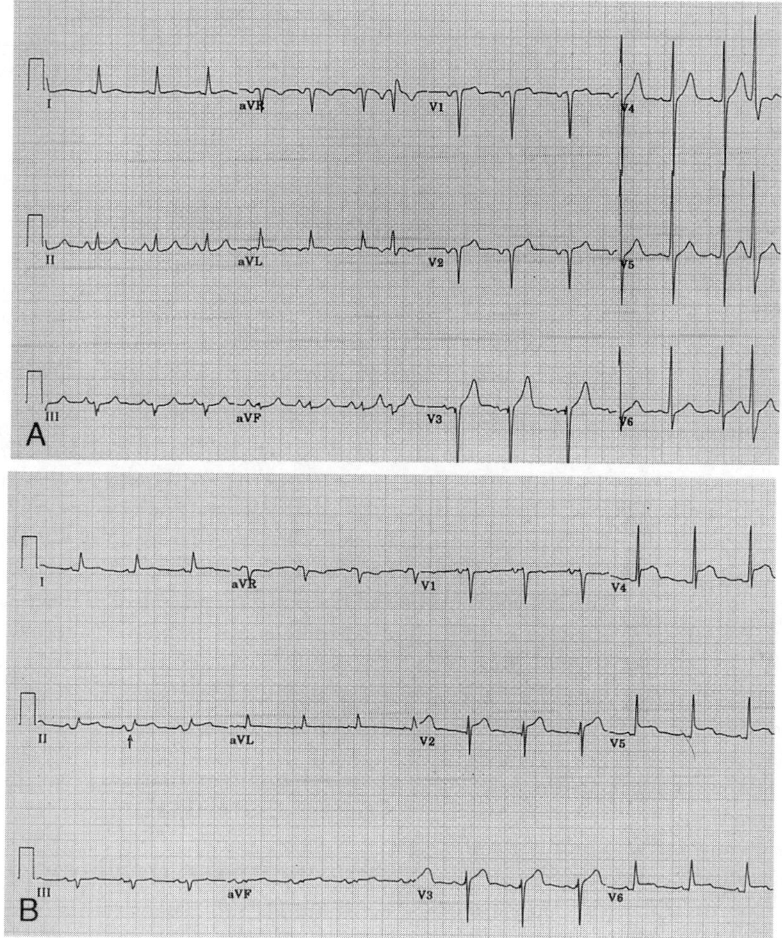

FIGURE 2.24.
A. Baseline electrocardiogram in man with lung cancer. **B.** Sudden development of ST-segment elevations and P-R depression caused by malignant pericardial effusion.

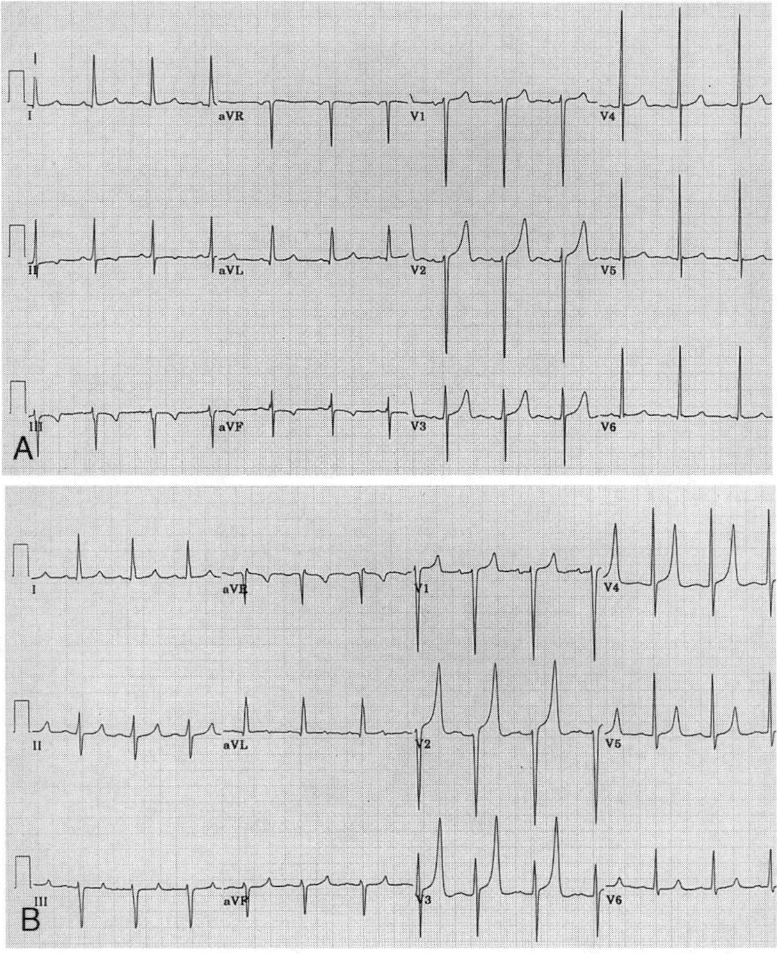

FIGURE 2.25.
A. Potassium level, 4.5 mEq/L. **B.** Potassium level, 7.3 mEq/L. The T waves are remarkably and symmetrically peaked.

infarction and acute pericarditis). Table 2.7 lists other ways to differentiate among these three causes of ST-segment elevation.

Acute pericarditis is associated with ST-segment elevation and, often, P-R-segment depression (Figs. 2.23, 2.24A, and 2.24B). In self-limited cases of acute pericarditis, such as viral or idiopathic, these changes may resolve within 2 weeks. As the ST-segment returns to the isoelectric line, T-wave inversion usually develops and persists for approximately another 2 weeks. As the pericarditis resolves, the T-wave abnormalities usually resolve. Large pericardial effusions may produce ECG criteria for low voltage and electrical alternans in addition to the ST-segment elevation. Sometimes, none or only one of these abnormalities may be present in large effusions. Electrical alternans is usually characterized by alternating heights of the QRS complex, although alternation in the height of the P wave, QRS complex, and T wave, occasionally occurs. Development of pericardial constriction may also cause low voltage in addition to diffusely inverted T waves. Atrial dysrhythmias are commonly found in pericardial constriction.

OTHER CONDITIONS

Potassium Abnormalities

Hyperkalemia and hypokalemia are two entities every primary care physician should be able to recognize and

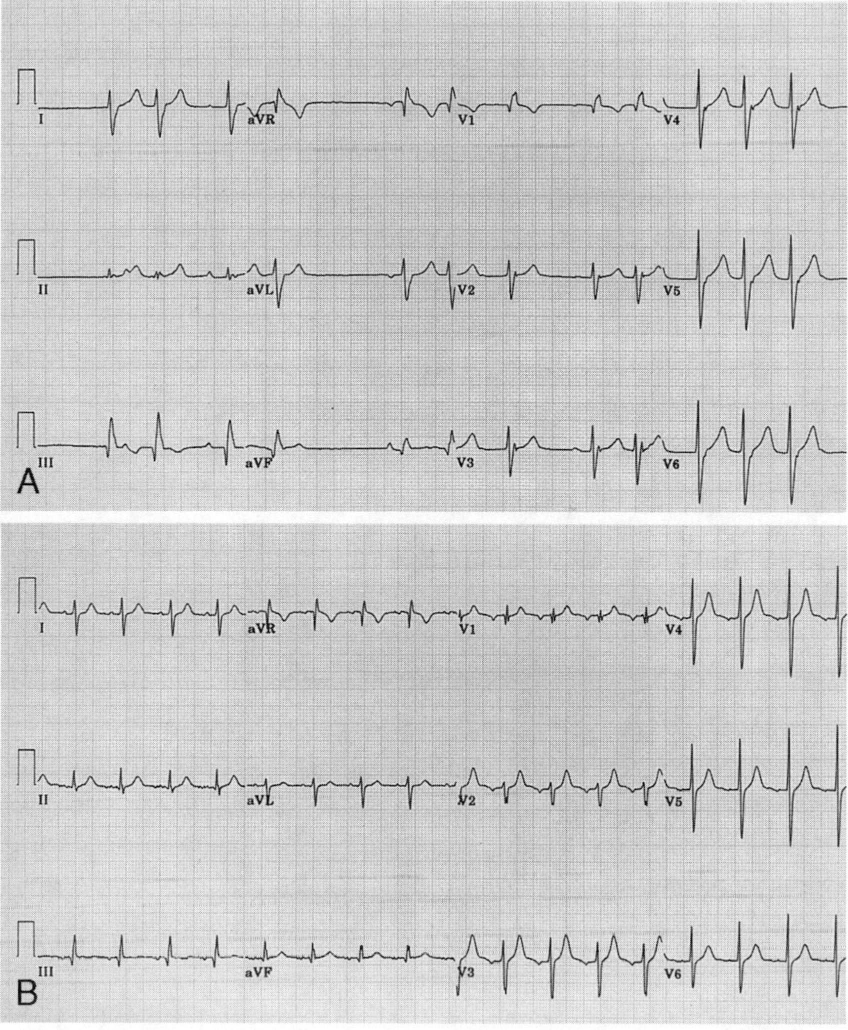

FIGURE 2.26.

A. Potassium level, 7.3 mEq/L. Occasional sinus complexes are present and the QRS is wide. **B.** Treatment of hyperkalemia restores normal sinus rhythm and narrows the QRS complex. Even the wide Q waves in inferior leads narrow.

treat. Both are commonly iatrogenic and potentially fatal and require rapid treatment.

The prominently peaked T waves of hyperkalemia (Figs. 2.25A and 2.25B) are well known to all clinicians and may appear at potassium levels greater than 5.5 mEq/L. As the hyperkalemia progresses, first-degree AV block may develop, the ST-segment may become depressed, and the QRS complex may lengthen (Figs. 2.26A and 2.26B). Even later, the P wave may disappear and the QRS widen further, ultimately culminating in ventricular fibrillation. Unexplained "idioventricular rhythm" should alert the physician to the possible presence of severe hyperkalemia.

On an ECG, low potassium levels are characterized by flattening of the T wave, increasing prominence of the U wave, and development of a U wave that is greater in amplitude than the T wave and that merges with the T wave (Fig. 2.27). As is seen with hyperkalemia, the P-R interval in hypokalemia may prolong and the QRS widen as the ST-segment depresses. Development of fatal ventricular dysrhythmias may supervene.

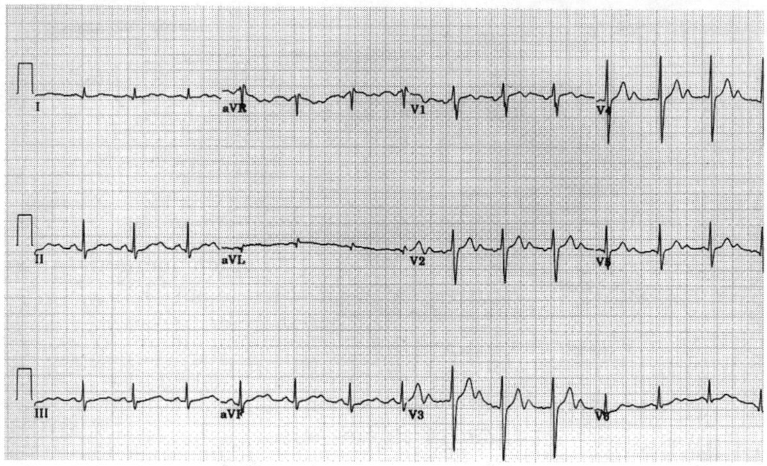

FIGURE 2.27.
Potassium level, 2.4 mEq/L. In limb leads, the T and U waves merge, leading to a long Q-T measurement. In the precordial leads, the T and U waves can be easily separated.

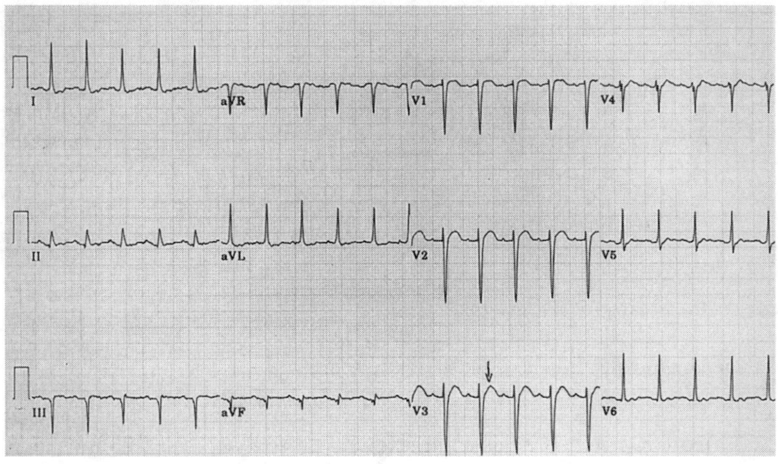

FIGURE 2.28.
The arrow points to early peaking of the T wave, followed by a more gradual sloping off. This patient's calcium level is 15.7 mg/dL.

Hypercalcemia

The ECG suggests hypercalcemia if the Q-T interval is shortened. The shortening, however, occurs during the early part of repolarization, such that the Q-T interval is disproportionately shortened from the end of the QRS complex to the peak of the T wave. This creates the appearance of a steep and rapid slope to the peak of the T wave (Fig. 2.28). Such changes should alert the physician to the possibility of hyperparathyroidism or cancer.

KEY POINTS

Atrioventricular Conduction Abnormalities

- First-degree AV block: Prolongation of the P-R interval > 0.2 seconds. Usually benign or drug-induced (e.g., digoxin, β-blockers, calcium-channel blockers).
- Type I second-degree AV block (Wenckebach phenomenon): Progressive lengthening of the P-R interval; then a P wave not followed by a QRS complex. Usually benign, may be seen in well-conditioned persons, drug-induced, or accompanying acute inferior-wall infarction.
- Type II second-degree AV block: Fixed P-R interval with sudden failure to be followed by a QRS. Wide QRS may be harbinger of complete heart block.
- High-grade second-degree AV block: Two or more successive P waves fail to conduct. Can be associated with acute anterior septal myocardial infarction.
- Third-degree AV block: Complete block in conduction from the atria to the ventricle. May be congenital, associated with increased vagal tone, myocardial infarction, and inflammatory causes, or drug-induced. Upon discovery, cardiology consultation should be obtained for consideration of temporary or permanent pacemaker.

Ventricular and Atrial Hypertrophy

- Right ventricular hypertrophy: found in association with congenital heart disease, mitral stenosis, pulmonary hypertension, and emphysema. May be associated with incomplete right bundle-branch block in patients who have atrial defects and with mitral stenosis. Right axis deviation, and low voltage in patients who have emphysema.
  Tip-off: Tall R wave in lead V1 and prominent S waves in leads V5 and V6.
- Left ventricular hypertrophy: found in patients with hypertension, aortic stenosis, and mitral and aortic regurgitation. Long-standing left ventricular hypertrophy may be associated with "strain pattern" (not to be confused with acute ischemia).
  Tip-off: S wave in lead V1 plus R wave in leads V6 or V6 ≥ 35 mm. More complex diagnosis can be made with point grade system of Romhilt and Estes.
- Right atrial hypertrophy: found in association with congenital heart disease, primary pulmonary hypertension, or intrinsic pulmonary disease.
  Tip-off: Tall, peaked (≥2.5 mm) P waves in leads II, III, and aVF.
- Left atrial hypertrophy: found in association with mitral stenosis and mitral regurgitation, hypertension, and long-standing congestive heart failure.
  Tip-off: Biphasic P wave in V1, negative deflection ≥2–5 mm-sec.

Intraventricular Conduction

- Right bundle-branch block: May be congenital or found in association with right ventricular hypertrophy, atrial septal defects, cardiomyopathies, or coronary artery disease.
  Tip-off: QRS "rabbit ears" in lead V1 (RSR) with inverted T waves in leads V1, V2, and V3. Ensure that the right bundle is *not* initiated by a Q wave, which may indicate anterior septal-wall myocardial infarction.
- Left bundle-branch block: Almost always signifies significant pathologic abnormality. Most commonly seen in advanced hypertensive heart disease, coronary heart disease, and cardiomyopathy.
  Tip-off: QRS > 0.12 seconds in lead I with "rabbit ears" in lead V6. Associated with abnormal ST-T wave changes precluding the diagnosis of ischemia. When associated with left axis deviation, prognosis is much worse.
- Left anterior hemiblock: Frontal axis ≥ −45°. Leads II, III, and aVF: small R wave, large S wave.
- Left posterior hemiblocks: Frontal axis ≥ 120°. Usually in association with right bundle-branch block and extensive coronary artery disease.

Atherosclerotic Heart Disease

- Myocardial ischemia: ST-segment depression and T-wave inversion (especially with exercise), which may return to normal as ischemia resolves.
- Myocardial injury due to prolonged ischemia: ST-segment elevation over the ischemic area producing a current of injury that may resolve if ischemia resolves. Upon discovery in a patient with chest pain, immediate hospitalization with consideration of thrombolytic therapy is warranted.
- Myocardial infarction, which produces tissue necrosis: Tip-off: Appearance of new Q waves in the affected area lasting > 0.03 seconds. May be proceeded by the appearance of tall "hyperacute" T waves, followed by the transient appearance of ST-segment elevation. Reciprocal ST-segment depression confirms the diagnosis of acute myocardial infarction. Right ventricular infarction should be suspected in the presence of an inferior-wall infarction with shock, hypotension, or heart block. Supported by ST-segment elevation in leads V3R or V4R.

Pericarditis and Electrolyte Abnormalities

- Pericarditis: Diffuse ST-segment elevation in all leads except aVR and V1.
  If patient is suspected of having an acute, inferior, anterior, lateral-wall myocardial infarction, pericarditis should be considered. May be associated with P-R depression.
- Hyperkalemia: ECG may be life-saving. Prominent "peaked" T waves with potassium levels > 5.5 mEq/L, followed progressively by first-degree heart block and then widening of the QRS complex. In patients with unexplained idioventricular rhythm, hyperkalemia should be considered.
- Hypokalemia: Flattening of the T wave and the appearance of U waves that merge with the T wave. May be harbinger of ventricular fibrillation.
- Hypercalcemia: Suspect when the Q-T interval is shortened. Appears as steep and rapid upward slope to the peak of the T wave. ECG should be done in patients with cancer and hyperparathyroidism, conditions that may be life-threatening.

SUGGESTED READINGS

Goldschlager N, Goldman N. Principals of clinical electrocardiography. 13th ed. San Mateo, CA: Appleton & Lange, 1989.

Marriott HJL. Practical electrocardiography. 8th ed. Baltimore: Williams & Wilkins, 1988.

Wagner GS. Marriott's practical electrocardiography. 9th ed. Baltimore: Williams & Wilkins, 1994.

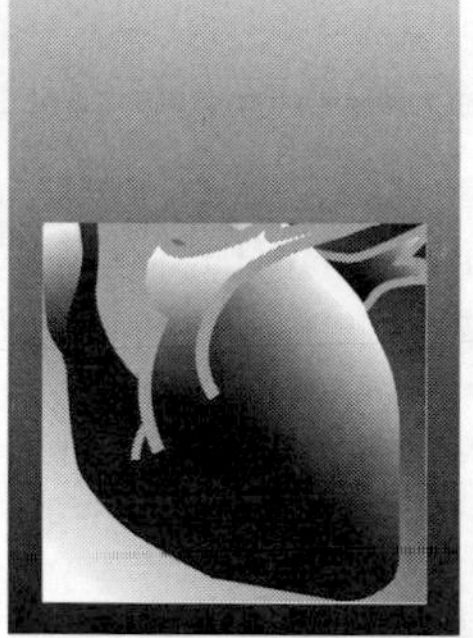

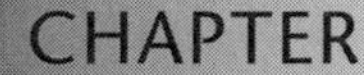

CHAPTER 3

Cardiac Arrhythmias

Mark A. Wood
Kenneth A. Ellenbogen

BACKGROUND

Cardiac arrhythmias are a common problem in clinical practice; presentations range from no symptoms to sudden cardiac death. The recognition and diagnosis of arrhythmias are very important to the primary care physician charged with the efficient management of these diverse entities. Toward this end, a basic understanding of the mechanisms underlying common arrhythmias and the drugs used in therapy makes rational clinical decision possible.

MECHANISMS OF CARDIAC ARRHYTHMIAS

All cardiac arrhythmias are caused by reentry or abnormal automaticity.

Reentry

In general, reentrant arrhythmias result from repeated, self-propagating electrical conduction around a discrete "circuit" in the heart. Such a reentrant circuit can involve only a few square millimeters of cardiac tissue (as in ventricular tachycardia) or several heart chambers (as in Wolff-Parkinson-White syndrome). Therapeutically, reentry may be terminated and prevented by creating conduction block anywhere along the circuit. This block can be mechanically created with catheter ablation or can be the result of the actions of antiarrhythmic drugs on the electrophysiologic properties of the circuit. By prolonging the refractory period (the time needed for tissue to regain excitability) of cardiac tissues with antiarrhythmic drugs, the reentry impulse meets unexcitable tissue and cannot propagate further.

Automaticity

In contrast, automaticity results from abnormal spontaneous activation (depolarization) of a discrete focus of myocardial tissue. Multifocal atrial tachycardia is an example of enhanced automaticity. Increased automaticity frequently results from injured or abnormal myocardial tissue, electrolyte imbalance, or metabolic abnormalities. Automatic rhythms can be suppressed with drug therapy; in addition, the discrete foci is sometimes destroyed by radiofrequency catheter ablation.

Antiarrhythmic Drugs

An understanding of the actions of common antiarrhythmic drugs allows the physician to make rational selections of therapies for the multitude of cardiac arrhythmias. To best match these agents with appropriate arrhythmias, the effects of these drugs on atrioventricular (AV) nodal function, myocardial conduction and refractoriness, and myocardial automaticity should be understood.

Digoxin

Digoxin is commonly used for most supraventricular arrhythmias because of its ability to prolong the refractory period and slow conduction in the AV node. Its effect is due to enhancement of vagal tone to the AV node and is typically modest and easily overridden by increased sympathetic tone. Clinically, digoxin has a slow onset of action that is often delayed for several hours. Digoxin enhances myocardial automaticity by increasing intracellular calcium. The stimulation of myocardial contractility is a useful property in patients with congestive heart failure, and the drug has no clinical effects on blood pressure. Toxicity is possible, especially in the setting of renal dysfunction.

β blockers

The β blockers slow AV nodal conduction, prolong the refractory period by blocking sympathetic tone, and have immediate onset of action. These agents effectively suppress myocardial automaticity and may also slow myocardial conduction and prolong the refractory period. A variety of β blockers are available, ranging from once-daily oral preparations to ultra–short-acting intravenously administered esmolol. The tendency of these agents to exacerbate congestive heart failure, obstructive pulmonary disease, and hypotension may limit their use.

Calcium Channel Blockers

The calcium channel blockers (diltiazem and verapamil) directly slow AV nodal conduction and prolong the refractory period independently of autonomic tone to the heart. As a result, these agents are additive to digoxin and β blockers in AV nodal blocking effects. The onset of action is rapid, occurring within minutes. These agents may reduce automaticity but have little effect on myocardial conduction or the refractory period. Both diltiazem and verapamil can produce hypotension and exacerbate heart failure, but this effect is uncommon with diltiazem. Both intravenous and oral preparations are available.

True Antiarrhythmic Agents

The true antiarrhythmic agents are classified according to their effects on ventricular conduction velocity and refractory period. All antiarrhythmic drugs have the potential for proarrhythmic effects. These agents should be administered only under appropriate ECG monitoring and by persons familiar with their use. Class I (Vaughan-Williams classification) agents slow ventricular conduction by blocking sodium channels during depolarization. The class I drugs are further subclassified as class IA, IB, and IC.

The class IA agents include quinidine, procainamide, and disopyramide. These agents slow atrial and ventricular conduction and prolong the refractory period by increasing the time necessary for tissue repolarization. Clinically, these effects manifest as QRS widening and QT prolongation. Polymorphic ventricular tachycardia (torsade de pointes) complicates the use of these agents in up to 5% of patients. These drugs enhance AV nodal conduction by way of anticholinergic effects.

Class IB drugs, such as lidocaine, mexilitene, and tocainide, act to slow ventricular conduction primarily in injured tissue; the drugs have lesser effects on normal myocardium. These agents have no clinical effects on atrial tissue or AV nodal function. Because the drugs do not significantly affect the QT interval (repolarization), torsade de pointes is rarely a complication. Moricizine is a class I antiarrhythmic agent with both IA and IB activities, which are more pronounced in ventricular tissue than in atrial tissue.

Class IC drugs include flecainide and propafenone. These agents dramatically slow atrial and ventricular myocardial conduction in both normal and diseased tissue. Propafenone may slow AV nodal conduction because of its additional β blocking effects. Class IC agents can increase mortality rates in patients with impaired left ventricular function and should not be used in patients with structural heart disease. These drugs can be used in patients with normal hearts (e.g., patients with Wolff-Parkinson-White syndrome or lone atrial fibrillation), although exercise-induced ventricular tachycardia has been reported.

Class III antiarrhythmic drugs prolong myocardial repolarization, thereby extending the refractory period. These agents are primarily potassium-channel blockers and include sotalol, bretylium, amiodarone, and ibutilide. With the exception of bretylium, all class III agents have both atrial and ventricular effects, and all are associated with a significant incidence of proarrhythmia (torsade de pointes). Sotalol and amiodarone slow AV nodal conduction and prolong the refractory period.

Sotalol has β blocking effects that may worsen heart failure and obstructive pulmonary diseases. The drug is not metabolized and undergoes only renal clearance. Its proarrhythmic potential increases with higher doses.

Bretylium has strong sympatholytic activity; it displaces norepinephrine from cardiac nerve terminals, leading to a "chemical sympathectomy." A significant hypotensive effect may limit the tolerability of this drug in many patients.

Amiodarone is an extremely complex pharmacologic agent that has strong class III activity (prolonging repolarization) but also has significant class I action (slowing conduction), β blocking activity, and calcium channel blocking activity. Amiodarone is the most effective antiarrhythmic agent known and is useful for a vast array of arrhythmias. Oral loading requires weeks to achieve full beneficial effects, but recently available intravenous amiodarone may have salutary effects within minutes. Most side effects, such as photosensitivity, hepatitis, thyroid dysfunction, and pulmonary fibrosis, occur with long-term use. Remarkably, amiodarone can often be used safely in patients experiencing torsade de pointes during therapy with other antiarrhythmic agents.

Ibutilide is an intravenous class III agent used only for the acute termination of atrial fibrillation and flutter. As is seen with other antiarrhythmic agents, ibutilide must be given only during continuous cardiac monitoring because of a 2 to 5% risk for torsade de pointes.

Adenosine is an endogenous compound that markedly depresses sinus node and AV nodal function. These effects are extremely brief (half-life, 6 seconds). The transient complete heart block that follows use of this drug is therapeutic for many reentrant supraventricular tachycardias: For other such tachycardias, adenosine is diagnostic because of its ability to unmask atrial activity. Table 3.1 summarizes the electrophysiologic effects of these antiarrhythmic agents.

SUPRAVENTRICULAR TACHYCARDIAS

Supraventricular tachycardias are a diverse group of arrhythmias that require an accurate differential diagnosis to manage appropriately. This section discusses the individual arrhythmias separately and features suggestions for differential diagnosis by ECG (Fig. 3.1).

Premature Atrial Contractions

Premature atrial contractions are ubiquitous in both healthy and sick persons and carry no clinical significance. The frequency of premature atrial contractions can be increased by caffeine, alcohol, sympathomimetic drugs, and adrenergic states.

Treatment

Treatment of premature atrial contractions is indicated only to relieve troubling palpitations and should first be directed toward removing offending causes. Therapy with β blockers or calcium channel blockers to decrease atrial automaticity is rarely necessary.

Sinus Tachycardia

Sinus tachycardia is identified by a normal P-wave axis (upright in leads I and II and inverted in aVR [i.e., axis of 0 to 90°]), gradual (nonparoxysmal) onset and termination, and typical slowing to vagal maneuvers.

TABLE 3.1. Electrophysiologic Effects and Uses of Common Antiarrhythmic Drugs

Drug	AV Node Refractoriness	AV Node Conduction	Myocardial Refractoriness	Myocardial Conduction	Automaticity	Rhythms Treated	Comments
Digoxin	Prolongs	Prolongs	No change	No change	Increases	AVNRT, AF, AFL, or EAT	Avoid in WPW, MAT
Calcium channel blockers Verapamil Diltiazem	Prolongs	Slows	No change	No change	Decreases	AVNRT, AVRT, AF, AFL, MAT, EAT	Avoid in WPW with AF
β blockers	Prolongs	Slows	No change	No change	Decreases	AVNRT, WPW, AVRT, AF, AFL	May worsen hypotension and heart failure
Class IA Quinidine Procainamide Disopyramide	Shortens	Enhances	Prolongs	Slows	Decreases	WPW, AF, AFL, VT	Risk for torsade de pointes; use with caution in CHF
Class IB Lidocaine Mexilitene Tocainide	No change	No change	No change	Slows	No change	VT	No atrial effects
Class IC Flecainide Propafenone	No change	No change	No change	Slows	Decreases	WPW, AF, AFL, VT	Use only in normal hearts; increased mortality with structural heart disease
Class III Sotalol Amiodarone Ibutilide* Bretylium	Prolongs	Slows	Prolongs	Slows	Decreases	WPW, AF, AFL, EAT, MAT, VT	Risk for torsade de pointes

AV, atrioventricular; AVNRT, AV nodal reentry tachycardia; AVRT, AV reciprocating tachycardia; AF, atrial fibrillation; AFL, atrial flutter; EAT, ectopic atrial tachycardia; MAT, multifocal atrial tachycardia; WPW, Wolff-Parkinson-White syndrome; VT, ventricular tachycardia; CHF, congestive heart failure.
*Ibutilide only for AF/AFL conversion

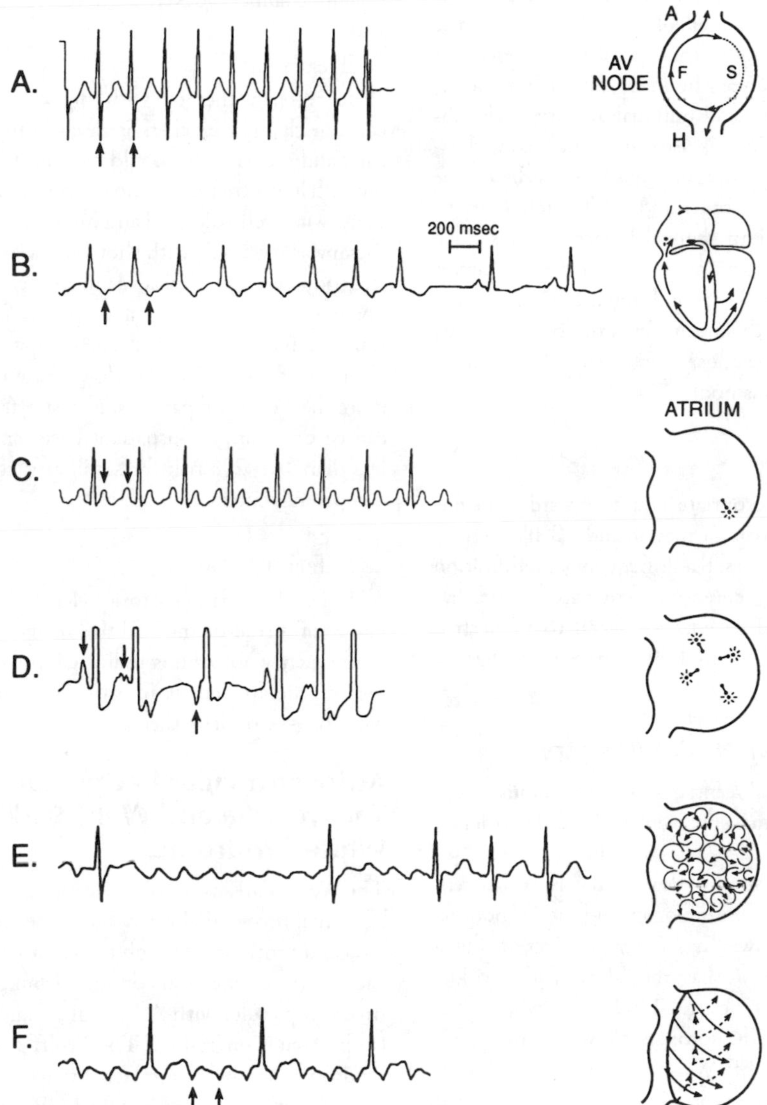

FIGURE 3.1.

Electrocardiographic appearance of common supraventricular tachycardias (*left*) with schematic representation of tachycardia mechanism (*right*). Arrows show the location of P waves. **A.** Atrioventricular (*AV*) nodal reentry tachycardia. Because of reentry within the AV node, atrial and ventricular activation occur simultaneously. **B.** Atrioventricular reciprocating tachycardia. Retrograde P waves in the ST segment are seen because of obligatory ventricular activation before retrograde atrial activation through an accessory pathway. **C.** Ectopic atrial tachycardia. A single ectopic focus activates the atrium, producing discrete P waves. **D.** Multifocal atrial tachycardia. Multiple ectopic atrial foci are active, independently producing at least three P-wave morphologies and an irregularly irregular rhythm. **E.** Atrial fibrillation. Multiple reentrant wavefronts with chaotic atrial activation produce no discrete P waves and an irregularly irregular rhythm. **F.** Atrial flutter. A discrete reentrant circuit in the right atrium produces the saw-tooth pattern of atrial activity. Note that the continuous atrial activity differentiates atrial flutter from ectopic atrial tachycardia (*part C*).

Sinus tachycardia is a physiologic response to stress and requires no therapy. Rarely, the syndrome of inappropriate sinus tachycardia results from enhanced intrinsic automaticity or autonomic tone of the sinus node. This syndrome is characterized by inappropriately rapid sinus heart rates at rest and minimal activity in the absence of any underlying disease state associated with sinus tachycardia. Inappropriate sinus tachycardia can be confused with panic disorder and is often refractory to β blockers and calcium channel blockers. Sinus node reentrant tachycardia can arise from a reentry circuit within the sinus node. This condition is uncommon and is easily confused with sinus tachycardia because of its normal P wave axis, response to vagal stimuli, and drugs that suppress the sinus node.

Treatment

Therapy for inappropriate sinus tachycardia or sinus node reentrant tachycardia may include β blockers or calcium channel blockers. Radiofrequency modification of the sinus node has cured inappropriate sinus tachycardia and sinus nodal reentry. Referral to an electrophysiologist is often required for management of these rare conditions.

Atrioventricular Nodal Reentry

Atrioventricular nodal reentry is the most common regular type of paroxysmal supraventricular tachycardia reported in clinical practice. The reentrant circuit involves two anatomically distinct pathways that have different conduction properties within or around the AV node itself. The "fast" pathway has faster conduction but a longer refractory period than the "slow" pathway. The fast pathway is located near the His bundle, whereas the slow pathway is near the coronary sinus ostium.

The typical form of AV nodal reentry occurs with conduction toward the ventricle (antegrade) down the slow pathway and retrograde conduction toward the atria by way of the fast pathway. In this rhythm, the atria and ventricle are activated nearly simultaneously, resulting in P waves concealed within the QRS complex.

The atypical form of AV nodal reentry can occur by reversal of the reentry circuit with retrograde conduction up the slow pathway and antegrade conduction down the fast pathway. This prolongs the interval between the QRS complex and retrograde P wave to produce an inverted P wave and a relatively normal PR interval. Because AV nodal conduction is essential to these rhythms, agents prolonging AV nodal conduction or the refractory period can be useful. Acute termination of sustained AV nodal reentry can frequently be accomplished with vagal maneuvers, adenosine, β blockers, or calcium channel blockers.

Treatment

Long-term therapy with digoxin, β blockers, or calcium channel blockers is rarely completely satisfactory, and recurrences should be expected (albeit possibly with lower frequency and shorter durations). For patients with well-tolerated and infrequent episodes, drug therapy as required (with short-acting verapamil) or instruction on the Valsalva maneuver can be used. For patients with frequent or poorly tolerated symptoms despite a trial of drug therapy, radiofrequency ablation of the AV nodal slow pathway is curative in more than 95% of patients, is cost-effective because it can be done on an outpatient basis, and should carry less than 1 to 2% risk for significant complications at competent centers.

Referral

Referral of patients to an electrophysiologist after failure of a trial of medical therapy is appropriate. Radiofrequency ablation is indicated in patients in whom medical therapy fails or in patients unwilling to comply with long-term drug therapy.

Atrioventricular Reciprocating Tachycardia and Wolff-Parkinson-White Syndrome

The Wolff-Parkinson-White syndrome results from an abnormal myocardial electrical connection between the atria and ventricles through the AV annulus. When this "accessory" connection conducts from the atria to ventricles in parallel with AV nodal conduction, ventricular preexcitation results. The Wolff-Parkinson-White syndrome can be recognized by a short PR interval, slurred delta wave, and widened QRS complex. Preexcitation can be intermittent. If the accessory pathway conducts only from the ventricle to the atria, a "concealed" pathway is present; technically, this does not indicate true Wolff-Parkinson-White syndrome.

The most common arrhythmia associated with accessory pathways is reentry in which a circuit is used antegrade through the AV node and ventricle, retrograde through the accessory pathway and atrium, and back to the AV node (orthodromic reciprocating tachycardia). Reversal of the circuit—down the accessory pathway to the ventricle and up the AV node to the atrium—produces a wide-complex, preexcited antidromic reciprocating tachycardia. Orthodromic tachycardias typically have a narrow QRS complex (because of normal AV nodal conduction) and a retrograde P wave after the QRS in the ST segment or T wave (because of retrograde atrial activation after obligatory conduction through the ventricle). Orthodromic reciprocating tachycardia using an accessory bypass tract is the second most common form of regular paroxysmal supraventricular tachycardia in clinical practice.

Treatment

Patients with asymptotic Wolff-Parkinson-White syndrome that is found incidentally do not require therapy; however, an echocardiogram is suggested to exclude the occasional associated congenital anomaly (e.g., Ebstein anomaly). Treadmill exercise testing should be considered in athletic persons to evaluate for provocable arrhythmias. Therapy for acute episodes of reciprocating tachycardia is directed toward prolonging the refractory period of the AV node with vagal maneuvers, β blockers, or adenosine. Intravenous digoxin, verapamil, and adenosine can acutely enhance accessory pathway conduction; these therapies are contraindicated only if atrial fibrillation or flutter is precipitated (this is a distinct possibility with large adenosine boluses). For acute episodes that are refractory, block can also be produced in the accessory pathway with intravenous procainamide or quinidine because the pathway is composed of typical myocardial tissue. Rarely, pace termination or direct-current cardioversion is necessary for highly symptomatic episodes. Recurrence of the tachycardia, a potentially problematic event, can be prevented by intravenous β blockers, calcium channel blockers, or procainamide infusions.

Long-term therapy can consist of AV nodal blocking drugs or class IA, IC, or III antiarrhythmic agents. As with AV nodal reentry, tachycardia recurrences are common if the patient is receiving drug therapy alone.

Referral

Before use of class IA, IC, or III antiarrhythmic agents is considered, an electrophysiologist should evaluate patients for radiofrequency ablation of the accessory pathway. Radiofrequency ablation is curative in 85 to 90% of patients in experienced centers and carries a 2 to 4% risk for complications. As with AV nodal reentry, radiofrequency ablation is indicated for patients in whom drug therapy fails or who are unwilling to comply with long-term medical therapy. For patients with frequent symptoms, catheter ablation is cost-effective and is the treatment of choice for life-threatening arrhythmias associated with Wolff-Parkinson-White syndrome.

The most serious rhythm disturbance in Wolff-Parkinson-White syndrome is atrial fibrillation or flutter with rapid conduction over the accessory pathway that results in sustained, extremely rapid ventricular rates greater than 250 beats/min or ventricular fibrillation. Patients with severe symptoms require immediate direct-current cardioversion to restore sinus rhythm. Accessory pathway conduction can be slowed acutely or blocked by intravenous procainamide or quinidine (or intravenous amiodarone for dire cases). Atrioventricular nodal blocking agents play no role in this condition and may actually accelerate accessory pathway conduction.

After stabilization, patients with atrial fibrillation and Wolff-Parkinson-White syndrome require immediate evaluation by an electrophysiologist for radiofrequency catheter ablation. Patients unresponsive to catheter ablation may warrant surgical pathway interruption. Long-term antiarrhythmic therapy with class IA, IC, or III drugs should be reserved for patients unresponsive to (or refusing) catheter ablation or those in whom such intervention is contraindicated.

Ectopic (Paroxysmal) Atrial Tachycardia

Ectopic atrial tachycardia frequently arises from enhanced focal atrial automaticity or small foci of atrial reentry. The ectopic P wave can assume any morphology according to the site of activation but typically differs from sinus P waves. Ectopic atrial tachycardia has atrial rates less than 340 beats/min and isoelectric intervals between P waves in all ECG leads; these characteristics differentiate it from atrial flutter. Diagnostically, AV block without tachycardia termination can often be induced with vagal maneuvers, calcium channel blockers, or β blockers or with adenosine. Atrial tachycardias frequently occur in patients with severe pulmonary disease, hyperadrenergic states, digoxin or theophylline toxicity, or severe metabolic derangements.

Treatment

Short-term therapy is directed toward slowing ventricular rates with β blockers or calcium channel blockers. These agents may also depress atrial automaticity. In contrast, digoxin enhances automaticity and should be avoided. For patients presenting with ectopic atrial tachycardia who are already taking digoxin, digoxin toxicity should be considered as a cause. Adenosine sometimes terminates ectopic atrial tachycardia.

Long-term management is often difficult. β blockers and calcium channel blockers both increase AV nodal block and depress automaticity and are the mainstays of therapy. Correction of complicating drug and metabolic derangements may be helpful.

Referral

Radiofrequency ablation of atrial foci has moderate to high success rates, and referral to an electrophysiologist is appropriate before trials of specific antiarrhythmic agents begin (class IA, IC, or III).

Multifocal Atrial Tachycardia

Multifocal atrial tachycardia is a variant of ectopic atrial tachycardia in which multiple sites of enhanced atrial automaticity are active simultaneously. Multifocal atrial tachycardia is diagnosed by the presence of three distinct P-wave morphologies, atrial rates greater than 100 beats/min, and predominance of no single P wave morphology. The P-P, PR, and R-R intervals vary continuously, producing an irregularly irregular rhythm that must be distinguished from atrial fibrillation to be managed appropriately.

Treatment

Multifocal atrial tachycardia is usually an acute disturbance that occurs in patients with severe pulmonary, metabolic, or pharmacologic derangements. The goal of therapy is to correct metabolic abnormalities and drug toxicities; β blockers are administered if possible (contraindications to β blockers are usually present, however). High-dose diltiazem or verapamil may be helpful. Class IA or III antiarrhythmic drugs can be tried in refractory cases, but responses are rare. Rhythm control usually follows correction of the underlying cause.

Referral

Chronic multifocal atrial tachycardia is rare and requires referral to a cardiologist.

Atrial Fibrillation

Atrial fibrillation, the most common rhythm disturbance requiring therapy, affects 4% of persons older than 60 years of age. Atrial fibrillation results from multiple chaotic wavefronts of reentry throughout the atria, producing an absence of discrete P waves on ECG, a continuous and constantly changing baseline of atrial activity, and an irregularly irregular ventricular rate. Atrial fibrillation almost always occurs in patients with cardiovascular disease, most often hypertension, coronary artery disease, or valvular heart disease.

Treatment

Heart rate control is the first goal in the short-term management of atrial fibrillation. If the patient has hemodynamic compromise, urgent cardioversion is indicated. Pharmacologic therapy is directed toward enhancing AV block to reduce the ventricular rate to 90 beats/min to 110 beats/min in most patients. Digoxin, although traditionally used, requires hours to work and has limited usefulness in patients with enhanced sympathetic tone for any reason. Intravenous diltiazem is now the drug of choice for short-term heart rate control. This drug is remarkably fast, safe, and effective; heart rate decreases by approximately 25% within 7 to 10 minutes after a 20-mg bolus. Hypotension and worsening of congestive heart failure are infrequent, and heart rate control is maintained by continuous infusion. β blockers are also highly effective for short-term heart rate control but are frequently contraindicated because of heart failure, hypotension, or pulmonary disease. Combination therapy with one or more agents may be necessary.

After short-term rate control, anticoagulation before cardioversion is recommended for patients with atrial fibrillation lasting 48 hours or longer. Four weeks of anticoagulation with warfarin is recommended (target international normalized ratio, 1.5 to 2.5) before elective direct-current cardioversion. Transesophageal echocardiography to exclude atrial thrombi has been used in patients with contraindication to anticoagulation.

For elective cardioversion to sinus rhythm, common practice is to begin oral antiarrhythmic loading on telemetry immediately before direct-current cardioversion. After cardioversion, the patient is monitored on telemetry for five drug half-lives to follow the QT interval and watch for the development of proarrhythmia (torsade de pointes). Acute conversion with drugs alone is more likely with atrial fibrillation lasting less than 24 to 48 hours. Intravenous ibutilide is more efficacious for chemical conversion than intravenous procainamide. Anticoagulation is maintained for 4 weeks after conversion if sinus rhythm persists. Cardioversion is often futile in patients with chronic atrial fibrillation of more than 1 year's duration or those with markedly dilated atria (> 5 cm). Maintenance of sinus rhythm averages about 50% at 1 year with all antiarrhythmic agents except amiodarone, which is associated with a 50% recurrence rate by 5 years. In patients with congestive heart failure, amiodarone may be safer than class IA drugs. Flecainide and propafenone should be used only in patients with structurally normal hearts.

For patients with atrial fibrillation that is refractory

to drug therapy, heart rate control with digoxin, calcium channel blockers, or β blockers is necessary. Resting heart rates of 50 to 70 beats/min and less than 120 beats/min with brief, low-intensity exercise (e.g., a short walk) are the goals of therapy. For patients with chronic, rapid ventricular rates despite drug therapy, radiofrequency AV nodal ablation and pacemaker therapy may dramatically relieve symptoms, frequency of hospitalization, and drug burden.

Long-term anticoagulation with warfarin to an international normalized ratio of 2.0 to 2.5 is recommended for all patients with chronic or paroxysmal atrial fibrillation and risk factors for thromboembolism (e.g., age older than 60 years, hypertension, coronary artery disease, previous embolic event, heart failure, or mitral valve disease). Patients younger than 75 years of age with no risk factors do not appear to require full anticoagulation but may be treated with aspirin. Recommendations for anticoagulation are listed in Table 3.2. Serious bleeding complications can be minimized by maintaining the international normalized ratio below 3.0 (especially in patients older than 75 years of age) and the systolic blood pressure less than 160 mm Hg.

TABLE 3.2. Guidelines for Anticoagulation in Patients with Atrial Fibrillation

	Therapy	
Age	**Risk Factors Present**	**Risk Factors Absent**
<60 years	Warfarin	No therapy
60–75 years	Warfarin	Aspirin
>75 years	Warfarin	Warfarin

Data obtained from Albers, et al, Arch Intern Med 1994;154: 1443–1448.

Referral

Referral to a cardiologist is appropriate for acute management of hemodynamically unstable atrial fibrillation or for determination of long-term therapy with antiarrhythmic drugs. Patients with chronic atrial fibrillation and consistently rapid ventricular rates should be referred for evaluation of AV node ablation and pacemaker implantation.

Atrial Flutter

Atrial flutter results from a discrete reentry circuit around the tricuspid valve annulus. As such, the atrial activity on the ECG is a continuous saw-tooth pattern best seen in leads II, III, and aVF. The ventricular response is typically regular with 2:1 block, but variable AV conduction can produce irregularity.

Treatment

In general, the causes, presentations, and management of atrial flutter are similar to those of atrial fibrillation. One exception is that in atrial flutter, ventricular rate control may be more difficult to achieve. Ventricular rates greater than 300 beats/min can result from anticholinergic class IA drug effects if these drugs are given before AV nodal block is achieved. Again, intravenous diltiazem is the agent of choice for acute heart rate control. Because of the low incidence of thromboembolism in patients with atrial flutter, anticoagulation is not routinely recommended, regardless of the duration of flutter. If chemical conversion fails, atrial flutter can be pace-terminated by transvenous or transesophageal techniques; these techniques spare the patient direct-current cardioversion.

Referral

Atrial flutter can be terminated and recurrences can be prevented by radiofrequency catheter interruption of the reentry circuit; this therapy should be considered in patients with recurrent atrial flutter and no history of atrial fibrillation.

Differential Diagnosis of Supraventricular Tachycardia

The central feature of the differential diagnosis of supraventricular tachycardia is the presence or absence of P waves and their relation to the QRS complex (Fig. 3.2). If distinct P waves cannot be identified on a 12-lead ECG during regular tachycardia, AV nodal reentry is the most likely diagnosis. If discrete P waves are absent during irregularly irregular tachycardia, atrial fibrillation is the most likely diagnosis. If P waves are present and have normal axis (0 to 90°; i.e., upright in leads II and aVF and negative in lead aVR), a sinus node origin of the P waves can be diagnosed. If more P waves than QRS complexes are noted (i.e., if AV nodal block occurs without tachycardia termination), the rhythm *cannot* be a reciprocating tachycardia. Under these circumstances, AV nodal reentry is also extremely unlikely, leaving ectopic atrial tachycardia, multifocal atrial tachycardia, or atrial flutter as possible diagnoses. For 1:1 P to QRS ratios, ectopic atrial tachycardia, multifocal atrial tachycardia, and atypical AV nodal reentry have a "normal" PR interval because atrial activation precedes ventricular activation. This is also called "long R-P tachycardia" because the P wave typically occurs more than half of the R-R interval after the preceding QRS complex. If retrograde P waves are present in the ST or T wave, reciprocating tachycardia using an accessory pathway is most likely, producing a short R-P tachycardia (i.e., P wave occurs less than half of the R-R interval after the preceding QRS complex). Variations and exceptions to these general rules can occur, but this algorithm may be useful for most supraventricular tachycardias.

VENTRICULAR TACHYCARDIA

Ventricular tachycardia can arise from either reentrant or automatic mechanisms, although the former is much more common in clinical practice. Clinically, it is useful to classify ventricular tachycardias into three categories, each of which has different evaluations and managements (Fig. 3.3).

Polymorphic Ventricular Tachycardia

Polymorphic ventricular tachycardia results from chaotic and multiple reentrant circuits within the ventricle and includes ventricular fibrillation and torsade de pointes. On ECG, ventricular fibrillation has no distinct QRS complexes but instead has a continuously changing electrical waveform. Torsade de pointes also shows a continuously changing waveform, but with sinusoidal oscillations in the

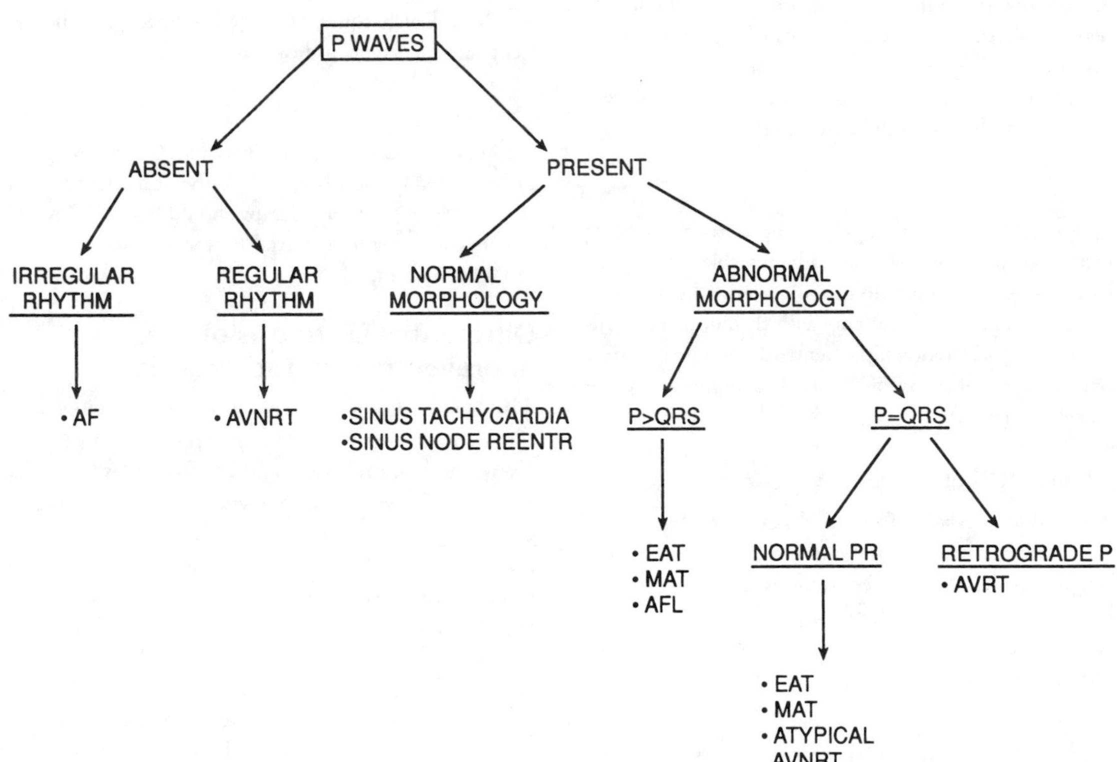

FIGURE 3.2.

Algorithm that uses P wave morphology and the relation of the P wave to the QRS complex to differentiate among common supraventricular tachycardias. *Normal morphology* is a P-wave axis of 0 to 90° (i.e., P upright in leads I, II, and inverted in lead aVR). *P > QRS* indicates more P waves than QRS complexes. *P = QRS* indicates an equal number of P waves and QRS complexes. *Normal PR* interval indicates a P wave occurring less than 50% of the R-R interval before each QRS complex (i.e., long R-P tachycardia). *Retrograde P* indicates a P wave occurring in the ST segment or T wave of the QRS complex (i.e., short R-P tachycardia). *AF,* atrial fibrillation; *AFL,* atrial flutter; *AVNRT,* AV nodal reentry tachycardia; *AVRT,* AV reciprocating tachycardia; *EAT,* ectopic atrial tachycardia; *MAT,* multifocal atrial tachycardia.

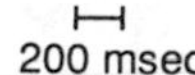

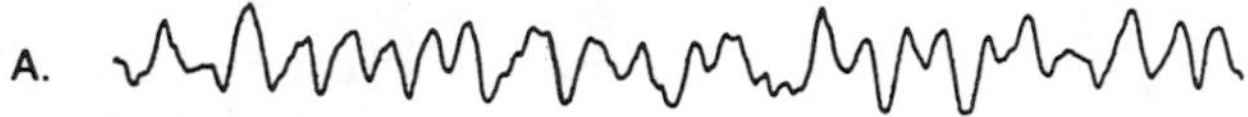

B.

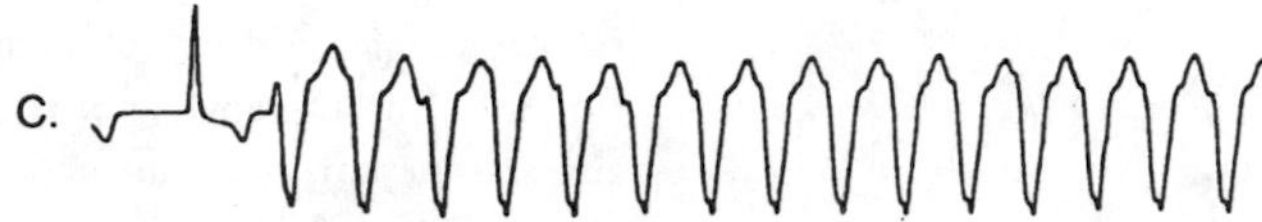

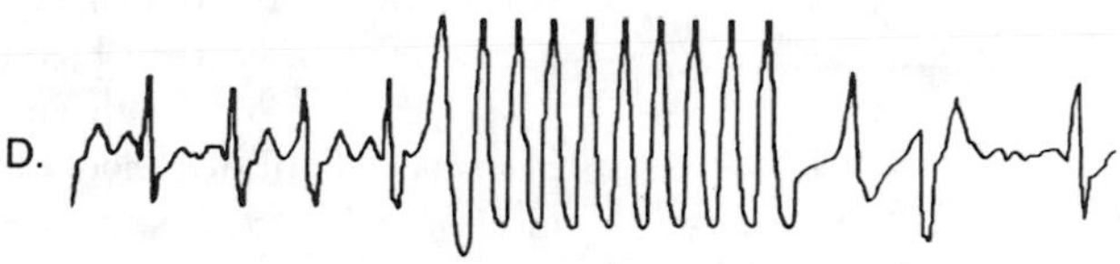

FIGURE 3.3.
Morphologies of common ventricular tachycardias. **A.** Ventricular fibrillation with no discrete QRS complexes and constantly changing waveform. **B.** Torsade de pointes characterized by sinusoidal oscillations in amplitude of the QRS complex and alternating electrical axis between oscillations. **C.** Monomorphic ventricular tachycardia demonstrates uniform QRS morphology for all beats. **D.** Nonsustained monomorphic ventricular tachycardia. Monomorphic ventricular tachycardia lasts less than 30 seconds and by definition is not associated with hemodynamic collapse.

waveform amplitude and a characteristic alternation of electrical axis between the oscillations. Torsade de pointes is typically preceded by QT prolongation in sinus rhythm. An important feature of polymorphic ventricular tachycardia is that it frequently arises from reversible and treatable causes, such as use of antiarrhythmic drugs, electrolyte derangements, or acute ischemia (Table 3.3). Evaluation is directed toward exclusion of these potential causes. The congenital form of the long QT syndrome should be considered in patients with no other causes of QT prolongation or in patients with no other causes for polymorphic ventricular tachycardia.

Treatment

Sustained polymorphic arrhythmias must be terminated by emergency direct-current cardioversion. Prevention of recurrences includes discontinuation of therapy with offending drugs, correction of electrolyte abnormalities, and anti-ischemic therapy if ischemia is suspected. β blocker therapy is useful for ischemia and congenital long QT syndrome. Drug-induced polymorphic ventricular tachycardia and torsade de pointes respond well to intravenous magnesium sulfate (2 g administered over 5 to 10 minutes, then 2 to 4 g administered in 15 minutes if needed). Polymorphic ventricular tachycardia is aggravated by bradycardia. Increasing heart rates to 100 to 120 beats/min by using isoproterenol, temporary cardiac pacing, or atropine may be helpful. Administration of class IA or III antiarrhythmic drugs is contraindicated in these patients.

TABLE 3.3. Causes of Polymorphic Ventricular Tachycardia

Drugs
- Class IA or III antiarrhythmic agents (e.g., quinidine and sotalol)
- Phenothiazines and derivatives (e.g., thioridazine)
- Antibiotics (e.g., intravenous erythromycin and pentamidine)
- Miscellaneous (e.g., terfenadine)

Myocardial ischemia or infarction

Electrolyte abnormalities
- Hypokalemia
- Hypocalcemia
- Hypomagnesemia

Bradycardia

Long-QT syndrome

Miscellaneous
- Subarachnoid hemorrhage
- Lithium
- Organophosphates
- Starvation or liquid-protein diets
- Radical neck surgery

Referral

Unless the polymorphic ventricular tachycardia is unquestionably related to drugs or electrolyte abnormalities, evaluation by a cardiologist is warranted in all cases, whether sustained or nonsustained.

Sustained Monomorphic Ventricular Tachycardia

Sustained monomorphic ventricular tachycardia usually represents a discrete reentry circuit within the myocardium and almost always arises in the setting of structural heart disease with reduced left ventricular function. Coronary artery disease with previous infarction is the most common cause. Sustained monomorphic ventricular tachycardia is typically caused by a fixed anatomic or electrical substrate in the heart and should *not* be considered as being secondary to stress, electrolyte abnormalities, or drug effects (although these factors can be triggers). Monomorphic ventricular tachycardia shows a widened (> 0.12 seconds) QRS structure at heart rates greater than 100 beats/min that is uniform within each ECG lead. The presence of atrioventricular dissociation is diagnostic.

Treatment

The short-term management of sustained monomorphic ventricular tachycardia depends on the patient's hemodynamic stability. If the patient is in arrest or is hemodynamically unstable, advanced cardiac life support protocols should be followed, including frequent attempts at direct-current cardioversion.

If the patient is hemodynamically stable, pharmacologic conversion with lidocaine or procainamide can be attempted; however, full resuscitation equipment should be in readiness. Intravenous amiodarone can be administered for recurrent or refractory ventricular arrhythmias.

Referral

After stabilization, evaluation by a cardiologist or electrophysiologist is required for all patients with sustained monomorphic ventricular tachycardia. Long-term therapy with antiarrhythmic agents requires electrophysiologic guidance to define safety and efficacy. Empiric drug therapy (with the possible exception of amiodarone) may actually increase the mortality rate and is not acceptable management. Patients in whom effective drug therapy cannot be defined may require an implantable cardioverter defibrillator. Patients who survive a cardiac arrest or hemodynamically unstable ventricular tachycardia are at high risk for recurrence even when "effective" drug therapy is defined. The implantable defibrillator should be considered the treatment of choice for these patients.

Nonsustained Ventricular Tachycardia

Nonsustained ventricular tachycardia can arise from reentry or enhanced automaticity; it has the same ECG characteristics as sustained ventricular tachycardia but lasts less than 30 seconds and is not associated with hemodynamic collapse. Although this rhythm is often interpreted as a harbinger of sustained ventricular tachycardia, the clinical significance is not always so clear, and the guidelines for therapy are not universally accepted. The primary goal in the evaluation of nonsustained ventricular tachycardia is to determine the patient's risk for future malignant arrhythmic events or sudden death. Left ventricular function is the strongest independent predictor of sudden death. Patients with left ventricular ejection fraction greater than 40% have a low risk for sudden death, regardless of the degree of ventricular ectopy. For patients with ejection fraction less than 40% and coronary artery disease, an abnormal signal-averaged ECG is another independent predictor of sustained arrhythmic events. The combination of low ejection fraction, abnormal signal-averaged ECG, and nonsustained ventricular tachycardia (or >10 premature ventricular contractions per hour) can identify patients with up to 40% risk for sudden death within 2 to 3 years. Patients with these risk factors, as well as those with nonsustained ventricular tachycardia and history of syncope or presyncope, should be referred to a cardiologist or electrophysiologist for further evaluation. The empiric suppression of ventricular ectopy with antiarrhythmic drugs can increase mortality rates by twofold to threefold in these patients and is not acceptable management. Formal electrophysiologic testing for inducible sustained ventricular arrhythmias is typically the next step in evaluation.

Treatment

The optimal treatment of nonsustained ventricular tachycardia is not fully known. Patients with ejection fraction greater than 40% have good survival even without therapy and require treatment only for symptomatic palpitations. β blockers are the first choice in these patients. Patients with coronary artery disease, ejection fractions less than 40%, and inducible ventricular tachycardia on electrophysiologic studies have improved survival with implantable defibrillators. The benefit of antiarrhythmic drug therapy in patients with reduced ejection fractions and nonsustained ventricular tachycardia has not been determined.

Referral

Patients with nonsustained ventricular tachycardia and ejection fractions less than 40% should receive electrophysiologically guided therapy. All patients with nonsustained ventricular tachycardia and a history of syncope, presyncope, or symptomatic palpitations should be evaluated by a cardiologist.

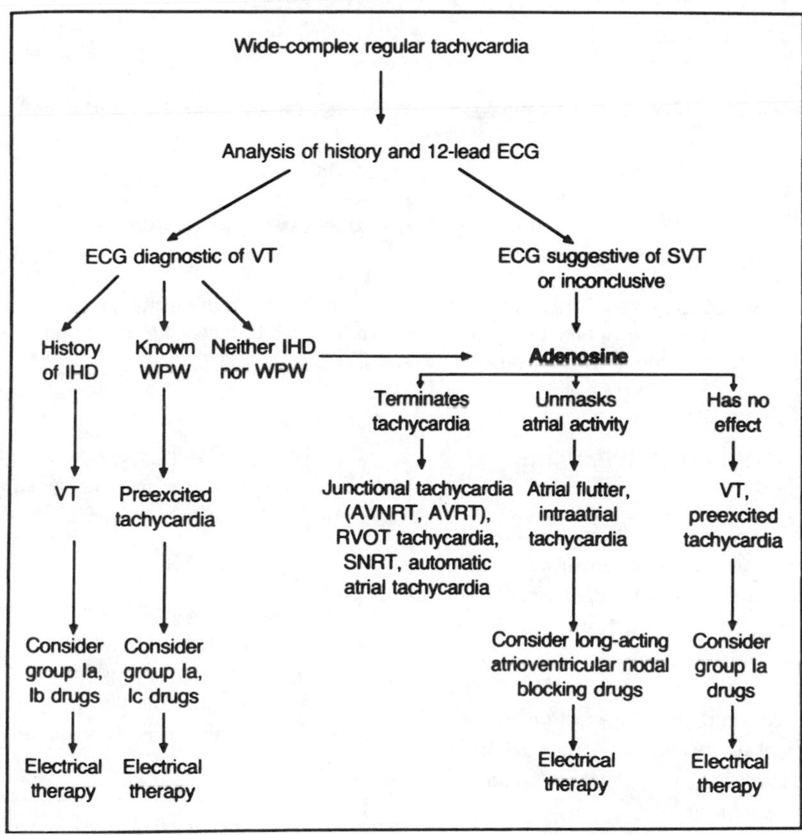

FIGURE 3.4.

Algorithm for differential diagnosis of wide-complex tachycardia, including appropriate use of adenosine. *AVNRT,* AV node reentry tachycardia; *AVRT,* AV reciprocating tachycardia; *ECG,* electrocardiogram; *IHD,* ischemic heart disease; *RVOT,* right ventricular outflow tract; *SNRT,* sinus node reentry tachycardia; *SVT,* supraventricular tachycardia; *VT,* ventricular tachycardia; *WPW,* Wolff-Parkinson-White syndrome. Reprinted with permission from Oates JA, et al. N Engl J Med 1991;325:1621–1629.

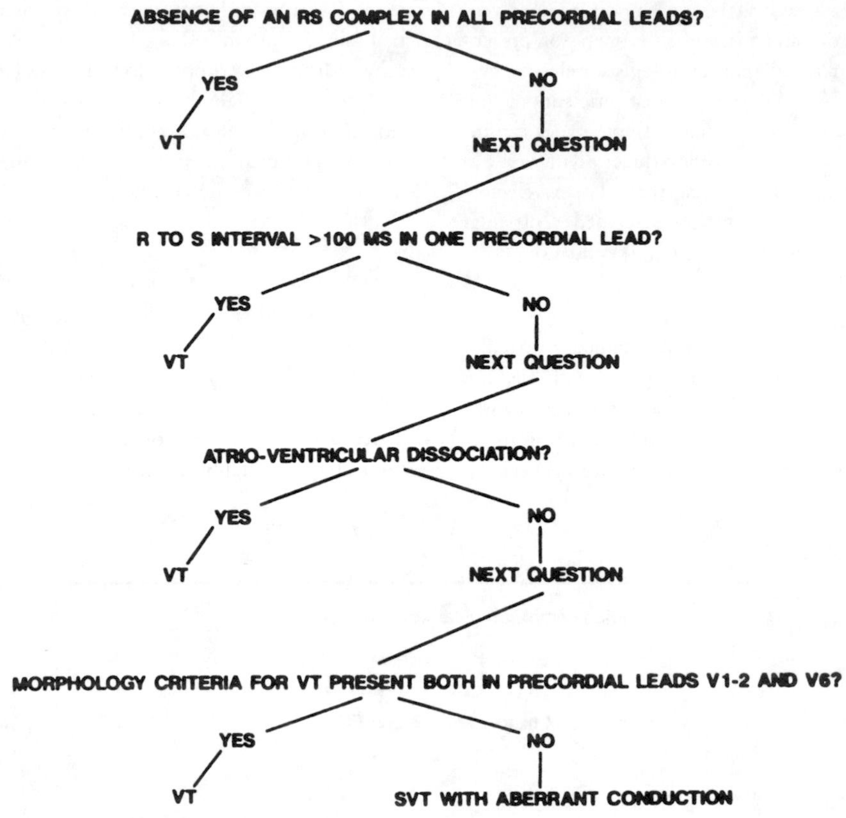

FIGURE 3.5.

Useful algorithm to differentiate ventricular from supraventricular tachycardia using simple surface electrocardiographic criteria. *SVT,* supraventricular tachycardia; *VT,* ventricular tachycardia. Reprinted with permission from Brugada P, et al. Circulation 1991;83:1649–1659.

Ventricular Tachycardia with the "Normal" Heart

Ventricular tachycardia rarely occurs in patients with structurally normal hearts. These "idiopathic" ventricular tachycardias can often be subclassified according to ECG morphology and characteristic features at electrophysiologic testing. Abnormal automaticity or focal reentry is believed to be the mechanism for most cases. Collectively, right ventricular outflow-tract tachycardia, left ventricular apical tachycardia, and repetitive monomorphic tachycardia can be asymptomatic or cause syncope or palpitations.

Treatment

Ventricular arrhythmias in structurally normal hearts may respond clinically to adenosine, β blockers, or calcium channel blockers; this confounds the differentiation from supraventricular tachycardia with aberrancy. Therapy with β blockers or calcium channel blockers can be effective, and cure by radiofrequency ablation is possible in most patients.

Referral

Patients presenting with these rare clinical syndromes should be evaluated by a cardiologist or electrophysiologist to optimize therapy and to exclude the more malignant syndrome of arrhythmogenic right ventricular dysplasia. This condition is a genetically based, often progressive infiltration of the right ventricular wall and septum by fatty tissue that results in multiple reentry circuits. The disorder is recognized by sustained or nonsustained ventricular tachycardia, baseline T wave inversion in leads V_1 to V_3, and a markedly abnormal signal-averaged ECG. Although the echocardiogram is frequently unremarkable, cardiac magnetic resonance imaging demonstrates right ventricular structural abnormalities. This disorder can be malignant, progressive, and refractory to drug therapy. Referral to an electrophysiologist is needed to define drug, ablation, or defibrillation therapy.

DIFFERENTIAL DIAGNOSIS OF VENTRICULAR TACHYCARDIA VERSUS SUPRAVENTRICULAR VENTRICULAR TACHYCARDIA

The differential diagnosis of tachycardia with a wide QRS complex on ECG testing is frequently difficult. Exclusion of ventricular tachycardia is usually the pressing clinical issue. In general, ventricular tachycardia should be suspected in older patients with any history of heart disease or reduced left ventricular function. The presence of atrioventricular dissociation, fusion beats, or capture beats is pathognomonic for ventricular tachycardia. A monophasic or biphasic left or right bundle-branch structure in leads V_1 or V_6, "northwest" QRS axis (−90 to 180°), concordance of precordial leads (all upright or all inverted), QRS width greater than 0.14 seconds, and more than a 0.10-second interval between peak of the R wave and peak of the S wave in the QRS complex all suggest the diagnosis of ventricular tachycardia. The hemodynamic stability of the rhythm should have little influence on the diagnosis because supraventricular tachycardia can be poorly tolerated and ventricular tachycardia can be well tolerated, depending on the clinical situation.

Supraventricular tachycardia is suggested by the absence of structural heart disease, presence of classic triphasic bundle-branch block patterns, QRS width less than 0.14 seconds, tachycardia initiation by a premature atrial contraction, or QRS structure identical to previous baseline conduction abnormalities. The response to adenosine can also be diagnostic for supraventricular tachycardia (Fig. 3.4). A useful algorithm for differentiating ventricular tachycardia from supraventricular tachycardia is shown in Figure 3.5.

KEY POINTS

Arrhythmia Medications

- Digoxin is used for most supraventricular arrhythmias and acts by slowing AV nodal conduction and prolonging the AV nodal refractory period.
- β blockers slow AV nodal conduction and prolong its refractory period.
- Calcium channel blockers such as diltiazem and verapamil slow AV nodal conduction and prolong its refractory period, independently of autonomic tone.
- Antiarrhythmic drugs (class I, II, and III) may be proarrhythmic.
- Class IA drugs include quinidine, procainamide, and disopyramide. They act to slow atrial and ventricular conduction and prolong the myocardial refractory period.
- Class IB drugs include lidocaine, mexilitine, and tocainide. They act to slow ventricular conduction.
- Class IC drugs include flecainide and propafenone. They dramatically slow atrial and ventricular conduction.
- Class III drugs include sotalol and amiodarone. They prolong myocardial repolarization and the refractory period.
- Adenosine drastically prolongs the AV nodal refractory period and has a short intravenous half-life of 6 seconds.

Superventricular Tachycardia

- For patients experiencing premature atrial contractions, discontinue offending causes (caffeine, alcohol, etc.). No drug treatment.
- Sinus tachycardia is usually physiologic; address the underlying mechanism. Sinoatrial node reentrant tachycardia is uncommon.
- Atrioventricular node reentry may require vagal maneuvers, adenosine (acutely), β blockers, or calcium channel blockers. Refer patients resistant to drugs for radiofrequency ablation.
- For acute episodes associated with Wolff-Parkinson-White syndrome, use vagal maneuvers, β blockers, calcium channel blockers, or adenosine. Radiofrequency catheter ablation is curative.
- Long-term therapy with class IA, IC, or III agents is now rare. For recurrent tachycardia, refer for radiofrequency ablation.
- Ectopic atrial tachycardia (acute) requires calcium-channel blockers, β blockers, or adenosine. Refer patients with refractory ectopic paroxysmal atrial tachycardia for radiofrequency ablation.
- Multifocal atrial tachycardia requires correction of underlying problems such as theophylline toxicity. High-dose diltiazem or verapamil can be tried.
- For atrial fibrillation, use intravenous diltiazem for short-term rate control. Anticoagulation is needed before conversion if rhythm occurs for 48 hours or more. Use direct-current cardioversion if the patient is unstable. Long-term therapy requires antiarrhythmic agents.
- For atrial flutter, use intravenous diltiazem, pace termination by the cardiologist, and direct-current cardioversion. Prevention and cure can be achieved by radiofrequency ablation.

Ventricular Tachycardia

- Mechanism is either reentrant (common) or automatic (rare).
- Use direct-current cardioversion for sustained polymorphic ventricular tachycardia or torsade de pointes.
- Treatment of polymorphic ventricular tachycardia includes discontinuing therapy with offending drugs, correcting electrolyte imbalance, and pacing to heart rates of 90 to 100 beats/min. Magnesium sulfate is useful for drug-induced ventricular tachycardia.
- Refer patients with polymorphic ventricular tachycardia to a cardiologist.
- For ventricular tachycardia that is hemodynamically unstable, follow advanced cardiac life support guidelines.
- For hemodynamically stable monomorphic ventricular tachycardia, procainamide can be used, followed by referral to a cardiologist.
- For nonsustained ventricular tachycardia, empiric therapy is not indicated. Referral to an electrophysiologist or cardiologist is necessary.
- Ventricular tachycardia with a "normal" heart is rare; refer these patients to an electrophysiologist.
- Treatment of ventricular tachycardia in patients with a "normal heart" is radiofrequency ablation, adenosine, β blockers, or calcium channel blockers.

SUGGESTED READINGS

Akhtar M. Clinical spectrum of ventricular tachycardia. Circulation 1990;82:1561–1573.

Albers GW. Atrial fibrillation and stroke. Ann Intern Med 1994;154:1443–1448.

Atrial Fibrillation Investigators. Risk factors for stroke and efficacy of antithrombotic therapy in atrial fibrillation. Arch Intern Med 1994;154:1449–1457.

Camm AJ, Garratt CJ. Adenosine and supraventricular tachycardia. N Engl J Med 1991;325:1621–1629.

Chou T-C. Electrocardiography in clinical practice. Orlando, FL: Grune and Stratton, 1986.

Garratt CJ, Griffith MJ. Electrocardiographic diagnosis of tachycardias. In: Camm AJ, ed. Clinical approaches to tachyarrhythmias. Armonk, NY: Futura Publishing Co., 1994.

Golschlager N, Goldman M. Principles of clinical electrocardiography. 13th ed. San Mateo, CA: Appleton & Lange, 1989.

Marriott, HJL. Practical electrocardiography. 8th ed. Baltimore: Williams & Wilkins, 1988.

Messerli FH, ed. Cardiovascular drug therapy. Philadelphia: W.B. Saunders, 1990.

Murgatroyd FD, Camm JA. Atrial arrhythmias. Lancet 1993;341:1317–1322.

Shenasa M, Haverkemp W , Borggrefe M, et al. Ventricular tachycardia. Lancet 1993;341:1512–1519.

The Cardiac Arrhythmia Suppresion Trial (CAST) Investigators. Preliminary report: effect of encainide and flecainide on mortality in a randomized trial of arrhythmia suppression after myocardial infarction. N Engl J Med 1989; 321:406–412.

Waldo AL, Wit AC. Mechanisms of cardiac arrhythmias. Lancet 1993;341:1189–1193.

Wood M, Ellenbogen K, Stambler B. Radiofrequency catheter ablation for the management of cardiac tachyarrhythmias. Am J Med Sci 1993;306:241–247.

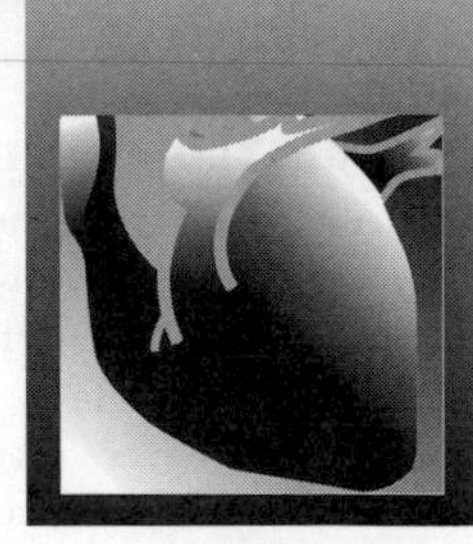

4

CHAPTER

Cardiac Pacing and Implantable Cardioverter Defibrillators

Richard K. Shepard
Kenneth A. Ellenbogen
David Gilligan
Mark A. Wood

BASIC ASPECTS OF CARDIAC PACING

A pacemaker senses intrinsic cardiac electrical events and provides electrical stimuli to excite the myocardium when they are absent. The pacemaker system consists of a pulse generator containing a battery and logic circuits and leads for electrical continuity between the pulse generator and the heart. A pacemaker may be single chamber, with a single lead to either the atrium or the ventricle, or dual chamber, with leads to both the atrium and ventricle. The sensing threshold of a pacemaker is the amplitude (in mV) of sensed intracardiac events. The pacing threshold is the minimum energy required to stimulate the myocardium.

The pacemaker coordinates sensed and paced cardiac events by means of an internal clock; thus, timing intervals between events is important to understanding pacemaker function. The lower-rate interval is the time the pacemaker "waits" after sensed or paced events before emitting a pacing stimulus. The upper-rate interval is the fastest the pacemaker will pace in response to sensed events (e.g., atrioventricular [AV] sequential pacing) or to sensor input in rate-responsive pacemakers. The AV delay establishes the electronic P-R interval in dual-chamber pacing.

The programmed pacemaker mode is described with a four-letter identification code according to the site of the electrodes and the mode of pacing (Table 4.1). The following abbreviations are used: V, ventricle; A, atrium; D, dual (atrium and ventricle); I, inhibited; T, triggered; and O, none. The first letter describes the chamber or chambers paced, and the second letter describes the chamber or chambers sensed. The third letter describes the response to sensing. "I" (inhibited) indicates that the pacemaker output will be suppressed by a sensed event. "T" (triggered) indicates that the pacemaker will discharge in response to a sensed event. "D" (dual) indicates both inhibited and triggered functions. The fourth letter describes programmability and rate modulation functions. It is most commonly "R," standing for rate responsiveness.

A pacemaker may be programmed to different modes depending on the clinical situation. Asynchronous modes (AOO or VOO) represent continuous pacing without sensing. This mode is activated in most pacemakers when an external magnet is applied. Pacemakers are also frequently programmed in this mode during surgery in which electrocautery might interfere with sensing. Single-chamber pacing modes are usually AAI or VVI and pace only when the patient's intrinsic heart rate falls below the pacemaker's lower rate. A dual-chamber pacemaker (e.g., DDD) may pace both atrium and ventricle when the intrinsic heart rate is below the programmed lower rate. It may pace the atria and sense the ventricle if AV conduction is intact and the P-R interval is shorter than the programmed AV delay. A dual-chamber pacemaker may also follow sensed atrial events with paced ventricular events when the intrinsic atrial rate is between the lower and upper programmed rates (atrial tracking). Rate-responsive pacemakers have sensors that respond to body movement, respiratory rate, minute ventilation, or Q-T interval. The pacing rate can change in response to sensed activity. These pacemakers are useful in patients who cannot increase their heart rate in response to exertion.

INDICATIONS FOR PERMANENT AND TEMPORARY PACING

In general, pacemakers are indicated in patients with symptomatic bradyarrhythmias or with heart rhythms

TABLE 4.1. Identification Code for Programmed Pacemaker Mode

Variable	Position I	II	III	IV
Category	Chambers paced	Chambers sensed	Response to sensing	Programmability, rate modulation
Letter designations	**O** = none	**O** = none	**O** = none	**O** = none
	A = atrium	**A** = atrium	**T** = triggered	**P** = simple programmable
	V = ventricle	**V** = ventricle	**I** = inhibited	**M** = multiprogrammable
	D = dual (A+V)	**D** = dual (A+V)	**D** = dual (T+I)	**C** = communicating
				R = rate modulation

TABLE 4.2. Indications for Permanent and Temporary Pacing

Needs Pacemaker	Refer for Evaluation	Does Not Need Pacemaker
Symptomatic sinus bradycardia	Asymptomatic bradycardia with heart rate < 40 beats/min	Asymptomatic bradycardia
Neurocardiogenic syncope with > 3-second pause	Neurocardiogenic syncope with bradycardia	Neurocardiogenic syncope without bradycardia
Acquired AV block with Symptomatic bradycardia Congestive heart failure Pauses > 3 seconds Escape rhythm < 40 beats/min Wide-complex escape rhythm Other evidence of decreased cardiac output (e.g., confusion)	Asymptomatic acquired AV block with Heart rate >40 beats/min Mobitz type II block Wenckebach phenomenon with wide QRS complex	Acquired AV block with Wenckebach phenomenon and narrow QRS complex
Symptomatic bradycardia caused by drugs to treat other cardiac problems		

AV, atrioventricular.

that may rapidly progress to profound bradycardia or asystole. Specific indications are given in this section and are listed in Table 4.2.

Sick Sinus Syndrome

Pacemakers are indicated for sinus node dysfunction with symptomatic sinus bradycardia. In some patients, this abnormality may occur as a consequence of essential drug therapy (e.g., antiarrhythmic therapy for atrial fibrillation). Asymptomatic patients with sinus heart rates less than 40 beats/min may require referral to a cardiologist for formal evaluation. In patients with neurocardiogenic syncope, pacemakers may be indicated if pauses longer than 3 seconds are associated with syncope.

Atrioventricular Block

Patients with acquired complete AV block almost always require permanent pacing, especially if they have any of the following:

- Symptomatic bradycardia
- Congestive heart failure
- Documented periods of asystole lasting longer than 3.0 seconds or an escape rate less than 40 beats/min in an asymptomatic patient
- Wide-complex escape rhythms
- Confusional states that clear with temporary pacing
- Medical conditions requiring drugs that suppress the automaticity of escape pacemakers and cause symptomatic bradycardia

Patients with asymptomatic complete heart block and a ventricular rate greater than 40 beats/min, asymptomatic Mobitz type II second-degree AV block, and asymptomatic type I second-degree AV block (Wenckebach phenomenon) with wide QRS complexes are best referred for cardiology evaluation.

PROBLEMS IN PATIENTS WITH PACEMAKERS

Modern pacing systems work reliably, and pacemaker malfunction or failure is rare; however, all physicians seeing patients with pacemakers should be familiar with potential pacemaker problems.

Loss of Capture

Loss of capture is defined as the presence of an electrical output from the pacemaker without capture of the myocardium (Fig. 4.1). Loss of capture may occur soon after pacemaker implantation because of lead dislodgment (partial or complete) or transient increases in pacing thresholds resulting from tissue reaction at the myocardial lead interface. Loss of capture with long-term pacing leads usually implies lead fracture, insulation failure, or depletion of the pacemaker battery. Electrolyte abnormalities or drug therapy can sometimes cause loss of capture because of elevation of pacing thresholds. Patients demonstrating failure to capture should be evaluated immediately by physicians trained in pacemaker management.

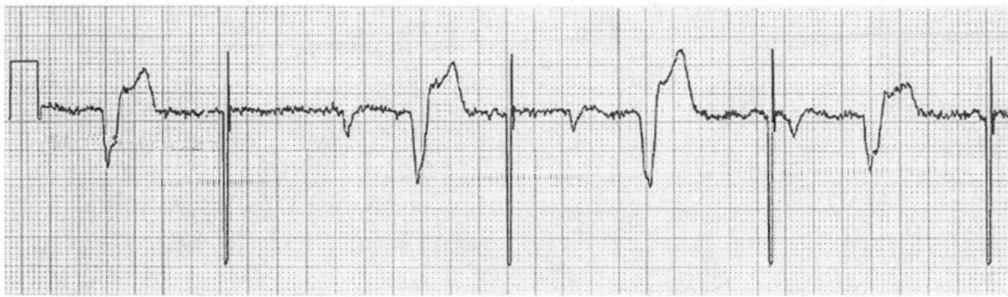

FIGURE 4.1.
Loss of capture. Pacemaker spikes are not followed by QRS complexes. An underlying rhythm is observed. This patient had lead dislodgement.

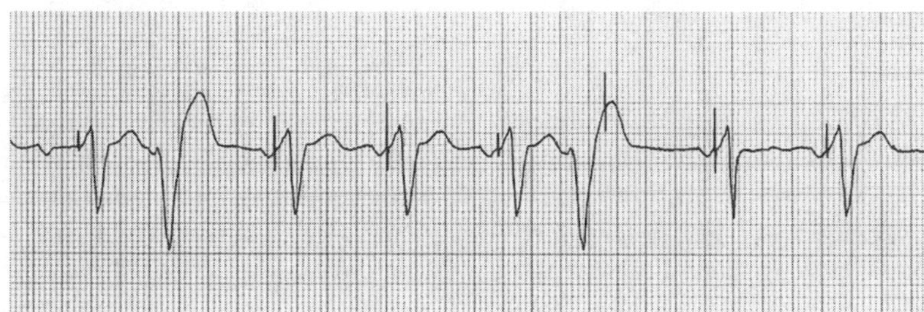

FIGURE 4.2.
Failure to sense. The second premature ventricular contraction is not sensed by the pacemaker, and a pacemaker spike is seen in the T wave.

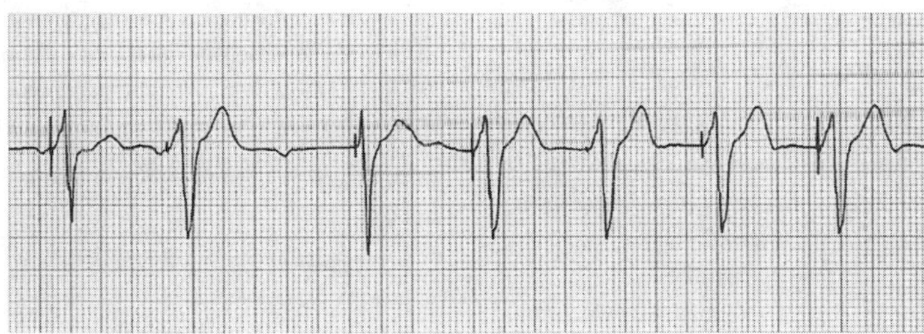

FIGURE 4.3.
Oversensing. The T wave of the second QRS complex is sensed by the pacemaker as a ventricular beat. The next pacemaker spike is inhibited and comes late.

Abnormal Sensing

Abnormal sensing may be manifest as undersensing or oversensing. Undersensing is failure to sense myocardial depolarizations (Fig 4.2). It is apparent as inappropriate pacing after intrinsic myocardial events or as failure to track the atrial events in DDD pacing. Common factors leading to undersensing include the following:

- Small intracardiac signals (e.g., P or R waves)
- Fibrosis at the lead tip
- Lead dislodgment
- Metabolic derangement
- Drug therapy
- Insulation defects and conductor fractures
- Inappropriate pacemaker programming
- Pacemaker battery depletion
- Response to electrical noise, such as Bovie electrocautery, direct-current cardioversion, or magnet application

Oversensing is usually due to sensing of signals other than true intracardiac depolarizations (Fig. 4.3). This is seen as failure to pace or pacing at a rate below the pacemaker-programmed lower rate resulting from inhibition of pacemaker output by these signals. Oversensing may be caused by the following:

- Pectoral muscle potentials
- Strong electrical fields
- Pacemaker stimuli from opposing chambers
- Lead malfunction

Intermittent lead fracture may cause chaotic pacing from oversensing during specific patient movements. Erratic pacing with variable pauses strongly suggests a lead problem. Undersensing and oversensing problems can often be alleviated or corrected by reprogramming. Patients with these problems should be referred to physicians experienced in pacemaker management.

Tachycardias

Pacemaker-mediated tachycardia, or endless-loop tachycardia, is a complication seen with dual-chamber pacemakers. This condition starts with atrial sensing of a retrograde P wave, usually caused by a premature ventricular contraction. This triggers a ventricular paced beat that produces another retrograde P wave, and so on. Asynchronous pacing, produced with a magnet application, will terminate pacemaker-mediated tachycardia. Reprogramming can prevent this condition in most patients. Affected patients should be referred to physicians experienced in pacemaker management.

Dual-chamber pacemakers can track the atria and pace the ventricle up to the maximum programmed rate in response to supraventricular rhythms such as atrial fibrillation, atrial flutter, sinus tachycardia, or atrial tachycardia. These rapid paced rates can be prevented by treating the primary arrhythmia (e.g., atrial fibrillation) or by reprogramming the pacemaker.

In rate-adaptive pacemakers, rapid ventricular pacing may be induced by abnormal sensor input. The most common sensors are vibration sensors and minute ventilation sensors. Body tremors, upper body activity, or external vibration (such as riding in a car on a rough road or dental drilling) may inappropriately stimulate vibration sensors and thereby cause tachycardia. Minute ventilation sensors may be overstimulated in mechanically ventilated patients during elective surgical procedures or in the intensive care unit. Pacemakers should be reprogrammed to prevent inappropriate rapid pacing.

OUTPATIENT FOLLOW-UP AND EVALUATION OF PATIENTS WITH PACEMAKERS

Routine follow-up of patients with pacemakers is mandatory because pacemaker complications are not uncommon and all pacemaker batteries eventually become depleted. Thorough follow-up ensures appropriate programming and reprogramming of the pacemaker for changing clinical conditions and identifying impending depletion of the pacemaker battery.

Before discharge after initial implantation, all patients should have 12-lead electrocardiography, wound and generator assessment, and posteroanterior and lateral chest radiography to confirm lead placement and rule out such operative complications as pneumothorax or lead malposition.

The patient should be seen 1 to 2 weeks after implantation for inspection of the operative site, general physical assessment, and pacemaker evaluation. A complete pacing evaluation is done 1 to 3 months after implantation, when pacing and sensing thresholds have stabilized. The pacemaker can then be reprogrammed for long-term function to optimize battery life. Full assessment of battery life, by measurement of sensing and pacing thresholds, should be done at 3- to 12-month intervals in most patients. For pacemaker-dependent patients or those who are remote from health care facilities, transtelephonic monthly documentation of pacemaker function is recommended.

At each clinic visit, a history should be taken to discover any possible problems related to the pacemaker (Table 4.3) and to determine whether a patient's original symptoms were relieved by the pacemaker. It is also important to include questions about symptoms that reflect diminished cardiac output. Such symptoms should lead to consideration of the following:

- Pacing at rapid ventricular rates
- Pacemaker syndrome
- Oversensing with pauses in paced rhythm or with triggering of ventricular pacing
- Undersensing with resultant competitive rhythms
- Failure to capture because of threshold elevation, conductor fracture, or lead break

Pacemaker Syndrome

Pacemaker syndrome refers to multiple symptoms and signs in patients in whom the atrial rhythm is dyssynchronous with the ventricular rate. Pacemaker syndrome is seen predominantly in VVI-paced patients who have intact retrograde ventriculoatrial conduction, but it is also seen in DDD-paced patients who have inappropriate AV pacing. Symptoms of pacemaker syndrome include the following:

- Weakness
- Breathlessness
- Orthopnea

Common Symptoms in Patients with Pacemakers — TABLE 4.3.

Symptoms	Causes
Palpitations	Rapid paced ventricular rates
	Normal tracking of sinus tachycardia, atrial tachycardia, atrial flutter, atrial fibrillation
	Pacemaker-mediated tachycardia
	Retrograde ventricular arrhythmia conduction
	Myopotential triggered
	Electromagnetic triggered
	Spontaneous tachycardia
	Spontaneous extrasystole
Weakness, fatigue	Pacemaker syndrome
	Inappropriately programmed, rate-responsive parameters
	Underlying cardiopulmonary and systemic disease
	Failure to capture
Breathlessness, orthopnea, paroxysmal nocturnal dyspnea	Pacemaker syndrome
	Underlying cardiac disease
Hiccups	Diaphragmatic stimulation
Muscle twitching	Insulation break
Syncope, presyncope, dizziness	Underlying cardiac disease
	Pacemaker syndrome
	Failure to capture
	Oversensing with pacemaker inhibition

- Paroxysmal nocturnal dyspnea
- Pulmonary edema
- Presyncope and syncope
- Awareness of neck palpitations

Treatment may require upgrading a VVI pulse generator to DDD or reprogramming of a dual-chamber device.

The Physical Examination

The physical examination at follow-up should include a thorough assessment of the pacemaker pocket site and the area overlying the leads. The pulse generator should be slightly movable. Signs of infection, such as pain and swelling, are abnormal and demand immediate attention. The firmness of the pocket site should also be noted. This may aid in the assessment of the causes of erosion through the skin or rotation of the pulse generator causing lead dislodgment, whether spontaneous or by the patient ("twiddler's syndrome"). During manipulation of the pocket, muscle stimulation may indicate an insulation break, and intermittent loss of capture may indicate a loose connection (e.g., between the pacing lead and the battery) or a conductor fracture. The jugular venous pulse should be examined for cannon A waves indicating atrial contraction against closed AV valves. Signs of venous thrombosis of the ipsilateral subclavian vein should be noted. Patients with any sign of pacemaker complication should be referred for expert management. Empiric therapy for suspected pacemaker infections is not accepted management.

SPECIAL CONSIDERATIONS IN PATIENTS WITH PACEMAKERS

All pacemaker interrogations and reprogramming must be clearly documented to avoid "phantom" reprogramming—unexplained reprogramming of a pacemaker that may be inappropriate. Pacemakers may be reprogrammed inadvertently for many of the following reasons.

Cardioversion and defibrillation may lead to undersensing, increases in pacing threshold, and pacemaker reprogramming. Pacemakers should always be fully interrogated before and after cardioversion. Electrocautery used in surgery may cause pacemaker inhibition, reprogramming, or damage. Patients with pacemakers who require electrocautery should be evaluated before and after the procedure by physicians experienced in pacemaker management. Magnetic resonance imaging exposes the patient to strong electromagnetic fields. This test is contraindicated in patients with pacemakers because permanent pacemaker damage or induction of arrhythmias could result.

A lithotriptor induces electromagnetic and mechanical forces that may influence pacing system function. Lithotripsy is generally safe in paced patients, but the pacemaker should be programmed in VVI mode with rate sensors turned off and the lithotriptor synchronized to the QRS complex. Transcutaneous electric nerve stimulation (TENS) is considered safe to use in patients with pacemakers. Ionizing radiation, as used in radiation therapy, may cause short-term or long-term cumulative damage to pulse generators. The pacemaker should be checked regularly in patients undergoing radiation therapy.

Airport metal detectors are safe for patients with modern pacemakers, as are microwave ovens. Patients should be warned to avoid any strong magnetic fields, such as power transformers or arc welding. Prophylaxis of endocarditis is not routinely recommended for patients with pacemakers.

IMPLANTABLE CARDIOVERTER DEFIBRILLATORS

Implantable cardioverter defibrillators (ICDs) are devices designed to treat recurrent malignant ventricular arrhythmias by delivering an electric shock or antitachycardia pacing. The ICD system is composed of defibrillation electrodes, sensing leads, and a generator battery and circuitry. The sensing and pacing lead is similar to that for a bradycardia ventricular pacemaker. Defibrillation therapy is delivered between two or more electrodes through the myocardium. The electrodes may consist of epicardial patches, subcutaneous patches, endocardial leads, or the defibrillator generator itself. Most ICDs also have VVI bradycardia pacing features. The ICD generator may be implanted in abdominal or pectoral positions. An ICD senses the cardiac rhythm and delivers therapy when tachycardia is present for a programmed duration of time or number of beats. After tachycardia detection, therapy consists of antitachycardia pacing or low- and high-energy shocks delivered in a programmed sequence.

An ICD is generally indicated for patients at risk for recurrent sustained malignant ventricular tachyarrhythmias that are resistant to drug therapy or for patients who have survived cardiac arrest. An ICD is not recommended for patients with less than 6 months' survival because of comorbidity, incessant ventricular tachycardia, or tachycardia with acute myocardial infarction. An ICD should be prescribed by a trained cardiac electrophysiologist after formal electrophysiology evaluation. Follow-up of patients with ICDs is similar to that of patients with permanent pacemakers. In general, patients should be seen every 3 to 6 months by physicians trained in ICD therapy.

The primary care physician may be required to intervene in a patient with an ICD in the situation of recurrent ICD shocks. These shocks can be appropriate for incessant ventricular tachycardia or can be inappropriate because of supraventricular tachycardia or electrical malfunction. Appropriate ICD shocks may be lifesaving but if recurrent over a short period may cause severe discomfort and ICD battery depletion. Frequent appropriate shocks should be managed acutely by trying to pharmacologically suppress the tachycardia and treat its underlying causes.

Reversible causes of worsening arrhythmias include the following:

- Electrolyte abnormalities (especially hypokalemia and hypomagnesemia)
- Heart failure
- Myocardial ischemia
- New antiarrhythmic drugs that may be proarrhythmic

In the emergency department or office setting, intravenous lidocaine, procainamide, bretylium, or amiodarone may suppress episodes of ventricular tachycardia. Long-term treatment may require initiation of new antiarrhythmic medications under the direction of physicians trained in electrophysiology.

Inappropriate firing by ICDs may be due to supraventricular arrhythmias, including atrial fibrillation, or electrical noise interpreted by the device to be ventricular tachycardia.

Because most ICDs use heart rate as the sole criterion for detecting tachyarrhythmia, any supraventricular rhythm with a ventricular response faster than the programmed detection rate may be detected as ventricular tachycardia; as a result, the patient may receive inappropriate shocks for these rhythms. This is not a device malfunction because the device is detecting the ventricular rate as programmed. Treatment involves preventing or slowing the supraventricular tachycardia or increasing the detection rate of the ICD. Calcium-channel blockers or β blockers will help prevent or slow the ventricular rate during supraventricular tachycardia. Short-term delivery is inhibited as long as a

TABLE 4.4. Evaluation of the Patient with Asymptomatic Intracardiac Cardioverter Defibrillator Shocks

Causes
- Oversensing
  - Wire fracture
  - T-wave sensing
  - Sensing of pacemaker spike
- Generator failure
- Atrial fibrillation
- Nonsustained ventricular tachycardia
- Supraventricular tachycardia
- Rate cutoff below exercise heart rate
- "Asymptomatic" or minimally symptomatic ventricular tachycardia above rate cutoff

Management
- Turn off device
- Treat arrhythmia
- Replace sensing leads if broken
- Implant a noncommitted device (for frequent nonsustained ventricular tachycardia)

pacemaker magnet is applied over the ICD. Some devices are programmed "off" by prolonged magnet exposure.

If the ICD fires in the absence of a rapid ventricular rate, device malfunction must be evaluated. Possible causes are lead fracture or loose electrical connections leading to oversensing of electrical noise. The ICD may fire when the patient moves in a certain position that strains a lead or connector. The device may sense pacing artifacts from a temporary or permanent implanted pacemaker causing inappropriate firing. Any patient receiving a shock in the absence of ventricular tachyarrhythmias must be evaluated immediately by an electrophysiologist (Table 4.4).

An ICD may fail to respond to ventricular tachyarrhythmia for several reasons. If patients are receiving new drugs, their ventricular tachycardia rate may have slowed to below the device programmed cutoff rate. This requires reprogramming. Interactions with permanent or temporary pacemakers may also inhibit therapy for ventricular tachycardia. An ICD may have been turned off by careless programming or by a strong magnet, either intentionally or inadvertently. Patients should be warned to avoid magnetic resonance imaging, power transformers, and industrial magnets (Table 4.5). Any such patient must be evaluated immediately by an electrophysiologist.

TABLE 4.5. Common Sources of Electromagnetic Interference

- Endogenous
  - Myopotential
- Medical equipment
  - Magnetic resonance imaging
  - Cardioversion, defibrillation
  - Transcutaneous pacing
  - Electrocautery
  - Lithotripsy
  - Diathermy
  - Ionizing radiation
  - Electrotherapy
    - Transcutaneous nerve stimulation
    - Implanted neuromuscular stimulation
- Ambient
  - Radiofrequency emissions
  - High tension lines
  - Arc welding
  - Rotating radar detectors
  - Induction furnaces

If an arrhythmia is not terminated after four to seven shocks, ICDs will not deliver further therapy until a rhythm other than ventricular tachycardia or ventricular fibrillation is sensed for a period of time. Failure of the ICD to sense previous shocks may be diagnosed as failure to respond. Patients in whom arrhythmias do not respond to ICD therapy should be treated as any other patient and given external defibrillation and standard cardiopulmonary resuscitation.

Special Circumstances

An ICD can be temporarily deactivated by placing a strong magnet over the device. This may be useful whenever the patient is receiving inappropriate or incessant shocks. Bradycardia pacing is not affected by the magnet in most devices. General surgery, radiotherapy, lithotripsy, and electroconvulsive therapy can be safely performed in patients with ICDs. The devices should be deactivated before the procedure and reactivated afterward with clear documentation of the changes in programming. Infections may be a serious life-threatening problem with ICDs. Patients suspected of having an infection should be referred to an electrophysiologist for treatment and for determination of whether device explantation is required.

In summary, ICD therapy is effective but complex. More than 20,000 patients per year receive ICDs. A basic understanding of the devices and skills used in the short-term management of patients with ICDs is important for all physicians caring for these patients.

KEY POINTS

Pacemakers

- Pacemaker function may be classified by four-letter typing: 1) chamber(s) paced (A, atria; V, ventricle; D, dual), 2) chambers sensed, 3) response to sensing, and 4) programmability and modulation functions (e.g., DDDR: dual-chamber paced, dual-chamber sensed, both inhibited and triggered responses [dual], and rate responsiveness).
- Indications for pacemaker include sick sinus syndrome; high-degree, symptomatic AV block; symptomatic bradycardia; and complete heart block.
- Pacemakers may be indicated for asymptomatic complete heart block, asymptomatic Mobitz type II second-degree heart block, and asymptomatic type I (Wenckebach) block with wide QRS complex.
- Problems with pacemakers include loss of capture, abnormal sensing, and pacemaker-mediated tachycardia. In any of these situations, refer back to the electrophysiologist.

Implantable Cardiac Defibrillators

- Indications for automatic internal cardiac defibrillators Include risk for recurrent sustained malignant ventricular tachyarrhythmias resisting during therapy.
- Consider ICD therapy in consultation with a cardiac electrophysiologist.
- If a patient experiences recurrent, frequent shocks, begin intravenous pharmacologic suppression (e.g., lidocaine). Check potassium and magnesium and supplement if necessary. Check for decompensated heart failure, drug interaction, or myocardial ischemia in the presence of recurrent shocks.
- Inappropriate ICD shocks may be caused by atrial fibrillation, lead fracture, or loose connections. Refer back to the electrophysiologist.
- Magnetic resonance imaging is contraindicated in patients with ICDs or pacemaker.

SUGGESTED READINGS

Belz MK, Wood MA, Ellenbogen KA. Pacemakers and implantable cardioverter defibrillators in the intensive care unit setting. In: Ayers SM, ed. Textbook of critical care. Philadelphia: WB Saunders, 1995.

Dreifus LS, Fisch C, Griffin JC, et al. Guidelines for implantation of cardiac pacemakers and antiarrhythmia devices. J Am Coll Cardiol 1991;18:1–13.

Ellenbogen KA. Cardiac pacing. Oxford: Blackwell Scientific, 1992.

Garson A. Stepwise approach to the unknown pacemaker ECG. Am Heart J 1990;119:924–941.

Hayes DL, Vlietstra RE. Pacemaker malfunction. Ann Intern Med 1993;119:828–835.

5 CHAPTER

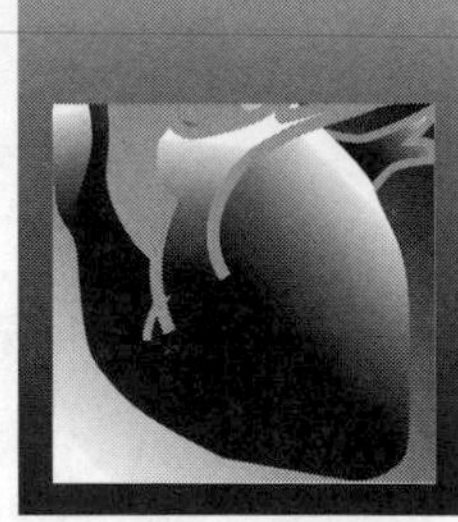

Hypertension

Elizabeth B. Ripley
Domenic A. Sica

BACKGROUND

Hypertension is defined as systolic blood pressure of at least 140 mm Hg or diastolic blood pressure of at least 90 mm Hg. It affects more than 43 million people in the United States, most of whom have mild to moderate (stages I and II) hypertension. The most recent National Health and Nutrition Examination Survey (1988–1991) found the prevalence of hypertension to be 23% in white persons, 32% in African-American persons, and 23% in Hispanic persons. Hypertension is more prevalent in men than in women, although these differences decrease after menopause. The incidence increases with age.

The recognition that hypertension is linked with increased risk for heart disease, stroke, and death emerged in the 1920s. The first successful trials used diastolic blood pressure as the "efficacy" end point, leading to an emphasis on the diastolic blood pressure as the primary focus for therapy. It has been only in the past 30 years that systolic blood pressure has been recognized as an equal, if not better, indicator of morbidity and death from hypertension. Although the deleterious effects of systolic hypertension have been recognized for some time, it was not until the 1980s that clinical trials focused specifically on the merits of treating systolic hypertension.

The treatment of hypertension has also progressed from the earliest available agents, which appeared in the 1950s, to the currently available pharmacologic stable of effective and well-tolerated medications. During the 1960s, it was proven that treatment of nonmalignant hypertension significantly reduced the incidence of cardiovascular events. Encouraged by these data, the High Blood Pressure Education Program, established in 1972, began to publicize the importance of diagnosing and treating hypertension. Since then, the benefits of treating even milder forms of hypertension in a wide range of ages has been demonstrated.

Since the establishment of the High Blood Pressure Education Program in 1972, the mortality rate in the United States from coronary heart disease has declined by approximately 50%; the rate of death from stroke has decreased by approximately 60%. Much of this improvement relates to the aggressive treatment of hypertension. Even with this dramatic decrease in cardiovascular and stroke incidence achieved in large populations, it is important to underscore the necessity of evaluating each patient's risk for hypertension in light of other coexisting medical illnesses and cardiovascular risk factors. Thus, the treatment of hypertension is only one of several strategies to be considered to further reduce end-organ damage, including stroke, cardiovascular disease, and renal failure.

TABLE 5.1. Classification of Blood Pressure for Adults 18 years of Age and Older

Category*	Systolic Blood Pressure (mm Hg)	Diastolic Blood Pressure (mm Hg)
Normal	<130	<85
High-normal	130–139	85–89
Hypertension		
Stage 1	140–159	90–99
Stage 2	160–179	100–109
Stage 3	180–209	110–119
Stage 4	≥210	≥120

Adapted from The Fifth Report of the Joint National Committee on Detection, Evaluation, and Treatment of High Blood Pressure (JNC V). Arch Intern Med 1993;153:154–183.
*When systolic and diastolic blood pressures fall into different categories, the higher category is used.

CLASSIFICATION

The traditional classification of hypertension was purely descriptive, conveying the notion that a certain blood pressure denoted mild, moderate, or severe risk for end-organ disease. The most recent classification for hypertension (Table 5.1) now stages hypertension by absolute diastolic or systolic blood pressure values. This staging system more accurately reflects that all levels of hypertension, either systolic or diastolic, are associated with increased risk.

DETECTION AND DIAGNOSIS OF HYPERTENSION

Elevated blood pressure is often inadvertently discovered in otherwise asymptomatic patients under casual circumstances (e.g., in a community blood pressure screening) or during the evaluation of another problem. Hypertension should not be diagnosed on the basis of a single measurement unless significantly elevated blood pressure (i.e., > 200/120 mm Hg) coexists with end-organ damage.

Elevated blood pressure should be confirmed on at least two occasions after the initial high measurement. The rapidity with which initial blood pressure elevations are confirmed and treatment initiated should be determined by the presenting blood pressure and the extent of any end-organ damage. Blood pressure readings should also be obtained in standardized ways so that the results are reproducible and most accurately re-

TABLE 5.2. Techniques for the Measurement of Arterial Pressure

1. The patient should be seated with feet flat on the floor and the arm supported at the level of the heart.
2. The patient should refrain from consuming caffeine and smoking cigarettes for 30 minutes before measurement.
3. The patient should rest for 5 minutes before the first reading.
4. The appropriate cuff size must be used; a cuff that is too small may exaggerate the blood pressure reading. The bladder should nearly or completely encircle the arm.
5. Measurement should be obtained with a well-functioning mercury sphygmomanometer, calibrated aneroid manometer, or calibrated electronic device.
6. Systolic and diastolic blood pressure should be recorded: the first Korotkoff sound (the first detectable heart beat) as systolic; the fifth Korotkoff sound (the disappearance of sound) as diastolic. If the sound is heard to 0 mm Hg, then the fourth Korotkoff sound (the muffling of the sound) should also be recorded.
7. Two or more readings separated by 2 minutes should be averaged. If the first two readings differ by more than 5 mm Hg, additional readings should be obtained.
8. During the initial assessment, blood pressure should be measured in both arms and the highest value subsequently used for treatment decisions. A thigh blood pressure should also be measured.
9. Standing blood pressure should be obtained after the patient has stood for at least 2 minutes. The arm should be supported at the level of the heart.

Adapted from The Fifth Report of the Joint National Committee on Detection, Evaluation, and Treatment of High Blood Pressure (JNC V). Arch Intern Med 1993;153:154–183.

flect the patient's true intraarterial pressure. Table 5.2 describes the correct technique for measuring blood pressure.

Ambulatory Blood Pressure Monitoring

Many diagnostic and therapeutic difficulties in hypertension can be resolved by the use of home blood pressure monitoring. Technically accurate blood pressure monitoring devices are now economically feasible for most patients. Monitoring of blood pressure using a 24-hour ambulatory blood pressure monitor (ABPM) has become increasingly popular. In particular, this technology has expanded our understanding of the circadian pattern of blood pressure, wherein blood pressure reaches its nadir in the early morning. Many subsets of hypertensive patients, including African-American persons, transplant recipients, and patients with renal failure, exhibit smaller decrements in blood pressure at night. This failure to "dip" and the consequent constant pressure load on the heart has been proposed as a contributing factor to the increased risk for cardiovascular and renal disease observed in these hypertensive patients.

In clinical practice, 24-hour ABPM can be of assistance. In patients with white-coat hypertension (i.e., an exaggerated increase in blood pressure in medical settings), 24-hour ABPM may determine whether episodic increases in blood pressure are occurring in more than simply a medical setting, as may be the case in someone with stressful work conditions. In patients thought to be drug resistant, 24-hour ABPM can help determine whether blood pressure truly is decreasing after dosing and for what portion of a dosing interval control exists.

Many patients with noniatrogenic experiences are also candidates for extensive monitoring. The use of ABPM may simplify the care of patients who report symptoms compatible with hypotension after ingestion of antihypertensive medications or in relation to autonomic dysfunction. In addition, in patients prone to episodic blood pressure elevations with or without flushing, headache, or palpitations, 24-hour ABPM may help characterize these elevations. In these cases, a diary is extremely useful in correlating symptoms with blood pressure values and in determining the likelihood that such symptoms were triggered by panic attacks. When used in conjunction with electrocardiographic monitoring, ABPM may also aid in the diagnosis of carotid sinus syncope and pacemaker syndromes.

Evaluation of Patients with Diagnosed Hypertension

The primary goal in treating hypertension is to decrease the end-organ damage that results from chronic hypertension. Therefore, the initial assessment of a hypertensive patient should answer three key questions.

1. Does the patient have essential hypertension or a secondary and, therefore, possibly reversible cause of hypertension?
2. Is there evidence of target-organ damage (Table 5.3)?
3. What other cardiovascular risk factors does the patient have?

The answers to these questions, in conjunction with the actual blood pressure, determine a patient's absolute cardiovascular risk and how aggressively blood pressure should be reduced.

A thorough medical history is important in the evaluation of hypertension (Table 5.4). The physical examination (Table 5.5) looks for evidence of target-organ damage or signs of secondary hypertension (Table 5.6). The initial laboratory evaluation is also designed to look for evidence of target-organ damage (e.g., elevated

Manifestations of Target-Organ Disease **TABLE 5.3.**

Organ System	Clinical Findings
Retinal	Hemorrhages or exudates, with or without papilledema
Cardiac	Clinical, electrocardiographic, or radiologic evidence of coronary artery disease
	Left ventricular hypertrophy or strain on electrocardiography, or left ventricular dysfunction on echocardiography
Cerebrovascular	Transient ischemic attack or stroke
Peripheral vascular	Absence of one or more major pulses in the extremities, claudication or rest pain, presence of aneurysm
Renal	Microalbuminuria or proteinuria
	Serum creatinine level > 1.5 mg dL

Adapted from The Fifth Report of the Joint National Committee on Detection, Evaluation, and Treatment of High Blood Pressure (JNC V). Arch Intern Med 1993;153:154–183.

Medical History **TABLE 5.4.**

1. Duration and level of blood pressure. In women, include blood pressure history during pregnancies.
2. History of antihypertensive therapy, including drug names, efficacy, and side effects.
3. Full medication review, including prescribed and over-the-counter drugs. Particular drugs of interest are oral contraceptives, steroids, nonsteroidal anti-inflammatory drugs, nasal decongestants, cold remedies, appetite suppressants, cyclosporine, erythropoietin, tricyclic antidepressants, and monoamine oxidase inhibitors.
4. History of cardiovascular, cerebrovascular, and renal diseases.
5. History of diabetes, dyslipidemias, and gout.
6. Review of systems to include symptoms of secondary hypertension, such as tachycardia, tremor, orthostatic hypotension, sweating, and pallor.
7. Family history of hypertension, including age of onset, history of cardiovascular disease, stroke, diabetes mellitus, and dyslipidemia.
8. History of recent weight gain.
9. Social history, including physical activity, smoking, and alcohol intake.
10. Dietary assessment emphasizing intake of sodium, cholesterol, and saturated fat.
11. Psychosocial and environmental factors, such as family situation, employment status, and education level, that may influence compliance or coping skills.

Adapted from The Fifth Report of the Joint National Committee on Detection, Evaluation, and Treatment of High Blood Pressure (JNC V). Arch Intern Med 1993;153:154–183.

TABLE 5.5. Initial Physical Examination

1. Two or more blood pressure measurements separated by 2 minutes with the patient either supine or seated and after the patient has stood for at least 2 minutes.
2. Height and weight.
3. Fundoscopic examination for arteriolar narrowing, arteriovenous nicking, hemorrhages, exudates, or papilledema.
4. Examination of the neck for carotid bruits, jugular venous distention, and thyroid gland enlargement.
5. Examination of the heart for rhythm, displaced point of maximal impulse, murmur, or gallops.
6. Examination of the abdomen for bruits, large kidneys, masses, or abdominal aortic pulsations or enlargement.
7. Examination of the extremities for decreased or absent pulses, bruits, or edema.
8. Neurologic assessment for signs of previous cerebrovascular disease.

Adapted from The Fifth Report of the Joint National Committee on Detection, Evaluation, and Treatment of High Blood Pressure (JNC V). Arch Intern Med 1993;153:154–183.

TABLE 5.6. Physical Findings Suggestive of Secondary Hypertension

Cause	Finding
Polycystic kidney disease	Abdominal or flank masses
Renovascular hypertension	Abdominal bruits, particularly those that lateralize or have a diastolic component
Aortic coarctation	Delayed or absent femoral arterial pulses and decreased blood pressure in lower extremities compared to the upper extremities
Cushing's syndrome	Truncal obesity, purple striae
Pheochromocytoma	Tachycardia, tremor, orthostatic hypotension, sweating, and pallor

Adapted from The Fifth Report of the Joint National Committee on Detection, Evaluation, and Treatment of High Blood Pressure (JNC V). Arch Intern Med 1993;153:154–183.

TABLE 5.7. Laboratory Evaluation of Hypertensive Patients

Laboratory Test	Results
Urinalysis	Evidence of parenchymal renal disease (proteinuria, hematuria)
Fasting glucose	Assistance in diagnosis of diabetes mellitus
Blood urea nitrogen and creatinine	Indices of baseline renal function
Potassium	Hypokalemia, suggesting search for primary hyperaldosteronism
Calcium	Hypercalcemia, which can cause hypertension
Uric acid	Establishment of baseline; may be a predictor of cardiovascular disease
Cholesterol and triglyceride profile	Evidence of risk for heart disease
Electrocardiography	Evidence of left ventricular hypertrophy, ischemia, and arrhythmias

Adapted with permission from Moser M. Initial workup of the hypertensive patient. In: Izzo J, Black H, eds. Hypertension primer. Dallas: American Heart Association, 1993:223.

creatinine levels) or clues to secondary forms of hypertension (e.g., hypokalemia) (Table 5.7).

WHITE-COAT HYPERTENSION

The blood pressure readings of hypertensive persons are traditionally higher in clinic settings when obtained by a physician. A subset of patients have been labeled as having white-coat hypertension; these patients are characterized by a persistently elevated blood pressure in a medical setting and a normal ambulatory blood pressure. This condition is seen in approximately 20% of patients with high-normal blood pressure and those with stage I hypertension. It occurs in both men and women and may be more common in older than in younger patients. The pathophysiology is uncertain, and although a genetic component has been postulated, most evidence suggests that it is an acquired behavior pattern. The diagnosis is suspected in patients who do not have signs of target-organ damage and have consistently elevated blood pressure at the clinic and normal pressure when measured outside the clinic or by a nonphysician. The prognosis for white-coat hypertension is debatable, suggesting that patients in this category are at lower cardiac risk than patients with other forms of hypertension.

Treatment

An emphasis on lifestyle modification and other cardiac risk factors remains the mainstay of treatment. It should be remembered, however, that normalizing clinic blood pressures with medications may lead to significant hypotension in nonoffice settings.

ISOLATED SYSTOLIC HYPERTENSION

Isolated systolic hypertension is a systolic blood pressure of 160 mm Hg or greater and a diastolic blood pressure of 90 mm Hg or less. This condition is rare before 44 years of age, but its prevalence increases with age and is more common in women and African-American persons.

Treatment

Definitive studies, including the Systolic Hypertension in the Elderly Program (SHEP), have shown significant reduction in the rate of stroke and a trend toward decreased incidence of cardiac events in elderly patients treated for isolated systolic hypertension. This study, as well as several other large studies, used diuretics and β-blockers as first-line treatment. Smaller, shorter studies have shown that other classes of drugs, such as calcium-channel blockers and angiotensin-converting enzyme (ACE) inhibitors, are effective in treating systolic hypertension. However, the role of these drugs in decreasing the rate of cardiovascular events has not been proven. It should be remembered that these studies have routinely involved relatively healthy older patients. In more debilitated patients, in whom life expectancy is considerably shortened, the benefit of treating systolic hypertension may not justify the potential risks of drug side effects or drug interactions.

SECONDARY HYPERTENSION

Hypertension can be caused by several medical conditions that can be corrected or treated, thereby curing or significantly improving the elevated blood pressure. The incidence of secondary hypertension is lower than that of essential hypertension. The most common clinical conditions causing secondary hypertension are the following:

- Renovascular hypertension
- Coarctation of the aorta
- Thyroid disease
- Primary hyperaldosteronism
- Cushing's syndrome
- Pheochromocytoma

Renovascular Hypertension

Renovascular hypertension is defined by an elevation in diastolic blood pressure and an absence of isolated systolic hypertension. The diagnosis is often confirmed retrospectively if angiographic or surgical relief of a stenosis results in decreased blood pressure or a decrease in the number of antihypertensive drugs required. Renovascular hypertension is primarily caused by fibromuscular dysplasia (which primarily occurs in young women) or atheromatous vascular disease. Table 5.8 shows clinical characteristics suggestive of renovascular

TABLE 5.8. Clinical Characteristics Associated with Renovascular Hypertension

Malignant or accelerated hypertension
Abdominal or flank bruit
Progression in the severity of chronic hypertension
Severe or difficult-to-control hypertension
Recent onset of hypertension
Onset at a young age (<25 years) or at an older age (>60 years)
Hypotension or renal failure with angiotensin-converting enzyme inhibitor treatment

Adapted with permission from Svetkey L. Renovascular hypertension. In: Greenburg A, ed. Primer on kidney disease, National Kidney Foundation. San Diego: Academic Press, 1994:353.

TABLE 5.9. Diagnostic and Screening Tests for Renovascular Hypertension

Conventional renal arteriography: the gold standard
Intravenous digital subtraction renal angiography
Captopril-stimulated peripheral renin activity
Captopril-stimulated renography
Duplex ultrasonography: sensitivity is operator dependent
Magnetic resonance imaging and angiography

Adapted with permission from Svetkey L. Renovascular hypertension. In: Greenburg A, ed. Primer on kidney disease, National Kidney Foundation. San Diego: Academic Press, 1994:353.

hypertension, which should prompt consideration for screening. Table 5.9 lists screening and diagnostic tests commonly used for renovascular hypertension.

Treatment

Treatment of renovascular disease requires lessening or elimination of the stenosis through the use of renal artery bypass or, more commonly, by percutaneous transluminal coronary angioplasty. When technically feasible, angioplasty is preferred because it requires neither general anesthesia nor a prolonged hospital stay. Angioplasty is least successful for ostial lesions and most successful for resolution of fibromuscular dysplasia.

In patients unsuitable for angioplasty or surgical revascularization, medical management with antihypertensive agents becomes necessary. These patients are typically sensitive to volume depletion, which occurs with excessive diuretic therapy or interruption of the renin-angiotensin-aldosterone axis, by means of ACE inhibitors or angiotensin II receptor blockers. With either therapy, creatinine values can increase disproportionately to the observed decrease in blood pressure. Although blood pressure can usually be controlled medically, renal artery stenosis increases the risk for development of primary chronic renal insufficiency or accelerating the rate of functional decline from other diseases (e.g., diabetic nephropathy).

Coarctation of the Aorta

Coarctation of the aorta is a relatively common cause of hypertension in children. Although familial cases have occurred, the condition is usually sporadic. It is more common in males. The pathognomonic physical findings associated with coarctation are decreased femoral pulses and a systolic pressure gradient between the arms or between the right arm and right leg blood pressures. A systolic murmur, heard best in the posterior left interscapular area, is often present. The diagnosis can be made noninvasively by chest radiography and echocardiography. A discrete thoracic coarctation may show a "3 sign" on chest radiography. This "3" consists of the proximal aorta, coarctated segment, and poststenotic dilatation. Echocardiography is useful in localizing the site of the coarctated segment, assessing the anatomy of the aortic arch, and estimating the pressure gradient across the coarctation. Cardiac catheterization is now reserved for patients in whom the echocardiogram suggests an abdominal location of the coarctation, associated cardiac abnormalities, or an abnormal arch anatomy.

Treatment

Treatment options are surgical repair or angioplasty, and the prognosis of untreated patients with coarctation of the aorta is poor.

Hypertension seen in patients with coarctation follows three clinical patterns:

- Prerepair hypertension, which is poorly understood but most likely reflects renal underperfusion and stimulation of the renin-angiotensin-aldosterone system.
- Postrepair hypertension, a paradoxical, severe hypertension that occurs only after surgical repair. This form of hypertension is thought to be caused by the sympathetic nervous system or renin-angiotensin-aldosterone activation and can be prevented with β-blocker pretreatment or with blockade of the renin-angiotensin-aldosterone system.
- Late hypertension, which is also poorly understood, occurs in patients despite apparently successful hemodynamic repairs. This upper-extremity hypertension occurs during leg, but not arm, exercise. Patients with persistent hypertension at rest or during exercise should be treated with antihypertensive medications.

Thyroid Disease

Both hyperthyroidism and hypothyroidism have been associated with hypertension. Hyperthyroidism is characterized by increased cardiac output, heart rate, stroke volume, and systolic pressure and by decreased peripheral vascular resistance and decreased diastolic pressure. Plasma renin activity is generally increased. Hypothyroidism often features cardiac output, decreased stroke volume, increased peripheral vascular resistance, and diastolic hypertension.

Treatment

Although the prevalence of hypertension in patients with hypothyroidism remains uncertain, most authors report that thyroid hormone replacement improves blood pressure control in up to 30% of patients. Thyroid hormone replacement is less likely to have clinically significant effects on blood pressure in older patients and in patients with longer durations of hypertension.

Primary Hyperaldosteronism

Primary hyperaldosteronism usually results from the autonomous secretion of aldosterone from an adrenal adenoma or adrenal hyperplasia. The clinical clues to the presence of primary hyperaldosteronism are spontaneous hypokalemia, diuretic-induced hypokalemia (serum potassium levels < 3.0 mEq/L), difficulty maintaining a normal serum potassium level during diuretic therapy despite apparently adequate supplementation, and refractory hypertension.

The presence of hypokalemia in primary hyperaldosteronism is critically linked to dietary sodium intake and thus can be "normal" in many patients. Peripheral plasma renin activity is routinely suppressed (<2 ng/mL per hour), and plasma aldosterone levels are increased (>20 ng/dL). When the ratio of plasma aldosterone level to plasma renin activity exceeds 30, primary hyperaldosteronism is strongly suggested. In the presence of suggestive plasma hormonal changes, evaluation for hyperaldosteronism typically requires an attempt to demonstrate the suppressibility of aldosterone production. Results of such testing are more readily interpreted for patients who have not received ACE inhibitors, diuretics, and β-blockers for 1 to 2 weeks.

Various tests have been designed to suppress aldosterone production by saline infusion or sodium loading, with dietary maneuvers and supplementation. The most common approach is an infusion of 2 L of normal saline over 2 hours, with serum aldosterone levels measured before and after the salt loading. Failure of aldosterone to be suppressed (serum aldosterone level > 10 ng/dL) suggests the presence of hyperaldosteronism. If intravenous saline infusion is not feasible, an oral 5-day sodium load can be used (nonrestricted sodium intake and, if necessary, sodium chloride tablets to achieve a daily sodium intake of 220 mEq/d). A 24-hour urine test for aldosterone, creatinine (to verify adequacy of collection), and sodium should be done. A 24-hour urinary aldosterone excretion greater than 10 to 14 μg/24 hours with evidence of adequate salt loading (urinary sodium level > 120 mEq/d) is considered a positive test result. In patients with primary hyperaldosteronism, this sodium loading can result in significant potassium wasting; thus, patients should not be receiving a low-potassium diet and should have serum potassium levels measured.

Suggestive biochemical indices should prompt an attempt to localize an adrenal mass by computed tomography. Identifying an adrenal mass by computed tomography is considered diagnostic. If imaging results are inconclusive, adrenal vein sampling for aldosterone can be attempted.

Treatment

If an adenoma is found and the patient is a suitable surgical candidate, surgical removal becomes the treatment of choice. This method usually results in normalization of blood pressure or at least improvement in blood pressure control. If hyperplasia is present or the patient is not a surgical candidate, spironolactone should be used for treatment.

Spironolactone, which blocks the aldosterone receptor, typically normalizes the serum potassium and can often be used as monotherapy if the dosage is appropriately titrated (≥100 to 200 mg/d) and if no permanent vascular changes have resulted from long-standing hypertension. Gynecomastia, a troublesome side effect of spironolactone in dosages greater than 100 mg/d, may require dosage reduction or addition of other agents, such as ACE inhibitors or thiazide diuretics.

Cushing's Syndrome

The typical clinical presentation of Cushing's syndrome includes truncal obesity, moon facies, hypertension, plethora, muscle weakness and fatigue, hirsutism, emotional disturbances, and purple striae. Other clinical findings are carbohydrate intolerance or diabetes, amenorrhea, loss of libido, easy bruising, and spontaneous fractures of the ribs and vertebrae.

The typical manifestations of cortisol excess may not be present in patients with ectopic adrenocorticotropic hormone (ACTH) excess. These patients may present with hyperpigmentation of the skin, severe hypertension, and marked hypokalemic alkalosis. Causes of Cushing's syndrome include Cushing's disease, ectopic ACTH excess, adrenal adenoma, carcinoma, and hyperplasia.

Diagnosis of Cushing's syndrome begins with evaluation of 24-hour urinary cortisol excretion (≥100 μg/24 hours suggests excessive cortisol production). False-negative results almost never occur; however, false-positive results may be obtained in non-Cushing's hypercortisolemic states such as stress, long-term strenuous exercise, glucocorticoid resistance, and malnutrition. If the 24-hour urinary cortisol level is increased, plasma

ACTH should be measured. A low ACTH level suggests adrenal tumor or hyperplasia; thus, adrenal computed tomography should be done. A normal level suggests a pituitary tumor and should prompt computed tomography or magnetic resonance image of the head. Because a high ACTH level suggests an ectopic syndrome, chest and abdominal computed tomography should be done in patients with this finding.

Treatment

The treatment of choice for Cushing's syndrome is surgical resection, whether the ACTH originates from the pituitary, ectopically, or from a cortisol-producing adrenocortical tumor. Radiation therapy of the pituitary bed has also been successful for pituitary tumors. Ketoconazole, an inhibitor of several steroid biosynthetic pathways, has been used to rapidly correct hypercortisolism.

Pheochromocytoma

Pheochromocytoma is a neuroectodermal tumor that produces excessive amounts of catecholamines, resulting in hypertension and an array of signs and symptoms (Table 5.10) that can mimic other medical or surgical disorders (Table 5.11). Although a pheochromocytoma has classic symptoms, 30% of tumors are found at autopsy or are discovered during surgery for an unrelated problem. The early recognition, localization, and appropriate management of benign pheochromocytomas almost always result in complete cure; if unrecognized, however, these tumors can lead to significant cardiovascular morbidity and death, including sudden death during surgical and obstetric procedures.

The definitive diagnosis of pheochromocytoma rests primarily on laboratory test results. The recommended screening test is determination of urinary total

TABLE 5.10. **Signs of Pheochromocytoma**

Labile hypertension associated with diaphoresis, headaches, and tachycardia with or without palpitations
Family history of pheochromocytoma
Patients with multiple endocrine adenomatosis syndrome, neurofibromatosis, or von Hippel–Lindau disease
Adverse cardiovascular responses to anesthesia or surgery
Adverse cardiovascular response to certain drugs (e.g., tricyclic antidepressants, thyrotropin-releasing hormone, naloxone, antidopaminergic agents, guanethidine)

Adapted with permission from Bravo E. Secondary hypertension: adrenal and nervous systems. In: Hollenberg N, ed. Atlas of heart diseases, hypertension: mechanisms and therapy. Philadelphia: Current Medicine, 1994:6.16.

TABLE 5.11. **Medical and Surgical Conditions That Can Be Confused with Pheochromocytoma**

Anxiety
Hyperthyroidism
Idiopathic orthostatic hypotension
Autonomic dysfunction
Acute withdrawal of clonidine, β-adrenergic blockers, α-methyldopa, or alcohol
Vasodilator therapy with hydralazine or minoxidil
Factitious administration of sympathomimetic agents
Tyramine ingestion in patients receiving monoamine oxidase inhibitors
Menopausal syndrome with migraine headaches
Angina pectoris
β-adrenergic hyperresponsiveness
Cerebellopontine angle tumors
Acute hypoglycemia

Adapted with permission from Bravo E. Secondary hypertension: adrenal and nervous systems. In: Hollenberg N, ed. Atlas of heart diseases, hypertension: mechanisms and therapy. Philadelphia: Current Medicine, 1994:6.16.

Pharmacologic Treatment of Hypertension in Pregnancy **TABLE 5.12.**

Angiotensin converting enzyme inhibitors and Angiotensin receptor blockers:	Contraindicated. These agents are associated with renal agenesis, infant renal failure, and skeletal abnormalities.
β-blockers	Atenolol, pindolol, and metoprolol have been used.
α_1- and β-blockers	Labetalol, either intravenously or orally, has been used.
Calcium-channel blockers	Nifedipine has been used. Calcium-channel blockers should not be used with magnesium sulfate infusions.
Diuretics	Although intuitively decreasing plasma volume would seem contrary to events in normal pregnancy, diuretics have been used successfully.
Vasodilators	Hydralazine has been used both intravenously and orally. Patient headaches and tachycardia can occur. Neonatal thrombocytopenia has been reported.
Central α-adrenergic agonists	Methyldopa has been used but may cause maternal somnolence.
Clonidine	Should be avoided must be tapered and not abruptly discontinued. It has been associated with embryotoxicity in rats and behavioral abnormalities in infants.

metanephrine levels. A level less than 1.3 mg/24 hours has resulted in the fewest false-negative results. Values exceeding the normal range in "normal" patients are often associated with interference by drugs or atypical urinary pigments. A positive screening test result should be followed by determination of fractionated catecholamines; more than 95% of patients with pheochromocytoma have positive urinary results. Plasma catecholamines, which are chemically labile and require careful handling, are profoundly affected by many physiologic and pathologic states. Therefore, plasma measurements of norepinephrine and epinephrine are not as sensitive as urinary measurements for the detection of pheochromocytoma.

Although these tumors may exist anywhere from the base of the brain to the scrotum and may be multicentric, most pheochromocytomas arise in or close to the adrenal glands; almost all are located within the abdomen. Computed tomography and magnetic resonance imaging are the recommended imaging techniques. The latter is preferable for both extraadrenal and adrenal locations, as well as for pregnant patients. Percutaneous biopsy should not be performed because it has been associated with cardiovascular crises. If initial abdominal scans are unrevealing, scintigraphy with ^{131}iodine-labeled metaiodobenzylguanidine (MIBG) can help localize the pheochromocytoma.

Treatment

Surgical excision of catecholamine-producing tumors is the definitive treatment. It is imperative that careful preparation be made for this surgery and that an experienced surgeon perform the procedure. Careful attention to anesthesia, cardiovascular hemodynamics, and blood volume are key to decreasing surgical mortality rates. Preoperative medical treatment involves initiating α-blockade with phenoxybenzamine, prazosin, doxazosin, or phentolamine. Patients should be normotensive for 1 week before surgery. β-Adrenergic blockade should be added several days before the operation, particularly if the patient has had arrhythmias. Labetalol, an α-blocker–β-blocker, can be effective despite the rather modest α-blockade achieved in comparison with β-blockade. To avoid precipitous increases in blood pressure, it is important to establish α-blockade before initiating β-blockade. After surgical resection, the tumor recurs in approximately 10% of patients. Catecholamine and metabolite levels should be measured after surgery and then annually to detect recurrence. For inoperable or metastatic tumors, surgical intervention and therapeutic embolization to reduce tumor load and catecholamine production have been considered. Radiation therapy and chemotherapy have also been used. The effects of excess circulating catecholamines can be controlled by α- and β-blocking agents.

PREGNANCY

Pregnancy is associated with many hemodynamic and hormonal changes (see Chapter 14). Vasodilation occurs early, with increased cardiac output, glomerular filtration rate, renal blood flow, and plasma volume. Blood pressure normally decreases, reaching a nadir during the second trimester. Hypertension is one of the most common medical complications of pregnancy. Although a blood pressure greater than 140/90 mm Hg occurs in 10% of patients, even normal blood pressure readings may be abnormal in pregnant women.

Hypertension during pregnancy can be divided into four categories:

- Gestational hypertension
- Chronic hypertension
- Preeclampsia
- Chronic hypertension complicated by preeclampsia

Key points in the pharmacologic treatment of hypertension in pregnancy are shown in Table 5.12.

Gestational Hypertension

Gestational hypertension is a blood pressure greater than 140/90 mm Hg developing during pregnancy or in the first 24 hours postpartum without other signs of preeclampsia or preexisting hypertension. Although gestational, or transient, hypertension resolves within 4 weeks of delivery, it predicts eventual development of essential hypertension.

Chronic Hypertension in Pregnancy

Chronic hypertension is present before pregnancy or is diagnosed before the 20th week of gestation.

Treatment

Management of chronic hypertension includes the following:

- Restricted activity
- Proper diet with a modest restriction in sodium intake
- Home blood pressure monitoring when possible
- Avoidance of alcohol and cigarettes

Preeclampsia

It is important to instruct patients about the warning signs of preeclampsia, such as hand or periorbital edema, headaches, and altered vision. Preeclampsia is an increase in systolic blood pressure of at least 30 mm Hg or an increase in diastolic blood pressure of at least 15 mm Hg from the average of values taken before the 20th week of gestation or b) blood pressure of 140/90 mm Hg occurring after the 20th week if previous readings are unknown. Predisposing factors for preeclampsia include the following:

- Primigravida
- Preeclampsia with previous pregnancy
- Chronic hypertension
- Family history of preeclampsia
- Twins
- Diabetes
- Large hydatiform mole
- Fetal hydrops

The pathophysiology of preeclampsia is thought to stem from uterine hypoperfusion, with resulting endothelial cell dysfunction. Increased angiotensin sensitivity leads to hypertension, decreased glomerular filtration rate, and proteinuria, with subsequent heightened sodium reabsorption and edema. Unlike lower-extremity edema, which is common in normal pregnancies, the edema in preeclampsia tends to be angioneurotic, affecting the periorbital area as well as the extremities. Eclampsia is defined as the development of seizures in a patient with preeclampsia.

Prevention

Attempts to prevent preeclampsia have centered on the use of aspirin, 60 mg/d, to decrease platelet thromboxane activity without affecting vasodilatory prostaglandin production. This therapy has been associated with a decreased rate of preeclampsia but also has a primary side effect of abruptio placenta. The use of aspirin therapy has therefore been reserved for women at high risk for preeclampsia. Calcium supplementation has also been tried with some success, but this treatment is limited because pregnant women have hypercalciuria; the addition of calcium supplements can increase the risk for nephrolithiasis.

Treatment

Management of preeclampsia once it develops is aimed at maternal protection and fetal protection, depending on the duration of the pregnancy. Close communication between the obstetrician and primary caregiver is crucial.

The treatment for preeclampsia is delivery. If delivery is to be delayed because of fetal development, close monitoring is essential; immediate delivery is necessary if fetal or maternal deterioration occurs. Use of intravenous hydralazine, labetalol, or diazoxide can help control blood pressure in the peridelivery period. Intravenous magnesium sulfate has been used to decrease the risk for seizures. Magnesium helps decrease motor activity and causes vasodilation, in part by stimulating prostaglandin synthesis. Calcium-channel blockers have been used successfully during pregnancy; however, their use should be discontinued during magnesium sulfate infusion because of their additive effect on depressing muscle activity and the occasional precipitous hypotension, which has accompanied simultaneous use. Sodium nitroprusside should also be avoided because of the risk for fetal cyanide poisoning.

TREATMENT OF HYPERTENSION

Once hypertension has been diagnosed, treatment must be determined. Lifestyle modification should be initiated for patients with high-normal blood pressure and for those with all stages of hypertension. The general goal of blood pressure reduction is a pressure less than or equal to 140/90 mm Hg. In patients who do not have evidence of target-organ damage, have a systolic blood pressure of 140 to 149 mm Hg, and have a diastolic blood pressure of 90 to 94 mm Hg, some physicians may choose to delay antihypertensive therapy with close (every 3 months) monitoring of blood pressure. In such patients, treatment should be initiated if blood pressure increases or if signs of target-organ damage develop. In patients with isolated systolic hypertension, reduction of systolic blood pressure to less than 160 mm Hg is recommended. In patients with renal insufficiency and hypertension, particularly African-American patients, it has been suggested that sustained reductions in blood pressure below 140/90 mm Hg may actually be more desirable. Diabetic patients, who are particularly prone to vascular disease, should have a blood pressure goal that averages 130/85 mm Hg.

Lifestyle Modification

"Lifestyle modification" is now the term preferred over "nonpharmacologic therapy." Recent emphasis on the treatment of hypertension to decrease cardiovascular morbidity and mortality rates has helped to underscore the primary or adjunctive importance of lifestyle modification. Some patients with high-normal blood pressure or stage I hypertension can be managed exclusively with lifestyle modification. Most persons with stage II to IV hypertension require pharmacologic therapy, but many can gain a "medicine-sparing" effect with properly maintained lifestyle modifications.

Stress can increase blood pressure acutely; thus, techniques such as biofeedback and relaxation therapies would seem appealing. To date, however, no definitive large-scale population study has shown that these techniques prevent or effectively treat hypertension. Although dietary fat intake is not directly linked to blood

Summary of Diagnosis

- Hypertension is diagnosed when systolic blood pressure is ≥140 mm Hg or diastolic pressure is ≥90 mm Hg on three occasions. One occasion of significantly elevated (e.g., >200/120 mm Hg) blood pressure is also diagnostic.
- Once hypertension has been diagnosed, the question of whether the hypertension is primary (essential) or secondary needs to be answered.
- Primary hypertension

  Physical examination very important, including examination of the following:

  Retina for atrioventricular nicking, hemorrhage, exudates, papilledema

  Neck for carotid bruits, thyroid

  Heart for S_4 sounds, murmurs

  Extremities for presence or absence of pulses

  Nervous system for a previous cerebrovascular accident

  Abdomen for bruits

  Kidneys for enlargement

  Aorta for aneurysm

  Laboratory tests include electrolysis, blood urea nitrogen concentration, creatinine levels, hemoglobin concentration, and hematocrit.

  Electrocardiography is used to help diagnose left ventricular hypertrophy, left atrial enlargement, and ischemia.

  Chest radiography is done to determine cardiomegaly.

  - **Isolated systolic hypertension** is important, especially in the elderly. It is an independent risk factor for stroke, and treatment decreases the incidence of fatal and nonfatal stroke.
- **Secondary hypertension** is associated with the following:

  Renovascular hypertension
  Coarctation of the aorta
  Thyroid disease
  Primary hyperaldosteronism
  Cushing's syndrome
  Pheochromocytoma
  Pregnancy

pressure, dyslipidemia poses a major cardiovascular risk. Patients with dyslipidemias not responding to decreased fat intake, such as a heart-healthy diet as recommended by the American Heart Association, should be considered for drug therapy.

Weight Reduction

Increased weight is associated with hypertension, diabetes, heart disease, and dyslipidemias. Blood pressure usually improves early in a weight-loss program, and loss of as little as 10 pounds can improve blood pressure control and enhance the efficacy of antihypertensive agents. Regular physical activity can be beneficial for both preventing and treating hypertension. This activity also enhances weight loss while reducing cardiovascular risk.

Sodium Intake

Epidemiologic studies have demonstrated a correlation between sodium intake and blood pressure; populations that have the highest dietary sodium intake display the highest blood pressures. In clinical trials that limited dietary sodium, modest reductions in blood pressure (reduction in diastolic pressure of 2 to 7 mm Hg) have been observed. Individual patients vary in their salt sensitivity (i.e., higher blood pressure with increased salt intake and lower blood pressure with decreased salt intake), with African-American and elderly patients tending to be the most salt-sensitive. Modest reductions in salt intake (diet with daily sodium intake of 2 g) can control blood pressure in select patients with high-normal blood pressure and those with stage I hypertension. In patients who require antihypertensive medication, pharmacologic therapy supported by modest sodium restriction can result in lower doses or fewer medications.

Potassium Intake

High dietary intake of potassium is associated with lower blood pressure; conversely, hypokalemia is associated with sodium retention and increased blood pressure. Normal serum potassium levels should be maintained in diuretic-treated patients with hypertension. Maintenance in such patients may require potassium supplementation or treatment with potassium-sparing diuretics. In patients with a propensity for hyperkalemia, such as those with renal insufficiency and diabetes, potassium supplementation or increased dietary intake should be closely supervised.

Calcium Intake

Most epidemiologic studies have observed an inverse correlation between calcium intake and blood pressure. However, calcium supplementation has not consistently resulted in improved blood pressure control. Hypertensive persons should maintain the recommended daily calcium allowance of 800 to 1200 mg. Supplementation beyond these amounts may prove useful in salt-sensitive persons with hypertension (e.g., African-American persons); more likely than not, however, supplements merely serve an important adjunctive role in osteoporosis management.

Cessation of Smoking

Cigarette smoking has clearly been established as a risk factor for cardiovascular disease. Continuing to smoke, even with well-controlled blood pressure, limits the benefit otherwise obtained from controlled blood pressure. Smoking cessation groups, counseling, and, for some patients, nicotine patches or gum can facilitate discontinuation of smoking. In addition, transdermal clonidine may lessen the withdrawal symptoms that are associated with nicotine withdrawal while simultaneously effecting a reduction in blood pressure.

Reduction of Alcohol Intake

Excessive alcohol intake can cause acute elevations in blood pressure and cause resistance to antihypertensive therapy. Discontinuation of heavy alcohol intake can also be associated with significant increases in blood pressure. This pressor effect usually reverses a few days after alcohol intake has been reduced. Patients who drink alcohol should be counseled to limit their daily intake to no more than 1 ounce of ethanol, which corresponds to 2 ounces of 100-proof whiskey, 8 ounces of wine, or 24 ounces of beer. Abstinence from alcohol intake by an "unrecognized" alcoholic sometimes results in excessive decreases in blood pressure because the blood pressure elevation that necessitates treatment is no longer supported by the pressor influences of ethanol intake.

Reduction of Caffeine Intake

Caffeine can acutely increase blood pressure and may inadvertently influence therapeutic decisions; thus, blood pressure readings should be measured at least one-half hour after caffeine consumption. Tolerance to this pressor effect develops quickly and, unless other symptoms are attributable to caffeine intake, no specific limitations need to be placed on intake.

Pharmacologic Treatment

Important developments in drug treatment of hypertension have occurred in the past few years. There has been a growing appreciation of the heterogeneous mechanisms underlying the pathophysiology of essential hypertension. It has become apparent that many factors can contribute to the increased blood pressure, including enhanced activity of the sympathetic nervous system, stimulation of the renin-angiotensin-aldosterone axis, variations in the body's handling of sodium, and an alteration in plasma volume. Although it may not be possible to pinpoint the exact cause of hypertension in any one patient, knowledge of the varying causes can help tailor a rational approach to therapy. Each patient has unique reasons for hypertension, but patients can be stratified into treatment groups according to age, race, weight, and comorbid conditions.

The Joint National Committee on the Detection, Evaluation, and Treatment of High Blood Pressure (JNC), sponsored by the National High Blood Pressure Education Program, provides a consensus report on the care of hypertensive patients every 4 years. The fifth report, JNC V, was published in 1993 and has sparked heated debates. The first three reports advocated a stepped-care approach to treatment. It was recommended that after lifestyle modification was initiated, drug therapy should be started with a diuretic or β-blocker; if hypertension was not controlled with these agents, other classes of drugs should be added in a stepwise manner to control blood pressure. The fourth JNC report offered a broader approach, recognizing that varied classes of antihypertensive agents were effective first-step treatment, including the following:

- Diuretics
- β-blockers
- Calcium-channel blockers
- α-blockers
- Central α-agonists
- Vasodilators

This strategy allowed the physician to choose a first-line drug from among any of the classes depending on a patient's characteristics. Some experts considered the fifth JNC report a step backward, whereas others believed that it was a more puristic approach to treatment: the committee emphasized that large-scale trials had proven that diuretics and β-blockers were primarily beneficial in reducing cardiovascular and cerebrovascular morbidity and mortality. The cost differential between diuretics and the newer classes of medications was also stressed. With these points in mind, the JNC V suggested the use of diuretics or β-blockers as first-line therapy unless comorbid conditions indicated the use of other classes of drugs.

Perhaps a less legislated approach would be the recommendation that unless the clinician believes that other classes of drugs can simultaneously either treat comorbid conditions or are better tolerated with the existing problems, diuretics and β-blockers should be used as first-line choices.

Add-on Therapy

The hypotensive effect of nondiuretic antihypertensive agents can set off a series of reflex responses that ultimately attenuate the ability of the agents to decrease blood pressure. It has been suggested that sodium retention is the principal factor that limits the antihypertensive effect of many nondiuretic agents. This phenomena of resistance is manifested clinically by weight gain and a shift in blood pressure toward pretreatment values. In such instances, the addition of a diuretic represents a logical therapeutic step that produces a marked decrease in blood pressure.

In practice, when monotherapy proves insufficient for normalization of blood pressure, combinations of drugs acting at different sites are used. This allows rational therapeutic regimens to be tailored to an individual patient, prevents the intolerable side effects that may be encountered when large doses of a single drug are given, and allows unwanted reflex responses to certain drugs to be counterbalanced. Particularly useful and commonly employed combinations include sympatholytics–diuretics; sympatholytics–vasodilators–diuretics; and either calcium-channel blockers, ACE inhibitors, or angiotensin II inhibitors with diuretics. To decrease side effects, using small doses of two medications is often more advantageous than escalating monotherapy to maximum doses.

Diuretics (Table 5.13)

The actual mechanism by which thiazides decrease blood pressure remains uncertain; however, the initial obligatory sodium and water loss associated with use reduces extracellular fluid volume. This probably activates a series of mechanisms that culminate in a long-term reduction in total peripheral resistance. The immediate effect of diuretics is to cause a renal loss of salt and water. This in turn decreases extracellular volume, reduces cardiac output, and, at least initially, increases total peripheral resistance. Ultimately, however, plasma volume returns to pretreatment values, and the persistence of the antihypertensive effect now results from a reduction in peripheral vascular resistance. The importance of the initial salt and water depletion in the long-term reduction in total peripheral resistance is underscored by the fact that a high-sodium diet can reverse the antihyper-

TABLE 5.13. Clinical Highlights of Diuretics

1. The **mechanism of action** involves an initial obligatory sodium and water loss, with resultant decreased extracellular fluid volume. This culminates in long-term reduction in total peripheral resistance, although plasma volume returns to normal.
2. Because the compensatory response to most other classes of antihypertensive medications involves sodium retention, the addition of a diuretic can lead to improved blood pressure control.
3. The **greatest antihypertensive effects occur at low doses.** At higher doses, there is a profound increase in side effects with only modest increase in efficacy.
4. The greatest clinical **utility as monotherapy** is seen in patients with low or normal renin levels, elderly patients, black patients, and individuals with congestive heart failure.
5. **Thiazides** are more effective antihypertensive agents than loop diuretics, except in patients with a serum creatinine level greater than 2.5 mg/dL.
6. The **primary side effects of thiazide diuretics** are hypokalemia, hypomagnesemia, hyponatremia, hyperuricemia, hypercalcemia, hyperglycemia, hypercholesterolemia, hypertriglyceridemia, sexual dysfunction, and weakness.
7. **Side effects of loop diuretics** (e.g., furosemide) are similar to those of thiazide diuretics, with the exception that loop diuretics cause hypercalciuria.
8. **Potassium-sparing diuretics** (amiloride, spironolactone, triamterene), when used in combination with other diuretics, can help minimize hypokalemia. They may cause hyperkalemia when combined with an angiotensin-converting enzyme inhibitor or potassium supplements.
9. **Spironolactone** can cause gynecomastia, mastodynia, menstrual irregularities, and diminished libido.
10. **Triamterene** can cause renal calculi.

tensive effect of diuretics and by the observation that in patients undergoing hemodialysis (a group unable to develop a natriuresis), diuretics do not decrease blood pressure.

The greatest clinical utility for diuretics as monotherapy can be found in the following groups: patients with low or normal renin levels, elderly patients, African-American patients, and patients with congestive heart failure. It should be remembered that the greatest antihypertensive effect is seen with low doses of diuretics. Higher doses lead to a profound increase in side effects, with only modest additional decrements in blood pressure. For example, hydrochlorothiazide in dosages greater than 25 mg/d has minimal additional effects on blood pressure but continues to increase kaliuresis and thereby increases the incidence and severity of hypokalemia.

β-Blockers (Table 5.14)

The use of β-blockers has been a major therapeutic advancement in clinical medicine. There are two subtypes of β-receptors: β_1 and β_2. The former are located in the heart and brain and, when stimulated, increase cardiac output. The latter are located in smooth muscle and the kidney and, when stimulated, lead to bronchodilation, vasodilation, and an increase in plasma renin activity. Antagonism of either of these receptors can inhibit their unique actions. The exact mechanism by which β-receptor antagonists decrease blood pressure remains unclear. Multiple physiologic actions have been attributed to β-receptor blockade, including a decrease in cardiac output, a putative direct central nervous system action, decreases in plasma renin activity, and an effect on presynaptic β-receptors.

Pharmacologic Differences among Agents The available β-blocking agents differ pharmacologically in ways that provide a framework for predicting their individual effects and side effects. These differences do not completely distinguish the compounds (considerable overlap exists) but rather permit the same overall physiologic outcome without certain undesirable side effects. The pharmacologic characteristics that differentiate the available β-blockers include the following:

- Cardioselectivity
- Lipid solubility
- Duration of action
- Intrinsic sympathomimetic activity

CARDIOSELECTIVITY Cardioselectivity does not imply cardiospecificity because drugs in this group also exhibit dose-dependent β_2-inhibitor activity. When hypertension coexists with asthma, peripheral vascular disease, or insulin-dependent diabetes and when β-blocker therapy is necessary, use of a cardioselective compound (e.g., atenolol, acebutolol, metoprolol) is preferable. Caution must still be exercised with these compounds because very little β_2-blockade is needed to precipitate problems in susceptible patients.

LIPID SOLUBILITY Lipophilicity determines whether a β-blocker crosses the blood–brain barrier. Lipid-soluble drugs are more readily metabolized by the liver and have shorter half-lives. Although the lipid-soluble β-blockers seem to produce a higher incidence of central nervous system side effects, merely switching to a more hydrophilic β-blocker does not ensure relief of central nervous system symptoms.

DURATION OF ACTION The duration of action of the available β-blockers varies widely. Although several of the β-blockers have short half-lives, their durations of action exceed their half-lives by several hours, suggesting that the hypotensive effect of these agents does not correlate with drug levels as much as it does with the duration of pharmacologic β-receptor blockade.

INTRINSIC SYMPATHOMIMETIC ACTIVITY The intrinsic sympathomimetic activity of an agent refers to its partial agonist activity. This property confers many theoretical advantages. For example, pindolol, which has significant intrinsic sympathomimetic activity, decreases blood pressure in a fashion equivalent to that of other β-blockers but with less reduction in cardiac output and heart rate and negligible peripheral vasoconstriction. It has also been suggested that withdrawal reactions associated with β-blockers that have intrinsic sympathomimetic activity are less common and not as severe as those associated with agents that lack intrinsic sympathomimetic activity.

β-Blockers as Monotherapy β-Blockers have been proposed as effective monotherapy for most hypertensive patients. However, the older the population, the less likely it is that blood pressure will be controlled with β-blockers alone. This decreased responsiveness relates to either an age-related decrease in the number of β-receptors or diminished renin levels. Diminished responsiveness to β-blockers has also been reported in African-American populations; this finding may reflect the lower renin levels observed in this group. β-Blockers may induce a state of paradoxical hypertension, resulting from fluid retention and β-adrenergic–mediated peripheral and renal vasoconstriction associated with

TABLE 5.14. Clinical Aspects of β-blockers

1. Agents that block β-adrenergic receptors can be **classified by their pharmacologic characteristics,** which include cardioselectivity, lipid solubility, duration of action, and intrinsic sympathomimetic activity.
2. β-blockers are less effective in older patients and black hypertensive patients.
3. **Cardioselective drugs** (atenolol, metoprolol, betaxolol, and acebutolol) are recommended for use in patients with coexisting asthma, peripheral vascular disease, and insulin-dependent diabetes. Caution must still be exercised: Although these drugs are cardioselective, they are not cardiospecific.
4. β-blockers with **intrinsic sympathomimetic activity** have partial agonist activity. These agents (acebutolol, carvedilol, penbutolol, pindolol) cause smaller decreases in cardiac output, heart rate, and peripheral vasoconstriction.
5. A **paradoxical pressor effect** may occur, particularly in patients with low renin levels. This effect is thought to be caused by fluid retention and α-adrenergic–mediated peripheral and renal vasoconstriction in the presence of β_2-receptor blockade.
6. β-blocker **withdrawal symptoms** can occur in hypertensive patients with coexisting coronary artery disease. These symptoms are associated with suprasensitivity and increased numbers of β-receptors that develop during active treatment. Withdrawal of β-blockade leads to excessive catecholamine response.
7. **Primary side effects** are bronchospasm, aggravation of peripheral arterial insufficiency, fatigue, insomnia, exacerbation of congestive heart failure, masking of symptoms of hypoglycemia, hypertriglyceridemia, and decreased levels of high-density lipoprotein cholesterol (except in the case of drugs with intrinsic sympathomimetic activity).

β_2-receptor blockade in the vascular beds of the respective receptors.

Complications Abrupt withdrawal of β-blockers causes symptoms consistent with sympathetic overactivity. This phenomenon partly relates to the suprasensitivity of β-receptors because β-receptor numbers upregulate in response to long-term β-blockade. Once β-blockade is stopped, the sudden exposure of this increased receptor population to endogenous catecholamines leads to an excessive catecholamine response. This is not as much of a problem in the general hypertensive population as it is in hypertensive patients with coexisting coronary artery disease.

α–β-Blockers (Table 5.15)

Labetalol is an interesting pharmacologic agent, which blocks both α- and β-receptors, thereby averting the paradoxic hypertension occasionally observed in patients taking β-blockers alone. Labetalol blocks postsynaptic α_1-receptors, producing vasodilation, whereas its nonselective β-blockade prevents a reflex increase in heart rate. Interestingly, the reduced antihypertensive response to β-blockers noted in elderly and African-American patients is much less apparent in patients taking labetalol.

Peripheral-Acting Adrenergic Antagonists (Table 5.16)

Reserpine Reserpine belongs to the class of drugs termed rauwolfia alkaloids and has enjoyed a colorful history in the management of both psychotic illness and hypertension. Reserpine is generally effective for hypertension, particularly in combination with a diuretic. A positive feature of this drug is its ease of administration, with once-daily dosing. Reserpine causes marked depletion of catecholamines from their storage granules in peripheral sympathetic neurons, the central nervous system, the heart, and, to a lesser extent, the adrenal medulla. The result is depletion of norepinephrine stores. This depletion of monoamines within the brain accounts for reserpine's sedative and depressant effects; a similar phenomenon within the myocardium decreases cardiac output and, in susceptible patients, can precipitate congestive heart failure.

A small (0.05 to 0.1 mg/d) dosage of reserpine alone has minimal effect on blood pressure; however, the addition of a diuretic to this low dose results in significant lowering of blood pressure and limits the undesirable side effects.

ADVERSE EFFECTS The most common adverse effects of reserpine are nasal congestion and lethargy. Less common than lethargy is true emotional depression, which fortunately is seldom observed with dosages lower than 0.2 mg/d. Because of its ability to increase both the volume and acidity of gastric secretions, reserpine may also exacerbate or even produce ulcers or gastrointestinal hemorrhage. A final issue is the purported link between reserpine and breast cancer in women. Although initial retrospective studies supported the possibility of such an association, more carefully controlled observations have been unable to confirm it.

Guanethidine Guanethidine is a member of a class of agents, the adrenergic neuron blocking drugs, that in-

TABLE 5.15. Clinical Aspects of α–β-Blockers

1. **Mechanism of action. Labetalol** blocks postsynaptic α_1-receptors, causing vasodilation, while its nonselective β-blockade prevents reflex increases in heart rate.
2. Labetalol can be administered orally or intravenously.
3. Because of the dual blockade, labetalol is more effective than β-blockers in black hypertensive patients.
4. Labetalol **may cause postural hypotension;** thus, dosing should be based on standing blood pressures.
5. Side effects are similar to those of both α- and β-receptor blockers.

TABLE 5.16. Clinical Aspects of Peripheral-Acting Adrenergic Antagonists

1. **Mechanism of action.** Guanadrel and guanethidine inhibit catecholamine release from neuronal storage sites. Reserpine causes depletion of tissue stores of catecholamines.
2. Guanadrel and guanethidine can cause diarrhea and orthostatic and exercise hypotension. Reserpine can cause lethargy, nasal congestion, and depression.
3. Reserpine should be avoided in patients with a history of mental depression or with active peptic ulcer disease.

hibit the function of postganglionic sympathetic neurons. Other agents in this class include bethanidine, debrisoquine, and guanadrel. Guanethidine is uniquely targeted for the sympathetic nervous system and produces few, if any, pharmacologic effects unrelated to sympathetic blockade. Guanethidine blocks the release of norepinephrine, which accompanies sympathetic nerve stimulation. After its incorporation into the neuron, guanethidine binds to storage vesicles, where it eventually depletes their granular contents of norepinephrine. Because guanethidine does not cross the blood–brain barrier, there is little if any depletion of central catecholamine content; this explains why the drug has no sedative or depressive effects.

Guanethidine has a steep dose–response relationship: the more of a drug given, the greater the effect. Although supine blood pressure is decreased somewhat by guanethidine, the drug's greatest effect occurs in the upright position. When sympathetic activation is a prerequisite for maintenance of blood pressure (i.e., upright posture), the effects of guanethidine become particularly apparent. The resultant orthostatic hypotension characterizes guanethidine's action and ultimately serves as one of the major limiting factors associated with this drug.

The amount of guanethidine required to decrease standing blood pressure to an acceptable level ranges from 25 to 300 mg/d. Guanethidine need only be given once daily because it has a long elimination half-life; dosage should be increased only after several days. The addition of small doses (10 mg to 20 mg) to a regimen consisting of a diuretic and dietary sodium control may produce a gratifying blood pressure response in patients with mild to moderate hypertension.

DRUG INTERACTIONS Because guanethidine is actively transported to its site of action, agents that compete for transport can limit guanethidine's access to its site of action within adrenergic nerves. Examples of such drugs include the tricyclic antidepressants, chlorpromazine, ephedrine, and phenylpropanolamine. If one of these interacting drugs is added to a successful regimen that includes guanethidine, blood pressure control will be lost within several days. In a similar fashion, if guanethidine is added to a regimen already containing one of these competing agents, a hypotensive response is unlikely. Of additional concern is the fact that amphetamines and amphetamine-like drugs (e.g., ephedrine, phenylpropanolamine) not only block the uptake of guanethidine but also cause the release of the drug already encapsulated within the neuron, resulting in a rapid reversal of guanethidine's effects. The ready availability of ephedrine and phenylpropanolamine in over-the-counter preparations makes this a potentially significant drug–drug interaction.

Centrally Acting α_2-Agonists (Table 5.17)

The centrally acting agents include clonidine, guanfacine, guanabenz, and α-methyldopa. These agents influence central adrenergic mechanisms in such a way that efferent sympathetic outflow is effectively limited by certain agonist properties. When given in low doses, these agents stimulate α_2-receptors within the brainstem vasomotor centers, leading to a decline in sympathetic outflow and, with that, peripheral vasodilation. As the dose is increased, peripheral α_2-receptors are also stimulated; thus, these agents have a narrow therapeutic margin and can promote an actual pressor response.

Clinical Aspects of Centrally Acting α_2-Agonists **TABLE 5.17.**

1. **Mechanism of action.** Centrally acting $\alpha_2$agonists (clonidine, guanabenz, guanfacine, and methyldopa) stimulate central α_2-receptors, which inhibit efferent sympathetic activity.
2. The **primary side effects** are drowsiness, sedation, dry mouth, fatigue, and orthostatic hypotension. The clonidine patch can cause local skin irritation. Methyldopa can cause elevated liver enzyme levels, fever, and Coombs-positive anemia.
3. A **withdrawal syndrome,** characterized by hypertension, anxiety, sweating, and tremors, can occur with the abrupt withdrawal of clonidine, although it is rarely seen with the discontinuation of a clonidine patch. Use of clonidine pills should be avoided in patients with questionable compliance.
4. These medications have a **narrow therapeutic margin** and can provoke a pressor effect with increasing doses as the central agonist action is counterbalanced by increasing stimulation of peripheral α_2-receptors.
5. Clonidine has been used to decrease the symptoms of narcotic or cocaine withdrawal.

Clonidine given in dosages greater than 0.9 mg/d (0.3 mg three times daily) may cause a pressor effect. Because clonidine has partial renal clearance, pressor effects can be seen in patients with renal failure at lower doses.

The hemodynamic and pharmacodynamic properties of these agents are highlighted by a decrease in total peripheral vascular resistance with an accompanying decline in heart rate and cardiac output. Renal blood flow and glomerular filtration rate are preserved, whereas renin secretion diminishes. In many instances, these agents can be successfully used as monotherapy; as with most antihypertensive agents, however, salt and water retention can follow from the decrease in blood pressure. Addition of a diuretic achieves a better response.

Adverse Effects A potentially dangerous adverse effect of clonidine is the withdrawal, or rebound, hypertension that accompanies abrupt discontinuation of clonidine therapy. This withdrawal syndrome is characterized by hyperactivity of the sympathetic nervous system with hypertension, anxiety, sweating, and tremors. Upon discontinuation of therapy, the ensuing withdrawal syndrome results from the surge of sympathetic activity. The dose of oral clonidine should therefore be tapered before therapy is discontinued. Clonidine patches can be removed abruptly, and the residual drug in the skin provides an adequate taper. Particular caution should be exercised in patients receiving high doses of clonidine and in those concurrently receiving a β-blocker. Discontinuation of clonidine therapy while β-blocker therapy is continued may lead to profound unopposed α-mediated vasoconstriction because β-receptors are blocked and prevented from mediating vasodilation.

Discontinuation of α-methyldopa therapy only occasionally results in rebound hypertension.

α-Receptor Blockers (Table 5.18)

α_1-Receptors are vascular postsynaptic receptors that mediate vasoconstriction. Phenoxybenzamine and phentolamine are two classic α-blockers that have achieved widespread use for the diagnosis and management, respectively, of pheochromocytoma. The prominent side effects of these agents hampers their routine use in the management of essential hypertension.

The first α-blocker to be seriously considered as antihypertensive agent for long-term use was the quinazoline derivative prazosin. Prazosin and other drugs of this class, such as terazosin and doxazosin, are modestly effective in decreasing blood pressure. These drugs neither block baroreceptors nor suppress renin and aldosterone release. Thus, once blood pressure has been reduced, both sympathetic activation and plasma volume expansion can be expected. The consequence of these sequelae is an attenuation of any initial antihypertensive effect.

The trend in antihypertensive product development has been toward longer-acting medications. The α-blocker medications clearly show the advantages to this approach. Prazosin is more lipid soluble and has a higher affinity for the α_1-receptor, thereby producing a more rapid and profound decrease in blood pressure than doxazosin or terazosin. With its shorter duration of action, prazosin requires twice-daily dosing, whereas doxazosin and terazosin lead to sustained reduction in blood pressure over 24 hours. Prazosin has the highest rate of orthostatic hypotension and a higher occurrence of a first-dose response with marked hypotension. This occurs particularly in patients receiving a low-sodium diet or diuretic therapy and in those who are simultaneously taking a β-blocker. This phenomenon is also both postural and dose-dependent and has led to the recommendation that therapy with these compounds be started at low doses and be given at bedtime. Although

TABLE 5.18. Clinical Aspects of α-Receptor Blockers

1. **Mechanism of action.** α-receptor blockers (doxazosin, prazosin, and terazosin) block postsynaptic α_1-receptors and cause vasodilatation.
2. α-receptor blockers are effective for the **symptomatic treatment of benign prostatic hypertrophy.**
3. These drugs **may cause postural hypotension,** and titration should be based on standing blood pressures.
4. The first dose should be given at bedtime, particularly in patients receiving diuretics or β-blockers to avoid symptomatic hypotension.
5. Other **side effects** include syncope, weakness, palpitations, and headache.
6. This class of drugs has **a positive effect on lipid metabolism and insulin resistance.**

Clinical Aspects of Direct Vasodilators **TABLE 5.19.**

1. **Mechanism of action.** Hydralazine and minoxidil cause direct, primarily arterial, smooth-muscle vasodilation. Minoxidil is a more potent vasodilator.
2. Hydralazine is subject to phenotypically determined metabolism (acetylation).
3. Both agents cause fluid retention and reflex tachycardia and usually require concomitant treatment with a diuretic and an agent for heart rate control, such as a β-blocker.
4. Both agents can cause headache, tachycardia, and fluid retention. Hydralazine can cause positive results on an antinuclear antibody test, but a lupus syndrome is uncommon at lower doses (<200 mg/d). Minoxidil is associated with hypertrichosis and may aggravate pleural and pericardial effusions.
5. Both agents can worsen angina in patients with coronary artery disease.

doxazosin and terazosin have less prominent orthostatic changes, nighttime dosing can still be of benefit. Because blood pressure control tends to wane near the end of the 24-hour dosing schedule, a secondary reason for nighttime dosing is to help control blood pressure during the normal morning surge.

The α-blockers have also gained favor for the treatment of symptomatic benign prostatic hypertrophy. Normotensive men have few symptomatic decreases in blood pressure. In hypertensive men with benign prostatic hypertrophy, the use of an α-blocker can be of benefit for both problems. A positive effect of α-blockers on lipid metabolism and insulin resistance has also been seen with monotherapy and in combination with a diuretic or β-blocker.

Direct Vasodilators (Table 5.19)

Vasodilator drugs reduce arterial pressure through a direct relaxant effect on vascular smooth muscle. These agents considerably differ from each other in their overall hemodynamic properties because they may act as arteriolar dilators, venodilators, or both. Ultimately, the effects on arterial dilatation make this class of agents a logical treatment option for hypertension because peripheral vasoconstriction is a primary associated defect.

Hydralazine was the first of the arterial dilators to be introduced. Although this drug gained widespread use in the 1960s and 1970s, excessive side effects and blunting of the drug's initial hypotensive effect curtailed its popularity. It was not until a broader perspective was gained on the physiologic control of blood pressure and the importance of compensatory reflex responses that the use of hydralazine was revived.

The vasodilatation of resistance vessels that accompanies the use of hydralazine is accompanied by a series of reflex mechanisms that lessen the initial decrease in blood pressure. As a result of the decrease in blood pressure, a baroreceptor-mediated reflex increase in sympathetic discharge occurs. This, in turn, is accompanied by an increase in heart rate, stroke volume, cardiac output, and myocardial oxygen requirements. In addition, the surge of sympathetic activity and the decrease in blood pressure activate the renin-angiotensin-aldosterone axis, thereby mediating sodium retention in the kidney. An antihypertensive regimen that includes an adrenergic inhibitor and diuretic to complement a vasodilator clearly potentiates any blood pressure decrease achieved from a vasodilator alone.

Adverse Effects Minoxidil, a more potent vasodilator than hydralazine, has been used primarily in patients with stage III and IV hypertension. Either hydralazine or minoxidil may precipitate a series of cardiovascular side effects, including palpitations, angina, marked fluid retention, and headaches. In addition, hydralazine may precipitate a drug-induced lupus syndrome, which is related to both dose and acetylator phenotype. It is most typically seen in patients (many of whom are white and slow acetylators) receiving continuous therapy with dosages exceeding 400 mg/d. A curious side effect of prolonged use of minoxidil is facial and upper-arm hypertrichosis, perhaps related to cutaneous vasodilatation. The topical preparations of minoxidil used for baldness do not significantly affect blood pressure.

Calcium-Channel Blockers (Table 5.20)

Calcium-channel blockers are a pharmacologically heterogeneous group of drugs that inhibit the entry of calcium into vascular smooth muscle. Three subclasses of calcium-channel blockers are available:

- Dihydropyridines (amlodipine, nifedipine, felodipine, isradipine, and nicardipine)
- Benzothiazepines (diltiazem)
- Phenylalkylamines (verapamil)

TABLE 5.20. Clinical Aspects of Calcium-Channel Blockers

1. **Mechanism of action.** Calcium-channel blockers block the inward movement of calcium ions across cell membranes and cause smooth-muscle relaxation.
2. Calcium-channel blockers are a **heterogeneous class of drugs,** with primary differences between **dihydropyridines** (nifedipine, felodipine, isradipine, nicardipine, and amlodipine), **benzothiazepines (diltiazem),** and **phenylalkylamines (verapamil).**
3. There is **little clinical indication for** the use of short-acting **nifedipine.**
4. **Dihydropyridines** primarily cause vasodilation with minimal inotropic effect and, by reflex mechanisms, have a tachycardic response. **Diltiazem** causes an intermediate vasodilation with a negative inotropic and chronotropic effect. **Verapamil** causes the smallest degree of vasodilation but is associated with the most negative inotropic and chronotropic effects.
5. All three groups are **effective treatments for angina.**
6. **Side effects,** such as headache, dizziness, and gingival hyperplasia, are associated with all three groups. Dihydropyridines more commonly cause peripheral edema, flushing, and tachycardia. Verapamil and diltiazem can cause atrioventricular block and bradycardia. Verapamil is associated with constipation.
7. Dihydropyridines should be used with caution in patients with congestive heart failure; the exception is amlodipine, which has been used successfully in these patients.
8. Diltiazem and verapamil have been shown by some studies to be of benefit in decreasing morbidity and mortality after infarction.

Dihydropyridines primarily cause vasodilatation with minimal inotropic effect and, by reflex mechanisms, produce a tachycardic response. Benzothiazepines cause an intermediate vasodilatation with a negative inotropic and chronotropic effect. Phenylalkylamines cause the smallest degree of vasodilatation but are associated with the most negative inotropic and chronotropic effects. Dihydropyridines have clinically significant differences from benzothiazepines and phenylalkylamines.

The calcium-channel blockers generally have dual effects: they decrease both blood pressure and angina. Unlike the other dihydropyridines, amlodipine has been shown to have a positive effect in the treatment of congestive heart failure. Diltiazem and verapamil have shown positive results in patient care after a myocardial infarction. Both of these agents are available in extended-release forms, which can improve compliance and consistency of control.

Adverse Effects Side effects of calcium-channel blockers include headache, dizziness, and gingival hyperplasia. Dihydropyridines are also associated with flushing and tachycardia, although these effects are less common with long-acting formulations. Peripheral edema can occur with any of the drugs but is more common with dihydropyridines. This edema is not the result of fluid retention and therefore is not treated with diuretics; rather, it results from increased hydrostatic pressure in the lower extremities caused by precapillary vasodilatation and reflex postcapillary constriction. Dose can be adjusted or therapy discontinued if edema is clinically significant. Of interest, calcium-channel blockers facilitate natriuresis by improving renal blood flow, diminishing renal tubular sodium reabsorption, and interfering with aldosterone secretion. Clinically, it has been shown that calcium-channel blockers are most effective in salt-replete states. Therefore, sodium restriction is less vital with calcium-channel blockers, and the combination of this class with a diuretic is less beneficial.

Unlike dihydropyridines, diltiazem and verapamil are also associated with atrioventricular block and bradycardia. Constipation is a relatively common side effect of verapamil.

Calcium-channel blockers, particularly the dihydropyridines with the prototype nifedipine, have recently received negative attention with regard to potentially deleterious effects on morbidity and mortality. These studies, which have been widely publicized in the lay press, primarily dealt with the short-acting forms. Longer-acting dihydropyridines, such as Procardia XL (nifedipine) and amlodipine, are not associated with rapid decreases in blood pressure or dramatic hormonal changes, as is the case for short-acting nifedipine. Therefore, the mechanism for the theoretic risk on cardiovascular disease is less apparent. The benefit of calcium-channel blockers to decrease blood pressure has been clearly documented. However, the correlation between the surrogate end point of lowered blood pressure with a calcium-channel blocker therapy and decreased morbidity and mortality has not been proven.

Angiotensin-Converting Enzyme Inhibitors (Table 5.21)

The ACE inhibitors are used with increasing frequency in the management of all stages of hypertension. Unlike direct vasodilators, these agents do not precipitate reflex tachycardia or any meaningful sodium and water retention. The antihypertensive effect of an ACE inhibitor is not solely limited to its ability to interrupt the renin-angiotensin-aldosterone system but also relates to its ability to increase bradykinin levels. The accumulation of bradykinin enhances synthesis of vasodilatory prostaglandins and thereby provides a second mechanism for decreasing blood pressure.

In patients with high renin levels, volume contraction, or both, blood pressure is greatly reduced more often with these agents than with others. Therefore, care should be taken when an ACE inhibitor is added to existing diuretic therapy. The ACE inhibitors in usual doses exhibit only a modest antihypertensive effect in hypertensive patients with low or normal plasma renin activity.

Although African-American hypertensive patients have been believed to respond poorly to ACE inhibitors, recent studies have shown that either increased doses of the ACE inhibitor or usual doses with the addition of a diuretic can provide blood pressure control equivalent to that seen in other populations.

Several of the ACE inhibitors have been marketed in fixed-dose combinations with diuretics. The synergistic effect of combining these two classes of medications has made the inability to independently titrate the doses less of an issue when a fixed-dose combination product is administered.

Therapy with ACE inhibitors has several special uses. First, it has been shown that the use of ACE inhibition in patients with insulin-dependent diabetes and proteinuria helps not only to decrease proteinuria but also to decrease the rate of decline in renal function. The ACE inhibitors have decreased proteinuria in patients with non–insulin-dependent diabetes and in patients with other proteinuric renal diseases; as a result of this effect, reduction in the rate of decline in renal function has been extrapolated. However, the benefit of using ACE inhibition to reduce the rate of renal function decline has not been proven. The use of ACE inhibition has also been shown to be beneficial for reducing morbidity and mortality in patients after myocardial infarction and in patients with congestive heart failure.

A pharmacologic action of ACE inhibition is the decrease in aldosterone biosynthesis. In patients with renal insufficiency and patients with type IV renal tubular acidosis, this can lead to symptomatic hyperkalemia. On the other hand, this property can help attenuate the diuretic-induced hypokalemia in some patients.

Clinical Aspects of Angiotensin-Converting Enzyme Inhibitors **TABLE 5.21.**

1. **Mechanism of action.** ACE inhibitors block the formation of angiotensin II, promoting vasodilation, and reduce the secretion of aldosterone. They also increase levels of bradykinin and vasodilatory prostaglandins.
2. ACE inhibitors **slow the progression of renal insufficiency** in patients with insulin-dependent diabetes and macroalbuminuria (>500 mg/24 hours).
3. ACE inhibitors are beneficial in **decreasing morbidity and mortality** in patients after myocardial infarction and in patients with congestive heart failure.
4. **Excessive hypotension** can occur when an ACE inhibitor is added to their diuretic regimen. When possible, the diuretic dose should be decreased or stopped before initiation of ACE inhibitor therapy.
5. These agents **may cause hyperkalemia** in patients with renal impairment and in those receiving potassium-sparing agents.
6. **Acute renal failure** can occur in patients with bilateral renal artery stenosis or stenosis in the artery to a solitary kidney.
7. **Side effects** include cough, rash, angioneurotic edema (may occur after first dose or after years of therapy), hyperkalemia, dysgeusia, and, rarely, neutropenia.
8. ACE inhibitors are **contraindicated in the second and third trimesters of pregnancy.**

ACE, angiotensin-converting enzyme.

Adverse Effects The major hemodynamic hazard of ACE inhibitors occurs in patients with severe bilateral renal artery stenosis or stenosis of the renal artery to a solitary kidney. Under these circumstances, oliguric acute renal failure can occur even if blood pressure is not substantially reduced. In patients with renal artery stenosis, afferent or preglomerular vasoconstriction leads to a decrease in pressure across the glomerulus and a compensatory increase in efferent vasoconstriction in order to maintain glomerular pressure and glomerular filtration rate. The ACE inhibitors selectively decrease efferent (postglomerular) vascular resistance, causing an abrupt decline in transglomerular pressure and filtration. Patients should have their electrolytes checked within 2 weeks of initiating ACE inhibitor therapy to ensure that hyperkalemia or worsening renal function has not occurred. If renal function worsens, ACE inhibitor therapy should be stopped; renal function usually returns to baseline after discontinuation of therapy. Worsening renal function in a patient receiving an ACE inhibitor should be taken as clinical evidence for significant renal artery stenosis, and this diagnosis should be pursued.

As a class, ACE inhibitors are also associated with the development of angioneurotic edema. Although this condition was initially believed to occur with the first doses, it has now been shown to occur even years after therapy begins. Unfortunately, this relatively rare but potentially life-threatening side effect cannot be predicted. Patients should be warned and given instructions, including discontinuing use and seeking medical care if facial, perioral, or tongue swelling occurs.

Renal failure and skeletal abnormalities have occurred in infants of women taking ACE inhibitors. Deleterious effects occur during the second and third trimesters of pregnancy, after renal development. The effects of ACE inhibition on renal function and continued development results in oligohydraminos, which in turn is thought to contribute to the skeletal abnormalities. Therefore, ACE inhibitors are contraindicated in pregnant women, and young women should be questioned about their plans for pregnancy before therapy begins. If pregnancy occurs, ACE inhibitor therapy should be stopped immediately.

Angiotensin II Receptor Blockers (Table 5.22)

Losartan is the first drug of the angiotensin II receptor blockers, a new class of medications, to reach the market in the United States. Other similar drugs, such as valsartan and irbesartan, are now available. Angiotensin receptors are located in the vascular smooth muscle, adrenal glands, kidneys, myocardium, brain, liver, uterus, and gonads. Angiotensin II is produced by conversion of angiotensin I by ACE and, possibly, non-ACE pathways. Angiotensin II is a potent pressor agent that mediates vasoconstriction in the peripheral vasculature, increases the secretion of aldosterone, and facilitates sympathetic activity. It also is important in angiogenesis and remodeling. Unlike the ACE inhibitors, which block the production of angiotensin II, losartan directly blocks the angiotensin AT_I receptor, thereby blocking the action of angiotensin II. Losartan has no antagonistic effect on the bradykinin system and reactively increases angiotensin II and renin levels. To date, these hormonal changes have not led to clinically significant side effects.

Losartan has a relatively flat dose–response curve, although some patients show increased blood pressure reduction with an increase in the dose from 50 to 100 mg or increasing the dosing to twice daily. The addition of a diuretic does enhance the efficacy of losartan. Adjustment of dosing is not necessary in patients with renal failure, but the dose should be decreased to 25 mg in patients with liver disease.

The primary patient population for angiotensin II receptor blockers is similar to that for whom ACE inhibitors are considered (i.e., diabetic patients and pa-

TABLE 5.22. Clinical Aspects of Angiotensin II Receptor Blockers

1. **Mechanism of action.** These agents work by directly blocking the receptor for angiotensin. Unlike angiotensin converting enzyme inhibitors, they have no effect on the kinin system.
2. There are three drugs in this class: losartan, valsartan, and irbesartan. Several other drugs are expected to be marketed in the next few years.
3. Cough, a problem seen with angiotensin-converting enzyme inhibitors, is not a side effect. These agents are rarely associated with angioneurotic edema.
4. Angiotensin II receptor blockers are **contraindicated in pregnancy.**

tients with congestive heart failure). These agents should be reserved for the treatment of hypertension because formal indications for treatment of other end-organ conditions, such as diabetes and heart failure, are not available. An angiotensin II receptor blocker may be an effective substitute for patients unable to tolerate an ACE inhibitor. Angioneurotic edema is rare in patients receiving an angiotensin blocker. Cross-reactivity in patients who previously developed angioedema with an ACE inhibitor has not been documented, however, caution should be exercised when treatment with an angiotensin II blocker is initiated in this group of patients.

Adverse Effects Unlike ACE inhibitors, losartan is not associated with a cough (coughing develops in 3 to 10% of patients receiving ACE inhibitors). Like ACE inhibitors, losartan should not be used in pregnant women.

LACK OF RESPONSE TO THERAPY

With the variety of antihypertensive agents having different mechanisms of action and side effect profiles, patients with essential hypertension should be able to obtain and maintain controlled blood pressure. When patients do not seem to respond to a medication in a predictable manner, several causes should be considered: nonadherence to therapy, drug-related causes, associated conditions, presence of secondary hypertension, and initiation of compensatory mechanisms. Table 5.23 lists potential causes of apparent drug resistance.

ECONOMICS OF HYPERTENSION

The treatment of stroke, cardiovascular disease, and renal failure costs Americans billions of dollars not only in medical care but also in loss of patient productivity and income. Likewise, the cost of outpatient treatment of hypertension in 1996 was estimated to be $7.5 billion. The goal from an economic standpoint is to use cost-effective medications to decrease blood pressure and risk for cardiovascular morbidity and death, thereby decreasing the cost of treating end-organ disease.

In comparisons of the cost of medications, it is important to assess not only the cost for the actual medication (i.e., the cost for each pill and the number of pills required each day) but also the costs of office visits, extra laboratory tests needed to check for side effects, treatment of side effects, and determination of whether monotherapy is adequate.

Strategies to decrease the cost of medication include using older and usually cheaper medications, such as diuretics, β-blockers, or reserpine. Prescribing a higher-strength tablet and having the patient take half of the tablet at a time may be cost-effective because some of the medications have a fixed cost that is independent of increasing strength of tablets. For patients without payment sources for medications, several drug companies have established programs to supply medication, guarantee stable pricing, or provide vouchers to decrease cost.

Summary of Treatment

- There are few medical conditions that affect as many patients or have as readily available and routinely performed measurement as blood pressure. The goal of therapy is to decrease the morbidity and mortality from end-organ damage; therefore, care should be taken to decrease all modifiable risk factors.
- **Lifestyle modification** is extremely important; the nonpharmacologic therapy may be difficult to achieve. These include the following:
  - Weight reduction
  - Exercise
  - Decrease in salt intake
  - Cessation of cigarette smoking
  - Moderate alcohol consumption
- Pharmacologic therapy includes the following:
  Diuretics and β-blockers, which are the mainstay of therapy
  Add-on therapy:
  - Labetalol, which blocks both α- and β-receptors
  - Reserpine
  - Guanethidine

  Centrally acting adrenergic inhibitors (e.g., clonidine)
  α-Receptor blockers (e.g., prazosin)
  Calcium-channel blockers
  - Short-acting calcium-channel blockers are to be avoided.
  - Long-acting calcium-channel blockers and second-generation calcium-channel blockers are preferred.

  ACE inhibitors
  - ACE inhibitors may be of additional benefit in the presence of congestive heart failure and diabetic neuropathy.
  - ACE inhibitors are dangerous in the presence of renal artery stenosis.
- Angiotensin receptor blockers (e.g., losartan)
  - Losartan does not have the side effect profile of ACE inhibitors.
  - Losartan may be of benefit in patients with congestive heart failure.

TABLE 5.23. Potential Causes of Drug Resistance

Nonadherence to therapy
- Cost of medication
- Inability to understand or remember instructions
- Side effects of the medication
- Inconvenient dosing
- Inadequate patient education

Drug-related causes
- Inadequate doses
- Inappropriate combinations
- Rapid inactivation
- Drug interactions
  - Concomitant medications, including:
    - Nonsteroidal anti-inflammatory drugs, oral contraceptives, sympathomimetics, antidepressants, nasal decongestants, cocaine, cyclosporine, erythropoietin

Associated conditions
- Obesity
- Excessive alcohol intake

Secondary Hypertension
- Renal insufficiency
- Renovascular hypertension
- Pheochromocytoma
- Primary aldosteronism
- Cushing's syndrome

Volume expansion
- Excessive sodium intake
- Inadequate diuretic therapy
- Fluid retention from reduction of blood pressure
- Progressive renal damage

Adapted from The Fifth Report of the Joint National Committee on Detection, Evaluation, and Treatment of High Blood Pressure (JNC V). Arch Intern Med 1993;153:154–183.

HYPERTENSIVE CRISES: EMERGENCIES AND URGENCIES

Hypertensive emergencies are clinical situations that require immediate blood pressure reduction to prevent or limit end-organ damage. These clinical events include the following:

- Hypertensive encephalopathy
- Intracranial hemorrhage
- Acute left ventricular failure
- Dissecting aortic aneurysm
- Preeclampsia
- Unstable angina
- Acute myocardial infarction

Hypertensive urgencies require the reduction of blood pressure gradually over a 24-hour period. Hypertensive urgencies include accelerated or malignant hypertension without severe symptoms, progressive target-organ complications, and severe perioperative hypertension.

Nifedipine had gained popularity as a quick and easy way to decrease blood pressure acutely. However, nifedipine in a non–extended-release formulation is associated with rapid and dramatic increases in catecholamine levels and frequently precipitous decreases in blood pressure. Some reports have suggested that angina and myocardial infarction develop after use in this manner. In actuality, if blood pressure is elevated to the extent that a decrease in pressure is urgent, use of a medication whose dosage cannot be titrated can be counterproductive. Use of intravenous medications, such as labetalol or nitroprusside, permits titration of blood pressure to assure appropriate decreases. In asymptomatic hospitalized patients or in patients seen in clinic with diastolic blood pressure less than 120 mm Hg, the goal is to improve overall control rather than to decrease blood pressure acutely.

It is important to remember that the goal of therapy is to *treat the patient, not the number.* Current regimens should be adjusted, and compliance should be verified. Patients should then be asked to return for repeated blood pressure measurements. If the patient is symptomatic, more aggressive care may be indicated. Oral agents that might decrease blood pressure with less rapid or often unpredictable results are clonidine, captopril, and minoxidil. Table 5.24 lists available drugs and routes of administration.

Drug Management of Hypertensive Crises **TABLE 5.24.**

Drug	Comments
Parenteral vasdilators	
Sodium nitroprusside	Onset of action immediate May cause nausea, vomiting, and muscle twitching May cause thiocyanate intoxication Should not be used in pregnant women
Nitroglycerin	Onset of action, 2–5 minutes May cause headache, tachycardia, vomiting, and flushing
Diazoxide	Onset of action, 1–2 minutes May cause hypotension, tachycardia, aggravation of angina, nausea, vomiting, and hyperglycemia with repeated doses
Hydralazine	Onset of action, 10 minutes with intravenous administration; 20–30 minutes with intramuscular administration May cause tachycardia, headache, vomiting, and aggravation of angina
Enalaprilat	Onset of action, 15–60 minutes May cause renal failure in patients wIth bilateral renal artery stenosis
Parenteral adrenergic inhibitors	
Phentolamine	Onset of action, 1–2 minutes May cause tachycardia, orthostatic hypotension
Labetalol	Onset of action, 5–10 minutes May cause bronchospasm, heart block, and orthostatic hypotension
Oral agents	
Captopril	Onset of action, 15–30 minutes May cause hypotension, renal failure in bilateral renal artery stenosis
Clonidine	Onset of action, 30–60 minutes May cause hypotension, drowsiness, and dry mouth
Labetalol	Onset of action, 30 minutes–2 hours May cause bronchoconstriction, heart block, and orthostatic hypotension
Nifedipine	Onset of action, 15–30 minutes May cause rapid and uncontrolled reduction in blood pressure May precipitate circulatory collapse in patients with aortic stenosis Safer medications are available

Adapted from The Fifth Report of the Joint National Committee on Detection, Evaluation, and Treatment of High Blood Pressure (JNC V). Arch Intern Med 1993;153:154–183.

KEY POINTS

- Patients with hypertension represent a very large and important population for the primary care physician.
- The history, physical examination, and initial laboratory evaluation should be used to exclude secondary, curable forms of hypertension from the diagnosis.
- Treatment decreases the incidence of stroke, renal failure, and nonfatal myocardial infarction. β-Blockers and diuretics have been shown to increase survival.
- The entire primary care team should be recruited to reinforce lifestyle modifications.
- Resistance to therapy is common. The practitioner should look for noncompliance and should always aim for monotherapy.
- It is important to watch the cost of hypertensive drugs, especially that of the newer agents—can the patient afford the drug 365 days of the year?

SUGGESTED READINGS

Braunwald E. Atlas of heart disease: hypertension management and therapy. Philadelphia: Current Medicine, 1994.

Izzo J, Black H. Hypertension primer. Dallas: American Heart Association, 1993.

Greenburg A, ed. Primer on kidney disease. San Diego: Academic Press, 1994.

SHED Cooperative Research Group. Prevention of stroke by antihypertensive drug treatment in older persons with systolic hypertension. JAMA 1991;268:3255.

The Fifth Report of the Joint National Committee on Detection, Evaluation, and Treatment of High Blood Pressure (JNC V). Arch Intern Med 1993;153:149–183.

CHAPTER 6

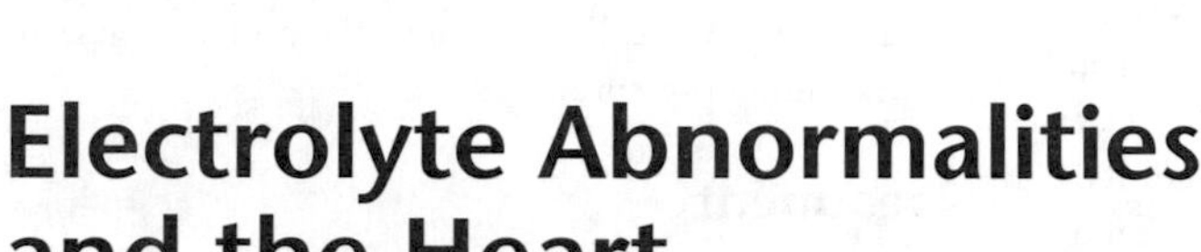

Electrolyte Abnormalities and the Heart

Domenic A. Sica
Elizabeth B. Ripley

INTRODUCTION

Electrolyte disturbances are a frequent occurrence in cardiovascular-renal disease. These disturbances arise either as the result of the underlying disease state (e.g., congestive heart failure [CHF]) or as a consequence of the medications (e.g., diuretics) needed to treat these conditions. The kidney has a central role in the pathogenesis and expression of these abnormalities. The kidney is not the cause but rather responds appropriately to signals from the failing heart or the therapies inevitably needed to treat circulatory congestion. Congestive heart failure is characterized by retention of salt and water; potassium, calcium, or magnesium deficiencies; and diminished glomerular filtration rate and renal blood flow. Electrolyte or volume divergences can indicate the severity of the underlying illness or can themselves further exacerbate the cardiac maladies. This is the case with the decreased cardiac contractility or the fatal arrhythmias associated with hypokalemia.

VOLUME STATUS

Background

Optimizing volume status in patients with cardiovascular-renal disease is vital because doing so maintains adequate tissue perfusion and suppresses congestive symptoms. The importance of a thorough history and physical examination and of comparing the findings to those of previous examinations cannot be overemphasized. In particular, a careful interpretation of changes in total body weight and lean body weight can establish the need for earlier intervention with intensified diuretic therapy before symptoms intervene.

Volume overload causes exacerbated loading conditions in CHF and is best managed by the use of loop or thiazide diuretics. Concomitant dietary sodium restriction is imperative under these circumstances. When sodium intake is not curtailed, unremitting urinary sodium loss in response to diuretic therapy fuels additional urinary loss of potassium, magnesium, or calcium. Despite careful attention to the proper use of diuretics, individual patients may still "escape" control and require hospitalization for more intensive intervention (see the section on diuretics in this chapter).

Symptoms

Individual patients may undergo excessive diuresis and thereby present with signs and symptoms of volume contraction. Volume contraction at its extreme may be marked by hypotension, prerenal azotemia, hyponatremia, and hypokalemia or hyperkalemia. Volume contraction can also present with more subtlety, with lethargy and fatigue out of proportion to the level of heart failure. Volume contraction predictably alters ventricular filling pressures, departing from "optimum" filling pressures for a specific level of myocardial function. As a result of this alteration, cardiac output diminishes; this in turn worsens the symptoms of decreased tissue perfusion. Furthermore, patients who have had a myocardial infarction are frequently "volume contracted" upon presentation and should not be routinely given potent diuretics until the physician assesses central filling pressures.

Treatment

When fluid replacement is warranted in a patient with CHF, purely hypotonic fluids should be avoided. Administering hypotonic fluids to such patients significantly increases the risk for development of dilutional hyponatremia; alternatively, overzealous administration of normal saline may trigger congestive symptoms, sometimes even before the volume deficit has been completely repaired. Regardless of the cause of volume contraction, a mild dilutional acidosis often results from the sudden increase in the bicarbonate space during rapid reexpansion with saline or other fluids that lack bicarbonate or other base. Such an "expansion" acidosis is self-limited and typically requires no therapy. Once a volume deficit has been corrected, subsequent recurrences should be anticipated and steps taken to avoid repeated development. For example, readjustment of the diuretic dose or liberalization of sodium intake may lessen the risk for additional such episodes.

ACID-BASE ABNORMALITIES

Background

Cardiovascular illnesses, especially CHF, rarely disturb acid-base balance. If respiratory acid-base disturbances develop, they are specific to the status of the underlying disease and thus can widely vary.

Respiratory alkalosis can develop in the hypoxic patient with CHF. If the volume overload state and lung compliance are sufficiently abnormal, effective alveolar ventilation may be compromised and respiratory acidosis develops.

Metabolic acidosis is uncommon in CHF unless tissue perfusion is severely limited, at which time lactic acidosis can develop. The major acid-base abnormality in patients with CHF is metabolic alkalosis. Metabolic alkalosis typically derives from diuretic therapy, often has a "contraction alkalosis" component, and is more likely with the ever-present renal dysfunction that is characteristic of advanced CHF. Despite the extracellular fluid volume expansion that is characteristic of CHF, the plasma bicarbonate concentration stays within normal limits despite the total-body increase of bicarbonate levels. With the contraction of extracellular fluid volume, as occurs with diuretic therapy, the remaining bicarbonate has a smaller space to occupy and its concentration increases. This phenomenon contributes to the typical processes by which metabolic alkalosis occurs after diuretic therapy.

Metabolic alkalosis in the range of 30 mEq/L is generally of little consequence in CHF. Higher values can lead to clinically relevant compensatory hypoventilation. The ensuing increase in PCO_2 results in an inverse change in alveolar oxygen concentration, with sometimes telling physiologic consequences in the marginally compensated patient with CHF.

Treatment

The simplest treatment of diuretic-induced metabolic alkalosis involves temporary discontinuation of therapy with the drug. Administration of sodium chloride then allows reexpansion of the extracellular fluid space and dilution of the bicarbonate concentration. Correction of hypokalemia or hypochloremia bolsters the effects of volume expansion and minimizes the renal production of bicarbonate. If diuretic therapy cannot be safely discontinued, metabolic alkalosis may be treated by routine administration of potassium chloride, although the large amounts of potassium chloride required for this form of therapy may prove hazardous in patients with underlying renal insufficiency. Additional approaches may include the administration of potassium-sparing diuretics such as spironolactone or amiloride or, on a temporary basis, the carbonic anhydrase inhibitor acetazolamide.

CARDIOVASCULAR MEDICATIONS ASSOCIATED WITH ELECTROLYTE AND VOLUME ABNORMALITIES

Many medications with a recognized ability to modify electrolyte profiles are commonly used in patients with cardiovascular abnormalities:

- Nonsteroidal anti-inflammatory drugs (NSAIDs)
- Diuretics
- Angiotensin-converting enzyme (ACE) inhibitors
- Angiotensin II receptor antagonists

Nonsteroidal Anti-Inflammatory Drugs

NSAIDs and Hyponatremia

Patients with severe CHF and an activated renin-angiotensin-aldosterone system usually have increased levels of vasodilatory prostaglandins. These increased levels correlate with the severity of hyponatremia. Renally derived prostaglandins help maintain glomerular filtration rate, enhance sodium excretion, and attenuate the action of antidiuretic hormone on renal tubular permeability to water. Altering prostaglandin production with NSAIDs may increase the likelihood of hyponatremia by interfering with each of these adaptive mechanisms.

NSAIDs and Hyperkalemia

The use of NSAIDs increases the risk for hyperkalemia, which is particularly likely to develop in elderly patients with cardiovascular disease. Renin release by the kidney partly depends on the presence of prostaglandins. Because NSAIDs diminish prostaglandin production, they then exaggerate or produce hyporeninemic-hypoaldosteronism. This diminishes the kidney's ability to dispose of potassium loads. This problem is particularly exaggerated in diabetic patients with CHF.

NSAIDs and Glomerular Filtration Rate

The NSAIDs play a pivotal role in CHF because they alter "baseline" glomerular filtration rate. In patients with CHF, glomerular filtration rate depends heavily on an adequate supply of prostaglandins to effectively counterbalance the vasoconstrictor effects of the excess angiotensin II, endothelin, and catecholamines that are characteristically present in CHF. A decrease in prostaglandins, as may occur with a therapy as innocuous as daily aspirin, may disrupt the balance of renal forces in favor of vasoconstriction, with a resultant decline in glomerular filtration rate. This decline can be precipitous, particularly if the patient is absolutely or "relatively" volume-contracted.

NSAIDs with Other Medications

The use of NSAIDs can alter the response to many medications commonly used in CHF. For example, loop diuretic response in CHF is pharmacodynamically impaired when NSAIDs are coadministered. This blunted diuretic response makes volume overload more likely. In addition, NSAID therapy can increase systemic vascular resistance and mean arterial and left ventricular filling pressures, thereby decreasing the cardiac index. This

TABLE 6.1. Urinary Responses to Various Types of Diuretic Therapy

Drug	Diuresis	Potassium	Magnesium	Calcium
Thiazide diuretics	XX	X	XX	–
Loop diuretics	XXX	XX	XX	XX
Combination therapy	XXXX	XXXX	XXX	X
Potassium-sparing diuretics	X	–	–	–

X, relative potency; –, decreased excretion.

altered hemodynamic profile diminishes diuretic response and reduces the blood pressure–lowering response to several antihypertensive medications. In particular, the favorable systemic or renal effects of ACE inhibitors can be blunted by the coadministration of aspirin or NSAIDs. The impact of NSAIDs has increased with the availability of several over-the-counter drugs that permit self-medication without physician supervision. Because many patients with cardiovascular disorders have musculoskeletal symptoms, exposure to such medication is likely to be significant. In addition, patients are often prescribed aspirin because of its antithrombotic action, which may also increase the risk for electrolyte and volume abnormalities in patients with cardiovascular disorders. If NSAID therapy is imperative, the possibility of diminished drug effect (e.g., antihypertensive agents, loop diuretics, and ACE inhibitors) should be entertained and dosage should be modified. As an alternative, NSAID therapy can be temporally distanced from the time at which necessary vasodilator drugs are administered, thereby minimizing the unwanted physiopharmacologic interaction.

Diuretics

Thiazide or loop diuretics are commonly used in such cardiovascular illnesses as hypertension and CHF. Combination diuretic therapy with a loop diuretic and metolazone is typically reserved for the management of diuretic-resistant conditions, whereas potassium-sparing diuretics are frequently used with either loop or thiazide diuretics to conserve urinary potassium and magnesium. Adverse effects of diuretics are a function of properties of their drug classification effect and the magnitude of the ensuing diuretic response (Table 6.1); the diuretic response relates to many pharmacokinetic or pharmacodynamic features (Table 6.2). Whether given orally or administered intravenously, diuretics must reach the tubular lumen to effect a diuretic response. Thus, vital to a diuretic response are selection of a dose that is adequate to achieve a threshold diuretic response and then repeated administration of this dose that is frequent enough to achieve the body weight goal.

TABLE 6.2. Determinants of Diuretic Response

- Pharmacokinetic factors
  - Total amount of drug entering the urine
    - Dose
    - Amount absorbed if given orally
    - Protein binding
    - Renal blood flow
    - Tubular capacity for organic acid secretion
  - Time course of urinary drug delivery
    - Capacity for active secretion
- Pharmacodynamic factors
  - Inherent dose-response relationship
  - Salt intake

Diuretic resistance frequently masquerades as an inappropriate dosage or inappropriate frequency of administration. With the former, careful attention should always be directed toward the absorption of diuretics (e.g., furosemide is poorly and unpredictably absorbed) as an indicator that the dose of diuretics may be inappropriate. In general, reduced gastric emptying in CHF prolongs the phase of drug absorption and reduces peak plasma concentrations, although overall absorption of diuretics is generally not changed. Finally, unrecognized excessive salt intake may result in the perception of a blunted diuretic response; if the true cause is not recognized, diuretic doses may be unnecessarily increased when simple restriction of sodium intake might suffice.

Combination Diuretic Therapy

Combination diuretic therapy is commonly administered for treating advanced CHF. This strategy uses diuretics of different classes to effect sequential nephron blockade and create a synergistic diuretic response. The most common diuretic combination is that of metolazone and furosemide. With this combination, the proximal and distal tubular actions of metolazone are supported by the loop blockade accomplished by furosemide. Although knowledge of the mechanisms of combination therapy is limited, certain practical considerations are important to the proper use of combination therapy:

- Diuretic-diuretic interaction requires the presence of both drugs because neither drug alone can establish the same magnitude of diuresis.
- Metolazone is slowly and erratically absorbed; thus, synchronization of its administration to subsequent loop diuretic treatment is less important than the actual decision to administer metolazone.
- Because of metolazone's poor absorption, the drug's synergism with furosemide may require multiple doses; thus, several hours to days are needed before effects are evident. This lag in response time relates to both the absorptive peculiarities of metolazone and the time required for sufficient drug to have accumulated in plasma to effect adequate tubular delivery of the diuretic under circumstances in which tubular drug delivery is generally compromised.
- Because the half-life of metolazone in patients with CHF is prolonged, therapy with metolazone and the accompanying loop diuretic must be completely discontinued in patients undergoing rapid diuresis. A continuing diuresis should be anticipated over the next several hours to days.
- Upon reinitiation of therapy, the metolazone and furosemide doses can generally be decreased and dose titration reattempted.
- Upon reinitiation of therapy, the final dosing usually requires that metolazone be administered only every second or every third day.

Diuretics in Edema

The edematous patient undergoing active diuresis is at particular risk for the development of electrolyte abnormalities. The risk is linked to the "degree" of volume contraction. For example, hyperuricemia is commonly observed with extracellular fluid volume contraction but rarely requires specific therapy unless a predilection for gout is present. Patients with mild edema reach target weight quickly and thus have a shortened exposure to an aggressive diuretic regimen. In contrast, the more severe edematous conditions require a more protracted diuresis, which creates greater likelihood of significant electrolyte losses. The more prolonged the presentation of sodium to the distal tubule, the more severe the losses of sodium, potassium, and magnesium. This provides a mechanism for the severe electrolyte disturbances that sometimes accompany successful combination therapy.

Urinary Electrolyte Losses

Urinary electrolyte losses with diuretics sometimes have a positive effect. Thiazide diuretics, whether given alone or in conjunction with loop diuretics, diminish urinary calcium excretion and thereby increase serum calcium concentrations. Potassium-sparing diuretics not only limit urinary potassium losses but also restrict urinary magnesium losses. Urinary magnesium losses are of particular importance to the patient with a cardiovascular disorder because magnesium depletion or hypomagnesemia is associated with the sudden death syndrome and other lethal arrhythmias.

Angiotensin-Converting Enzyme Inhibitors

Angiotensin-converting enzyme inhibitors are used frequently in cardiovascular disease, particularly for treating CHF, hypertension, and post–myocardial infarction ventricular remodeling. Because of the underlying pathophysiology of these disease states, treatment with ACE inhibitors can provoke many fundamental renal and electrolyte complications, including hypotension, diminished renal function, and hyperkalemia (Table 6.3). Angiotensin II receptor antagonists produce renal effects similar to those seen with ACE inhibitors, but the exact frequency with which they induce renal complications is unknown.

HYPOTENSION

Pathophysiology

The mechanisms by which ACE inhibitors induce hypotension in advanced CHF are incompletely defined. In addition to the drugs' ability to precipitate a sudden decline in angiotensin II concentrations and a decrease in sympathetic outflow, other potential factors include an increase in vasodilatory prostaglandins and a decline in total peripheral resistance that is disproportionate to the increase in cardiac output. In addition, hypotension is concomitant with a reduction in glomerular filtration rate, which reduces the excretion of most ACE inhibitors and thereby prolongs the hypotensive effect of the drug.

Blood pressure in supine patients commonly declines when an ACE inhibitor is administered (especially if it is coupled with diuretic administration or dietary sodium restriction). Organ blood flow is generally well-maintained unless the hypotensive response is extreme. The incidence of overtly symptomatic hypoten-

TABLE 6.3. Electrolyte and Volume Abnormalities Commonly Seen With Drug Therapy for Cardiovascular Disease

Drug	Magnesium	Sodium	Potassium	Calcium	Glomerular Filtration Rate
Diuretics	Decrease	Decrease	Decrease	Decrease	Decrease
NSAIDs	–	Decrease	Increase	—	Decrease
ACE inhibitors	Increase	Decrease or Increase	Increase	—	Decrease
Angiotensin II receptor antagonist	Increase	Dec/Inc	Increase	—	Decrease
β-blockers	—	—	Increase	—	Decrease

ACE, angiotensin-converting enzyme; NSAIDs, nonsteroidal anti-inflammatory drugs.

sion is relatively low in carefully monitored patients with CHF who are receiving ACE inhibitors.

If volume status is regulated to avoid predictable episodes of volume contraction and if the blood pressure response to selected dosages of ACE inhibitors is periodically reviewed, undesirable decreases in blood pressure can generally be avoided. This phenomenon varies among ACE inhibitors that have different pharmacologic half-lives; it is more conspicuous with long-acting ACE inhibitors.

The risk for hypotension in patients treated with ACE inhibitors is increased by any condition that activates the renin-angiotensin-aldosterone axis. Such is the case for hyponatremic patients with CHF, who are highly prone to develop hypotension when receiving ACE inhibitors. In such patients, the risk for hypotension is reduced, but not eliminated, by beginning ACE inhibitor therapy at low doses. Unless marked, persistent, or symptomatic, hypotension does not absolutely contraindicate further use of an ACE inhibitor. Hypotension observed within the first days of treatment with an ACE inhibitor may be best managed with temporary reduction in dosage. Hypotension occurring after several weeks of treatment generally responds to a liberalization of dietary sodium intake in conjunction with temporary reduction in diuretic dose. If concomitant therapy with vasodilator agents, such as hydralazine or isosorbide dinitrate, is being used, the doses of these agents can be reduced. Although hypotension may be viewed as a relative contraindication to the continued use of an ACE inhibitor, the ACE inhibitor should be cautiously reintroduced as soon as is feasible.

RENAL DYSFUNCTION

Pathophysiology

The renal effects of ACE inhibitors in patients with severe CHF probably derive from variable degrees of inhibition of both the circulating and tissue renin-angiotensin systems. The renal response to an ACE inhibitor depends largely on the preexisting state of renal perfusion. For example, approximately 35% of patients with severe CHF who are given an ACE inhibitor (a circumstance in which renal perfusion is expected to be compromised) experience a decrease in glomerular filtration rate. In turn, the probability of experiencing a decline in glomerular filtration rate is associated with the presence or absence of volume contraction, such as that stemming from excessive diuretic therapy or severely restricted dietary sodium. Patients experiencing the most extreme renal changes (e.g., diabetic patients with autonomic neuropathy) also tend to have a slower heart rate.

In CHF, renal plasma flow or the glomerular filtration rate tends to decrease with the initial doses of an ACE inhibitor. This decrease typically correlates with a decrease in blood pressure. With long-term dosing, renal blood flow may increase and the glomerular filtration rate may remain stable. The latter sometimes declines excessively during long-term ACE inhibitor treatment, particularly if blood pressure decreases below the autoregulatory range or if the patient has significant microvascular renal disease. Three pathophysiologic factors encourage development of renal insufficiency in patients with CHF given an ACE inhibitor:

1. Excessive reduction in renal perfusion pressure
2. Excessive activation of the renin-angiotensin-aldosterone axis
3. Extent of occurrence of efferent arteriolar dilatation

Because decompensated CHF can markedly decrease the glomerular filtration rate, it may be impossible to know whether a patient's renal insufficiency is due to CHF, an ACE inhibitor, or some combination of both. Renal insufficiency in patients with severe CHF who are receiving ACE inhibitors may present suddenly as symptomatic acute renal failure, a phenomenon more likely if the patient is on a salt- restricted diet or has renal artery stenosis. Renal insufficiency can also develop insidiously over weeks to months. Typically, the renal insufficiency induced by ACE inhibitors is neither progressive nor symptomatic and corrects or stabilizes itself despite continued use of the medication.

Treatment

Risk for ACE inhibitor–associated renal insufficiency may be lessened by reducing the dosage of or temporarily discontinuing therapy with coadministered diuretics, liberalizing dietary sodium intake, and carefully titrating the ACE inhibitor dose. Therapy with ACE inhibitors is most innocuous when started in a euvolemic patient. If possible, the clinician should avoid permanent discontinuation of ACE inhibitor therapy in patients experiencing renal insufficiency because these patients often derive the most benefit from ACE inhibitors. Considering the morbidity and mortality of CHF, a moderate increase in the serum creatinine level may be a clinically acceptable tradeoff if the patient has no clinical evidence of uremia. In general, reduction of the ACE inhibitor dosage should be considered in patients in whom serum creatinine levels have not decreased with liberalization of sodium intake or a decrease in diuretic dose.

HYPERKALEMIA

Pathophysiology

By decreasing plasma aldosterone levels and thereby reducing urinary potassium excretion, ACE inhibitor therapy may lead to hyperkalemia. Fortunately, severe hyperkalemia with ACE inhibitors is uncommon; increases in plasma potassium levels are generally fairly modest (approximately 1.0 mEq/L). Patients receiving ACE inhibitors typically also receive diuretics; this combination further lessens the risk for severe hyperkalemia. In fact, ACE inhibitors are likely to offset the hypokalemia that might otherwise accompany diuretic therapy and therefore may spare the need for exogenous administration of potassium.

Treatment

Hyperkalemia with ACE inhibitors is more common when other risk factors for the development of hyperkalemia are present. Diabetic patients with hyperglycemia or persons receiving potassium supplements or potassium-sparing diuretics are particularly prone to the development of hyperkalemia. In these patients, potassium supplements or potassium-sparing agents should be avoided (even if digitalis or loop diuretics are being administered) until potassium balance can be assessed. On the other hand, there are certain patients in whom the combined effects of inadequate potassium intake and ongoing diuresis make cautious potassium supplementation a necessity.

HYPONATREMIA

Pathophysiology

Hyponatremia frequently complicates the clinical course for patients with CHF, especially in its later stages. The hyponatremia of CHF is characterized by total-body sodium and water excess; the excess of water predominates over that of sodium, generating a variant of dilutional hyponatremia. Sodium retention is a primary process in CHF and stems from combined renal and cardiac mechanisms fueled by the neurohumoral abnormalities characteristic of CHF. The decline in renal blood flow and glomerular filtration rate in CHF amplifies this existing overactivity in the renin-angiotensin-aldosterone and sympathetic nervous system axes (Table 6.4). The resultant trend toward sodium retention is ineffectively stemmed by counterbalancing natriuretic forces, such as atrial natriuretic peptide and renal prostaglandins, and sodium retention results. Congestive heart failure may compromise any or all of the requirements for excretion of a dilute urine, a problem only further exacerbated by poor regulation of thirst.

Water retention parallels, but ultimately must exceed, the extent of sodium retention in the hyponatremic patient. Much of the excessive total-body water consists of "obligatory" water absorbed with sodium. Further water gain is coupled with the effects of excessive concentrations of angiotensin II or antidiuretic hormone. Angiotensin II stimulates central thirst mechanisms, promotes release of antidiuretic hormone, and augments proximal tubular reabsorption of sodium and water. The concentrations of antidiuretic hormone are either absolutely or relatively (normal values despite plasma hypo-osmolality) increased in CHF. Inappropriate suppression of antidiuretic hormone release permits intensified distal-nephron water absorption, which uncouples the existing state of water and sodium excess in favor of a predominant water excess (dilutional hyponatremia).

Symptoms

The level of hyponatremia in advanced CHF (sodium level, approximately 125 mEq/L) is not sufficient to

TABLE 6.4. Clinical Implications of Hyponatremia in Congestive Heart Failure

RAA axis activity
  Hyponatremia correlates with activity in the RAA axis
Indication of CHF severity
  Decrease in serum sodium often associated with
    Elevated plasma renin activity and norepinephrine levels
    Regional blood flow derangements and impaired central hemodynamics
    Decreased renal function and diuretic resistance
Prognostication
  Independent determinant of survival
Prediction of pharmacodynamic responses to ACE inhibitors
  Often predicts hypotension and azotemia after ACE inhibitors
  Often predicts dramatic, favorable hemodynamic and clinical responses to ACE inhibitors

ACE, angiotensin-converting enzyme; CHF, congestive heart failure; RAA, renin-angiotensin-aldosterone. Adapted from Leier CV, Dei Cas L, Metra M. Clinical relevance and management of the major electrolyte abnormalities in congestive heart failure: hyponatremia, hypokalemia, and hypomagnesemia. Am Heart J 1994;128:564–574.

cause specific symptoms attributable to plasma hypo-osmolality; rather, the severity of the heart failure syndrome more typically dictates the level of symptoms. In particular, hyponatremic patients are relatively unstable hemodynamically, are prone to hypotension when administered ACE inhibitors, and generally lead a more tenuous existence.

Patients with serum sodium values less than 135 mEq/L have greater activation of their neurohumoral systems and more profound deviations in hepatosplanchnic and renal blood flow. In these patients, renal function is at least mildly abnormal and more susceptible to change if plasma volume or blood pressure decrease acutely. The degree of change in renal function seen under these circumstances is seldom sufficient to produce symptoms; rather, symptoms arise from either impaired elimination of renally cleared drugs that have side effects associated with drug accumulation or from cardiac effects of hyperkalemia. The prognosis for patients with hyponatremia is worse than that for patients with "higher" serum sodium concentrations.

Treatment

Patients with CHF and hyponatremia are more sensitive to the hypotensive and azotemic effects of ACE inhibitors. These patients are typically more debilitated and rely heavily on the markedly activated renin-angiotensin-aldosterone axis for the support of systemic blood pressure. Hyponatremia has proven to be one of the clinical situations in CHF wherein ACE inhibitor therapy should be initiated cautiously at low doses in order to prevent a decrease in blood pressure. If blood pressure declines excessively, renal function also tends to deteriorate and hyperkalemia becomes more likely. On the other hand, hyponatremic patients with CHF often exhibit the most dramatic clinical response to ACE inhibitors. Serum sodium values often substantially improve when such patients are given ACE inhibitors and return to normal when therapy with a loop diuretic is initiated.

Dilutional hyponatremia from hyperglycemia or overdiuresis with replacement of fluid losses by more hypotonic fluids as a cause of hyponatremia can be ascertained by a careful history and physical examination and review of laboratory studies. Overdiuresis is somewhat more common in the beginning stages of heart failure treatment, particularly if thiazide diuretics are being used. Thiazide diuretics work in the cortical portion of the kidney and fail to alter urinary concentrating ability compared with loop diuretics. This characteristic permits maximal water conservation with thiazide diuretics and thereby increases risk for dilutional hyponatremia. Patients can be treated with water restriction, discontinuation of therapy with or decreases in the dose of diuretic, or conversion to a loop diuretic.

Most patients with hyponatremia and CHF are classified as functional class III or IV and have significant volume overload. If feasible, diuretic therapy should be temporarily discontinued in such patients and fluid intake restricted to less than 1000 mL/d. However, this conservative form of therapy is rarely successful. If it fails, fluid restriction can be continued and loop diuretic therapy intensified, with care taken to avoid prerenal azotemia. Use of NSAIDs should be temporarily discontinued because these drugs may modify the ability to eliminate an ingested water load or may exaggerate the already-present decrease in glomerular filtration rate. The efficacy of measures designed to inhibit the release or action of vasopressin is unproven. Diuretic therapy and fluid restriction may still prove inadequate for the normalization of serum sodium levels, often because of the development of prerenal azotemia. If this condition develops, inotropic support (e.g., dobutamine or milrinone) is warranted.

Administration of hypertonic saline to edematous hyponatremic patients can be dangerous and ultimately counterproductive, posing the risk for increasing the state of congestion. This maneuver should be reserved for life-threatening hyponatremia. The patient with hyponatremic edema is best managed by hemodialysis or hemofiltration; either method quickly and safely corrects severe hyponatremia. Similarly, ACE inhibitors provide a form of inotropic support by diminishing afterload and thereby improving cardiac output. This approach is a cornerstone of therapy for hyponatremia, and regimens that include an ACE inhibitor have repeatedly corrected dilutional hyponatremia. If hyponatremia ranges from sodium levels of 130 to 135 mEq/L, merely increasing the dose is often adequate to normalize the serum sodium level; however, fluid restriction and provision of loop diuretics will accelerate the recovery process. Hyponatremic patients are particularly susceptible to the hypotensive and azotemic effects of ACE inhibitors. Therapy with these drugs must be initiated at low doses and slowly titrated upward while systemic hemodynamics is preserved (systolic blood pressure > 80 mm Hg). Diuretic therapy should be tempered as the ACE inhibitor dose is being titrated upward. If congestive symptoms dictate, diuretic treatment should be administered early in the process of upward titration of an ACE inhibitor dose; otherwise, loop diuretic therapy should be withheld or kept at a low dose until a near-maximal ACE inhibitor dose has been reached. The loop diuretic can then be adjusted to an optimally effective oral dose. The addition of a loop diuretic to the treatment regimen is often the final step necessary for the normalization of the serum sodium level (Table 6.5).

HYPOKALEMIA

Pathophysiology

Congestive heart failure provides an optimal milieu for the development of hypokalemia and a pathophysiolgic environment conducive to detrimental consequences. Many potential mechanisms exist for the development of hypokalemia in CHF. These mechanisms can be separated into external deficits, which occur primarily through urinary losses, and internal translocation, which is a function of transcellular shifts mediated by β_2-agonism, hyperglycemia, or acid-base changes (Table 6.6).

The most important of these causative mechanisms is evoked by a summed activation of the renin-angiotensin-aldosterone axis and the ensuing expected increase in plasma aldosterone levels. This axis is variably activated in the pretreatment phases of CHF and is further stimulated by the volume-depleting properties of diuretics. Once this axis is aroused, increased quantities of circulating aldosterone promote tubular sodium-potassium exchange; this, in turn, causes increased uri-

TABLE 6.5. Management of Hyponatremia in Congestive Heart Failure

Exclude redistributional hyponatremia from hyperglycemia
Exclude overdiuresis with hypotonic fluid replacement as cause; temporarily discontinue diuretic therapy or decrease dose
Hyponatremia in decompensated congestive heart failure
- Limit oral or intravenous intake of hypotonic fluid
- Discontinue therapy with thiazide or potassium-sparing diuretics
- Substitute or initiate intravenous loop-diuretic therapy in symptomatic and volume-overloaded patients
- Determine need for temporary inotropic support in severely decompensated patients
- Begin low doses of ACE inhibitors and cautiously increase the dose
- While optimizing the dosing schedule of ACE inhibitors, initiate or establish a loop diuretic maintenance dose

ACE, angiotensin-converting enzyme. Adapted from Leier CV, Dei Cas L, Metra M. Clinical relevance and management of the major electrolyte abnormalities in congestive heart failure: hyponatremia, hypokalemia, and hypomagnesemia. Am Heart J 1994;128:564–574.

TABLE 6.6. Mechanisms Causing Hypokalemia in Congestive Heart Failure

External deficit
- Activation of the RAA axis with increased tubular exchange of sodium for potassium
- Diuretics
  - Increased distal tubular delivery of sodium
  - Further activation of the RAA axis by diuretic-induced volume depletion
  - Metabolic alkalosis
- Diminished dietary intake
- Magnesium depletion

Internal translocation
- Systemic alkalosis
- Hyperglycemia
- β_2-agonism from endogenous catecholamines

RAA, renin-angiotensin-aldosterone.

nary potassium loss. Magnesium deficiency, which is common in either untreated or diuretic-treated CHF, can also increase the chances of developing hypokalemia. Adequate magnesium stores are necessary for the renal conservation of potassium; accordingly, refractory hypokalemia in a patient with CHF (that is, >60 mEq of potassium chloride every 24 hours) should prompt immediate consideration of magnesium depletion. Dietary potassium intake is sometimes insufficient for maintenance of potassium balance but rarely is an independent cause of hypokalemia.

Although much of the hypokalemia in CHF can be attributed to external renal losses of potassium, this is not the only factor influencing serum potassium concentration. The risks attendant with external potassium losses are further compounded by periodic transcellular shifts of potassium, which can occur in response to varied stimuli. Thus, β_2-agonism, insulin or glucose, and alkalemia can trigger the inward migration of potassium against its concentration gradient. Transcellular shifts are particularly important with β_2-agonism: Elevated basal levels of catecholamines, accompanying superimposed "stress states" (i.e., pain, myocardial infarction, and pulmonary edema), may initiate a process whereby a decrease in potassium levels of approximately 1.0 to 1.5 mEq/L occurs. This change is evanescent and resolves within hours once the stimulus (e.g., catecholamine excess) has subsided.

Neglect of several aspects of the measurement of potassium can conceal clinically relevant hypokalemia. The process of blood clotting releases potassium from platelets and erythrocytes; as a result, plasma potassium values are slightly lower (approximately 0.2 to 0.4 mEq) and less variable than serum potassium values. Hemolysis spuriously increases potassium values, whereas prolonged and repetitive fist-clenching can markedly elevate serum potassium levels. Finally, diuretic-associated hypokalemia has a circadian pattern: Potassium values are lower (approximately 0.5 mEq/L) in the evening.

Hypokalemia and Congestive Heart Failure

At some stage of their disease, patients with CHF inevitably develop total-body potassium depletion or hypokalemia, an association in contradistinction to the much weaker association between thiazide treatment and potassium depletion in essential hypertension. For the purpose of treating hypokalemia, the correlation between serum potassium and total-body potassium depletion is limited and offers only relative guidance as to the amount of supplemental potassium that should be provided. Despite the fickle nature of this relationship, almost all patients with CHF should receive some form of potassium replacement, either hypokalemia treatment or as presumptive therapy for losses that should be anticipated as a consequence of diuretic therapy. Replacement can occur by dietary supplementation, the administration of potassium chloride or potassium-sparing diuretics, or ACE inhibitor therapy.

Hypokalemia represents a significant risk factor for sudden death or serious arrhythmias. The association of sudden death with thiazide diuretic treatment in hypertensive patients without evidence of heart disease is questionable.

Hypokalemia and Acute Myocardial Infarction

In the setting of acute myocardial infarction, the association of fatal ventricular arrhythmias with hypokalemia is widely accepted. In such patients, the incidence of ventricular tachycardia or ventricular fibrillation is clearly greater when the serum potassium value is less than 3.5 mEq/L. The incidence increases as the degree of hypokalemia becomes more pronounced. Under these circumstances, the hypokalemia observed after myocardial infarction is probably caused by high circulating levels of catecholamines. The ventricular fibrillation observed under these conditions could be triggered by hypokalemia, high epinephrine levels, or the extent of the myocardial infarction; in this setting, hypokalemia is an epiphenomenon.

Hypokalemia and Arrhythmia

Congestive heart failure is characterized by a significantly arrhythmogenic environment. In addition, the inherent arrhythmogenic qualities of long-term drug therapies for CHF (such as digitalis or antiarrhythmic agents known to prolong the Q-T interval) may be intensified in the presence of hypokalemia. A prolonged Q-T interval is associated with a tendency to develop polymorphic ventricular tachycardia; this propensity is exaggerated by diuretic-induced hypokalemia. The role of electrolyte disturbances in the genesis of torsade de pointes is clearly demonstrated in the case of sotalol. When given alone, sotalol lengthens the Q-T interval without usually causing Q-T dispersion (a factor that increases the risk for torsade de pointes). Syncope developed in a series of 13 patients taking sotalol, all of whom had a prolonged Q-T interval. Twelve of the 13 patients had been treated with diuretics and had low serum potassium values. The prudent therapeutic choice under any of these circumstances is to bring the serum potassium level into the 4.0 to 5.0 mEq/L range. Effective management of potassium abnormalities with properly targeted serum potassium concentrations and with eventual repletion of body stores is probably the most effective and safe antiarrhythmic intervention available.

Other Mechanisms of Hypokalemia

Severe or long-standing hypokalemia may exacerbate CHF by several proposed mechanisms, including defects in contractility of cardiac or skeletal muscle, a predisposition to vasoconstriction, and an acceleration of myocardial pathologic processes. Potassium also has direct tubular and glomerular effects to promote natriuresis; hypokalemia is a recognized source of sodium retention. Chronic hypokalemia has been associated with reversible changes in the glomerular filtration rate and with fixed structural changes paralleled by irreversible declines in the glomerular filtration rate (Table 6.7).

Treatment

The principles of treatment for hypokalemia are well-established. Eliminating the cause of potassium loss is often sufficient to permit dietary potassium to repair the potassium deficit. Unfortunately, this option is infrequently available in patients with CHF. In almost all patients with CHF who have reasonably good renal function, intervention should be directed toward maintaining serum potassium values between 4.0 and 5.0 mEq/L. The widespread practice of urging patients to ingest a high-potassium diet to prevent potassium depletion has not proven effective. Although bananas and oranges are enriched with potassium, their salt form of potassium (e.g., potassium citrate) is "nonchloride" and

TABLE 6.7. Clinical Issues and Relevance of Hypokalemia and Whole-Body Potassium Depletion in Congestive Heart Failure

Patients with congestive heart failure, elevated renin levels, and good renal function or those receiving diuretics have whole-body depletion of potassium (regardless of serum potassium levels)
Hypokalemia implicates whole-body potassium depletion; otherwise, serum potassium levels relate poorly to total-body potassium content
Hypomagnesemia often coexists with hypokalemia
Hypokalemia is arrhythmogenic and increases arrhythmogenicity of digitalis and medications that prolong the Q-T interval
Risk factor present for morbidity and mortality as relates to sudden death
May adversely influence vascular, renal, myocardial, and skeletal muscle function

Adapted from Leier CV, Dei Cas L, Metra M. Clinical relevance and management of the major electrolyte abnormalities in congestive heart failure: hyponatremia, hypokalemia, and hypomagnesemia. Am Heart J 1994;128:564–574.

therefore suboptimal for the correction process. Thus, therapy with potassium preparations that do not contain chloride (e.g., potassium acetate, potassium citrate, or potassium gluconate) will not correct metabolic alkalosis or the associated potassium deficit unless some independent source of chloride has been provided.

In patients with acute hypokalemia, serious dysrhythmias, or digitalis toxicity, potassium therapy is best achieved by the intravenous administration of potassium chloride. The rate of intravenous potassium administration should rarely exceed 20 mEq/h, unless the arrhythmias are life-threatening.

Refractory hypokalemia often requires simultaneous treatment with magnesium. Thus, the inclusion of an oral magnesium preparation in the treatment of any patient with CHF who has hypokalemia attributable to diuretic therapy is considered reasonable therapy.

Therapy with ACE inhibitors is the mainstay of long-term treatment, not only for the major clinical, hemodynamic, and hormonal derangements of CHF but also for restoration of electrolyte, potassium, and magnesium balance. Most patients with CHF, however, also require long-term oral potassium chloride supplementation or a potassium-sparing diuretic agent for optimization of serum potassium values. The aldosterone antagonist spironolactone may be particularly useful in this regard. However, its prolonged half-life increases the risk for developing hyperkalemia.

Hyperkalemia is an outcome of excessive potassium replacement with or without potassium-sparing diuretics or ACE inhibitors. Patients with renal dysfunction should receive potassium supplementation or potassium-sparing agents only under close laboratory and clinical surveillance. In patients with CHF and renal insufficiency who are receiving long-term ACE inhibitor therapy, the impact of potassium supplementation or potassium-sparing diuretics on serum potassium values must be followed even more carefully. Administration of supplementation or diuretics must be discontinued as soon as serum potassium levels arrive at the upper end of the optimal maintenance range.

In the authors' experience, the development of life-threatening hyperkalemia almost always involves an underappreciation of a patient's "real" level of renal function in conjunction with excessive use of supplemental potassium and potassium-sparing diuretics. Hyperkalemia can develop fairly quickly if ACE inhibitors have also caused acute or subacute renal dysfunction.

HYPOMAGNESEMIA

Pathophysiology

Magnesium is a ubiquitous divalent cation that strongly influences cardiac membrane function and is an important catalyst of many myocyte enzymatic reactions. Unfortunately, the presence or role of hypomagnesemia in cardiovascular disease remains somewhat controversial. Much of the uncertainty surrounding the importance of hypomagnesemia relates to the paucity of carefully conducted and well-controlled clinical investigations on its cardiovascular effects. Nonetheless, certain cardiovascular illnesses, such as CHF, are characterized by the development of whole-body magnesium deficiency, regardless of the serum magnesium value.

Several mechanisms contribute to the magnesium abnormalities found in CHF, the most important of which are the following:

- Exaggerated activity of the renin-angiotensin-aldosterone axis
- Diuretic therapy
- β_2-adrenergic stimulation (Table 6.8).

TABLE 6.8. Factors Promoting Hypomagnesemia in Congestive Heart Failure

Activation of the renin-angiotensin-aldosterone axis
Increased sodium delivery to distal nephron segments consequent to loop diuretic therapy
Combination diuretic therapy
Acid-base abnormalities
Metabolic alkalosis
Inadequate dietary intake and relative malabsorption
Long-term digitalis therapy
Transcellular shifts
Epinephrine-related β_2-agonism prompting transcellular shifts
Insulin effect

The latter effects a transcellular shift of magnesium and is nullified by nonselective β-blockade.

Diagnosis

Regardless of cause, the diagnosis of hypomagnesemia remains difficult because of a limited correlation between total-body magnesium deficits and measured plasma values. The measurement of intracellular magnesium (e.g., in lymphocytes, myocardium, or skeletal muscle) is not practical. In many instances, the presence of total-body magnesium deficiency is masked by a "normal" serum magnesium level. An additional clue to the presence of magnesium deficiency is the presence of hypocalcemia of unknown origin. Magnesium has a permissive effect on the release and action of parathyroid hormone release and, when deficient, precludes the body's normal corrective actions for "hypocalcemic circumstances" (e.g., hypercalciuria induced by loop diuretics). Accordingly, the presumption of magnesium deficiency is sufficient to dictate treatment. If a firm diagnosis of magnesium deficiency is desired, a magnesium retention test can be done. This test can be dangerous in patients with overt renal insufficiency and should not be done in patients whose magnesium deficiency is a consequence of primary renal magnesium wasting.

Symptoms

Many symptoms occur with hypomagnesemia; these can be confused with either the symptoms of CHF or medication effects. Symptoms include confusion and mental status changes, muscular weakness, and refractory hypokalemia or hypocalcemia. Several rhythm and conduction system abnormalities can occur with hypomagnesemia, including prolongation of the P-R interval, QRS complex, and Q-T interval; premature ventricular contractions; complex ventricular ectopy; atrial fibrillation; or torsade de pointes. Magnesium may have a limited influence on ventricular arrhythmias caused by reentrant mechanisms and may suppress ventricular arrhythmias that result from enhanced automaticity or triggered activity.

Hypomagnesemia can also heighten the proarrhythmic effect of antiarrhythmic medications. Digitalis-related arrhythmias are also seen more frequently in the presence of magnesium depletion. In addition, diuretic-induced hypomagnesemia and simple dietary deficiency of magnesium have been implicated in the sudden death syndrome. This association may have far-reaching implications because sudden death continues to be a major cause of cardiovascular death in the United States, accounting for more than 300,000 deaths annually.

Treatment

Treatment with magnesium in patients with CHF or myocardial infarction is not exclusively predicated on "normalization" of a low serum magnesium value; merely administering and increasing extracellular magnesium concentrations may favorably dispose the heart to fewer arrhythmias. Magnesium has several physiologic effects that could contribute to its antiarrhythmic effect, independent of the specific serum value at the start of treatment. These effects include positive influences on potassium homeostasis, coronary tone, ventricular afterload, and catecholamine release.

The mode of magnesium administration may cause different outcomes. For example, the positive effect of intravenous magnesium given after myocardial infarction can be ascribed to the development of a transient hypermagnesemia that corrects the hypomagenesemic state. Oral magnesium supplementation is more unpredictable in its absorption and subsequent retention and may not always result in a clearly detectable positive cardiovascular outcome.

Treatment of overt hypomagnesemia requires a magnesium dose of 1.0 to 1.5 mEq/kg of body weight. Typically, approximately 50 mEq is given in the first 24 hours; the rest of the dose is administered over the next 48 to 72 hours. Severe deficits are best treated intravenously because oral magnesium replacement often triggers osmotic diarrhea. This effect reflects the total osmotic load rather than the specific chemical nature of the accompanying anion. Although magnesium oxide is the preferred oral agent because of its better absorption, it too can provoke a diarrheal state in susceptible patients (Table 6.9).

Many replacement alternatives exist in the form of magnesium-containing antacids or other magnesium salts; unfortunately, the magnesium in these preparations is unpredictably absorbed. Whenever supplemental magnesium is provided, the salt form of the preparation should be considered because different milliequivalent amounts of magnesium are present in each. Ongoing magnesium losses should be considered in the course of replacement therapy (gastrointestinal magnesium losses associated with diarrhea or urinary magnesium losses from diuretic treatment). With regard to urinary magnesium losses, the potassium-sparing diuretics triamterene, spironolactone, and amiloride are also magnesium-sparing; thus, they can be considered as effective adjunctive therapy in patients with CHF who are receiving loop diuretics and are otherwise not prone to the development of hyperkalemia (Table 6.10).

TABLE 6.9. **Clinical Issues and Relevance of Hypomagnesemia and Whole-Body Magnesium Depletion in Congestive Heart Failure**

Serum levels poorly correlate with total body stores
Depletion occurs most typically in patients with class III or IV congestive heart failure undergoing aggressive diuretic therapy; postoperatively or in critically ill patients, and after cardiac transplantation
Implicated in the pathogenesis of hypertension, atherogenesis, and variant angina
Frequently accompanies and contributes to refractory hypokalemia or hypocalcemia
Heightened risk for arrhythmia
Probably increases risk for morbidity and death in certain disorders (e.g., digitalis toxicity, long Q-T interval, acute myocardial infarction, postoperative setting, critical illness)
Possibly contributes to widespread cellular dysfunction, impaired vasodilation, myocardial hypocontractility, and other derangements

Adapted from Leier CV, Dei Cas L, Metra M. Clinical relevance and management of the major electrolyte abnormalities in congestive heart failure: hyponatremia, hypokalemia, and hypomagnesemia. Am Heart J 1994;128:564–574.

TABLE 6.10. **Clinical Considerations and Indications for Magnesium Administration in Congestive Heart Failure**

- Acute intervention, intravenous administration
  - Threatening ventricular dysrhythmias in CHF with
    - Hypomagnesemia
    - Hypokalemia
    - Chronic decompensation with anticipated aggressive diuretic therapy
    - Digitalis toxicity
    - Long Q-T interval
    - Suspected whole-body magnesium depletion in presence of normal serum magnesium concentration
  - Problematic atrial dysrhythmias
    - Multifocal atrial tachycardia
    - Uncontrollable atrial fibrillation or flutter
- Long-term maintenance, oral adminstration
  - CHF with uncomplicated
    - Hypomagnesemia
    - Resistant or refractory hypokalemia or hypocalcemia
  - Class III and IV CHF requiring long-term, moderate- to high-dose loop diuretic treatment with or without thiazides

CHF, congestive heart failure. Adapted from Leier CV, Dei Cas L, Metra M. Clinical relevance and management of the major electrolyte abnormalities in congestive heart failure: hyponatremia, hypokalemia, and hypomagnesemia. Am Heart J 1994;128:564–574.

HYPERMAGNESEMIA

Pathophysiology

Hypermagnesemia generally results from an excessive intake of magnesium or overzealous replacement of presumed losses in the presence of advanced functional renal failure, as may be seen in class III and IV CHF. Excess oral intake is generally a consequence of the inappropriate use of magnesium supplements, magnesium-containing antacids, or cathartic agents.

Symptoms

The symptoms of hypermagnesemia sequentially occur as serum magnesium values increase. Neuromuscular effects dominate early, and deep tendon reflexes disappear at magnesium concentrations of approximately 4 mEq/L. Between values of 5 and 10 mEq/L, cardiac and, ultimately, respiratory function change; these changes include prolongation of the Q-T interval, arrhythmias, and diminished cardiac contractility. This last change, in conjunction with cutaneous vasodilation,

Summary of Diagnosis

- Electrolyte abnormalities must be sought by the company they keep: heart failure, diuretic therapy, intravenous fluid administration.
- Optimize fluid volume; the volume overload of CHF requires both diuretic therapy and sodium restriction.
- Diagnosis is made by physical examination (signs are rales, ascites, liver enlargement, peripheral edema, pleural effusions on chest radiograph).
- Watch for volume contraction: hypotension, prerenal azotemia (ratio of blood urea nitrogen to creatinine > 20:1), hyponatremia, and hypokalemia.
- Metabolic alkalosis (contraction alkalosis) is commonly seen in patients with CHF receiving diuretic therapy. HCO_3, > 30 mEq/L.
- Search carefully for the pharmacologic cause, such as NSAIDs (increased blood urea nitrogen, creatinine, and potassium levels) and diuretics. Note that both thiazides and loop diuretics "waste" potassium, magnesium, and calcium. Combination therapy consists of furosemide and metolazone; this is very effective but can produce marked loss of potassium, magnesium, and calcium; hyperuricemia; and clinical gout. Commonly seen in patients with CHF being treated with diuretics. An ACE inhibitor can produce hypotension, diminished renal function, and hyperkalemia. Ensure adequate volume (sodium level > 134 mEq/L and pressure (systolic blood pressure > 90 mm Hg) before the initiation of therapy. Start at low dose and titrate up.

may result in a life-threatening state of refractory hypotension.

Treatment

Treatment of hypermagnesemia entails increasing urinary losses of magnesium by inducing a natriuresis because magnesium losses can be expected to parallel urinary sodium excretion. Volume contraction indicates increased proximal tubular reabsorption of magnesium; thus, magnesuria is most readily achieved by saline-induced volume expansion, with or without loop diuretic therapy. A patient who ingests a massive overdose of magnesium in the presence of advanced renal insufficiency is best managed by hemodialysis that uses a magnesium-free dialysate. Preliminary management of such patients should include intravenous calcium (calcium gluconate, 1 g every 2 to 3 minutes) because calcium physiologically antagonizes the membrane-depressant effects of hypermagnesemia.

KEY POINTS

Hyponatremia (Sodium level < 125 mEq/L)

- Commonly seen in patients with CHF.
- Cause: Increase in total-body sodium level and water; water level is higher than sodium level.
- Symptoms: Proclivity for hypotension, renal function abnormalities, sensitivity to ACE inhibitors.
- Treatment: Look for excessive thiazide diuresis, restrict fluids, and switch to a loop diuretic. Discontinue NSAID therapy. Do *not* administer hypertonic saline. Add or increase the ACE inhibitor dose.

Hypokalemia (Potassium level < 3.5 mEq/L)

- Cause: Overdiuresis, activation of the renin-angiotensin-aldosterone axis. Depletion of magnesium.
- Symptoms: Risk factor for sudden death and ventricular dysrhythmias. Aggravated by concomitant digoxin and sotalol therapy. Muscle weakness, fatigue, and cramps.
- Treatment: Identify the cause. A high-potassium diet is not effective. Add supplemental potassium chloride and potassium-sparing diuretics. ACE inhibitors are mainstay of long-term therapy.

Hypomagnesemia (Magnesium level < 1.5 mEq/L)

- Cause: Activation of the renin-angiotensin-aldosterone axis, diuretic therapy (note similarity to hypokalemia).
- Diagnosis is difficult because of the poor correlation between total-body and plasma levels of magnesium.
- Significance of hypomagnesemia is controversial and not as well established. Look for concomitant hypocalcemia.
- Symptoms: Confusion, mental status changes, weakness, refractory hypokalemia or hypocalcemia, ventricular dysrhythmias.
- Treatment: Oral magnesium supplementation can be unpredictable. Dosage, 1.0 to 1.5 mEq/kg of body weight over 72 hours. Consider using potassium-sparing diuretics.

SUGGESTED READING

Gettes LS. Electrolyte abnormalities underlying lethal and ventricular arrhythmias. Circulation 1992;85(Suppl 1):170–176.

Leier CV, Dei Cas L, Metra M. Clinical relevance and management of the major electrolyte abnormalities in congestive heart failure: hyponatremia, hypokalemia, and hypomagnesemia. Am Heart J 1994;128:564–574.

Oster JR, Materson BJ. Renal and electrolyte complications of congestive heart failure with angiotensin-converting enzyme inhibitors. Arch Intern Med 1992;152:704–710.

Sica DA. Renal disease, electrolyte abnormalities, and acid-base imbalance in the elderly. Clin Geriatr Med 1994;10:197–211.

Sica DA, Gehr TWB. Diuretics in congestive heart failure. Cardiol Clin 1989;7:87–97.

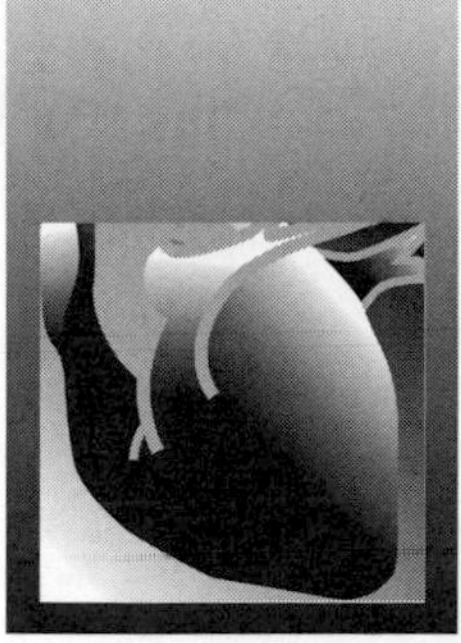

CHAPTER 7

Chest Pain

Yves Janin
Michael L. Hess

INTRODUCTION

Chest pain is a common symptom in any primary care practice and is one of the most frequent symptoms for which patients seek medical attention. The differential diagnosis of chest pain is extensive and consists of disorders of all thoracic structures and contiguous areas, including the neck and upper abdomen.

Chest pain can be the initial manifestation of a life-threatening condition that, if promptly and properly treated at its onset, can be reversed. A patient presenting shortly after the onset of the chest pain caused by acute myocardial infarction, could, if promptly reperfused, have only minimal myocardial damage and well-preserved systolic function. However, should this patient's pain be misdiagnosed as musculoskeletal in origin or secondary to some gastroesophageal condition, severe and irreversible cardiac damage may ensue and the patient's survival may be significantly compromised. Chest pain should always be seriously evaluated and never dismissed as trivial. In the evaluation of a patient with chest pain, the primary consideration should be to exclude life-threatening conditions. A patient who presents to an emergency facility with chest pain should not be discharged without a diagnosis. A high index of suspicion is necessary for the diagnosis of chest pain, and most diagnoses can be made, or at least strongly suspected, solely on the basis of the history and physical examination.

CHEST PAIN DUE TO CORONARY ARTERY DISEASE

Angina Pectoris

Angina pectoris is a manifestation of myocardial ischemia resulting from an imbalance between myocardial oxygen demand and myocardial oxygen supply. Myocardial oxygen demand is determined by the heart rate, inotropic state of the myocardium, and systolic ventricular wall stress. Myocardial oxygen supply depends on the oxygen-carrying capacity of the blood and coronary blood flow, which is itself determined by coronary vascular resistance and coronary perfusing pressure. In the presence of a significant coronary artery stenosis and the pressure gradient across the lesion blood flow across the stenotic area will depend on the perfusing pressure proximal to the lesion, the intraventricular pressures achieved during diastole, and the length of diastole. Tachycardia, a significant decrease in systolic blood pressure, and high intraventricular pressures reduce coronary blood flow across a significantly stenotic area and result in ischemia of the myocardium in the territory of that coronary artery. This is exacerbated by any decrease in the oxygen-carrying capacity of the blood, which could be secondary to anemia, hypoxia, or an increase in carboxyhemoglobin levels.

Signs and Symptoms

Angina pectoris is a heterogenous symptom complex. Anginal pain most commonly originates in the chest and then radiates to the neck, jaw, throat, shoulders, arms, elbows, or wrists. It usually has a retrosternal component. Anginal pain may begin in any of the secondary radiation sites and usually recurs in the anginal pattern typical for the particular patient.

Anginal pain usually originates in the retrosternal area and radiates across the precordium and bilaterally. Location of the pain in a different area does not exclude the diagnosis of angina. In some patients, especially women and patients who have previously had coronary interventions, anginal pain may start in atypical locations, such as the right precordium, the left suprascapular area, the left shoulder, and the left auricular area. A patient's report that "since my coronary artery bypass graft surgery, I get pain on the right of the chest" should not be dismissed but rather should be thoroughly investigated.

Although anginal pain secondary to myocardial ischemia never starts in the abdomen, patients with inferior myocardial ischemia may present with pain in the lower sternum, xiphoid, and epigastric areas; may point to the upper epigastrium when asked to localize their pain; and sometimes may be unable to state whether they are having chest pain. When anginal pain radiates to the upper extremity, left more often than right, it does so along the ulnar aspect and may extend to the ulnar fingers (but seldom involves the thumb). Pain may be absent in some patients with myocardial ischemia; such patients have sudden dyspnea, weakness, or fatigue as their anginal equivalent. Anginal pain may be accompanied by the onset of the following symptoms:

- Fatigue
- Weakness
- Dyspnea
- Palpitations
- Nausea
- Dizziness
- Lightheadedness

Patients with new onset of angina may be anxious; this anxiety should not lead to an erroneous diagnosis of psychogenic chest pain or the so-called hyperventilation syndrome. Anginal pain is diffuse and is not localized to a well-circumscribed area.

Stable angina is precipitated by exertion, be it ordinary physical activity or more strenuous exertion, such as the following:

- Climbing stairs
- Doing yard work
- Physical training
- Sexual intercourse
- Emotional or mental stress
- Exposure to temperature extremes
- Postprandial period

Unstable angina may occur at rest. Anginal pain does not start immediately after a sudden movement of the trunk or arm and is not pleuritic. Anginal pain may be associated with chest-wall tenderness.

The threshold for angina differs among patients. Patients with a fixed anginal threshold have pain after the same amount of activity, such as walking half a block or climbing a flight of stairs. Patients with variable-threshold angina have other concomitant factors in addition to significant coronary artery disease, including the following:

- Hypertension or fluid overload
- Arrhythmias
- Obesity
- Respiratory insufficiency with variable arterial hypoxemia
- Anemia
- Chronic gastrointestinal bleeding
- Thyroid disease
- Coronary spasm

Unlike myocardial infarction pain, which may have a sudden and severe onset, anginal pain has a crescendo pattern, gradually building up to its maximal intensity if not interrupted by an intervention. Anginal pain is frequently described by patients in the following ways:

- Pressure or heaviness, "like a weight sitting on my chest"
- Burning sensation
- An ache, "like a toothache"
- Squeezing sensation, "like a vise"
- Tightness, "like a fist holding me here"
- Ill-defined, uncomfortable feeling that the patient cannot properly describe, "like a misery in my chest"

Anginal pain is not sharp or stabbing (i.e., not "like a pin" or "like a knife"). It is not fleeting, does not last for a few seconds, but does not usually last longer than 15 minutes unless it becomes complicated by a myocardial infarction or is precipitated by a tachyarrhythmia or bradyarrhythmia. It is gradually relieved by cessation of the precipitating activity and rest or by the administration of sublingual nitroglycerin. Anginal pain takes a few minutes to subside. Some patients exhibit the phenomenon of walk-through angina, in which anginal pain subsides when the patient continues the activity that precipitated the anginal episode. This is attributed to the recruitment of the collaterals of circulation in the ischemic territory of the heart.

During the anginal episode, patients may have tachycardia or bradycardia, tachypnea, hypertension that may be secondary to the anxiety and pain, or a significant decrease in blood pressure secondary to ischemia-induced myocardial dysfunction. During systole, an abnormal precordial thrust may be palpated because of dyskinesia of the ischemic myocardium. Decreased ventricular diastolic compliance may result in a new third or fourth heart sound. If the ischemia affects the base of a papillary muscle, a transient mitral regurgitation murmur may be detected. Ischemia, decreased myocardial compliance, and ventricular hypokinesia or dyskinesia may precipitate the onset of heart failure.

Diagnosis

The electrocardiogram (ECG) may reveal ST-segment depression and T-wave inversion in a coronary territory or may be unremarkable. The diagnosis of angina pain is based on the history and its association with known risk factors of coronary artery disease. Age should not be used as a diagnostic criterion because adolescents or young adults may present with acute coronary spasm and myocardial ischemia secondary to the use of cocaine or metamphetamines (use that the patients may firmly deny). Young adults with a strong family history of coronary artery disease or hyperlipidemia may have premature coronary artery disease, and elderly patients may have new onset of angina in the presence of persistently tender costochondral joints and various rheumatologic diseases (Table 7.1).

Variant Angina Pectoris

Prinzmetal's angina, or variant angina, is angina at rest; it is not precipitated by exertion or emotional stress and is associated with ST-segment elevation that subsides as the pain is relieved. Although patients with Prinzmetal's angina have a well-preserved exercise capacity, exertional angina coexists with variant angina in more than half of affected patients. Variant angina may be associated with myocardial infarction and ventricular tachyarrhythmias, resulting in syncope and sudden death.

Signs and Symptoms

Variant angina is caused by a sudden, transient, severe coronary artery spasm that is focal; involves one or, occasionally, more than one site; and usually occurs at the site of a coronary stenosis, although it may also occur in normal coronary arteries. Most episodes of variant angina tend to occur in the early morning hours. Most patients tend to be heavy smokers. Patients with normal coronaries are more often younger and tend to

TABLE 7.1. Angina

Causes	Exertion—mental, physical, emotional
Symptoms	Pressure, weight, tightness, indigestion Rarely described as pain
Suspicion of angina	Maintain high index of suspicion
Angina in women	Atypical chest pain may, in fact, be typical in women
Electrocardiogram	May be normal
Risk factors	Beware of overdiagnosis of chostochondritis or esophageal reflux in patients with risk factors

be female. Variant angina can occur after acute myocardial infarction, coronary angioplasty, or coronary bypass surgery. It may be precipitated by alcohol withdrawal. Variant angina may be associated with migraine and the Raynaud phenomenon and may be part of a generalized vasospastic disorder.

Diagnosis

The diagnosis of variant angina is suggested by the occurrence of angina at rest and syncope and by the demonstration of transient ST-segment elevation on the ECG obtained during the episode of pain (the elevations resolve as the pain subsides). In patients suspected of having variant angina, the possibility of cocaine use should be considered because cocaine can also induce coronary vasoconstriction and myocardial ischemia.

Myocardial Infarction

Acute myocardial infarction is three times more likely to occur in the morning than in the late evening. The increased likelihood in the morning results from an increase in events in the first 4 hours after awakening. This circadian pattern is not present in patients with diabetes mellitus, advanced age, a history of smoking, or a history of myocardial infarction. Most myocardial infarctions occur at rest. In about half of patients with myocardial infarction, a precipitating factor can be identified (primarily emotional stress, increased physical activity, or patients on chronic nitrate therapy or taking Viagra).

Signs and Symptoms

Most patients with acute myocardial infarction have prodromal symptoms, consisting mainly of unstable angina in the form of a new-onset angina or worsening of a preexisting anginal pattern occurring at rest or with minimal activity. Some patients who develop new onset of exertional chest pain or dyspnea attempt to "get back in shape" by increasing their physical activity, often with disastrous consequences.

The cardinal symptom of acute myocardial infarction is chest pain that usually has a retrosternal component. Myocardial infarction is usually due to acute coronary thrombosis; if the thrombus lyses and reforms, leading to periods of transient reperfusion, a waxing and waning pattern of the pain may become constant when coronary occlusion becomes complete. Chest pain from acute myocardial infarction is severe in most patients and radiates across the precordium to the neck, jaw, lower teeth, left shoulder, and ulnar aspect of the left arm and then down to the ulnar fingers. It may radiate to the interscapular area, where it may be most severe. The pain is described as a crushing, vise-like, tearing, or heavy pressure sensation that is best exemplified by patients by a clenched fist held over the precordium or is likened to pain caused by "an elephant sitting on my chest." In some patients, neck and throat pain are so severe that the patients have the impression of being choked or strangulated.

Patients with an inferior myocardial infarction may report lower retrosternal and epigastric pain. The pain is not pleuritic at its onset, but patients prefer to remain immobile with minimal respiratory excursions and to limit their speech to a minimum. Most patients have associated symptoms, including the following:

- Diaphoresis
- Nausea
- Weakness
- Dyspnea
- Tachypnea
- Sensation of being ready to faint
- Vomiting
- Hiccuping
- Lower abdominal cramps
- Urge to defecate

The pain of acute myocardial infarction is prolonged; it lasts more than 30 minutes and frequently lasts for several hours.

Acute myocardial infarction may not be accompanied by chest pain, especially in the elderly, but may manifest itself by a new onset of acute congestive heart failure or a worsening of preexisting heart failure, syncope, ventricular tachyarrhythmias, severe weakness (which may masquerade as a depressive state), or acute agitation in a senile or mentally disabled patient. Finally, a large percentage of acute myocardial infarctions are silent and not recognized by the patient, only to be discovered later by routine ECG.

Diagnosis

Electrocardiography is sensitive for detecting myocardial infarction. The ECG criteria for diagnosing an acute myocardial infarction include new Q waves, 0.30 ms wide and 0.20 v deep; a 1-mm (0.1 milli-volt) ST-segment elevation in two contiguous leads; or new onset of left bundle-branch block. More than 90% of patients in whom the ST segment is elevated by 1 mm in two contiguous leads are confirmed to have an acute myocardial infarction (see Chapter 2). However, in the hyperacute phase of an acute myocardial infarction, the ECG changes may be limited to a straightening of the ST segments and to increased amplitude of symmetrical T waves. Posterior myocardial infarctions are identi-

TABLE 7.2. Myocardial Infarction

Diagnosis	Maintain high index of suspicion for patient with multiple risk factors Rapid diagnosis required for timely thrombolytic therapy
Symptoms	Pain—severe and prolonged, retrosternal with radiation
Recurrent angina or previous coronary artery bypass grafting or percutaneous transluminal coronary angioplasty	Patient may present with "atypical" pain
Risk factors	Not applicable to cocaine abuser, patient with insulin-dependent diabetes (especially women), and older patients

fied by tall R waves and ST-segment depressions in the anteroseptal leads (Table 7.2).

Even in the absence of a diagnostic ECG, patients who have continued chest pain and who are suspected of having an evolving myocardial infarction should have ECGs performed frequently; the results should be compared with each other and with any other baseline ECG available. It is important that the baseline on those ECGs be isoelectric because minimal ST-segment elevation may escape detection with a "wandering" baseline.

Syndrome X

Up to one-third of patients who undergo coronary arteriography are found to have normal or almost normal coronary arteries. Although their prognosis is good in terms of life expectancy, most of these patients continue to report chest pain and thus believe that they have heart disease; as a result they seek further medical opinions and undergo repeated hospitalizations. Many patients with syndrome X develop a panic disorder.

Signs and Symptoms

Syndrome X is characterized by exercise-induced angina, a positive ECG response to exercise testing, and normal coronary arteries. It is a heterogeneous syndrome that is more common in women. Chest pain in patients with syndrome X is similar to that in patients with coronary artery disease. It is usually exertional and gradual in onset and may radiate to the neck or jaw. However, syndrome X has certain atypical features, including the following:

- Prolonged duration
- Angina at rest
- Poor response to sublingual nitrates
- Preponderance during waking hours
- Absence of left ventricular wall-motion abnormalities during the transient but prolonged episodes of chest pain.

Diagnosis

Ambulatory ECG monitoring reveals that these episodes of chest pain are accompanied by ST-segment changes similar to those seen during myocardial ischemia. Various pathogenetic mechanisms have been proposed, including

- Myocardial ischemia secondary to reduced coronary flow reserve
- Release of adenosine
- Myocardial metabolic abnormalities
- Estrogen deficiency
- Increased pain perception

CHEST PAIN DUE TO NONCARDIAC CONDITIONS

Esophageal Disorders

Shared innervation with the heart makes the neighboring esophagus a reasonable consideration in patients with chest pain and no coronary artery disease (esophagus, cervical vertebrae C8 to T10; heart, thoracic vertebrae T1 to T4). In addition, shared innervation of efferent vagal fibers explains the similar quality and distribution of cardiac and esophageal pain.

Signs and Symptoms

Esophageal pain may have characteristics of anginal pain. It may occur during exercise or stressful conditions, be described as a precordial tightness or pressure, radiate down the left arm, and be relieved by nitrates.

Dysphagia and oral regurgitation of liquid may occur in patients with esophageal chest pain and those with cardiac chest pain. Features occurring frequently with chest pain of esophageal origin include the following:

- Onset of severe chest pain that continues as a precordial ache for several hours
- Variations in the amount of exercise necessary to produce the pain
- Chest pain beginning up to 10 minutes after the cessation of exercise
- Pain awakening the patient from sleep at night

TABLE 7.3. Esophageal Pain

Characteristics	Anginal characteristics Several hours in duration Does not produce chest pressure Does not produce exertional pain No incidence of sudden death
Diagnosis	Avoid diagnosis of esophageal reflux in high-risk "cardiac" patient

Diagnosis

Gastroesophageal reflux disease is the most common esophageal disorder associated with chest pain and is most reliably evaluated by 24-hour esophageal pH monitoring. However, the association of increased gastroesophageal reflux and chest pain does not necessarily establish a direct cause-and-effect relationship. Indeed, most episodes of reflux do not produce chest pain; yet, in some hypersensitive patients, chest pain develops during the episodes of acid reflux in the absence of an increase in total esophageal acid exposure.

Esophageal motility disorders were found in 28% of a large series of patients with noncardiac chest pain; the nutcracker esophagus was the most common abnormality. Although these motility disorders are associated with chest pain, only a few patients have chest pain when the esophageal dysmotility is most marked (Table 7.3).

Even with prolonged esophageal pH and motility monitoring, a substantial proportion of episodes of chest pain are found to be associated with neither gastroesophageal reflux nor abnormal motility. Furthermore, follow-up studies show that variations in esophageal motility are not correlated with changes in chest pain. Yet, testing patients with noncardiac chest pain for gastroesophageal reflux and esophageal dysmotility is beneficial because it reassures patients that their pain is noncardiac.

"Linked Angina"

Esophageal disease may exacerbate myocardial ischemia in patients with established coronary artery disease, a phenomenon called "linked angina." Esophageal acid stimulation can cause anginal attacks and significantly reduce coronary blood flow in patients with angiographically documented significant coronary artery disease, probably through a neural reflex mechanism.

Panic Disorder

Chest pain typical of angina can occur in patients with panic disorder. In a prospective study of patients with chest pain and angiographically normal coronary arteries, approximately one-third of the patients met the DSM-IIIR criteria for panic disorder and had had at least one panic attack per week for the preceding 3 weeks. Furthermore, like psychiatric patients with panic disorder, medical patients had a high rate of concurrent depression. At follow-up, patients with panic disorder had more debilitating chest pain and lower exertional capacity, viewed themselves as more disabled, had more episodes of major depression, and had worse social adjustment and higher anxiety levels than patients who did not have panic disorder. These factors support the hypothesis that long-term disability in patients with chest pain and angiographically normal coronary arteries is associated with panic disorder.

Disorders of Visceral Pain Perception

Syndrome X, gastroesophageal reflux, esophageal dysmotility, and panic disorder seem to overlap and can be associated with chest pain that is indistinguishable from angina pectoris in patients with angiographically normal coronary arteries. Unlike superficial pain, visceral pain is characterized by tonic increases in muscle tone and is often accompanied by autonomic responses. As the intensity and duration of the noxious stimulus increases, the visceral pain becomes more diffuse and may be referred to areas far from the site of origin. Pain originating from the esophagus may eventually be perceived throughout the entire chest and may radiate to the arms. A patient's perception of this pain sometimes exceeds the intensity of the noxious stimulus and is influenced by cognitive and emotional factors.

Perception of abnormal visceral pain could explain the cardiac hypersensitivity observed in patients with syndrome X; the esophageal hypersensitivity to acid reflux noted in the subgroup of patients with no increase in total esophageal acid exposure; the esophageal dysmotility observed in some patients with noncardiac chest pain; and the similarity of the chest pain in patients with syndrome X, esophageal disorders, and panic disorder.

CARDIAC CAUSES OF ANGINA-LIKE CHEST PAIN

Mitral Valve Prolapse Syndrome

Signs and Symptoms

The mitral valve prolapse syndrome is one of the most prevalent cardiac valvular abnormalities, affecting 5 to 10% of the American population. It is more common in young women. Although most patients with mitral valve prolapse are asymptomatic, the following recurrent and disabling symptoms sometimes occur:

- Palpitations
- Light-headedness
- Dizziness
- Chest pain
- Dyspnea
- Fatigue
- Anxiety
- Syncope
- Transient neurologic signs
- Frequent occurrence of supraventricular and ventricular premature beats
- Tachyarrhythmias

Up to half of patients with mitral valve prolapse report chest pain. This pain can be located anywhere in the chest but is usually left precordial or infra-mammary; it rarely radiates to the neck or upper extremity. The pain is sharp or sticking in nature rather than dull or pressure-like, and it is not related to exertion. It is not relieved by nitroglycerin and can last from seconds to hours. It can be cyclic with exacerbations and remissions and can occur in clusters, particularly during periods of emotional stress. It is usually not accompanied by ST-segment elevation or depression. There are no consistent relieving factors. The cause of chest pain in mitral valve prolapse is unknown, although several potential mechanisms have been proposed, including coronary artery spasm, abnormalities of left ventricular structure and function, and metabolic abnormalities resulting in myocardial ischemia.

Diagnosis

Mitral valve prolapse is diagnosed by postural auscultation and is confirmed by transthoracic echocardiography. Prompt squatting from the standing position moves the nonejection click and the systolic murmur to late systole. Mitral valve prolapse is prevalent in the general population, but it should not be considered the cause of chest pain until other, more serious conditions have been eliminated.

Pericarditis

Signs and Symptoms

Chest pain is the cardinal symptom of inflammatory pericardial conditions. It may be retrosternal or located over the left precordium. It is pleuritic, increasing with motion, respiration, variations in body position, and swallowing. Typically, it is sharply accentuated in the supine position and is relieved by sitting and leaning forward. In fact, the pain can be so severe in the recumbent position that the patient may find it intolerable to sit up and may have to roll over the side of the bed in order to get up and seek help. Patients with acute pericarditis tend to remain motionless and have rapid and shallow respiration. The chest pain characteristically radiates to the trapezius ridge and may radiate to the neck, shoulders, or back. It does not, however, radiate to the ulnar aspect of the upper extremity, arm, elbow or wrist. Inconsistent with pericarditis are a history of viral illness and fever.

Diagnosis

A pericardial friction rub should be diligently sought in patients with chest pain. The rub is frequently evanescent and variable and is frequently discovered after changing the position of the patient. It varies with respiration and may have up to three components (see Chapter 12). The discovery of a pericardial friction rub in a patient with acute chest pain should not comfort the examiner because the condition may be associated with cardiac tamponade, acute myocardial infarction, acute myopericarditis, or acute aortic dissection. After examination of the ECG, transthoracic echocardiography should be rapidly performed and evaluated for the presence of a pericardial effusion, evidence of tamponade, left ventricular wall-motion abnormalities, aortic insufficiency, and aortic root intimal flaps. Elevations of the ST segment that are concave upward and occur over several coronary arterial territories, in the absence of left ventricular-wall motion abnormalities, should suggest a diagnosis of pericarditis (see Table 7.4 and Chapter 2).

Acute Myocarditis

Acute myocarditis is common in the general population but is frequently unrecognized. Its occurrence is often secondary to viral infections. The most common cause of viral myocarditis is the Coxsackievirus B group. Patients with myocarditis or myopericarditis may present with precordial chest pain and ECG and enzymatic features resembling acute myocardial infarction. These findings may be associated with a history of fatigue, dyspnea on exertion or at rest, fever, and features of a gastrointestinal infection. These patients usually have wall-motion abnormalities seen on echocardiography and have nonsignificant coronary artery disease seen on cardiac catheterization.

TABLE 7.4. Pericarditis

- Pleuritic and positional
- Sharp—worse in the supine position; relieved by sitting up and leaning forward
- Usually associated with pericardial friction rub
- Diffuse ST-segment elevations on the electrocardiogram with no recipient changes

Acute Aortic Dissection

Acute aortic dissection affects the ascending aorta in two-thirds of patients with aortic dissection. It occurs more frequently in men in the fifth or sixth decade of life.

Signs and Symptoms

Most patients with acute aortic dissection develop severe, excruciating, tearing precordial chest pain that may radiate to the interscapular area, neck, and shoulders. The pain of acute aortic dissection is maximal at its onset and follows the path of the dissecting hematoma. Nausea, vomiting, and diaphoresis frequently accompany the chest pain. Syncope occurs in approximately 10% of patients. Although most patients with acute aortic dissection have a history of hypertension, they may be normotensive on presentation. Hypotension or frank shock occurs in approximately 20% of patients. Extension to the aortic root may produce flail aortic leaflets and acute severe aortic insufficiency. These patients usually present with severe heart failure. The murmur of acute severe aortic insufficiency may not be detected because of the rapid equalization of diastolic pressures between the left ventricle and the aorta. The first heart sound, however, is greatly attenuated or absent.

Further progression of the dissection to involve the coronary ostia may compromise coronary blood flow and result in acute myocardial ischemia or infarction. The administration of thrombolytic agents to patients with aortic dissection can lead to death. Acute proximal aortic dissection should always be considered in any patient with acute myocardial infarction in the presence of a history of hypertension or with a presentation including syncope, severe acute congestive heart failure, cardiogenic shock, or severe aortic insufficiency.

Diagnosis

The dissection can rupture in the pericardial sac, at first presenting the picture of acute pericarditis (which may be accompanied by a pericardial friction rub) and then progressing to pericardial tamponade. Syncope has been found to be associated with cardiac tamponade. The recovery of bloody pericardial fluid during pericardiocentesis should alert the physician to the possibility of an acute aortic dissection. Involvement of the carotid artery or the right brachiocephalic trunk can result in acute ischemic stroke manifested by a variety of acute neurologic deficits. In addition, occlusion of the arterial supply to the spinal cord may result in acute paraplegia, paresthesias, and loss of sphincter control. In up to 60% of patients, progression to the subclavian arteries has resulted in a pulse deficit. Further distal extension of the dissection can lead to acute mesenteric ischemia or infarction, acute renal artery occlusion, or loss of the femoral pulses with acute lower-extremity ischemia.

The aforementioned presentations can confuse the clinical picture. In an unconscious patient, for example, an acute cerebrovascular accident in the presence of ECG evidence of an acute myocardial infarction may be erroneously attributed to embolization from a left ventricular thrombus. Certain conditions are associated with aortic dissection (Table 7.5), including the following:

- Cystic medial degeneration of the aorta
- Connective tissue disorders, especially Marfan's and Ehlers-Danlos syndromes
- Coarctation of the aorta and bicuspid aortic valve
- Pregnancy

Once the diagnosis of acute proximal aortic dissection is suspected, a cardiothoracic surgical consultation should be obtained immediately and transthoracic echocardiography should be performed. The echocardiogram may show a pericardial effusion with or without evidence of

- Hemodynamic compromise
- Normal or depressed left ventricular systolic function
- Left ventricular wall-motion abnormalities

TABLE 7.5. Aortic Dissection

One of the most commonly missed diagnoses in a coronary care unit
Severe excruciating pain
May be associated with the murmur of aortic insufficiency or pericardial friction rub
Most patients have a history of hypertension
Suspect dissection in high-risk patients, such as those with severe hypertension or a young patient with Marfan's syndrome

- Severe aortic insufficiency
- Intimal flap with a false lumen involving the aortic root

If the diagnosis is still equivocal, the patient should have transesophageal echocardiography, preferably after intubation and in the operating room. If the result is negative but doubt persists, the patient should undergo computed tomography.

Aortic Stenosis

Valvular aortic stenosis is the most common form of left ventricular outflow obstruction. It is secondary to degenerative changes, which lead to fibrosis and secondary calcifications of the aortic leaflets. Its hemodynamic consequence is a systolic overloading of the left ventricle, which results in compensatory left ventricular hypertrophy in an attempt to reduce left ventricular wall stress. This compensation, however, occurs at the cost of increased stiffness of the left ventricle and increased myocardial oxygen consumption. Prolongation of the systolic ejection period shortens diastole and, therefore, coronary blood flow. In addition, the intramyocardial blood vessels are compressed by the large mass of contracting myocardium and by the high left ventricular pressures developed during systole. This results in myocardial ischemia and angina pectoris, even in the absence of coronary artery disease.

Hypertrophic Cardiomyopathy

Signs and Symptoms

Hypertrophic cardiomyopathy can occur in children, adolescents, and adults and can present as chest pain or syncope (see Chapters 15 and 16). In most patients with obstructive hypertrophic cardiomyopathy, symptoms develop in early adulthood. These patients may present with dyspnea, chest pain, atrial fibrillation, presyncope, or syncope on exertion. Myocardial ischemia occurs in hypertrophic cardiomyopathy, and anginal chest pain is a frequent symptom. The left ventricular outflow tract obstruction in hypertrophic cardiomyopathy is a dynamic phenomenon. It is increased by any maneuver that increases myocardial contractility or decreases preload and thus reduces left ventricular end-diastolic dimensions. In the presence of an increased left ventricular outflow obstruction, the left ventricle must develop high intracavitary systolic pressures in order to maintain stroke volume. The high pressures cause generation of a high left ventricular wall stress and an increased myocardial oxygen demand that may exceed the capacity of the coronary arterial system. Other potential mechanisms of myocardial ischemia include the transient systolic obstruction of the epicardial coronary arteries by myocardial bridges, prolonged diastolic relaxation resulting in elevated myocardial wall tension, diastolic occlusion of the intramyocardial coronary arteries, and small-vessel disease of the small intramyocardial coronary arteries.

Diagnosis

Diagnosis of hypertrophic cardiomyopathy is suggested by the detection, along the left sternal border, of a systolic ejection murmur that typically increases during the Valsalva maneuver or after upright posture is assumed. The ECG may show a pseudoinfarction pattern with abnormal Q waves or giant T-wave inversions. The diagnosis is confirmed by transthoracic echocardiography. Magnetic resonance imaging is indicated if echocardiography cannot define the site and extent of hypertrophy.

PULMONARY CAUSES OF ANGINA-LIKE CHEST PAIN

Acute Pulmonary Embolism

Signs and Symptoms

Patients with acute pulmonary embolism may present with shock, with syncope or a supraventricular tachyarrhythmia, with new-onset isolated dyspnea that is worse on exertion, or with pulmonary infarction and chest pain that may be accompanied by hemoptysis. Pulmonary infarction occurs in 59% of all patients with acute pulmonary embolism, and chest pain occurs in 66%. Acute pulmonary embolism develops suddenly and may occur at rest or during minimal exertion. Pulmonary embolism is pleuritic and may be exacerbated by movement. It may be alleviated by decreasing respiratory excursions on the involved side. It is frequently accompanied by dyspnea, which is the most common symptom and which is increased on exertion. True anginal chest pain, however, occurs in ill patients with acute pulmonary embolism, secondary to the increased afterload of the right ventricle, which may become ischemic. Hemoptysis is rare. Most patients are tachypneic and tachycardic. Although an increased pulmonary component of the second heart sound and a right ventricular lift should attract the attention toward causes of acute pulmonary hypertension, these symptoms occur infrequently.

Diagnosis

Electrocardiography in patients with acute pulmonary embolism is nonspecific and usually reveals sinus rhythm or nonspecific ST-segment or T-wave changes. Left-axis deviation occurs as frequently as right-axis deviation. The SlQ3T3 or S1S2S3 patterns, although infrequent, should increase the suspicion of acute pulmonary embolism. The absence of hypoxemia or a normal alveolar-arterial oxygen gradient do not exclude the diagnosis. Although plain radiography of the chest may have normal results, it often reveals atelectasis, a blunted costophrenic angle, and an elevated diaphragm. Decreased pulmonary vascular markings occur in less than one-fourth of patients with acute pulmonary embolism. The diagnosis of acute pulmonary embolism should be suspected clinically. Before the patient undergoes ventilation-perfusion lung scanning, therapy with intravenous heparin should be instituted quickly if no major contraindications are present. Only 13% of patients with pulmonary embolism have a high-probability finding on the ventilation-perfusion scan; of the patients with a low-probability or near-normal scan, 16% and 9%, respectively, have angiographically demonstrable pulmonary emboli. Therefore, in the presence of a high clinical suspicion of pulmonary embolism, a near-normal ventilation-perfusion lung scan does not exclude the diagnosis. Rather, it should lead to pulmonary angiography or, in the presence of demonstrable deep venous thrombosis, to continued therapy for pulmonary embolism (Table 7.6).

Pulmonary Embolism — TABLE 7.6.

- Sudden-onset, pleuritic chest pain that may be associated with cough and hemoptysis
- Electrocardiography is generally nondiagnostic
- Suspect pulmonary embolism in high-risk patients, such as postoperative patients, women receiving oral contraceptives, and patients with severe heart failure
- Arterial hypoxemia is not always present

Acute Pulmonary Hypertension

In patients with heart disease, sharp increases in pulmonary venous pressure increase pulmonary blood volume, reduce lung compliance, increase airway resistance, increase microvascular filtration, and can lead to varying degrees of alveolar edema. These changes cause an increase in the effort of breathing and in the myocardial oxygen demand. In patients with coronary artery disease, an imbalance in myocardial oxygen demand or supply results in myocardial ischemia, angina, and, occasionally, infarction. In addition, the right ventricular stroke work and wall stress increase in order to maintain left ventricular preload in the presence of acute pulmonary hypertension. This may eventually lead to right ventricular ischemia and angina. Acute pulmonary hypertension can produce chest pain caused by acute distention of the pulmonary arteries with resultant stimulation of their adventitial nerve endings. The pain of acute pulmonary hypertension varies widely but rarely radiates to the upper extremities or neck.

Pleural Disease

Pleural disease is manifested by pleuritic chest pain that is localized over the involved hemithorax and increases with respiration, cough, and movements of the thorax. It is decreased by immobility and holding one's breath. It can radiate to the shoulder and neck or to the adjoining abdominal wall. Patients with pleural disease are usually quiet and tachypneic and have shallow respirations. The involved hemithorax is often splinted. Pleural disease is diagnosed by physical examination that reveals a pleural friction rub, which is heard during both inspiration and expiration and is often transient.

Pneumothorax

Spontaneous pneumothorax is almost always the result of rupture of subpleural blebs, which are located at the apex of the upper lobe or in the superior segment of the lower lobe. It typically occurs in young men and is much less frequent in women. The peak incidence is seen in persons between 20 and 40 years of age. Patients usually develop sudden sharp, pleuritic chest pain that radiates to the shoulder; it usually occurs at rest but may also develop during exertion. Chest pain is accompanied by dyspnea, splinting of the involved hemithorax, tachypnea, and shallow respirations. It tends to decrease as the collapse of the lung progresses.

Pneumothorax is diagnosed by physical examination that reveals an expanded tympanitic hemithorax with no breath sounds. It is confirmed by chest radiography.

CHEST-WALL PAIN SYNDROMES

Costochondral Syndrome

Inflammation of the second, third, fourth, or fifth costochondral joints may occur at any age and in both sexes. It is associated with anterior chest pain that may develop suddenly, may radiate to the upper extremities, and is exaggerated by movement. The involved costochondral joint is very tender and may be swollen.

Costochondral joint pain is such a common and benign condition that it should never be considered as the cause of the chest pain until all other causes have been ruled out. In addition, palpation of the costochondral joints frequently causes pain in the absence of any inflammation, especially in the elderly and in debilitated patients. Thus, costochondral joint pain is more often a companion of a variety of other causes of chest pain than the source.

Sternalis Syndrome

Pain occurs in the center of the chest and is associated with tenderness at the sternomanubrial junction.

Xiphoidalgia

Anterior chest pain may radiate to the shoulders, back, or epigastrium and is associated with tenderness over the xiphoid process.

Cervical Spine Disease

One of the most common causes of neck, shoulder, and arm pain is disc herniation in the lower cervical region. When the protruded disc lies between the sixth and seventh cervical vertebrae, the seventh cervical nerve root is compressed. This produces pain in the scapular area, pectoral region, medial axilla, posterolateral upper arm, elbow, dorsal forearm, and fingers. Coughing and sneezing exacerbate the pain.

Cervical spine disease is diagnosed by the dermatomal distribution of the pain and the associated neurologic deficits.

Thoracic Outlet Syndromes

The thoracic outlet syndromes include the cervical rib, scalenus anticus syndrome, costoclavicular syndrome, and hyperabduction syndrome. These physical abnormalities result in compression of the brachial plexus, the subclavian artery, or the subclavian vein near the first rib and the clavicle. Compression of the brachial plexus causes pain, paresthesias, and numbness; these symptoms are often most severe in the C8—TI distribution. The pain begins insidiously and involves the neck, shoulder, arm, and hand, with occasional radiation to the anterior chest. This chest pain may be associated with paresthesias along the ulnar distribution of the arm and forearm. It is induced by abduction of the arm or by working with the arms above the shoulders, but it is not precipitated by walking.

Thoracic outlet syndromes are diagnosed by detecting the neurologic signs and demonstrating a loss of the radial pulse with the Adson maneuver or with hyperabduction.

CHEST PAIN CAUSED BY INTRA-ABDOMINAL CONDITIONS

Acute Pancreatitis

The major symptom of acute pancreatitis is abdominal pain, which is located in the epigastrium and periumbilical region and typically radiates straight to the back. It may also radiate to the flanks, chest, and shoulders. Pain varies in intensity but is usually moderately severe. It is exacerbated by the supine position; most patients lie on their side with their trunk flexed and their knees drawn up. Nausea and vomiting are frequent. Changes in the ST segment and T wave may occur.

Acute pancreatitis is diagnosed clinically by documenting severe tenderness and rigidity of the mid-to-upper abdomen and epigastrium. Acute pancreatitis may be associated with a pericardial effusion that has a high amylase content.

Acute Cholecystitis

Acute cholecystitis is associated with right upper quadrant pain that may radiate to the interscapular area, right scapula, or shoulder. Splinting of the right hemithorax and right flank occurs. Nausea and vomiting are common, and ST-segment and T-wave changes may occur. Acute cholecystitis is diagnosed on the basis of the history and physical examination.

Peptic Ulcer Disease

Patients with peptic ulcer disease usually report epigastric burning or gnawing pain that often occurs 90 minutes to 3 hours after eating and often awakens patients from sleep. It is usually rapidly relieved by food or antacids. Perforation of a peptic ulcer irritates the diaphragm, resulting in pleuritic chest pain on the affected side that radiates to the shoulder.

Herpes Zoster

Before the development of a cutaneous eruption, herpes zoster may cause a sharp, burning pain accompanied by dyesthesias over the precordium along the distribution of the peripheral nerves whose dorsal ganglia are involved. This is most common in the elderly and may be associated with other systemic manifestations, including fever, constitutional symptoms, and neck stiffness.

CONCLUSION

Patients with chest pain should always be seriously evaluated. The primary consideration in the initial evaluation of patients with chest pain should be to exclude grave conditions that could be life-threatening rather than to make a definitive diagnosis. A high index of suspicion is necessary. All investigations should begin with a thorough history. Patients should be encouraged to describe their pain, without interruption from the physician. This rarely takes more than a few minutes but is crucially important because it usually includes most of the elements of the pain that are disturbing the patient. The chest pain should then be characterized by well-directed, nonsuggestive questioning. Particular emphasis should be given to the following:

- Time of onset of chest pain and the activity that the patient was engaged in at the time
- Character of the pain
- Intensity pattern of the pain
- Mode of onset and disappearance of pain
- Time of day when pain occurs
- Conditions, circumstances, or factors that induce pain, exacerbate it, and diminish it or make it subside
- Duration of the pain
- Symptoms associated with the pain
- Patient's medical history
- Associated comorbid conditions
- Presence of risk factors for coronary artery disease
- Possible use of recreational drugs

Most diagnoses of chest pain can be made or strongly suspected on the basis of the history alone. The physical examination can provide additional clues and can often prevent disastrous therapeutic interventions. For example, the detection of an aortic regurgitation murmur in a patient with an acute myocardial infarction should raise the possibility of an acute aortic dissection as the primary cause.

Electrocardiography should be performed on most patients with chest pain, and radiography of the chest should be done on all patients. Echocardiography, computed tomography of the chest, and other tests should be done as indicated on the basis of clinical suspicion.

KEY POINTS

Chest Pain Due to Coronary Artery Disease

- Rule in or rule out this diagnosis rapidly and efficiently. In general, death is not associated with noncardiac chest pain.
- Diagnosis of chest pain is a working diagnosis determined by history and physical examination.
- Stable angina, due to myocardial oxygen demand mismatch, is usually retrosternal, radiates bilaterally across the pericardium, and is relieved by rest and nitroglycerine.
- Women and patients with previous interventions (percutaneous transluminal coronary angioplasty or coronary artery bypass grafting) may have variations, wrongly labeled atypical.
  - Variant angina, or Prinzmetal's angina, occurs at rest, is associated with ST-segment elevation, and is generally due to coronary artery spasm. This type of angina tends to occur in the morning; is associated with heavy smoking; can occur after acute myocardial infarction, percutaneous transluminal coronary angioplasty, or coronary artery bypass grafting; and is seen with the Raynaud phenomenon and migraine.
- Unstable angina is a prodrome of myocardial infarction. Myocardial infarction pain is usually retrosternal and is characterized as crushing, vicelike, tearing, or heavy pressure-like pain that can radiate to the neck, throat, or arms. In elderly patients, unstable angina may present as heart failure. Rapid diagnosis is imperative.
- Patients with syndrome X present with typical exercise-induced angina, a positive ECG response to exercise testing, and normal coronary arteries. Medical therapy generally results in a good prognosis.

Noncardiac Causes of Angina-like Chest Pain

- Esophageal disorders may mimic angina because of shared nervous innervation.
- Gastroesophageal reflux can be characterized as prolonged, severe pain that begins after exercise and may awaken the patient from sleep.
- Esophageal spasm is not associated with exertion but with trigger foods. May occur in up to one-third of patients with noncardiac chest pain.
- "Linked angina" occurs in patients with both esophageal disease and coronary artery disease in which motility problems or reflex angina associated with exertion occurs in the supine position and is relieved by sitting up.
- Panic disorders are a common cause of chest pain, may last for minutes to hours, are not relieved with rest and nitroglycerin, and are associated with a "feeling of doom." Physical examination, ECG, and echocardiography have normal results. Treated not with cardiac medications but with tricylic antidepressants, benzodiazepines, or monoamine oxidase inhibitors.

Cardiac Causes of Angina-like Chest Pain

- Diagnosis is generally made by history and physical examination. Inquire about the use of both Viagra and nitrate in the male. Cardiac causes of angina-like chest pain can be associated with morbidity and death.
- Mitral valve prolapse is more common in women and is characterized by pain, dyspnea, and fatigue. Diagnosed by postural auscultation and transthoracic echocardiography. Generally not associated with morbidity or death.
- Pericarditis is retrosternal and pleuritic, is accentuated in the supine position, and is relieved by sitting up and leaning forward. The two- or three-component friction rub heard on auscultation is the hallmark of the physical examination. The ECG should show diffuse ST-segment evaluation with no reciprocal changes.
- Acute myocarditis may be viral in cause, especially in pediatric patients. Patients present with precordial chest pain that may be associated with enzymatic myocardial infarction. Echocardiography may show wall-motion abnormalities; results of coronary angiography are generally normal.
- Acute aortic dissection is an important, commonly missed diagnosis of acute chest pain syndromes. Patients have a history of hypertension, and most cases involve the ascending aorta. Severe excruciating precordial chest pain radiates to the back and is maximal in onset. May involve the aortic root and produce aortic insufficiency, rupture into the pericardial sac, lead to pericarditis with a friction rub, and progress to tamponade. May involve the coronary ostia and present as myocardial infarction. Requires a car-

KEY POINTS

diology consultation for diagnosis with transesophageal echocardiography and a cardiac surgical consultation (see Chapter 17).

- Aortic stenosis can produce effort angina independent of coronary artery disease. Diagnosis is suspected on detection of harsh, basilar systolic murmur with radiation to the neck and aortic calcification on chest radiography. Diagnosis is confirmed by echocardiography.
- Hypertrophic cardiomyopathy can produce effort angina independent of coronary artery disease. Diagnosis includes systolic ejection murmur at the left sternal border that increases with Valsalva maneuver. Diagnosis is confirmed by echocardiography.

Pulmonary Causes of Chest Pain

- Acute pulmonary embolism causes pulmonary infarction in 60% of patients with cough, hemoptysis, pleuritic chest pain, and pleural friction rub. In 66% of patients, chest pain is accompanied by dyspnea, tachycardia, tachypnea, and sinus tachycardia on ECG. The S1Q3T3 sign on ECG is rare. Diagnosis is confirmed by arterial hypoxemia, ventilation—perfusion scanning, and pulmonary angiography.
- Pulmonary hypertension can be both acute and chronic. Can produce effort angina, is relieved by nitroglycerin, and is independent of coronary artery disease. Cause is believed to be distention of the pulmonary arteries. Diagnosed by echocardiography or catheterization of the right side of the heart.
- Pleural disease: Pleuritic, localized chest pain over the affected area that increases with inspiration, cough, and movement. Not relieved by rest or nitroglycerin. To confirm diagnosis, search for underlying pulmonary or pleural process.
- Pneumothorax caused by rupture of subpleural blebs occurs in the young, especially males. Characterized by sharp, pleuritic pain radiating to the shoulder. Physical examination shows tachypnea, dyspnea, and splinting. Diagnosis is confirmed by chest radiography.

Chest-Wall Pain Syndromes

- Costochondral syndromes and Tietze syndrome: Signs and symptoms include anterior chest pain exaggerated by movement and point tenderness and swelling of the involved chostochondral point. Cause of costochondral syndromes and Tietze syndrome includes inflammation of two, three, four, or five chostochondral points occurring at any age in both sexes. These benign conditions are generally associated with a known diagnosis of arthritis.
- Sternalis syndrome and xizphoidalgia are associated with tenderness of the sternum and xiphoid process and muscle tenderness aggravated by coughing or sneezing.
- Cervical spine disease is associated with neck pain with radiation to the arm; sensory loss may be present.
- Thoracic outlet syndrome is caused by compression of brachial plexus with pain, paraesthesia, and numbness, usually with a C9–T1 distribution.

Chest Pain Caused by Intra-abdominal Conditions

- Signs and symptoms of acute pancreatitis include abdominal pain that may radiate to the chest wall and shoulders and is usually severe. Pain is exacerbated in the supine position.
- Signs and symptoms of acute cholecystitis include right-upper-quadrant pain that may radiate to the right scapular shoulder.
- Signs and symptoms of peptic ulcer disease include epigastric burning or gnawing pain.

SUGGESTED READING

Alban-Davies H, Jones DB, Rhodes J, et al. Angina-like esophageal pain: differentiation from cardiac pain by history. J Clin Gastroenterol 1985;7:477–481.

Beitman BD, Mukreji V, Lamberti JW , et al. Panic disorder in patients with chest pain and angiographically normal coronary arteries. Am J Cardiol 1989;63:1399–1403.

Chambers J, Bass C. Chest pain with normal coronary anatomy: A review of natural history and possible etiologic factors. Prog Cardiovasc Dis 1990;33:161–184.

Fuster V, Ip JH. Medical aspects of acute aortic dissection. SeminThorac Cardiovasc Surg. 1991;3:219–224.

Joy M, Cairns Aw, Sprigings D. Observations on the warm-up phenomenon in angina pectoris. Br Heart J 1987;58: 116–121.

Kaski JC, Rosano GMC, Nihoyannopoulos P, et al. Syndrome X. Clinical characteristics and left ventricular function. A long term follow-up study. J Am Coll Cardiol 1995;25: 807–814.

Sampson JJ, Cheitlin MD. Pathophysiology and differential diagnosis of cardiac pain. Prog Cardiovasc Dis 1971;13: 507–531.

Savage DD, Garrison RJ, Devereaux RB, et al. Mitral valve prolapse in the general population. I. Epidemiologic features. The Framingham Study. Am Heart J 1983;106: 571–576.

Semble EI, Wise CM. Chest pain: a rheumatologist's perspective. South Med J 1988;81:64–68.

Shabetai R. Acute viral and idiopathic pericarditis. In: Shabetai R, ed. The pericardium. New York: Grune and Stratton, 1981:349–350.

Shabetai R. Acute pericarditis. In: Diseases of the pericardium. Cardiol Clin 1990;8:639–644.

Sigle DE, Rakowski H, Kimball BP, et al. Hypertrophic cardiomyopathy. Clinical spectrum and treatment. Circulation 1995;92:1680–1692.

Stein PD, Terrin ML, Hales CA, et al. Clinical, laboratory, roentgenologic and electrocardiographic findings in patients with acute pulmonary embolism and no preexisting cardiac or pulmonary disease. Chest 1991;100: 598–603.

Viar WN, Harrison TR. Chest pain in association with pulmonary hypertension: its similarity to the pain of coronary disease. Circulation 1952;5:1–11.

Woodruff JF. Viral myocarditis. A review article. Am J Pathol. 1980;101:425–484.

Wynne J. Mitral valve prolapse. N Engl J Med 1986;314: 577–578.

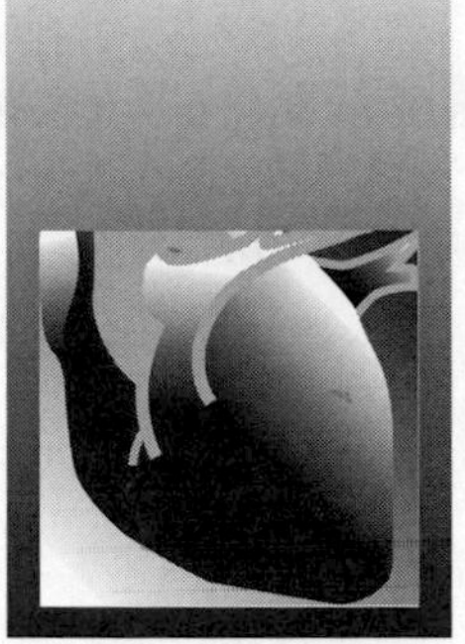

CHAPTER 8

Atherosclerotic Heart Disease

Yves Janin
Michael L. Hess

ATHEROSCLEROSIS

Pathology

Atherosclerosis is the most common cause of death in the western world. It is a focal disease of the arterial intima that is not uniformly distributed throughout the different arterial systems. Atherosclerosis begins in childhood with an accumulation of lipid in the intima. This results in a fatty streak that progresses and forms a fibrous plaque in early adulthood. New lesions are generated throughout life, and all stages of plaque development can coexist in the same artery.

The fibrous plaque consists of a connective tissue matrix and a lipid core, which are separated from the lumen of the vessel by a fibrous cap of variable thickness. Under the influence of various factors, including shear wall stress and the release of proteolytic enzymes by the inflammatory cells of the plaque, arterial plaque may become eroded or may fissure and rupture. Plaque rupture usually occurs at the junction between the fibrous cap and the adjacent vessel wall. The rupture results in the exposure of the lipid core, which is highly thrombogenic and triggers platelet aggregation and the coagulation cascade. This leads to the generation of thrombin and culminates in the formation of a thrombus at the site of plaque rupture, resulting in obstruction of the involved artery. The severity of the preexisting coronary arterial stenosis at the site of plaque rupture may be minimal or extensive. Depending on the integrity and activity of the intrinsic fibrinolytic system, the newly developed thrombus may quickly be totally or partially lysed or may be unaffected. Partial lysis of the thrombus leads to the accumulation of a fibrin coat on the fibrous cap of the plaque, resulting in increased thickness. As the atherosclerotic coronary arterial plaque grows, it increases the obstruction of blood flow to the dependent myocardium. The coronary arterial endothelium in areas of atherosclerosis is functionally abnormal, exhibiting an absence of vasorelaxation or even an abnormal vasoconstrictor response to vasodilator stimuli.

Pathophysiology

Myocardial oxygen demand is determined by the contractility of the myocardium, the afterload against which it has to work, and the wall stress to which it is submitted. Myocardial oxygen demand must be met by the myocardial oxygen supply to prevent the development of an oxygen debt and cellular ischemia. Myocardial oxygen supply is determined by the following:

- Oxygen-carrying capacity of the blood
- Length of diastole during which coronary perfusion occurs
- Coronary perfusion pressure, which depends on the diastolic aortic pressure
- End-diastolic intraventricular pressure
- Coronary vascular resistance

Coronary vascular resistance in turn depends on the following:

- Degree of atherosclerotic narrowing
- Severity of the luminal encroachment by the newly developed thrombus
- Degree of accompanying vasospasm
- Severity of endothelial dysfunction

Angina pectoris occurs when myocardial oxygen demand exceeds myocardial oxygen supply.

Unstable angina and myocardial infarction represent two ends of a spectrum caused by plaque rupture and superimposed platelet aggregation and thrombosis. Nonocclusive thrombi are generally manifested by unstable angina, whereas occlusive thrombi cause myocardial infarction. In unstable angina, there is a substantial amount of ischemic myocardium. Nonocclusive thrombi may, however, also lead to a myocardial infarction if

- There is a significant decrease in diastolic aortic root pressure and thus in coronary perfusion pressure.
- The coronary artery has a significant distal stenosis, causing a critical reduction in the perfusion pressure of the dependent myocardium.
- Coronary arterial spasm ensues.
- A coronary steal develops secondary to either local intramyocardial coronary flow characteristics or to therapy with potent arteriolar vasodilators.

In unstable angina, the thrombus consists primarily of platelets; in myocardial infarction, fibrin predominates. The presence of collaterals to the acutely jeopardized myocardial zone usually limits the amount of necrosis in the periphery of the ischemic territory.

ACUTE CHEST PAIN—EMERGENCY PRESENTATION

All patients presenting with chest pain must be evaluated thoroughly. Chest pain should never be dismissed, no matter how "atypical" the pain appears to be or how seemingly unrelated the history or the behavior of the patient. Musculoskeletal or costochondral chest pain should never be diagnosed without a previous complete and thorough investigation in order to rule out all other causes of chest pain. Chest pain is a serious symptom that has strong potential for morbidity and death.

History

The physician should obtain a history from the patient while the patient's vital signs are being recorded. If the patient presents to an emergency department, an intravenous line is started and supplemental oxygen is administered. After a patient is allowed to state in his or her own words the events that prompted the visit to the emergency department, the nature of the chest pain should be investigated.

Sample questions include the following:

- Does the patient have a history of cardiovascular disease?
- Is the chest pain still present, how long has it been present, and how severe is it?
- Is this the first episode of chest pain, or have there been any previous episodes of chest pain in the recent or distant past?
- How did the pain start?
- Was the onset of pain sudden and severe or did it gradually increase in intensity?
- What circumstances preceded or accompanied the onset of the pain?
- What was the quality of the pain?
- Did the pain radiate, and, if so, to what sites?
- Were there any associated symptoms?
- Did any factors or interventions decrease the intensity of the pain, relieve it, or exaggerate it?
- Is the pain similar to anginal pain or is it different, and in what way?
- Is the pain similar to the chest pain that accompanied a previous myocardial infarction?
- What risk factors for cardiovascular disease does the patient have? (Table 8.1)
- Does the patient have a history of drug use?
- Does the patient have a history of coronary artery disease? Is the patient taking nitrates and Viagra?

Through these questions, the physician must focus on determining whether

- Chest pain is life-threatening
- Pain is cardiac in origin
- Pain is due to atherosclerotic heart disease
- Patient is having unstable angina or an acute myocardial infarction.

Treatment

Because the incidence of ventricular fibrillation is highest in the first few hours after an acute myocardial infarction, the first therapeutic act for a patient presenting to an emergency facility with chest pain should be to place the patient on a cardiac monitor. This ensures the prompt recognition of any tachyarrhythmia or bradyarrhythmia and allows immediate initiation of the appropriate therapy.

TABLE 8.1. Major Risk Factors for the Development of Premature Coronary Artery Disease

Male sex (in persons younger than 60 years of age, disease occurs in 8 to 10 men for every woman)
Family history of premature coronary artery disease
Diabetes mellitus (a higher index of suspicion should be used for the younger patient, both male and female, with insulin-dependent diabetes)
Hypertension
Cigarette smoking
Hypercholesterolemia
Sedentary lifestyle

Cardioversion

Ventricular fibrillation and unstable ventricular tachycardia should be treated immediately by cardioversion, with no previous attempt to intubate or to start an intravenous line. Symptomatic, severe bradycardia; slow junctional rhythm; or complete heart block should prompt the physician to immediately apply the pads of the external pacer on the patient. No attempt should be made to place an internal pacemaker wire.

Electrocardiogram

If the patient reports chest pain, an electrocardiogram (ECG) should be immediately obtained while the history is being taken. The ECG should have an isoelectric baseline to allow detection of subtle changes in the ST segments that otherwise would be uninterpretable.

Patients with cardiac chest pain and ECG changes should not be sent to the radiology department for a chest radiography and should not have a blood gas determination or a central line placement in the event that they may become candidates for thrombolytic therapy. If there is any doubt about oxygenation, a pulse oximeter should be used. To minimize bleeding, nasotracheal intubation should not be attempted in patients who have received or may be eligible for thrombolysis or who will require intravenous heparin therapy.

Patients with ongoing cardiac chest pain should have repeated ECGs to detect any new changes. To detect any evolution, these ECGs should be compared to old ECGs and to previous ECGs obtained since the patient's arrival. A 0.5-mm ST-segment elevation is not an indication for thrombolysis, but a 1-mm elevation in two contiguous leads is diagnostic of an acute myocardial infarction and is an indication for thrombolysis.

Narcotics

Patients should not be administered heavy doses of narcotics in the absence of a diagnosis. As in the management of acute abdominal pain, patients should not be sedated if no working diagnosis has been established. A patient with new-onset chest pain and no ECG changes on arrival may become somnolent and quiet after the administration of a standard dose of narcotic while at the same time developing an acute myocardial infarction that may thus be undetected for several more hours. However, pain and anxiety should be relieved. Small doses of morphine are well tolerated. Morphine has a venodilator effect that may result in hypotension and a parasympathomimetic action. In the presence of bradycardia, meperidine is preferred.

Aspirin

All patients with cardiac chest pain should receive 160 mg of chewable, nonenteric, coated aspirin unless they are allergic to this drug. Nauseated or vomiting patients should receive a 325-mg suppository aspirin. Aspirin is a potent inhibitor of platelet aggregation. Inhibition of platelet function is evident in 1 hour after aspirin ingestion.

Nitroglycerin

After the institution of a peripheral intravenous line, 0.4 mg of nitroglycerin should be administered sublingually. The effect should be noted, and sublingual administration should be repeated every 5 minutes for a total of three doses or until a nitroglycerin infusion can be started (if indicated). Nitroglycerin dilates the coronary arteries and their collaterals. However, its primary action is venous dilatation, with a consequent decrease in preload that results in a reduction in end-diastolic ventricular volumes and wall stress. Nitroglycerin also decreases blood pressure and afterload. It is this decrease in preload and afterload that reduces myocardial oxygen consumption and, therefore, the ischemic burden on a myocardium with limited and compromised oxygen delivery.

Associated Conditions

Hypotension

Patients with acute myocardial infarction frequently have volume depletion secondary to diaphoresis, vomiting, no oral intake for several hours, or the use of diuretics. They may also become hypotensive after receiving nitroglycerin. In the presence of ischemia or infarction, the right ventricle becomes noncompliant and stiff and thus is greatly dependent on preload. By producing venous vasodilatation, nitroglycerin reduces preload and can lead to severe hypotension in patients with right ventricular ischemia or infarction.

Patients who develop hypotension after the administration of nitroglycerin should be immediately placed in a mild Trendelenburg position and receive an intravenous bolus of normal saline solution. If the patient does not promptly respond to fluids and is still hypotensive and reporting chest pain, dopamine should be administered rapidly. The dopamine dosage must be titrated carefully in order to achieve a systolic blood pressure of 90 mm Hg and to avoid excessive tachycardia, which exacerbates myocardial ischemia. During treatment, a right-sided ECG should be recorded in order to detect a right ventricular infarction.

Hypertension

Mild hypertension is usually secondary to the pain and anxiety associated with the chest pain syndrome. Severe hypertension, however, should be treated to decrease left ventricular afterload and myocardial oxygen demand. The drug of choice for treatment of hypertension in the context of cardiac chest pain is nitroglycerin, which can be administered by an intravenous drip. Care should be taken to avoid abruptly decreasing blood pressure to normotensive levels in order to avoid the development of an ischemic stroke in patients with cerebrovascular disease. Nitroprusside, although the drug of choice in patients with hypertensive emergencies and aortic dissection, is not recommended in acute cardiac ischemic syndromes because it may induce a coronary steal and a secondary exacerbation of the myocardial ischemia. Nifedipine should never be used in patients with myocardial ischemia because it can produce profound and unpredictable decreases in the arterial blood pressure, worsening the ischemia and extending the myocardial infarction by decreasing coronary perfusion pressure and collateral flow. In addition, nifedipine is associated with a reflex tachycardia.

ANGINA PECTORIS

All patients with angina pectoris (see Chapter 7) should be evaluated thoroughly for the risk factors of coronary heart disease that are amenable to interventions (Table 8.1). Risk factors include

- Cigarette smoking
- Hypercholesterolemia
- Diabetes mellitus
- Hypertension
- Morbid obesity
- Hypothyroidism (vis-à-vis its association with hypercholesterolemia and accelerated atherosclerosis)

The only independent absolute risk factor for atherosclerosis is an elevated total cholesterol or low-density lipoprotein (LDL) cholesterol level with or without a low high-density lipoprotein (HDL) cholesterol level. The higher the total and LDL cholesterol levels, and the lower the HDL cholesterol level, the greater the risk for an atherosclerotic event. Patients with diabetes mellitus who have an increased incidence of coronary heart disease develop an atherogenic lipoprotein profile consisting of

- Elevated triglyceride levels
- Decreased HDL cholesterol levels
- Small and dense LDL cholesterol
- Normal or elevated LDL cholesterol levels

Stable Angina

The cause of angina is a mismatch of myocardial oxygen delivery to myocardial oxygen demand.

Diagnosis

Stable angina is diagnosed by the history of exertional substernal chest "pain" (e.g., discomfort, burning, and pressure) relieved by rest or nitroglycerin. The ECG obtained at the time of examination may be normal or may demonstrate ST-segment depression or T-wave inversion. The physical examination may be normal in patients with coronary artery disease, but the physical examination equivalent of hypertension (fundoscopic excess, bruits, S_4 gallop) and hypercholesterolemia (e.g., xanthelasma) should be sought.

The diagnosis can be confirmed with stress or pharmacologic thallium scanning or echocardiography.

Summary of Diagnosis

- Exertional substernal chest "pain" (e.g., pressure, heaviness, soreness, and burning) is relieved by rest and lasts less than 5 minutes.
- Physical examination may be unrewarding except in cases of aortic stenosis, pulmonary hypertension, diabetes, or hypercholesterolemia.
- On the ECG, look for Q waves of previous myocardial infarction, ST-segment depression, or T-wave inversion in an anatomical lead system.
- Chest radiography may be normal.
- Confirm results with stress thallium scanning or stress echocardiography.
- Clearly search for all risk factors to identify the high-risk patient.
- Coronary angiography may be necessary for a definitive diagnosis

Treatment

Patients who have had an atherosclerotic event should be receiving a lipid-lowering drug in order to reduce the total cholesterol level to less than 150 mg/dL, reduce the LDL cholesterol level to less than 100 mg/dL, and increase the HDL cholesterol level to greater than 35 mg/dL (see Chapter 21).

Smoking Cessation Patients must be convinced to quit smoking. The cessation of cigarette smoking results in a decreased risk for overall cardiovascular death; this decrease is greatest in the first few months after cessation but continues more gradually over the subsequent years.

Nutrition and Exercise The control of diabetes mellitus and the treatment of hypertension should be optimized. The patient should be provided with nutritional counseling, and an attempt should be made to achieve ideal body weight and get the patient involved in a regular exercise program.

Aspirin Aspirin is one of the most important interventions in the treatment of patients with atherosclerotic coronary heart disease. In patients with angina pectoris, aspirin has been shown to significantly decrease the incidence of a first myocardial infarction. Aspirin, in a dosage of 160 or 325 mg/d, should be administered to all patients with angina pectoris in the absence of contraindications.

Nitrates Nitrates have been the traditional pharmacologic treatment for patients with angina pectoris. Administered over the short term sublingually as a tablet or as an oral spray containing 0.4 mg, nitroglycerin results in a rapid decrease in the chest pain of angina. Patients with frequent episodes of angina pectoris should use a long-acting nitroglycerin preparation in the form of isosobide dinitrate or mononitrate; 8

consecutive nitrate-free hours should be allowed to prevent the onset of nitrate tolerance. This nitrate-free period is usually taken at night. If the patient develops nocturnal angina, however, the nitrate-free period should occur during the evening. Patients who have a predictable onset of angina during certain activities, such as sexual intercourse, should take a short-acting nitroglycerin preparation before engaging in this activity. Nitrate therapy can result in severe headaches and may be associated with postural hypotension, making some patients intolerant of their use. Viagra therapy is contraindicated in patients taking oral nitrates.

β-Blockers β-Blockers are especially useful in patients with exercise-induced angina and those with hyperadrenergic states. They decrease the heart rate and myocardial contractility both at rest and during exercise, thus protecting the myocardium during periods of increased sympathetic activity. These drugs also reduce the arterial blood pressure and, therefore, the afterload. The cardioselective β-blockers with no sympathomimetic activity, metoprolol and atenolol, are preferred. The dose of the β-blocker should be titrated to achieve a resting heart rate of 50 to 60 beats/min and a 70 to 80% reduction in the amount of tachycardia expected during a treadmill stress test. Because β-blockers may adversely affect the lipoprotein profile, these values should be regularly followed. Although they are usually well tolerated, β-blockers may produce bronchospam, heart block, depression, fatigue, constipation, and sexual dysfunction.

Calcium-Channel Blockers Calcium-channel blockers are especially useful in the following patients:

- Patients with hypertension
- Persons with angina who remain symptomatic despite the use of appropriately dosed aspirin, nitrates, and β-blockers
- Patients with Prinzmetal's variant angina
- Patients suspected of having coronary arterial spasm because of the presence of variable-threshold angina
- Patients who have contraindications to or cannot tolerate β-blockers

Calcium-channel blockers should be used with caution in patients who are already receiving a β-blocker. The potent arterial vasodilator amlodipine should be preferred. This drug is a long-acting dihydropyridine with minimal inotropic, chronotropic, and cardiac conduction effects and has a slow onset of action and minimal side effects. (Table 8.2 summarizes pharmacology in stable angina.)

Patients with angina pectoris who continue to be symptomatic despite intensive risk factor modification and a good medical therapeutic regimen should undergo a noninvasive stress imaging study. Cardiac catheterization should be reserved for patients with reversible myocardial perfusion defects or wall-motion abnormali-

TABLE 8.2. **Pharmacologic Therapy for Stable Angina**

Aspirin, 325 mg/d
Hydroxymethylglutaryl coenzyme A inhibitors ("statin" drugs)
  Lovastatin, 20–40 mg/d
  Simvastatin, 10–20 mg/d
  Pravastatin, 10–20 mg/d
Nitrates—both prophylactic therapeutic
  Sublingual nitroglycerin, 0.3–0.4 mg
  Oral isosorbide dinitrates, 20–40 mg three times daily
  Isosorbide mononitrate, 30–60 mg/d
  β-Blockers
    Metropolol, 50–100 mg/twice daily; extended release, 50–100 mg/d
    Atenolol, 50–100 mg
Calcium-channel blockers
  Avoid the short-acting, first-generation calcium-channel blockers
  Amlodipine, 5–10 mg/d
  Extended-release preparations—diltiazem, 100–300 mg/d

Summary of Treatment

- Nonpharmacologic treatment consists of lifestyle modifications—cessation of primary and secondary cigarette smoking; weight reduction; low-cholesterol diet; regular, graded exercise program.
- Hypertension and elevated cholesterol levels unresponsive to diet should be aggressively treated, with a target total cholesterol level less than 180 mg/dL and LDL cholesterol level less than 100 mg/dL.
- Pharmacologic treatment consists of aspirin, 325 mg/d; β-blockers (e.g., metoprolol, 50 mg twice daily) (added benefit in the hypertensive patient); nitrates for prophylaxis; long-acting calcium-channel blockers; sublingual nitroglycerin.
- Aspirin, β-blockers, and simvastatin have been shown to increase survival rates in this patient population.

ties, especially in the presence of a reduced left ventricular systolic function. Figure 8.1 presents a suggested strategy and management plan for patients with chronic, stable angina.

Unstable Angina

Unstable angina is caused by plaque rupture, thrombus formation, or subtotal occlusion of a coronary artery. Unstable angina may present as a new onset of angina at rest or on exertion or as an exacerbation of a preexisting anginal pattern. New-onset angina is associated with significantly limited ordinary physical activity occurring within 2 months of presentation. Rest angina occurs within 1 week of presentation. Patients with a known history of angina may present with a change in their anginal pattern, with angina occurring with increased frequency, lower exercise thresholds, or increased duration within 2 months of presentation. The pain of unstable angina can be prolonged, lasting more than 20 minutes, but its course usually fluctuates.

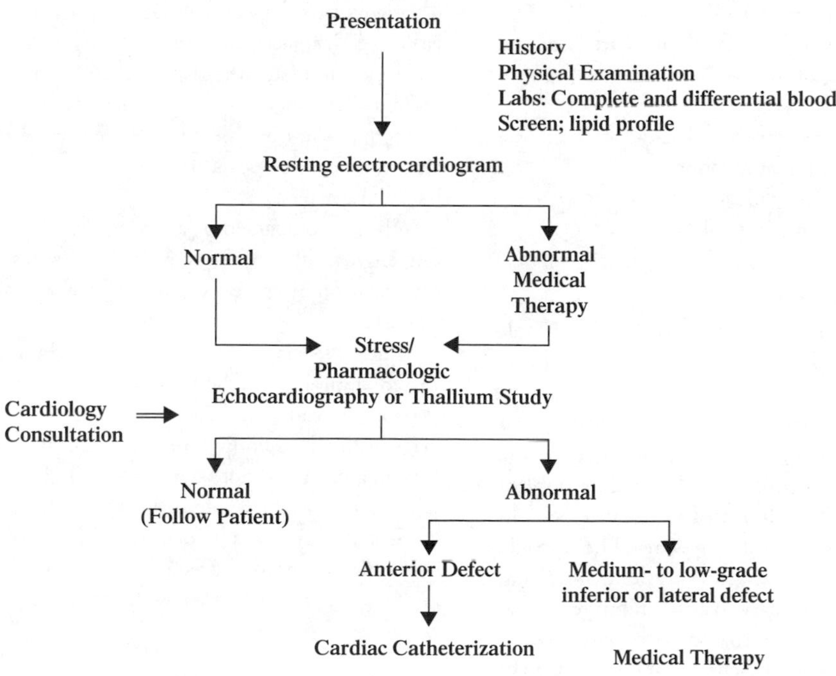

FIGURE 8.1.
Suggested strategy and management plan for chronic stable angina. CBC, complete blood count; Diff, differential; ECG, electrocardiography.

Unstable angina can be secondary to an increase in myocardial oxygen demand. The following conditions can manifest de novo in unstable angina or can be caused by unstable angina in patients with known coronary artery disease:

- Tachyarrhythmias
- Severe hypertension
- Anemia
- Hypoxia
- Exacerbations of chronic obstructive lung disease
- Pulmonary embolization
- Hyperthyroidism
- High output states
- Hyperadrenergic states
- Aortic stenosis
- Hypertrophic cardiomyopathy
- Cocaine abuse

Each of the aforementioned conditions must be ruled out in all patients presenting with angina.

Patients with unstable angina and the following conditions constitute a high-risk group:

- Known coronary artery disease
- Congestive heart failure
- Previous coronary angioplasty or bypass grafting
- Peripheral or cerebrovascular disease
- Diabetes mellitus at high risk for coronary artery disease
- Prolonged chest pain (lasting > 20 minutes)
- Rest pain
- ECG evidence of myocardial ischemia
- New onset of mitral regurgitation
- Acute congestive heart failure
- Develop hemodynamic instability

Physical Examination

The physical examination of patients with unstable angina may reveal a prominent A wave or Y descent on the jugular venous pulse, secondary to increased stiffness of the right ventricle induced by ischemia or a prominent V wave secondary to mitral regurgitation. There may be an S_3 or an S_4, which could be right or left sided, secondary to decreased ventricular compliance or increased end-diastolic pressures. The S_4 could be associated with a prominent presystolic apical impulse and could be secondary to acute mitral regurgitation. There may be a parasternal lift secondary to acute dilatation of either ventricle. The apical impulse may be diffuse. An early or mid-systolic murmur may end well before the aortic closure sound, which may radiate to the axilla or to the base of the heart, resulting from acute mitral regurgitation.

Summary of Diagnosis

- Frequency or severity of stable angina, new-onset rest angina, or nocturnal angina increases.
- The ECG shows new appearance of ST-segment depression or T-wave inversion in an anatomic lead system.
- Chest radiography may be normal.
- High index of suspicion should be engaged, especially in patients with several risk factors.
- Sestamibi scan is positive in the patient with chest pain.
- Stress thallium scanning or stress echocardiography should be done after pain resolves.

The ECG manifestations of unstable angina consist of the following:

- ST-segment depression
- T-wave inversion
- Tall, peaked, upright T waves
- Pseudonormalization of previously negative T waves

Multivessel coronary artery disease is more frequent in patients with ST-segment depressions than in those with no ST-segment changes. Deeply inverted T waves in anterior and lateral leads, with isoelectric or slightly elevated ST segments in leads V1 and V2, and depressed ST segments in leads V3 and V4 are usually associated with significant stenosis of the proximal left anterior descending artery.

When accompanied by a new onset of severely limiting angina, diffuse ST-segment depressions may be a manifestation of critical stenosis of the left main coronary artery.

When associated with prolonged chest pain, increased amplitude of the R waves and ST-segment depressions in leads V1, V2, and V3 represent the mirror image of the ECG findings of a posterior myocardial infarction and should not be misinterpreted as indicating ischemia or unstable angina.

Unstable angina is associated with a high risk for myocardial infarction; affected patients should be admitted to the hospital, preferably a coronary care unit, and treated aggressively.

Treatment

Aspirin Incidence of fatal and nonfatal myocardial infarctions is markedly decreased when the physician administers aspirin to patients with unstable angina. Aspirin should be given to all patients with unstable angina who have no contraindications to its use. Patients should receive 160 mg of soluble chewable aspirin during acute angina episodes and then 325 mg of enteric coated aspirin daily.

Intravenous Infusion of Nitroglycerin A continuous intravenous infusion of nitroglycerin should be started under the following circumstances:

- If the patient is still having chest pain after the first three tablets of sublingual nitroglycerin.
- If the chest pain is accompanied by significant ECG changes.
- If the patient is at high risk.

Nitroglycerin should be administered at 5 μg/min, and the dosage should be gradually increased every 5 minutes until the following occur:

- Chest pain has been relieved.
- Infusion rate of 300 μg/min has been reached.
- Severe intolerable headaches or hypotension develops.

Nitroglycerin decreases preload, ventricular end-diastolic wall tension, and coronary arterial spasm and inhibits platelet aggregation. Patients who are hemodynamically unable to tolerate nitroglycerin may benefit from the intravenous administration of normal saline before the reinstitution of the nitroglycerin drip. In previously normotensive patients, systolic blood pressure should be maintained above 90 mm Hg; in hypertensive patients, the mean arterial blood pressure should not be allowed to decrease by more than 30%. Tolerance to the effects of nitroglycerin depends on dose and duration of therapy and usually develops within 24 hours of the institution of the continuous infusion. Once the symptoms have been well controlled for 24 hours, the patient should be slowly weaned off intravenous nitroglycerin drip and should be administered an oral or topical nitrate preparation, with an 8-hour nitrate-free interval in dosing. If the symptoms are still not completely controlled at 24 hours or if the patient does not tolerate weaning from the nitroglycerin drip, continuous infusion should be continued at a higher dose to partially and transiently overcome the phenomenon of tolerance. In general, intravenous infusion of nitroglycerin should not last longer than 72 hours.

β-Blockers β-Blockers reduce the following:

- Heart rate
- Myocardial contractility
- Wall stress
- Sympathetic tone
- Blood pressure
- Afterload

In addition to their anti-ischemic effects, β-blockers have an antiarrhythmic effect secondary to an inhibition of pacemaker potentials and appear to stabilize unstable atherosclerotic plaques. However, because their use results in unopposed α-adrenergic vasoconstriction, they should not be used in patients with a history of cocaine abuse. β-Blockers significantly reduce the incidence of myocardial infarction in patients with unstable angina. The cardioselective β-blockers, metoprolol and atenolol, are preferred. These drugs can be used in patients with mild wheezing and chronic obstructive lung disease if the patients are carefully monitored for the onset of bronchospasm. In these patients, it is safer to start with half the usual dose of the β-blocker.

If there is any doubt about the safety of the longer-acting β-blockers (metoprolol has a half-life of 3 to 7 hours), a shorter-acting agent should be used. The effect of esmolol, which has a half-life of 9 minutes, resolves within 20 to 30 minutes after discontinuation of therapy. Patients with the following conditions should not receive β-blockers:

- Severe first-degree atrioventricular (AV) block with a P-R interval greater than 0.24 seconds
- Second- or third-degree AV block
- Severe left ventricular systolic dysfunction with congestive heart failure or shock

In patients with no contraindications, metoprolol should be administered intravenously over 1 to 2 minutes in three separate 5-mg doses administered 5 minutes apart. This should be followed 1 hour later by the institution of oral therapy with 25 to 50 mg of metoprolol administered every 6 hours. The target heart rate should be less than 60 beats/min.

Heparin Heparin therapy for unstable angina significantly reduces the rate of fatal and nonfatal myocardial infarctions, refractory angina, and death. Heparin forms a complex with antithrombin III, which markedly accelerates the inhibition of thrombin and therefore of fibrin formation and platelet activation. Heparin should be administered as an intravenous bolus of 5000 U, followed by a continuous infusion of 1000 U/h. An activated partial thromboplastin time should be obtained 6 hours after heparin therapy begins and 6 hours after each change in the infusion rate. The heparin infusion rate should be adjusted to achieve an activated partial thromboplastin time of 60 to 70 seconds.

Patients receiving infusions of heparin concomitantly with high doses of intravenous nitroglycerin develop a state of heparin resistance and require increasing amounts of heparin in order to maintain a therapeutic state of anticoagulation. When the nitroglycerin drip is discontinued in these patients, the extent of anticoagulation may significantly increase; this change must be carefully followed and corrected. The optimal duration of intravenous heparin therapy is unknown, although most available data show effective results with 3 to 5 days of therapy. Patients with unstable angina should continue to receive intravenous heparin for at least 3 days, preferably 5 days or until revascularization is performed. During the first 5 days of heparin therapy, platelet counts should be measured daily to monitor for heparin-induced thrombocytopenia. This condition occurs in up to 20% of patients but is severe in only 2%. Discontinuation of heparin therapy is associated with a significant increase in thrombin activity and a rebound in thrombotic and ischemic events. The heparin infusion may be gradually tapered over a period of several hours while the patient is being carefully observed for any manifestation of recurrent ischemia, although this has not been definitely proven to be effective. The following are not contraindications to heparin therapy:

- Recent surgery
- History of a bleeding peptic ulcer
- Peptic ulcer under therapy
- Menstruation

Calcium-Channel Blockers Calcium-channel blockers should be administered to the following patients:

- Patients who are still symptomatic despite all of the aforementioned measures
- Patients with Prinzmetal's variant angina
- Patients with a history of cocaine abuse
- Patients with persistent hypertension

Calcium-channel blocker with minimal negative inotropic effects, such as amlodipine, are recommended for patients with unstable angina.

Thrombolytic Therapy Thrombolytic therapy does not benefit and is not recommended for patients with unstable angina in the absence of an acute myocardial infarction with ST-segment elevations or left bundle-branch block.

To rule in or rule out the concomitant occurrence of a myocardial infarction, the total creatinine kinase, creatine kinase–MB, and troponin levels should be determined every 6 hours for the first 24 hours after admission of patients with unstable angina.

The following patients should have urgent cardiac catheterization and revascularization:

- Patients with persisting chest pain and accompanying ECG changes for more than 1 hour despite aggressive therapy that consisted of rapid and efficient implementation of all the therapeutic options described
- Patients with recurrent ischemic symptoms despite continuing intensive medical therapy
- Patients who respond to medical therapy but develop ischemic symptoms with minimal activity
- Patients who belong to the previously described high-risk group with unstable angina

The following patients have a nonurgent (intermediate) need for catheterization and revascularization:

- Patients with unstable angina who had prolonged rest or nocturnal chest pain or pain with minimal activity in the presence of a moderate or high probability of coronary artery disease
- Patients with ECG changes accompanying the anginal episode
- Patients with abnormal Q waves or ST-segment depressions in more than one coronary territory
- Elderly patients

Although patients in the intermediate-risk group could be managed conservatively and undergo noninvasive testing, they have such a high likelihood of coronary artery disease that they should undergo cardiac catheterization (see Table 8.3 for suggested management plan).

The low-risk group, which does not need catheterization, consists of the following:

- Patients who present with a new onset of angina
- Patients who present with an exacerbation of a preexisting anginal pattern, but without rest angina
- ECG changes or any feature of high or intermediate risk

Once stabilized and pain free while receiving oral therapy, low-risk patients can be referred after 48 to 72 hours for a noninvasive stress imaging study (see Table 8.3 for summary).

Summary of Treatment

- Rapid and efficient diagnosis is necessary for chest pain that lasts longer than 10 to 15 minutes and is not relieved by rest and nitroglycerin.
- Patients should be initially hospitalized, preferably in the coronary care unit.
- Morphine should be given to relieve pain, if still present.
- Systemic heparin therapy (with the activated partial thromboplastin time maintained between 60 and 75 seconds) should be given for at least 3 days.
- Nasal oxygen, β-blockers, and nitrates (cutaneous nitrate therapy initially) should be used. If the patient has never received nitrates, start low dosage because of the resultant headaches. Nitrate tolerance may be seen in patients receiving long-term oral nitrate therapy.
- Aspirin, 325 mg, should be given immediately (*regular* aspirin, not enteric coated aspirin).
- For recurrent pain, consider coronary angiography with possible percutaneous transluminal coronary angioplasty (PTCA) or coronary artery bypass surgery.

Management of the Patient with Unstable Angina — **TABLE 8.3.**

Admit to hospital
Bed rest, telemetry, nasal O_2, venous access
Aspirin, 160–325 mg immediately
Sublingual nitroglycerin, 0.4 mg three times, then as-necessary; intravenous nitroglycerin (5 μg/min)
β-Blockers if no contraindications are present (chronic obstructive pulmonary disease, asthma, wheezing)
  Metoprolol, 50–100 mg twice daily
  Atenolol, 50–100 mg twice daily
Intravenous heparin, 5000-U bolus followed by 1000 U/h. Maintained activated partial thrombolyplastin time between 60 and 70 seconds for 3–5 days
Persistent pain, consider amlodipine
Obtain total creatinine phosphokinase, creatine phosphokinase–MB, lactate dehydrogenase level, or troponin levels
With stabilization, schedule stress pharmacologic echocardiography or thallium scintigraphy
Cardiology consultation

MYOCARDIAL INFARCTION

Myocardial infarction is caused by plaque rupture, thrombus formation, and occlusion of a coronary artery.

Signs and Symptoms

Patients with acute myocardial infarction usually present with a sudden onset of severe precordial or substernal pain, which rapidly reaches its maximal intensity and is prolonged, lasting more than 20 minutes. Chest pain may be altogether absent. Some patients with acute myocardial infarction may present with:

- New onset of congestive heart failure
- Acute pulmonary edema
- Hypoxic respiratory failure requiring emergency intubation
- Syncope, which could be secondary to tachyarrhythmia or bradyarrhythmia

Other patients may present later with

- Cerebral or peripheral embolus
- Pericarditis
- Worsening congestive heart failure
- Severe weakness and fatigue

Patients with an acute inferior myocardial infarction may present with an epigastric and lower retrosternal–xiphoid discomfort, which they ascribe to "indigestion," associated with nausea, vomiting, and diarrhea.

The two principal questions to consider in any patient presenting with acute cardiac pain are the following:

1. Is this an acutely life-threatening condition, such as an acute aortic dissection with leakage in the pericardium?
2. Is the patient having an acute myocardial infarction? This event can be strongly suspected from the clinical presentation of the patient but can only be diagnosed by ECG.

ELECTROCARDIOGRAM

An ECG should be obtained with an isoelectric baseline. An ECG with a "wandering" baseline should not be accepted. The electrocardiograms should be repeated frequently in patients with nonspecific or nondiagnostic ECG changes, particularly in the presence of continued chest pain despite the implementation of therapy and in patients whose condition changes. It is helpful to procure previous ECGs, particularly in patients with known coronary artery disease. In the hyperacute phase of a myocardial infarction, the first ECG changes may consist of tall, peaked, symmetrical T waves and a straightening of the ST segments. However, the first ECG obtained after the patient's arrival may show nonspecific changes or minimal (< 0.5-mm) ST-segment elevations in one coronary territory, thus stressing the importance of frequently repeating the ECG. The ECG criteria for the diagnosis of acute myocardial infarction in a patient with chest pain are as follows:

- ST-segment elevation of at least 1 mm, measured 0.02 seconds after the J point, in two contiguous leads
- New pathologic Q waves, which must be at least 0.03 seconds wide and 0.2 mm deep
- New left bundle-branch block (more than 90% of the patients who had a 1-mm ST-segment elevation were proven to have a myocardial infarction; abnormal Q waves usually appear within 8 to 12 hours of symptom onset)

Patients with a posterior myocardial infarction present with an ECG mirror image of the ECG showing acute myocardial infarction, if it is recorded directly over the posterior left ventricular wall. The ECG criteria for a posterior myocardial infarction are

- R wave greater than or equal to 0.04 seconds in lead V1 and adjacent right precordial leads
- 1-mm or greater ST-segment depression in leads V1 and V2

Physical Examination

The cardiac examination may be normal or may reveal a diffuse apical impulse with a late systolic impulse produced by a dyskinetic or an akinetic myocardial region. There may be a parasternal heave secondary to ventricular dilatation. A presystolic apical impulse, reflecting atrial emptying in a stiff and noncompliant ventricle, may be detected. Particular attention should be paid to a decreased or absent S_1. This sound can be decreased by prolonged diastole secondary to bradycardia or by the presence of increased end-diastolic ventricular volumes secondary to left ventricular systolic dysfunction or to acute mitral regurgitation. It is decreased or absent in morbid or fatal conditions, such as acute dissection of the aortic root, whose diastolic regurgitation murmur may not have been systematically searched for and that may not be detected among the noise level generally present in the emergency department. An S_3 or S_4 may be detected, both secondary to increased stiffness of the ventricle. An early systolic to mid-systolic murmur, ending well before the aortic closure sound, is caused by acute mitral regurgitation secondary to papillary muscle dysfunction or rupture of a chorda tendinae. This murmur may radiate to the axilla or the base of the heart. In cases of right ventricular infarction, the stiff noncompliant right ventricle may be manifested by a prominent A wave or a prominent Y descent in the jugular venous pulse or by Kusmaul's sign. In addition, a right-sided S_3 or S_4 may be detected. A characteristic feature of patients with right ventricular infarction is presentation with cardiogenic shock in the absence of pulmonary edema and with increased jugular venous pressure.

Summary of Diagnosis

- History consists of prolonged chest pain that is unrelieved by rest and nitroglycerin and may be associated with diaphoresis, nausea, and vomiting.
- Physical examination reveals general "ill," diaphoretic appearance; patient reports "chest pain" (e.g., pressure and burning) with possible radiation to the jaw and left arm. Other findings are S4 gallop; basilar rales (rare); new murmur of mitral regurgitation; and S_3 gallop.
- The ECG shows ST-segment elevation in an anatomic lead with reciprocal ST-segment depression. The ECG is the cornerstone of diagnosis and must be performed and interpreted rapidly.
- Diagnosis is confirmed by serial enzyme levels: total creatine kinase, creatine kinase–MB, troponin, and lactate dehydrogenase.

Treatment

Because the left ventricular ejection fraction is the most important determinant of the long-term prognosis and survival of patients after an acute myocardial infarction, one of the main objectives in the treatment of patients with an acute myocardial infarction is to salvage as much myocardium as possible. This can be accomplished by early intravenous thrombolytic therapy or primary emergency coronary angioplasty. Therefore, once acute myocardial infarction has been diagnosed, the main issue to be resolved is whether the patient is a candidate for thrombolytic therapy.

Indications for Thrombolytic Therapy

Indications for thrombolytic therapy are chest pain lasting longer than 20 minutes and the following:

- ST-segment elevations of at least 1 mm in two contiguous leads
- Left bundle-branch block
- ST-segment depressions in leads V1 and V2 consistent with a posterior myocardial infarction
- Time : Onset of the pain to diagnosis of acute myocardial infarction
  - Less than 12 hours: all patients
  - Patients presenting 12 to 24 hours after the onset of pain
  - Patients with persistent chest pain and those at high risk.

Treatment Timing Because the evolution of myocardial necrosis in acute myocardial infarction and myocardial salvage after restoration of coronary blood flow are time dependent, thrombolytic therapy should be administered as soon as possible to patients who have no contraindication to this treatment. In a systematic overview of major trials, the Fibrinolytic Therapy Trialists' Collaborative Group reported that among 45,000 patients presenting with ST-segment elevation or left bundle-branch block, the relation between benefit and delay from symptom onset indicated a mortality reduction of about 30 per 1000 for patients presenting less than 1 to 6 hours after onset. The reduction was approximately 20 per 1000 for patients presenting 7 to 12 hours after onset, and a statistically uncertain benefit of about 10 per 1000 was seen for patients presenting at 13 to 18 hours. Although later treatment was associated with a larger excess of deaths on days 0 through 1, the mortality reduction on days 2 through 35 was little affected by the time of treatment.

During the evolution of acute myocardial infarction, a variable combination of coronary arterial thrombosis and vasoconstriction frequently results in spontaneous intermittent coronary artery recanalization and reocclusion. Spontaneous reperfusion of the occluded infarct-related artery occurs in 13 to 20% of patients and contributes to the limitation of the infarct size. These patients present with a longer duration of stuttering chest pain and may still have viable myocardium in the territory of the infarct-related artery. In the presence of collateral vessels to the infarct-related artery, the viability of the acutely ischemic myocardium may be preserved, especially at the periphery of the jeopardized territory. In these patients, the late administration of thrombolytic agents may salvage this ischemic but viable watershed zone.

Management of Patients with Acute Myocardial Infarction **TABLE 8.4.**

Acute management
- in the emergency department setting
  - Obtain ECG
  - Bed rest, telemetry, nasal O_2, venous access
  - Aspirin, 325 mg, and heparin
  - Intravenous morphine; nitroglycerin
- Obtain cardiology consultation
- Rapidly include or exclude the indications for thrombolytic therapy—ideal is less than 4–6 hours since the onset of pain
- Intravenous β-blockers
- Hospitalize, preferrably in a coronary care unit

Administration of thrombolytic combinations
- Accelerated tissue plasminogen activator: intravenous bolus of 15 mg followed by an infusion of 50 mg or 0.75 mg/kg of body weight over 30 minutes, then 35 mg or 0.5 mg/kg even 60 minutes for up to a total or 100 mg
- Intravenous heparin: 5000-U bolus followed by 100 U for 1 hour, with a target activated partial thromboplastin time of 60–70 seconds

Late restoration of the patency of the infarct-related artery is better than persistent occlusion. An open artery after a myocardial infarction is the most significant predictor of long-term survival in patients with single-vessel disease. Late administration of thrombolytic therapy in patients who continue to have chest pain with acute myocardial infarction involving a large territory will achieve the following by opening the infarct-related artery:

- Reduce the extent of left ventricular remodeling and cavity dilatation
- Decrease the electrical instability of the myocardium
- Provide a possible source of collateral flow to other coronary arterial territories

Table 8.4 describes suggested management plan of acute myocardial infarction.

Elderly Patients

The in-hospital mortality rate is much greater in older patients than in the overall group of patients with myocardial infarction; elderly patients have an approximately fourfold increased risk for death. The mortality rate in patients older than 80 years of age who are treated with streptokinase and aspirin decreases from 37 to 20%, a 46% reduction. The 30-day mortality rate in patients older than 75 years of age treated with accelerated tissue plasminogen activator (t-PA) and intravenous heparin is 19.1%, compared with a rate of 20.2% in those who received streptokinase and intravenous heparin. The respective 30-day mortality rates in patients 75 years of age or younger were 4.4% and 5.5%. Thus, although the relative mortality reduction after therapy with accelerated t-PA and intravenous heparin was smaller (6% compared with 20%) in patients older than 75 years of age, the absolute reduction was similar to that of patients 75 years or younger. Older patients receiving thrombolytic agents have an increased incidence of intracerebral hemorrhage and infarction compared with younger patients receiving accelerated t-PA and intravenous heparin. Patients older than 75 years of age have a 4% incidence of all strokes and a 2% incidence of hemorrhagic strokes, compared with the respective incidences of 1.2% and 0.5% in patients 75 years of age or younger. The incidence of combined 30-day mortality or nonfatal stroke in patients older than 75 years of age is 20.6% for those treated with accelerated t-PA and intravenous heparin and 21.5% for those treated with streptokinase and intravenous heparin. Among patients 75 years of age or younger, the combined incidence of death or nonfatal stroke was 5.2% for those treated with accelerated t-PA and intravenous heparin and 6.3% for those who received streptokinase and intravenous heparin, a 1.1% reduction. Thus, although the incidence of intracerebral hemorrhage and infarction is increased in patients older than 75 years of age who are treated with accelerated t-PA and intravenous heparin, there is a clear-cut favorable net clinical benefit, with fewer deaths and nonfatal strokes in patients 75 years of age (Table 8.5).

Contraindications to Thrombolytic Therapy

Absolute Contraindications

- Active internal bleeding
- Previous intracranial bleeding, cerebral neoplasm, or major intracranial abnormality
- Stroke or head trauma within preceding 6 months
- Known allergy to the thrombolytic agent

Relative Contraindications

- Surgery or gastrointestinal bleeding within preceding 2 months
- Pregnancy or within 1 month postpartum
- Severe, persistent hypertension (diastolic blood pressure > 100 mm Hg)
- Trauma, including cardiopulmonary resuscitation with rib fractures, within preceding 2 weeks
- Hemorrhagic retinopathy
- Bleeding diathesis or concurrent use of oral anticoagulants
- Active peptic ulcer disease

TABLE 8.5. Acute Myocardial Infarction in Older Patients*

Variable	> Age 75 Years	< Age 75 Years
Mortality rate	Accelerated t-PA plus intravenous heparin, 19.1%	Accelerated t-PA plus intravenous heparin, 4.4%
	Streptokinase plus intravenous heparin, 20.2%	Streptokinase plus intravenous heparin, 5.5%
Stroke Rate	Accelerated t-PA plus intravenous heparin, 4% of all strokes, 2% of hemorrhagic strokes	Accelerated t-PA plus intravenous heparin, 1.2% of all strokes, 0.5% of hemorrhagic strokes
30-day Mortality Rate with Stroke	Accelerated t-PA plus intravenous heparin, 20.6%	Accelerated t-PA plus intravenous, heparin, 5.2%
	Streptokinase plus intravenous heparin, 21.5%	Streptokinase plus intravenous heparin, 6.3%

t-PA, tissue plasminogen activator.
*Data taken from GUSTO (Global Utilization of Streptokinase and t-PA for Occluded Arteries) clinical trials.

HYPERTENSION Patients with acute myocardial infarction who present with hypertension should not be routinely excluded from thrombolytic therapy. Indeed, among patients who present with a systolic blood pressure greater than 175 mm Hg, streptokinase therapy results in a mortality rate of 5.7%; the rate was 8.7% in the placebo group.

Hypertensive patients whose systolic blood pressure decreases to less than 180 mm Hg and diastolic blood pressure decreases to less than 105 mm Hg after therapy with morphine, nitrates, and β-blockers should be considered for thrombolytic therapy. Those who remain severely hypertensive, with systolic blood pressure exceeding 200 mm Hg and diastolic blood pressure greater than 110 mm Hg, should be referred for cardiac catheterization and primary angioplasty.

CARDIOPULMONARY RESUSCITATION Patients who sustain a cardiac arrest and require less than 10 minutes of cardiopulmonary resuscitation should not be excluded from thrombolytic therapy, although they could be referred for primary angioplasty. Patients who had prolonged cardiopulmonary resuscitation or who have an altered mental state after cardiopulmonary resuscitation should be referred for primary angioplasty.

PEPTIC ULCER DISEASE A history of gastrointestinal bleeding in the preceding 2 months is a relative contraindication to thrombolytic therapy. However, because a well-treated peptic ulcer should heal within 1 month of initiation of therapy, patients with a treated peptic ulcer may be considered for thrombolytic therapy if they have had no evidence of bleeding in the preceding month.

OTHER RELATIVE CONTRAINDICATIONS Menstruation is not a contraindication to thrombolytic therapy. Puncture of a subclavian or jugular vein is not an absolute contraindication but can result in bleeding and airway compromise. Patients who have been receiving warfarin may be at increased risk for bleeding. In the presence of a left ventricular thrombus, thrombolytic therapy may result in embolization.

ACUTE MYOCARDIAL INFARCTION

Treatment

The initial management of patients with acute myocardial infarction should proceed according to the previously described initial management of the patient with chest pain, which should include the administration of oxygen, chewable aspirin, and sublingual nitroglycerin.

Thrombolytic Therapy

When an acute myocardial infarction is diagnosed by ECG, the first priority should be to determine whether the patient is a candidate for thrombolytic therapy. Before this is determined, morphine may be administered, nitroglycerin and heparin intravenous infusions should be started, and intravenous β-blocker therapy should be initiated as previously described for the treatment of unstable angina.

Aspirin reduces the incidence of reinfarction. During the first 6 weeks after myocardial infarction, β-blockers reduce the frequency of ventricular ectopy, atrial fibrillation, and nonfatal cardiac arrest; decrease the frequency of cardiac rupture; and reduce the incidence of recurrent myocardial ischemia and infarction. The prophylactic use of lidocaine is not recommended because it increases the risk for fatal asystolic events.

If contraindications to thrombolytic therapy exist, the patient should be immediately referred for emergency primary cardiac catheterization and angioplasty, if possible.

In the absence of contraindications to thrombolytic therapy, the accelerated t-PA regimen should be ordered and immediately administered. Accelerated t-PA is administered as an intravenous bolus of 15 mg, followed by an infusion of 50 mg or 0.75 mg/kg of body weight, over the next 30 minutes, and then by an infusion of 35 mg or 0.5 mg/kg, administered over 60 minutes, for a total of up to 100 mg given over 90 minutes. To ensure delivery of the thrombolytic agent to the thrombus in the infarct-related artery, adequate coronary perfusion pressure must be ensured and hypotension should be aggressively treated.

Heparin

Administration of the thrombolytic agent results in lysis of the thrombus and exposure of the various thrombogenic portions of the ruptured plaque, including its highly thrombogenic lipid core. Thrombolytic therapy also results in a marked activation of thrombin. Thus, the use of intravenous heparin is of paramount importance in inactivating the free thrombin formed in the vicinity of the lysing thrombus, thereby decreasing the incidence of reocclusion. Heparin should be administered as a 5000-U bolus, followed by an intravenous infusion of 1000 U/h. In patients who weigh less than 80 kg, the initial heparin infusion rate should be 800 U/kg. The activated partial thromboplastin time should be determined 6 hours after the initial infusion. The heparin infusion rate should be adjusted to achieve a target activated partial thromboplastin time of 60 to 70 seconds because at 12 hours from initiation of therapy, this range is associated with the lowest rates of death at 30 days, stroke, and bleeding. In patients who receive thrombolytic therapy, the lytic state can produce a transient coagulation defect that can prolong the activated partial thromboplastin time for up to 24 hours. Therefore, the heparin dose should be adjusted upward in the first 12 hours only if it is below the therapeutic range. The heparin infusion should be discontinued after 48 hours. However, certain indications dictate a prolonged course of heparin:

- Post–myocardial infarction angina
- Atrial fibrillation
- Left ventricular mural thrombus
- Severely depressed left ventricular systolic function
- Large anterior myocardial infarction
- Deep venous thrombosis

The main complication of thrombolytic therapy is bleeding, and the complication most likely to cause death is intracerebral hemorrhage. Stroke is associated with a mortality rate of 41% and a disability rate of 31%. The incidence of severe or life-threatening bleeding is significantly lower (0.9%) in patients administered accelerated t-PA and intravenous heparin than in those given streptokinase regimens (Table 8.5).

Concomitant Conditions

Right Ventricular Infarction

Patients with right ventricular infarction have a stiff, noncompliant ventricle that depends on high filling pressures; thus, these patients may not tolerate the reduction in preload induced by nitroglycerin. Cardiogenic shock associated with right ventricular infarction is characterized by high right atrial pressures and normal or low left ventricular filling pressures. Treatment involves the rapid administration of large volumes of fluid in order to achieve a pulmonary capillary wedge pressure of 18 to 20 mm Hg. Patients who remain hypotensive after volume loading may be treated with infusion of the inotropic agent dobutamine, insertion of an intraaortic balloon pump, and primary coronary angioplasty.

Previous Coronary Artery Bypass Grafting

Patients with acute myocardial infarction who previously had coronary artery bypass grafting (CABG) have significantly higher 24-hour, 30-day, and 1-year mortality rates than patients without previous CABG. Furthermore, patients who had previous CABG also have a significantly higher incidence of complications, including cardiogenic shock, pulmonary edema, recurrent ischemia, and reinfarction.

In about two-thirds of the patients with previous CABG who develop an acute myocardial infarction, the affected vessel is a vein graft, which is frequently occluded by a large thrombus. In a study of patients who had received intravenous thrombolytic therapy, successful reperfusion occurred in only two of eight grafts (25%) but intragraft thrombolysis or angioplasty restored flow in eight of 10 grafts (80%). In an acute myocardial infarction series of 130 patients with prior CABG, primary angioplasty had an 86% success rate in thrombosed vein grafts; the in-hospital mortality was similar in patients with or without previous CABG. If a cardiac catheterization laboratory can be quickly accessed, patients with acute myocardial infarction who have previously had CABG should undergo primary angioplasty. If no catheterization facilities are available, the patient should receive thrombolytic therapy.

Persistent Chest Pain

Persistence or recurrence of chest pain and the ECG manifestations of acute myocardial infarction after the administration of the thrombolytic agent and implementation of the adjunctive therapy is an indication for rescue angioplasty. Any occurrence of hemodynamic instability, cardiogenic shock, or acute pulmonary edema is an indication for emergency primary angioplasty or rescue angioplasty. (See Table 8.4 for a summary of the suggested management of patients with acute myocardial infarction.)

Complications

Heart Failure

The occurrence and severity of heart failure in patients with myocardial infarction is determined by the amount of ischemic dysfunctional myocardium and necrotic akinetic or dyskinetic myocardium and by the presence of an occluded infarct-related artery. Increasing left ventricular systolic dysfunction is associated with increasing mortality rates. In most patients, uncomplicated heart failure is transient and responds to a medical regimen consisting of intravenous nitroglycerin, diuresis, dobutamine, and angiotensin-converting enzyme inhibitors or angiotensin-receptor blockers. Invasive hemodynamic monitoring may be necessary in unresponsive patients and in those with pulmonary edema, hypotension, or evidence of systemic hypoperfusion.

Cardiogenic Shock

Cardiogenic shock is the leading cause of in-hospital death among patients with acute myocardial infarction. It is defined as systemic hypotension with evidence of end-organ hypoperfusion in the presence of elevated left ventricular filling pressures. Patients who present with or develop cardiogenic shock during their hospital stay should have an immediate cardiology consultation and be treated with vasopressors, inotropes, insertion of an intraaortic balloon pump, and emergency coronary arteriography and angioplasty. Cardiogenic shock could also be secondary to a mechanical complication of acute myocardial infarction.

Mechanical Complications

The appearance of any new systolic murmur should lead to a consideration of acute mitral regurgitation or ventricular septal defect. Although a precordial systolic thrill has been described in patients with ventricular septal ruptures, this sign should not be used as a criterion to differentiate between acute mitral regurgitation and a ventricular septal defect. Both of these conditions occur during the first week after myocardial infarction and may present as refractory acute pulmonary edema and cardiogenic shock.

Ventricular septal rupture and acute mitral regurgitation are more common with posterior myocardial infarctions, first infarctions, and single-vessel coronary artery disease. They are commonly associated with right ventricular infarction. Acute mitral regurgitation occurring during an acute myocardial infarction is usually secondary to papillary muscle dysfunction, although it can also be secondary to papillary muscle rupture, chordal rupture, or acute left ventricular dilatation. The posteromedial papillary muscle being supplied only by the posterior descending artery is more susceptible to ischemia and infarction than the anterolateral papillary muscle, which has a dual blood supply.

Although a systolic murmur can usually be heard by auscultation, in patients in shock the murmur may be undetectable. Both acute mitral regurgitation and ventricular septal rupture should be considered in any patient with myocardial infarction who presents with or develops congestive heart failure, acute pulmonary edema, or cardiogenic shock. Acute mitral regurgitation and ventricular septal rupture should be strongly suspected if cardiogenic shock is refractory to medical therapy, even in the absence of any systolic murmur. These patients should undergo emergency cardiology consultation, intraaortic balloon pump insertion, and cardiac catheterization and then should be promptly referred to surgery.

The occurrence of sudden electromechanical dissociation in the absence of any evidence of recurrent myocardial ischemia is the most common presentation of acute cardiac rupture. It occurs most commonly in elderly women, with small infarcts, first infarcts, and single-vessel disease within the first 2 weeks after myocardial infarction. The diagnosis requires a high index of suspicion. Emergency pericardiocentesis and thoracotomy offer the patient the only chance for survival; these patients have a poor outcome.

Pericarditis

Pericarditis can be secondary to inflammation of the pericardium overlying an area of transmural myocardial infarction or to an autoimmune reaction. It is usually transient and responds to aspirin therapy. Nonsteroidal anti-inflammatory drugs are not recommended for the pericarditis of acute myocardial infarction.

Left Ventricular Thrombus

Left ventricular thrombus is most common in large anterior myocardial infarctions and is most commonly located in the left ventricular apex, which is usually hypokinetic, dyskinetic, or aneurysmal. Patients with large anterior myocardial infarctions, severely reduced left ventricular systolic function, congestive heart failure or large aneurysmal or dyskinetic areas should receive anticoagulation for 3 to 6 months after myocardial infarction.

Electrical Complications

The most common rhythm seen after reperfusion with thrombolytic agents or angioplasty is an accelerated idioventricular rhythm, which is well tolerated in most patients, is transient, and does not require therapy.

Inferior myocardial infarctions are associated with an increased vagal tone resulting in conduction disturbances, which are usually transient and respond to atropine.

Sinus bradycardia and first-degree AV block are usually benign. Any bradycardia that is symptomatic and does not respond to atropine requires temporary transcutaneous or transvenous pacing.

Second-degree AV block type I is supranodal, whereas type II is infranodal and therefore associated with wide QRS complexes. Type I second-degree AV block should be treated only in the presence of hemodynamic compromise or severe bradycardia and worsening ischemia. Type II second-degree AV block progresses unpredictably to complete heart block in one-third of patients and thus requires the insertion of a temporary transvenous pacemaker in the presence of an anterior myocardial infarction.

The development of bundle-branch block in the setting of an acute myocardial infarction is usually associated with extensive myocardial damage. The occurrence of a right or left bundle-branch block with type II second-degree AV block in association with an anterior myocardial infarction is an indication for temporary pacing.

Complete heart block in the presence of an inferior myocardial infarction is usually transient and well tolerated and requires only that the patient be connected to a standby transcutaneous pacemaker. In the setting of an anterior myocardial infarction, however, complete heart block indicates extensive myocardial damage and requires a temporary transvenous pacemaker.

Atrial tachyarrhythmias may exacerbate myocardial ischemia and should be promptly treated. Atrial fibrillation or flutter associated with a rapid ventricular response and either hemodynamic compromise or increased myocardial ischemia should be treated with cardioversion. Ventricular premature beats do not need to be treated unless they become frequent, multiform and associated with short runs of nonsustained ventricular tachycardia. In this case, lidocaine should be administered.

The incidence of ventricular fibrillation is highest in the first hour after a myocardial infarction, and this event may occur without any warning arrhythmias. The patient should be immediately treated with cardioversion and administered lidocaine.

Torsade de pointes may occur in the setting of myocardial ischemia, especially in the presence of hypokalemia or hypomagnesemia. Torsade de pointes may terminate spontaneously or may require cardioversion or pace termination. The serum potassium level should be maintained at greater than 4.5 mEq/dL and additional magnesium should be administered intravenously, even in the presence of a normal serum magnesium level.

Summary of Treatment

- Immediate treatment consists of ECG; 325 mg of regular aspirin; nasal oxygen; and intravenous administration of morphine, 2 to 4 mg.
- The sooner thrombolytic therapy (e.g., t-PA and streptokinase) begins, the greater the success rate. Quickly check for contraindications.
- Emergency PTCA should be done if logistically possible.
- Patients should be transferred from the emergency department to a coronary care unit. Monitor patient carefully for supraventricular and ventricular rhythms.
- Intravenous lidocaine should be given for ventricular tachycardia. If patient is unresponsive, use direct-current cardioversion.
- Immediate defibrillation must be done for ventricular fibrillation. Institute cardiopulmonary resuscitation if necessary.
- For cardiogenic shock, cardiology consultation for consideration of emergency PTCA or intraaortic balloon counter-pulsation pump is necessary.
- In patients with recurrent pain, cardiology consultation for emergency coronary angiography for PTCA or coronary bypass surgery should be obtained.

KEY POINTS

Stable Angina

- Do not "underdiagnose" the condition. The perception of angina in women may be "atypical," varying from the textbook definition of angina.
- There is generally no risk for death in patients with costochondritis, esophagitis, or hiatal hernia.
- Lifestyle modifications require time and extensive education from the health care provider.
- Patients should be educated about the signs and symptoms progressing to unstable angina.
- Nitroglycerin administered sublingually can have a prophylactic benefit.
- Consider referral to the cardiologist for coronary angiography if the symptoms are not under control or if the symptoms progress or become intolerable; the goal is PTCA or coronary artery bypass surgery.

Unstable Angina

- The aim of the treatment of unstable angina is prevention of myocardial infarction. Unstable angina is not a "rule-out myocardial infarction" diagnosis but rather should be diagnosed to identify patients with unstable coronary artery anatomy and prevent the infarction.
- Present practice guidelines suggest stress thallium scanning or stress echocardiography at the completion of therapy. If no anterior perfusion defect is seen or if the result of an early exercise test is negative, these patients can be managed medically.
- An aggressive intervention with coronary angiography in this patient population may be considered.
- Begin therapy with lipid-lowering hydroxymethylglutaryl coenzyme A inhibitors ("statin" drugs) to prevent subsequent events.
- Patient education stressing lifestyle modification is crucial.

Myocardial Infarction

- Rapid diagnosis and initial therapy including thrombolytic agents should be started in the emergency department.
- Nursing staff in the coronary care unit should be trained in direct-current conversion, electrical defibrillation, and cardiopulmonary resuscitation.
- Minimal delay of thrombolytic therapy is critical because "Time is muscle loss."
- All patients with non–Q-wave and Q-wave myocardial infarctions probably deserve formal cardiology consultation.
- Length of stay in the coronary care unit depends on the presence or absence of complications: recurrent pain, ventricular tachycardia or ventricular fibrillation, mechanical problems for shock. If course is uncomplicated, length of stay should be 48 hours.
- An echocardiogram is recommended 7 to 13 days after myocardial infarction for evaluation of ventricular function: If left ventricular ejection fraction is less than 40%, begin angiotensin-converting enzyme inhibitor therapy (e.g., captopril, 50 mg three times daily).
- Medical education for a complex medical program after myocardial infarction: aspirin, β-blocker, angiotensin-converting enzyme inhibitors, long-acting nitrates, and "statin" drugs.
- Continue education regarding lifestyle modifications.

SUGGESTED READINGS

Abrams J, Vela BS, Coultas DB, et al. Coronary risk factors and their modification: lipids, smoking, hypertension, estrogen and the elderly. Curr Prob Cardiol 1995;20:533–610.

Ambrose JA. The open artery: beyond myocardial salvage. Am J Cardiol 193;72:85G–90G.

Brunwald E, et al. Unstable angina. Clinical practice guideline. Number 10. Washington, DC: U.S. Department of Health and Human Services. March 1994.

Cannon CP. Thrombin inhibitors in acute myocardial infarction. Cardiol Clin 1995;13:347–354.

Falk F, Fernandez-Ortiz A. Role of thrombosis in atherosclerosis. Am J Cardiol 1995;75:3B–11B.

Fuster V. Elucidating the role of plaque instability and rupture in acute coronary events. Am J Cardiol 1995;76:18C–23C.

Glentech, Inc. Summary of clinical data on accelerated dosing of activase (altephase, recombinant), a tissue plasminogen activator, in the treatment of acute myocardial infarction. The GUSTO Trial. March 1996;4:1–49.

Gotto AMJ. Lipid risk factors and the regression of atherosclerosis. Am J Cardiol 1995;76:3A–7A.

Kamat SG, Kleiman NS. Platelets and platelet inhibitors in acute myocardial infarction. Cardiol Clin 1995;13:435–447.

Moscucci M, Bates ER. Cardiogenic Shock. Cardiol Clin 1995;13:339–345.

Navab M, Fogelman AM, Berliner JA, et al. Pathogenesis of atherosclerosis. Am J Cardiol 1995;76:18C-23C.

O'Rourke RA. Management of patients after myocardial infarction and thrombolytic therapy. Curr Prob Cardiol 1964;19:179–226.

Simoons ML. Risk benefit of thrombolysis. Cardiol Clin 1995;13:391–406.

Theroux P, Lidon RM. Unstable angina: pathogenesis, diagnosis and treatment. Curr Prob Cardiol 1993;18:157–231.

Weitz JI. Activation of blood coagulation by plaque rupture: mechanisms and prevention. Am J Cardiol 1995;75: 18B–22B.

White HD. Selecting a thrombolytic agent. Cardiol Clin 1995; 13:421–433.

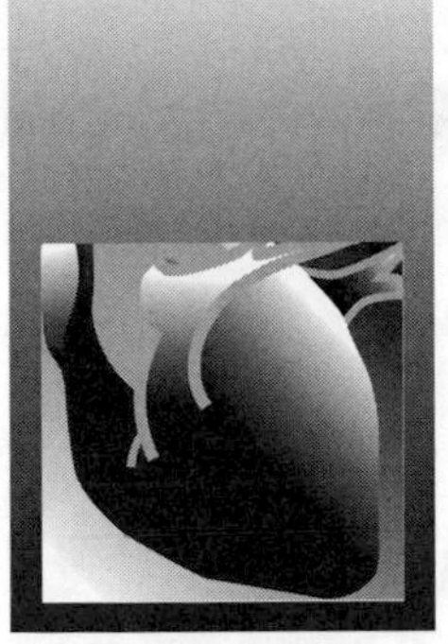

CHAPTER 9

Valvular Heart Disease

Walter H.J. Paulsen
James A. Arrowood

BACKGROUND

Members of a primary care team are in a unique position to apply their skills in the diagnosis and management of valvular heart disease. It is the primary care team who sees the patient, carefully evaluates the history, and auscultates a murmur. The team must then decide whether this murmur indicates disease (see Chapter 1, Physical Diagnosis), which evaluation should be done, how best to manage the patient, and when to refer the patient to a specialist. In this chapter, the authors focus on mitral and aortic valve disease and briefly discuss the less common tricuspid and pulmonic valve lesions.

AORTIC VALVE DISEASE

Left ventricular outflow may be obstructed above the aortic valve (supravalvular stenosis) or below the aortic valve (discrete subvalvular aortic stenosis). Obstruction may be caused by dynamic obstruction of hypertrophic obstructive cardiomyopathy (see Chapter 15) or may be localized at the aortic valve. The localized obstruction is the most common, followed by dynamic obstruction. All of the aforementioned present with a midsystolic ejection murmur but sometimes can be distinguished from the other obstructions by the location and other associated findings on auscultation and examination.

Aortic Stenosis

Causes

The most common cause of left ventricular outflow obstruction is valvular aortic stenosis, which may be acquired or congenital.

Acquired stenosis may be caused by commissural fusion and fibrosis of the valve cusps or by calcification of the cusps of the valve. Fusion and fibrosis are usually caused by inflammation. Calcification occurs when turbulent flow produced by abnormal valve architecture results in trauma to the cusps, leading to calcification and fibrosis and causing increased rigidity and narrowing of the orifice. From infancy through adolescence, aortic stenosis usually results from a congenital unicommissural, unicuspid valve. This condition is discovered in infancy in most patients with aortic stenosis, but some patients reach adulthood before marked signs or symptoms appear.

Calcification of a congenital bicuspid valve is the likely cause of aortic stenosis in persons 30 to 65 years of age. Beyond age 70 years, degenerative calcification of a tricuspid aortic valve is the most common cause. Rheumatic aortic valve disease is now a rare finding. In most persons older than 70 years, some degree of fibrosis and calcification of the valve cusps probably occurs because of years of normal mechanical stress. This usually does not cause significant stenosis but may result in a systolic murmur. In some patients, however, the cusps may become highly calcific, causing increased rigidity and symptom-producing stenosis. Calcific aortic stenosis is now the most frequently encountered type of aortic stenosis in patients requiring aortic valve replacement.

Pathophysiology

Gradually increasing obstruction to left ventricular ejection and its abnormal loading slowly causes changes to the left ventricle that eventually manifest in the symptoms associated with aortic stenosis. Increasing pressures in the left ventricle result in compensatory concentric hypertrophy of the left ventricle. This preserves systolic function and a normal cardiac output but increases left ventricular stiffness and abnormal diastolic filling. Elevated left ventricular end-diastolic pressures result; these increases, when transmitted back into the left atrium and lung vasculature, can cause symptoms of dyspnea. Because of difficulties in filling a stiffened ventricle with increased pressures, atrial contraction contributes an increasing percentage to filling the left ventricle and to the stroke volume compared with the normal ventricle. Loss of the normal, appropriately timed atrial contraction (atrial fibrillation) typically causes clinical deterioration.

Aortic stenosis also involves an imbalance between oxygen supply and demand to the myocardium. The hypertrophied left ventricle, the increased left ventricular systolic pressures, and the prolonged ejection time (it takes longer to eject a given stroke volume through a narrowed orifice) at the expense of diastolic filling time work together to increase myocardial oxygen consumption. In addition, because of the elevated left ventricular end-diastolic pressure, the pressure gradient between the aorta and the capillary bed is reduced, decreasing myocardial perfusion. As a result, the subendocardium may become ischemic; this may be responsible for the angina commonly observed in these patients. Left ventricular hypertrophy with a gradually increasing aortic gradient allows maintenance of cardiac output without left ventricular dilation or the development of symptoms. Systolic wall stress and contractility remain within the normal range during this compensated phase. Eventually, contractility of the myocardium decreases and systolic wall stress increases, producing a decrease in cardiac output and an elevation in left ventricular end-diastolic pressures. Corresponding elevations in pulmonary capillary pressures and eventual congestive heart failure result. When this occurs, the valve area is usually less than 0.4 cm^2 of body surface area and the mean transvalvular pressure gradient exceeds 50 mm Hg.

Signs and Symptoms

Patients with aortic stenosis remain asymptomatic until the valve orifice has become critically reduced (usually a valve area ≤ 1.0 cm^2). This occurs relatively late in the course of the disease, often in the sixth decade of life. Dyspnea and easy fatigabilty after unusual exertion are the most common initial symptoms. As the valve orifice narrows further, the left ventricle continues to become enlarged, pulmonary venous pressures increases, and the "terrible triad" of aortic stenosis develops: angina, congestive heart failure (dyspnea on usual effort), and syncope.

Exertional angina occurs in approximately two-thirds of patients with severe aortic stenosis and resembles that observed in patients with coronary artery disease. About half of the patients with severe aortic stenosis have concomitant significant coronary artery disease, which may contribute to chest pain. Syncope most often occurs with exertion and is caused by reduced cerebral perfusion when systemic vasodilation occurs in the presence of a cardiac output that cannot be increased because of the severe obstruction to outflow. In elderly patients with calcific aortic stenosis, coexisting cerebrovascular disease may also contribute to transient cerebral ischemia. These symptoms portend a poor prognosis unless the obstruction is relieved. Statistics indicate that the interval from onset of symptoms to death is approximately 5 years in patients with angina, 3 years in those with syncope, and 2 years in those with congestive heart failure. Patients with severe aortic stenosis may be asymptomatic for many years and have an excellent survival. Although the rate of sudden death in symptomatic patients approaches 15 to 20%, only about 4% of deaths occur suddenly in asymptomatic patients. One recent study followed 113 asymptomatic patients with moderate to severe aortic stenosis who ranged in age from 40 to 94 years (mean age, 70 years). Symptoms developed in 33% of patients within 2 years of diagnosis, and no sudden deaths occurred in 188 patient-years of follow-up. Finally, the obstruction of aortic stenosis tends to progress more rapidly in elderly patients who have degenerative calcific disease than in patients who have congenital or rheumatic disease.

Physical Examination

Physical findings in patients with aortic stenosis vary depending on the cause of the stenosis (rheumatic versus degenerative), the patient's age, and severity of the stenosis. Systemic systolic blood pressure may be elevated, especially in elderly patients who have inelastic arterial beds, but rarely exceed 180 mm Hg. The arterial pulse contour, best appreciated in the carotid arteries, increases slowly with delayed peak and is sustained (so-called pulsus parvus et tardus). When the stenosis is severe, systolic and pulse pressures are both reduced. The left ventricular apical impulse is usually not displaced beyond the midclavicular line except in the case of left ventricular failure; in this condition, it is displaced toward the anterior axillary line. A palpable systolic thrill, if present, is best elicited with the patient leaning forward in full expiration and is located in the right intercostal space or the supersternal notch.

The murmur of aortic stenosis is characteristically harsh, is crescendo–decrescendo in character, and is located at the base of the heart with transmission to the carotid arteries. The murmur usually terminates before A_2 (aortic component of the second heart sound); if the stenosis becomes severe and the valve cusps become less mobile, however, A_2 will diminish and may become inaudible, and the murmur may extend up to and through P_2 (pulmonary component of the second heart sound). In elderly patients with degenerative calcific aortic stenosis, the murmur may be more musical and higher pitched and more prominent at the apex or left sternal border. The murmur of aortic stenosis can be distinguished from the murmur of mitral regurgitation through its crescendo–decrescendo shape and its lack of radiation into the axilla. An aortic ejection sound (ejection click) very shortly after S_I occurs when the opening cusps are suddenly halted from their upward excursion. It is more likely to be heard when the cusps are mobile rather than rigid and thus is more likely to be present in children with congenital aortic stenosis than in elderly patients with the calcific degenerative form. One-third to one-half of patients with aortic stenosis have a blowing decrescendo diastolic murmur heard best at the left sternal border, indicating accompanying aortic insufficiency. With the onset of left ventricular failure after long-standing severe aortic stenosis, the cardiac output decreases and the murmur decreases in intensity and may disappear completely.

The clinical picture shifts to inadequate cardiac output and intractable heart failure. Critical aortic stenosis may not be easily recognizable with this presentation but should be actively sought in patients with severe heart failure of unknown cause because valve replacement may result in substantial clinical improvement.

Laboratory Testing

Electrocardiography With long-standing aortic stenosis, electrocardiography will probably show increased QRS amplitude and ST-segment and T-wave changes consistent with left ventricular hypertrophy. Conduction blocks ranging from first-degree atrioventricular block to left bundle-branch block may also be present if calcification of the valve has extended into the conduction system. This may occur from mitral annular calcification as well.

Chest Radiography Because left ventricular hypertrophy is concentric and occurs without chamber dilation, radiographically determined heart size is usually within normal limits. Calcification of the aortic valve, if present, cannot be identified with any certainty on plain films, but it may be seen with careful fluoroscopic examination. It is present in most patients older than 40 years of age who have severe valvular aortic stenosis. Long-standing aortic stenosis may also commonly produce post-stenotic dilation of the ascending aorta.

Echocardiography Echocardiography is the single most important examination that can be done in someone with a midsystolic ejection murmur and suspected aortic stenosis. Two-dimensional echocardiography can determine valve structure and leaflet mobility. It can also readily identify nonvalvular forms of aortic stenosis and the presence of hypertrophic obstructive cardiomyopathy. Estimates of end-diastolic and end-systolic chamber dimensions and ejection fraction can provide information about left ventricular function as well. Doppler techniques can accurately determine the severity of stenosis through measurement of transvalvular pressure gradients and valve areas and can identify and quantify concomitant mitral or aortic regurgitation. Serially obtained echocardiograms can provide information on disease progression in patients with nonsevere stenosis on initial examination.

Treatment

Echocardiography should be done in all patients in whom the initial history and physical examination suggest the possibility of aortic stenosis or other left ventricular outflow obstruction. Once aortic stenosis has been identified, the timing of surgery for relief of obstruction is of primary importance. In children and adolescents with noncalcific congenital aortic stenosis, commissural incision either under direct vision or with aortic balloon valvuloplasty may offer substantial hemodynamic improvement, with a mortality rate less than 1%. These procedures are indicated not only in symptomatic patients but also in asymptomatic patients with critical severe aortic stenosis (valve area < 0.75 cm^2/m of body surface area). Although hemodynamics are improved after surgery, the valve may remain anatomically abnormal, leading to restenosis after 10 to 20 years and necessitating reoperation.

Aortic Valve Replacement In symptomatic adults with severely reduced valve areas (< 0.70 cm^2 or < 0.4 cm^2/m of body surface area), valve replacement should be undertaken. This surgery should also be done in patients with severe aortic stenosis who are asymptomatic but have left ventricular dilation and dysfunction. In asymptomatic patients with severe aortic stenosis and no impairment of left ventricular function, studies have shown that survival is excellent as long as symptoms are absent. Because sudden death has been reported to occur in 3 to 5% of these patients, valve replacement in this group has been recommended. Asymptomatic patients with nonsevere aortic stenosis should be followed clinically for the development of symptoms or worse findings on examination, at which time echocardiography should be repeated. While under observation, these patients should be advised about appropriate antibiotic prophylaxis against bacterial endocarditis.

The surgical mortality rate for aortic valve replacement ranges between 2% and 8% in patients younger than 70 years of age who do not have left ventricular dysfunction. The risk increases with higher New York Heart Association class, increasing left ventricular dysfunction, age, and the presence of aortic insufficiency (Table 9.1). Long-term survival after surgery depends on similar factors and is generally excellent: survival rates of 80 to 85% at 5 years and 70 to 75% at 10 years. In most patients, symptoms and quality of life markedly improve. Aortic valve replacement in patients older than 70 or 80 years of age is being performed with increasing frequency because patients are living longer and the prognosis in patients who do not have surgery is so dismal. A Mayo Clinic study of 50 patients with a mean age of 77 years and critical aortic stenosis who refused surgery found that 57% were alive at 1 year and only 25% were alive at 3 years. Surgical mortality is higher in this group (10 to 15%), but long-term survival is not much different from that in younger patients (73% at 2 years). Thus, if the patient's general condition permits, aortic valve replacement is indicated for symptomatic elderly patients and age should not be considered a contraindication to operation.

Percutaneous Balloon Aortic Valvuloplasty In percutaneous balloon aortic valvuloplasty, one or more balloon dilation catheters are positioned across a stenotic aortic valve and then inflated. An attempt is made to fracture calcified nodules or to separate fused commissure to partially relieve the obstruction. Patient response varies, but the transaortic gradient initially decreases in most patients. Overall results have been poor because of high rates of restenosis (approximately 50% at 6 months) and high 1-year mortality rates (approximately 25%). In the adult, balloon aortic valvuloplasty is not a substitute for surgery and is indicated only in the following patients with critical aortic stenosis:

- Patients who require urgent noncardiac surgery
- Patients with severe heart failure or cardiogenic shock who have a high surgical risk, in whom valvuloplasty will be a bridge to aortic valve replacement
- Pregnant women with critical aortic stenosis
- Elderly patients in whom valvuloplasty will be a palliative measure because other organ system disease or life-threatening illness precludes surgery

Referral

In general, referral to a cardiologist is indicated if

- The patient is symptomatic.
- The patient is asymptomatic with severe stenosis.
- Diagnosis is unclear.

If surgery is indicated, coronary arteriography will be necessary in patients older than 40 years of age or those with angina. It is essential to determine coronary anatomy because coronary bypass surgery should be performed at the time of aortic valve replacement.

Discrete Subvalvular Aortic Stenosis

This lesion consists of a membrane of fibromuscular ring encircling the left ventricular outflow tract just beneath the base of the aortic valve. The lesion occurs twice as frequently in men as in women, and more than half of the patients have associated malformations. Patent ductus arteriosus, ventricular septal defect, and coarctation of the aorta are the most common malformations.

TABLE 9.1. New York Heart Association Classification for Patients with Congestive Heart Failure

Class	Description
I	Asymptomatic patients with ejection fraction $< 40\%$
II	Symptomatic patients with dyspnea on moderate exertion
III	Symptomatic patients with dyspnea on mild exertion
IV	Symptomatic patients with dyspnea at rest

Signs and Symptoms

Most patients present with symptoms similar to those of valvular aortic stenosis. The physical examination is also similar, except that an early systolic ejection click is usually absent and the early diastolic murmur of aortic regurgitation is more frequent. Aortic regurgitation is thought to occur because of trauma to the aortic valve cusps secondary to the high-velocity jet passing through the subvalvular obstruction.

Laboratory Testing

Echocardiography allows visualization of the obstruction and differentiation between valvular and subvalvular stenosis.

Treatment

Both the obstruction and the associated aortic regurgitation tend to be progressive, and the presence of even mild or moderate subaortic stenosis warrants consideration for elective excision of the membrane or fibrous ridge. Surgical outcome is usually excellent and totally curative in most patients, but progressive subaortic obstruction may recur, especially if residual tissue remains. Thus, long-term follow-up is necessary.

Supravalvular Aortic Stenosis

Usually unrecognized in children and young adults, supravalvular aortic stenosis is a congenital narrowing of the ascending aorta originating just superior to the sinuses of Valsalva, above the origins of the coronary arteries. It may be familial, may be transmitted as an autosomal dominant disorder with a variable expression, may be associated with elfin facies and mental retardation (Williams syndrome), or may be sporadic. All forms are usually associated with varying degrees of peripheral pulmonary artery stenosis. The form associated with mental retardation has been linked with idiopathic infantile hypercalcemia, but most patients recognized after infancy do not have hypercalcemia.

Signs and Symptoms

Presenting symptoms are similar to and have the same implication as symptoms of valvular aortic stenosis. Cardiac examination produces a midsystolic ejection murmur similar to that seen with valvular aortic stenosis, but no systolic ejection click is heard. There may also be a difference in pulses and arterial pressures between the two upper extremities, with systolic pressure in the right arm exceeding that in the left. This difference is attributed to selective streaming of blood into the inominate artery. If peripheral pulmonary artery stenosis coexists, a late systolic or continuous murmur may also be heard.

Laboratory Testing

Chest radiography and electrocardiography show no significant findings unless pulmonary artery stenosis has led to the development of right ventricular hypertrophy. Echocardiography can allow localization of the site of the obstruction, differentiation from valvular aortic stenosis, and estimation of the severity of the obstruction.

Treatment

With progressive obstruction, symptoms appear and sudden death becomes possible, a course similar to that of valvular aortic stenosis. The indications for cardiac catheterization in surgery are similar to those with valvular aortic stenosis.

Aortic Insufficiency

Causes

When the aortic valve becomes incompetent, blood regurgitates from the aorta into the left ventricle during diastole. Incompetence may be caused by disease of the aortic valve leaflets or the wall of the aortic root, or both. Acquired intrinsic diseases affecting the valve leaflets vary. Rheumatic fever results in inflammation of the cusps and then fibrosis, leading to cusp retraction and failure of opposition. Associated mitral valve involvement is common. Infective endocarditis may perforate or destroy a cusp or lead to a vegetation, thereby preventing proper cusp coaptation. A congenitally deformed bicuspid valve can result in incomplete closure and progressive regurgitation. Connective tissue diseases, such as Marfan's syndrome, Ehlers–Danlos syndrome, cystic medial necrosis, and myomatous degeneration, may directly affect the valve leaflets and have been observed with increasing frequency.

Diseases of the aorta may result in dilation of the aorta root and annulus, resulting in separation of the aortic cusps and regurgitation. These diseases include the following:

- Annuloaortic ectasia
- Cystic medial necrosis of the aorta (isolated or with Marfan's syndrome)
- Syphilitic aortitis

Connective tissue disorders that can be associated with aortic regurgitation include the following:

- Ankylosing spondylitis
- Systemic lupus erythematosus

- Reiter's syndrome
- Osteogenesis imperfecta
- Rheumatoid arthritis

Long-standing vascular disorders such as hypertension and atherosclerosis can also produce incompetence of the aortic valve. Acute regurgitation is most often caused by infective endocarditis, aortic dissection, or trauma to the aorta.

Pathophysiology

Chronic Aortic Regurgitation Regurgitation during diastole across an incompetent aortic valve increases filling of the left ventricle and imposes volume overload. The total stroke volume ejected by the ventricle (forward stroke volume plus volume that regurgitates back into the left ventricle) is increased in aortic regurgitation. In contrast to mitral regurgitation, in which a fraction of the stoke volume is directed into the low-pressure left atrium, in aortic regurgitation the entire stroke volume must be ejected into the high-pressure aorta. Because of the regurgitation, the aortic diastolic pressure is low (widened pulse pressure), thereby facilitating ventricular emptying. The major compensatory adaptation that allows ejection of an increased stroke volume, however, is left ventricular dilation. This increase in left ventricular end-diastolic volume allows this chamber to eject a larger stroke volume without requiring any increase in the relative shortening of each myofibril. Left ventricular dilation, however, increases the systolic wall tension required to develop a given level of systolic pressure to eject blood. As long as this wall tension is not too great, the ventricle remains compensated and forward stroke volume is maintained, with little increase in left ventricular end-diastolic pressure.

If the increased volume load on the ventricle continues or increases (worsening aortic regurgitation), left ventricular dilation increases, along with the requirement for an increase in systolic wall tension. When the myofibril cannot meet this demand, the ventricle begins to fail and forward stroke volume declines. This results in further left ventricular dilation and elevation in end-diastolic pressure. At first, left ventricular deterioration may precede the development of symptoms. With worsening function, pulmonary venous pressures may be highly elevated and forward cardiac output may be decreased. Symptoms ensue, first during the stress of exercise and then even at rest. Both left ventricular dilation and elevated systolic wall tension increase myocardial oxygen requirements. A major determinant of myocardial blood flow is the gradient between the aorta and coronary veins during diastole. Because aortic diastolic pressure is reduced in aortic regurgitation, coronary perfusion is reduced. This combination of increased oxygen demand and reduced supply may cause myocardial ischemia, which, in turn, may play a role in the deterioration of left ventricular function.

Acute Aortic Regurgitation Acute aortic regurgitation is usually caused by infective endocarditis (see Chapter 10), aortic dissection, and trauma to the aorta. With chronic aortic regurgitation, the left ventricle has had the opportunity to adapt slowly to the increased volume load, leading to the events described previously. With acute regurgitation, the volume overload is suddenly imposed on a normal-sized left ventricle, which cannot accommodate the large regurgitant volume. Marked elevation of left ventricular end-diastolic pressure with minimal left ventricular dilation occurs and may produce pulmonary venous hypertension and acute pulmonary edema. The pulse pressure is nearly normal, the heart rate is increased, forward cardiac output is reduced, and the left ventricular volume is only slightly increased.

Signs and Symptoms

Chronic Aortic Regurgitation With chronic aortic regurgitation and left ventricular volume overload, compensatory mechanisms allow the patient to remain asymptomatic for many years. As the left ventricle enlarges, patients may report uncomfortable sensations secondary to the ejection of a large left ventricular stroke volume with rapid diastolic run-off. Patients may describe prominent pulsations in the neck and awareness of the heart beat (especially when the patient lies on the left side) and disagreeable thoracic pain due to pounding of the heart against the chest wall. Tachycardia produced by exertion or emotional stress can produce palpitations and head pounding. Dizziness may be due to marked pressure changes with ejection and rapid diastolic run-off in the cerebral circulation. Syncope is rare, and angina is usually atypical. It may be prolonged or occur at rest or during the night because of the decreased coronary perfusion when the heart rate slows and arterial diastolic pressure decreases to extremely low levels. These symptoms may be present for many years before symptoms of overt left ventricular dysfunction develop. When frank symptoms do develop, exertional dyspnea, orthopnea, and paroxysmal nocturnal dyspnea are usually reported.

Acute Aortic Regurgitation With acute aortic regurgitation, patients most often develop sudden cardiovascular collapse with weakness, severe dyspnea, and hypotension.

Physical Examination

Findings on examination in chronic aortic regurgitation are due in part to the ejection of a large ventricular stroke volume with rapid diastolic run-off and are associated with many eponyms. The head may bob with each heart beat, and the peripheral pulse has a rapid rising upstroke followed by a quick collapse (Corrigan's or water hammer pulse). This pulse is readily apparent on inspection of the carotids but is also discovered by palpitation of the radial artery with the patient's arm elevated. Systolic blood pressure is elevated and diastolic pressure is abnormally low (usually < 50 mm Hg). A pulse pressure that does not exceed 50% of the peak systolic pressure or a diastolic pressure greater than 70 mm Hg usually indicates that the regurgitation is not severe unless left ventricular failure has developed. Several peripheral auscultatory findings confirm a widened pulse pressure:

- Traube's sign refers to the pistol shot-like systolic and diastolic sounds heard over the femoral or brachial artery.
- Müller's sign is credited with systolic pulsations of the uvula.
- Quincke's pulse is a systolic pulsation in the nail beds.
- Duroziez's sign is the systolic and diastolic murmur that can be created by compressing the femoral artery while auscultating in the groin.
- Hill's sign occurs when systolic pressure in the leg exceeds brachial artery pressure by more than 50 mm Hg.

The apical impulse is displaced inferiorally and laterally if severe regurgitation is present and the ventricle is dilated. If the apical impulse is not displaced, aortic regurgitation is usually mild. The murmur of aortic regurgitation is a high-frequency blowing decrescendo diastolic murmur. It is best heard along the left sternal border in the third and fourth intercostal space while the patient is sitting up and leaning forward with the breath held in expiration. The severity of the regurgitation correlates with the duration of the murmur rather than the intensity. A ventricular gallop heard at the apex may reflect an increased left ventricular end-systolic volume or left ventricular dysfunction. A mid or late diastolic rumble (low frequency) at the apex may be present. This murmur (Flint's murmur) occurs with severe aortic regurgitation and is generated when the mitral orifice is narrowed by impingement of the aortic regurgitant jet on the anterior mitral leaflet and the rapidly increasing left ventricular diastolic pressure caused by dual filling from the left atrium and aorta. A short midsystolic flow murmur may be audible along the left sternal border or primary aortic area and radiates to the carotids. It is probably related to the increased ejection rate and volume. With the acute onset of hemodynamically significant aortic regurgitation, patients are tachycardiac and hypotensive and exhibit signs of left heart failure. The pulse pressure is usually not as wide as that seen in chronic aortic regurgitation. The peripheral signs described previously are absent or significantly attenuated, usually because of intense vasoconstriction. The aortic diastolic murmur of acute aortic insufficiency is less audible than the murmur of chronic aortic regurgitation. Given that fact, the diagnosis may be overlooked or the severity underestimated. Bedside Doppler echocardiography is helpful in making this diagnosis.

Laboratory Testing

Electrocardiography With chronic aortic regurgitation, the electrocardiogram exhibits signs of left ventricular enlargement, including left axis deviation and left ventricular hypertrophy. In patients with acute aortic regurgitation due to bacterial endocarditis, the development of atrial ventricular block suggests a valve ring abscess. Periodic electrocardiography during the early stages of treatment is indicated to monitor the patient for this development.

Chest Radiography Cardiac enlargement, the most common finding with aortic regurgitation, is a function of the duration and severity of the regurgitation. Prominent dilation of the ascending aorta would suggest aortic root disease as the cause of the aortic regurgitation. Linear calcifications limited to the dilated ascending aorta should raise suspicion of syphilitic aortitis. In acute aortic regurgitation, heart size may be normal or only slightly increased despite marked pulmonary congestion and edema.

Echocardiography Two-dimensional Doppler echocardiography provides information to determine the causes of aortic regurgitation and aid in the management and follow-up of patients. This test provides an estimate of the severity of the regurgitation, along with left ventricular functions and end-systolic and diastolic dimensions. When Doppler echocardiography is performed serially, early changes in left ventricular dimensions and function can help determine the optimal time for aortic valve replacement. A prolapsed or flail cusp, vegetation, or dilated aortic root can suggest the cause of the aortic regurgitation. Transesophageal echocardiography can be helpful in identifying vegetations, valve ring abscesses (if conduction defects are present in the setting of endocarditis), or aortic dissection. This test can also help diagnose concomitant aortic stenosis or mitral valve disease.

Treatment

Chronic Aortic Regurgitation Mild or moderate chronic isolated aortic regurgitation is usually associated with a normal-sized left ventricle that has normal function, is well tolerated, and imparts an excellent prognosis. Eighty-five to 90% of patients with mild to moderate aortic regurgitation survive for 10 years after diagnosis. Even if severe or moderately severe, regurgitation with normal left ventricular size and function is well-tolerated and associated with a favorable prognosis for many years. Approximately 75% of patients survive for 5 years after diagnosis, and 50% survive for 10 years. When a patient becomes symptomatic, as in aortic stenosis, deterioration occurs rapidly and sudden death may occur. Survival without surgical treatment is usually less than 2 years after onset of congestive heart failure and less than 5 years after onset of angina.

A patient suspected of having aortic regurgitation requires a careful history, with attention paid to symptoms consistent with congestive heart failure (dyspnea, fatigue, angina), and a physical examination, with attention paid to a widened pulse pressure, peripheral signs, and signs of congestive heart failure. Echocardiography should be performed to quantify the regurgitation, determine left ventricular size and function, and aid in determining causes. This test will also serve as a baseline study for future follow-up should it be needed.

Determining the optimal time for aortic valve replacement or repair is the important clinical decision that must be made in patients with chronic aortic regurgitation. Three variables must be followed:

1. Severity of the regurgitation
2. Size and function of the left ventricle
3. Symptoms of the patient

Patients with moderate or less than moderate regurgitation almost always have a normal or mildly dilated left ventricle, are asymptomatic, and do not require surgery. They should be followed clinically and with echocardiography and require antibiotic prophylaxis against endocarditis.

Patients with severe or moderately severe regurgitation will need careful evaluation. If symptoms secondary to aortic regurgitation are present, aortic valve surgery will probably be necessary. If symptoms are absent but severe regurgitation is present, the state of the left ventricle determines when valve replacement is necessary. In these patients, the goal is to replace the valve before left ventricular dysfunction develops.

Acute Aortic Regurgitation When severe acute aortic regurgitation develops, patients often present with acute pulmonary edema and peripheral vascular collapse. Prompt aortic valve replacement is necessary. While the patient is being prepared for surgery, intravenous therapy with a positive inotropic agent (dobutamine or milrinone) or a vasodilator agent (nitroprusside) may be necessary. If infective endocarditis is diagnosed, blood cultures should be obtained and antibiotic therapy should be started immediately. If the patient is hemodynamically stable, surgery may be deferred for several days while these two measures are taken. At the earliest signs of hemodynamic deterioration, aortic valve replacement should be done.

The surgical treatment of aortic regurgitation and combined aortic stenosis and aortic regurgitation depends on the cause of the disease, the structure of the valve and aorta, and the age of the patient. Until recently, most patients underwent valve replacement with a mechanical or bioprosthetic valve, with the attendant risks of implantation of synthetic nonhuman material. Improved surgical options now include aortic valve repair, aortic homograft implantation, and aortic valve replacement with a pulmonary autograft. Because these surgical options involve only human material, they are expected to have a reduced incidence of valvular thrombosis and endocarditis and lower gradients compared with prosthetic valves. The feasibility of these options depends on the variables noted previously and the surgeon's experience.

The surgical risk for aortic valve replacement in patients with aortic regurgitation depends on the patient's age and general condition, whether left ventricular function is normal or depressed, the extent of coronary disease, and the skill and experience of the surgical team. The surgical mortality rate is low (1 to 2%) for uncomplicated cases with normal left ventricular function but increases with age and increasing left ventricular dysfunction. If endocarditis is present, surgical mortality rates may vary from 1 to 15% depending on the extent of annular destruction and the acuity of regurgitation. Long-term mortality rates increase if marked left ventricular enlargement and prolonged left ventricular dysfunction were present before surgery. This increase presumably results from an increased incidence of thromboembolic events, fatal arrhythmias, or chronic heart failure. Remodeling of the left ventricle (reduction in ventricular mass and fibrous content) takes place for up to 3 years after surgery, and improvement in function relates to the extent of preoperative compromise.

Referral

In general, patients should be referred to a cardiologist for the following indications:

- Confirmation of the diagnosis and assistance in determining cause
- Symptomatic chronic aortic regurgitation
- Asymptomatic patients with evidence of moderate to severe regurgitation
- Development of acute aortic regurgitation

MITRAL TRICUSPID AND PULMONIC VALVE DISEASE

Abnormalities of the mitral valve are due to congenital, rheumatic, connective tissue, degenerative, or infectious disease and range from minor distortion to severe stenosis or regurgitation. Complications are arrhythmias, thromboembolism, ventricular failure, and endocarditis.

Mitral Stenosis

Causes

The cause is rheumatic in 99% of mitral stenosis cases and congenital in 1%. It is the most common valve lesion caused by rheumatic fever and is four times as frequent in females as in males. Fifty percent of patients with mitral stenosis have no history of acute rheumatic fever; these patients experience a subclinical attack of the disease.

Pathophysiology

Rheumatic mitral stenosis leads to progressive thickening and fibrosis of the valve leaflets and chordae tendineae, resulting in significant stenosis (valve area < 1.5 cm^2) by the age of 30 to 40 years (earlier in developing countries). The hemodynamic consequences are as follows:

- Reduced cardiac output
- Diastolic gradient across the mitral valve
- Elevation of left atrial and pulmonary venous pressures leading to
  - Dyspnea
  - Pulmonary congestion
  - Edema
- Vascular changes in the lungs that lead to pulmonary arterial hypertension and to right ventricular failure

Signs and Symptoms

Cardiac auscultation typically reveals a loud S_1 and an opening snap, followed by a mid- to late-apical diastolic rumble with presystolic accentuation. If pulmonary hypertension has supervened, a loud P_2 emerges.

Laboratory Testing

Chest radiography reveals left atrial enlargement, pulmonary congestion, pulmonary hypertension, and right ventricular enlargement.

Electrocardiography may show left atrial enlargement, atrial fibrillation, and right ventricular enlargement. Transthoracic echocardiography allows reliable noninvasive evaluation of the following:

- Severity of mitral stenosis
- Left atrial size
- Degree of pulmonary hypertension
- Right ventricular function
- Suitability of the mitral valve for valvotomy (commissurotomy)
- Presence of coexisting valve lesions

Transesophageal echocardiography can detect left atrial thrombi and may provide additional information on valve structure.

Cardiac catheterization confirms the hemodynamic data provided by echocardiography and reveals the state of the coronary arteries.

Treatment

Management consists of the following:

- Prevention of recurrent rheumatic fever with penicillin or sulphonamides for at least 5 years after the last attack of rheumatic fever and preferably until age 35 years
- Control of tachycardia with digoxin, aided if necessary by β-blocker or calcium-channel blockers
- Control of pulmonary congestion with a diuretic
- Prevention of endocarditis using antibiotic prophylaxis
- Anticoagulation to prevent or treat thromboembolism. Unless specifically contraindicated, anticoagulants should be administered to all patients in atrial fibrillation and to all patients who have experienced an embolic phenomenon (regardless of rhythm); they should be seriously considered in patients in sinus rhythm with a significantly enlarged left atrium (transthoracic echocardiographic diameter > 55 mm). Patients who have experienced an embolic phe-

nomenon should have transesophageal echocardiography, which can detect left atrial thrombi with high sensitivity and may assist in optimizing management.

- Mechanical intervention is indicated in patients with New York Heart Association class III or IV symptoms (who invariably have a valve area ≤ 1.0 cm²). In active patients or large patients, somewhat larger valve areas (1.0 to 1.3 cm²) can produce substantial symptoms and morbidity. Intervention is indicated to relieve symptoms and improve survival. The procedure of choice is percutaneous valvotomy if the valve is morphologically suitable (pliable and noncalcified) and no more than minimal mitral regurgitation is present. The suitability for valvotomy can be reliably assessed by transthoracic echocardiography, but transesophageal echocardiography should be performed before percutaneous valvotomy to exclude the presence of left atrial thrombus. Patients whose mitral valves are not suitable for valvotomy should undergo valve replacement.

Chronic Mitral Regurgitation

Causes

The causes of chronic mitral regurgitation include congenital factors, rheumatic heart disease, myxomatous degeneration, connective tissue disorders, ischemic heart disease, and left ventricular dilation. The latter usually causes mild regurgitation but sometimes leads to severe regurgitation.

Pathophysiology

Mitral regurgitation leads to the loss of a portion of the left ventricular stroke volume into the left atrium, which should result in a decreased forward cardiac output. However, the ventricle compensates by becoming dilated and enlarged, which preserves the normal forward cardiac output. This, coupled with the development of an enlarged and compliant left atrium, allows patients to remain asymptomatic for many years. Eventually, however, left ventricular volume overload progresses to the point at which the ventricle can no longer compensate. As a result, left ventricular systolic function decreases, forward cardiac output falls, and left atrial and pulmonary venous pressures increase, leading to left heart failure. Pulmonary arterial hypertension may develop, resulting in right ventricular failure and the emergence of right heart failure.

Signs and Symptoms

Cardiac auscultation usually reveals an apical S_3 and a high-pitched apical pansystolic murmur that radiates to the left axilla.

Laboratory Testing

Electrocardiographic findings may include left atrial and left ventricular hypertrophy and atrial fibrillation. Chest radiography shows left ventricular and left atrial enlargement and evidence of pulmonary congestion or edema. Echocardiography provides important information on mitral valve structure that often reflects the cause of the regurgitation and provides reliable estimates of the degree of regurgitation, left ventricular and atrial sizes, left ventricular ejection fraction, and pulmonary artery systolic pressure. Cardiac catheterization confirms the echocardiographic data and reveals the presence or absence of coronary artery disease.

Treatment

Management consists of prophylaxis against endocarditis, vasodilators to reduce left ventricular afterload and improve forward stroke volume, diuretics to reduce left ventricular preload, and digoxin, antiarrhythmic agents, and anticoagulants for the management of atrial fibrillation and the appropriate timing of surgical intervention.

Indications for surgery are lack of symptom response to medical therapy and/or the development of left ventricular dysfunction. However, evaluation of left ventricular function in chronic mitral regurgitation is problematic when standard clinical estimates of left ventricular function, such as ejection fraction, are used.

Chronic mitral regurgitation is associated with loading conditions (increased preload and decreased afterload) that elevate the ejection-phase indices of left ventricular function. This obscures a true reduction of myocardial contractility before surgery. Reduction of contractility becomes evident only after surgical correction of the regurgitation. Because the run-off into the low resistance left atrium is abolished by surgery, left ventricular afterload is increased and the artificially elevated ejection fraction decreases to its true valve. It is therefore necessary to "correct" left ventricular ejection fraction for left ventricular afterload in order to properly gauge preoperative contractile function. In practice, the complex methods involved in performing this correction are too tedious and time-consuming to be easily clinically applicable. Therefore, retrospective studies have been used to identify preoperative measures of left ventricular dysfunction that can be used easily in clinical practice. Thus, low normal or mildly depressed left ventricular ejection fraction should signal the need for surgical intervention to prevent irreversible left ventricular dysfunction. The surgical treatment is mitral valve repair or replacement. If the valve is amenable to repair (i.e., mobile and noncalcified), then repair should be considered. Compelling evidence now suggests that repair in properly selected patients is associated with a lower surgical mortality rate, a lower rate of valve-related complications, and better long-term survival than valve replacement.

Acute Mitral Regurgitation

Pathophysiology

The causes of acute mitral regurgitation represent acute manifestations of disease processes that cause chronic regurgitation and commonly include disruption of valve leaflets or rupture of chordae tendineae due to endocarditis, ischemic dysfunction, or rupture of a papillary muscle. The sudden development of severe mitral regurgitation does not provide any time for the left heart to adapt to accommodate the augmented volume. The severe regurgitation into an unprepared nondilated and noncompliant left atrium markedly increases left atrial and pulmonary venous pressures and causes the abrupt onset of pulmonary edema. Because the left atrial pressure in late systole is markedly elevated as a result of the large systolic regurgitation, the pressure gradient in late systole between the ventricle and atrium declines and the systolic murmur may be decrescendo rather than pansystolic, as in chronic mitral regurgitation.

Signs and Symptoms

Electrocardiography or radiography may show no evidence of left heart enlargement. Echocardiography (transthoracic and transesophageal) reveals severe mitral regurgitation and can reliably evaluate valve structure, which usually clarifies the cause of the regurgitation. The left atrium and ventricle are not enlarged, and the left ventricular ejection fraction may be normal or even supranormal.

Treatment

Treatment consists of measures to reduce left ventricular afterload, such as vasodilators or the intraaortic balloon pump. Diuretics are used to reduce preload so that the patient is stabilized sufficiently to safely undergo cardiac catheterization, if necessary as a prelude to mitral valve repair or replacement.

TRICUSPID VALVE

Abnormalities of the tricuspid valve can be classified as functional or organic. In functional derangement, a common abnormality, the tricuspid valve is structurally normal but the dilation of the right ventricle from any cause is accompanied by dilation of the tricuspid annulus, which leads to regurgitation. Organic causes of tricuspid valve disease are uncommon and include congenital, infectious, rheumatic diseases, carcinoid syndrome, and trauma.

Tricuspid Stenosis

Causes

The most common cause of tricuspid stenosis is rheumatic, usually with concomitant involvement of the mitral valve. Carcinoid syndrome and congenital disorders are uncommon.

Pathophysiology

The tricuspid valve significantly obstructs right ventricular filling when the normal valve area (approximately 7.0 cm^2) is reduced to less than 1.5 cm^2. This leads to a reduction of forward cardiac output, an elevated right atrial pressure, and a diastolic gradient across the tricuspid valve. Patients present with fatigue (low cardiac output), systemic venous congestion, and atrial fibrillation.

Signs and Symptoms

Cardiac auscultation is remarkable for a diastolic rumble that is best heard at the left lower sternal border and that increases with inspiration.

Laboratory Testing

Electrocardiography and chest radiography reveal right atrial prominence. Echocardiography displays the valve structure and reliably estimates the degree of stenosis and right atrial dilation. Cardiac catheterization confirms the echocardiographic data and defines coronary anatomy.

Treatment

Management consists of appropriate antibiotic prophylaxis against recurrent rheumatic fever and endocarditis, diuretics and digoxin for control of systemic venous congestion, and appropriate drugs for control of tachycardia and management of atrial fibrillation. Mechanical intervention is indicated for New York Heart Association class III or IV symptoms, which are usually associated with a valve area less than 1.5 cm^2. Traditional intervention is surgical tricuspid valve valvotomy (commissurotomy) or valve replacement. However, recent preliminary work suggests that percutaneous valvotomy may be an option in selected cases.

Because tricuspid stenosis is commonly associated with lesions of the mitral and aortic valves, its management is frequently accompanied by management of the concomitant left heart abnormality.

Tricuspid Regurgitation

Causes

The cause of tricuspid regurgitation is usually functional (i.e., secondary to right ventricular failure of any cause), most commonly as a result of left heart abnormality or pulmonary hypertension. Other causes include rheumatic, infective, and congenital diseases and trauma.

Pathophysiology

The systolic regurgitation into the right atrium elevates right atrial and systemic venous pressure and reduces forward cardiac output. The adaptive mechanisms and the problems related to estimating right ventricular myocardial contractility are similar to those described for mitral regurgitation.

Signs and Symptoms

Patients present with fatigue (low cardiac output) and systemic venous congestion manifested as dependent edema, elevated jugular venous pressure, hepatic enlargement, and ascites. The tricuspid regurgitation results in the transmission of the right ventricular pressure pulse to the right atrium and the great veins imparting a prominent systolic wave to the jugular veins and liver. Auscultation is remarkable for a pansystolic murmur that is maximally heard at the lower end of the sternum and is louder on inspiration.

Laboratory Testing

Electrocardiography usually demonstrates right ventricular and atrial enlargement and, frequently, atrial fibrillation. Chest radiography typically reveals cardiomegaly with right atrial and ventricular prominence. Echocardiography shows the structure of the tricuspid valve, thereby allowing distinction between the structurally normal valve of functional regurgitation and the intrinsically abnormal valve of organic regurgitation. This test can also reliably estimate the severity of the regurgitation, the degree of dilation of right heart chambers, and the pulmonary artery systolic pressure; it can also provide useful information on right ventricular function. Cardiac catheterization provides information on coronary anatomy and confirms the echocardiographic findings.

Treatment

In the absence of increased pulmonary vascular resistance and in the presence of normal right ventricular function and sinus rhythm, tricuspid regurgitation is well tolerated and responds to medical therapy for long periods. Medical treatment consists of fluid restriction, diuretics, afterload-reducing drugs, management of atrial fibrillation, and prophylaxis against endocarditis. If pulmonary vascular resistance is elevated and right ventricular failure has supervened, however, functional tricuspid regurgitation leads to inescapable and progressive right heart failure that may only respond to correction of the left-sided abnormality that is the cause of the pulmonary hypertension. If tricuspid regurgitation is functional, the presentation and findings are intertwined with the antecedent left heart abnormality.

Indications for surgery (tricuspid valve annuloplasty or replacement) are symptoms of right ventricular failure unresponsive to optimum medical therapy. If the patient with functional tricuspid regurgitation is undergoing surgical correction of the left-sided lesion, the physician must decide whether to perform no procedure on the tricuspid valve, anticipating improvement with the expected decrease in pulmonary pressures, or to proceed with a tricuspid operation. Intraoperative transesophageal echocardiographic quantification of residual tricuspid regurgitation after correction of the left-sided abnormality can aid in determining the necessity of tricuspid valve surgery when the preoperative findings are ambiguous.

PULMONIC VALVE

Congenital abnormalities are the most common cause of pulmonic valve disease. Acquired causes are less common and include functional disorders, rheumatic heart disease, infective endocarditis, and the carcinoid syndrome.

Pulmonic Stenosis

Causes

The cause of pulmonic stenosis is usually congenital; rheumatic heart disease and the carcinoid syndrome are rare.

Pathophysiology

Stenosis of the pulmonic valve creates an obstruction to right ventricular ejection that the ventricle overcomes by generating a higher than normal pressure during systole. This results in a pressure gradient across the valve. The right ventricle compensates for the increased pressure load by developing concentric hypertrophy, which normalizes wall stress and thereby maintains a normal ejection fraction and forward cardiac output. Secondary hypertrophy of the right ventricle is particularly marked in the infundibular (subvalvar) region, resulting in dynamic narrowing of this area during systole and leading to a component of infundibular stenosis in addition to the valvular stenosis. As the pulmonic stenosis progresses, the increased right ventricular pressure outstrips the ability of the ventricle to enlarge, wall stress increases, ejection fraction and cardiac output decrease, and right ventricular failure and right heart failure result.

Signs and Symptoms

Clinical examination is remarkable for a parasternal (right ventricular) heave, a pulmonary ejection click, a pulmonary ejection murmur, and a delayed and soft P_2.

Laboratory Testing

Electrocardiography reveals right ventricular hypertrophy and right atrial hypertrophy. Chest radiography reveals a prominent pulmonary artery that results from post-stenotic dilatation distal to the valve. Echocardiography provides reliable information on pulmonic valve structure; severity of the stenosis; and estimates of right ventricular dimensions, function, and peak systolic pressure. Cardiac catheterization confirms the echocardiographic data and provides information on coronary anatomy.

Treatment

Mild pulmonic stenosis (peak systolic transvalvular pressure gradient < 50 mm Hg) is usually asymptomatic, whereas moderate (peak systolic pressure gradient, 50 to 79 mm Hg) and severe (peak systolic pressure gradient > 80 mm Hg) stenosis may be associated with exertional dyspnea, chest pain, atrial and ventricular arrhythmias, hypoxic spells, and right ventricular failure.

Medical management is indicated for patients with mild stenosis, who are usually asymptomatic or minimally symptomatic, and consists of prophylaxis against endocarditis and periodic surveillance. Mechanical intervention, consisting of percutaneous balloon valvotomy, surgical valvotomy, or valve replacement, is indicated in patients with symptomatic moderate stenosis and in all patients with severe stenosis, regardless of symptoms. The initial procedure of choice is percutaneous balloon valvotomy, which achieves results that are similar to those seen with traditional surgical valvotomy. Infundibular gradients usually resolve over time with either procedure.

Pulmonic Regurgitation

Causes

The cause of pulmonic regurgitation is commonly functional; a structurally normal valve is incompetent because of dilation of the pulmonic valve annulus, usually as a result of pulmonary hypertension from any cause or, less commonly, of idiopathic dilation of the pulmonary artery and annulus. Other causes include congenital absence of the pulmonic valve, major disruption of valve integrity as a result of valvotomy (for pulmonic stenosis), and destruction of the valve by infective endocarditis.

Pathophysiology

As a result of the incompetence of the pulmonic valve during diastole, the right ventricle fills with the regurgitant blood from the pulmonary artery plus the blood received from the right atrium. To accommodate this increased preload, the right ventricle dilates and enlarges, thereby maintaining normal systolic wall stress. The systolic stroke volume is increased to compensate for the proportion that regurgitates into the ventricle during diastole, thereby preserving a normal right ventricular forward output.

Signs and Symptoms

The increased stroke volume generates a systolic ejection murmur, and the regurgitation jet generates a short early diastolic murmur, both of which are heard maximally in the pulmonic area and are accentuated by inspiration. Right ventricular dilation may cause a right parasternal heave, and electrocardiography and chest radiography show the right ventricular hypertrophy and dilation.

Laboratory Testing

Echocardiography provides reliable information on pulmonic valve structure, the severity of regurgitation, estimates of right ventricular size and function, the severity of any concomitant tricuspid regurgitation, and an estimate of the right ventricular peak systolic pressure and pulmonary artery systolic pressure. Cardiac catheterization confirms the hemodynamic data and provides information on coronary anatomy.

Treatment

Isolated pulmonic regurgitation with a normal pulmonary artery pressure is well tolerated for long periods; in such cases, therapy consists of prophylaxis against prophylaxis and periodic surveillance. In contrast, the presence of pulmonary hypertension tends to increase the severity of pulmonic regurgitation, which exceeds the compensatory reserve of the right ventricle and leads to right ventricular and right heart failure. Surgical therapy, indicated for symptomatic right heart failure that is not readily amenable to medical therapy (diuretics, afterload reducing drugs, and digoxin), consists of pulmonic valve replacement with an homograft or xenograft and treatment of the underlying condition (often left heart abnormality) responsible for the pulmonary hypertension.

KEY POINTS

Aortic Stenosis

Causes: Congenital or acquired. Calcification of a congenital bicuspid valve is the most common cause of calcific aortic stenosis in the elderly.

Pathophysiology: Pressure overload of the left ventricle leading to left ventricular hypertrophy. Decrease in compliance. May lead to subendocardial ischemia. Maintenance of normal sinus rhythm is important.

Diagnosis: Harsh, basilar: systolic ejection murmur with radiation to the carotid arteries. May be associated with a thrill. May diminish or obliterate A_2.

Electrocardiography: Left ventricular hypertrophy with ST-segment and T-wave changes. May be associated with heart block.

Chest radiography: Normal heart (concentric left ventricular hypertrophy). Look for calcification in the aortic area on the lateral chest radiograph.

Echocardiography: Gold standard. All patients suspected of having aortic stenosis should have echocardiography. Can quantitate valve area and valve gradient.

Cardiac catheterization: Confirms aortic valve gradient and valve area and defines the coronary anatomy.

Treatment: Symptomatic children and adolescents: Refer to the pediatric cardiologist. Surgical balloon valvuloplasty or surgical excision of the cusps. Symptomatic adults: Refer to the cardiologist; aortic valve replacement. Palliative therapy, balloon valvuloplasty. Asymptomatic patients: Prophylaxis against subacute bacterial endocarditis.

Aortic Insufficiency

Causes: Primary (congenital, deformed bicuspid valve) Secondary (connective tissue disease, Marfan's syndrome) Acquired because of dilation of the aortic root or endocarditis

Pathophysiology: Volume overload of the left ventricle leading to ventricular dilation and increasing left ventricular end diastolic pressure.

Symptoms: Bounding pulse; signs and symptoms of congestive heart failure. Angina-like chest pain.

Diagnosis: Physical examination: Wide pulse pressure on auscultation. At the base, high-frequency blowing, decrescendo diastolic "blow." Associated with a systolic ejection murmur.

Electrocardiography: Left axis deviation, left ventricular hypertrophy.

Chest radiography: Cardiac enlargement. "Boot-shaped" heart. Look for dilation of the ascending aorta.

Echocardiography: All patients suspected of having aortic insufficiency should be referred for echocardiography. Can confirm the diagnosis, degree of regurgitation, and status of left ventricular function.

Cardiac catheterization: Refer to the cardiologist.

Treatment: Medical: Standard therapy for a heart failure program: prophylaxis against subacute bacterial endocarditis for all patients. Surgical: Refer to the cardiologist. Valve replacement in this condition requires judgment and experience. Valve replacement: mechanical versus homograft.

Mitral Stenosis

Causes: 99% rheumatic; 1% congenital.

Pathophysiology: Valve area less than 1.5 cm^2. Reduced cardiac output; elevated left atrial and pulmonary venous pressures progressing to pulmonary arterial hypertension.

Symptoms: Dyspnea on exertion. Shortness of breath, easy fatigability, orthopnea, paroxysmal nocturnal dyspnea, and pulmonary edema.

Diagnosis: Physical examination: Prominent S_1, opening snap following S_2, followed by a mid to late diastolic "rumble." Electrocardiography: Left atrial enlargement, atrial fibrillation, right ventricular enlargement.

Chest radiography: Left atrial enlargement, pulmonary congestion, pulmonary hypertension, and right ventricular enlargement.

Echocardiography: Gold standard for all patients suspected of having mitral stenosis. Can identify severity of stenosis, left atrial size, right ventricular function, and pulmonary artery systolic pressure.

Treatment: Medical: Prophylaxis against subacute bacterial endocarditis, management of atrial fibrillation and diuretics for volume control. Surgical: Refer to the cardiologist for consultation for mitral valvuloplasty or balloon valvuloplasty. Replacement of valve may be necessary.

Mitral Regurgitation

Causes: Primary (rheumatic heart disease, myxomatous degeneration, ischemic heart disease). Secondary (primary cardiomyopathy and ischemic heart disease with left ventricular dilatation).

Pathophysiology: Left ventricular volume overload; increasing end diastolic pressure, increasing left atrial and pulmonary venous pressure progressing to the signs and symptoms of congestive heart failure with hypertrophy and dilatation of the left ventricle.

Symptoms: Dyspnea on exertion, shortness of breath, easy fatigability, orthopnea, paroxysmal nocturnal dyspnea, and pulmonary edema.

Diagnosis: Physical examination: Typical S_3 and a high-pitched, apical pansystolic murmur that radiates to the axilla.

KEY POINTS

Electrocardiography: Left atrial enlargement, left ventricular hypertrophy and atrial fibrillation.

Echocardiography: A must in all patients with mitral regurgitation. The distinction between primary and secondary mitral regurgitation is important and at times difficult. Refer to the cardiologist.

Cardiac catheterization: Confirms the echocardiographic data and reveals the presence or absence of coronary artery disease.

Treatment: Medical: Prophylaxis against subacute bacterial endocarditis; warfarin in the presence of atrial fibrillation. Digoxin, diuretics, angiotensin-converting enzyme inhibitors, or angiotensin-1 receptor blockers in the presence of congestive heart failure. Surgical: Mitral valve repair preferred; mitral valve replacement if necessary.

Tricuspid Valve Disease

Causes: Tricuspid stenosis—rheumatic in association with mitral valve disease. Tricuspid regurgitation—primary (rheumatic, infective, congenital). Secondary is more common (secondary to right ventricular failure due to pressure or volume overload).

Pathophysiology: Tricuspid stenosis with valve area less than 1.5 cm^2: Elevated right atrial pressure, reduced forward flow, systemic venous hypertension. Tricuspid regurgitation: Volume overload of the right atrium and systemic venous volume overload.

Symptoms: Tricuspid stenosis: Low cardiac output (fatigue, dyspnea on exertion, shortness of breath, and atrial fibrillation). Tricuspid regurgitation: Low cardiac output in association with edema, right-upper-quadrant pain and tenderness (hepatic enlargement), and ascites.

Diagnosis: *Electrocardiography:* Tricuspid stenosis: Right atrial enlargement. Tricuspid regurgitation: Right atrial and right ventricular enlargement, atrial fibrillation.

Chest radiography: Tricuspid stenosis: May appear normal or may show right atrial and right ventricular enlargement. Tricuspid regurgitation: Right atrial and right ventricular enlargement.

Echocardiography: Confirms the diagnosis of tricuspid stenosis or regurgitation. Right atrial size, right ventricular function, and pulmonary hypertension.

Cardiac catheterization: Confirms the echocardiographic findings and presence or absence of coronary artery disease.

Treatment: Medical: Prophylaxis against subacute bacterial endocarditis; diuretics for volume controls. Surgical: Tricuspid stenosis: Tricuspid valvotomy preferred. Percutaneous tricuspid valvotomy in carefully selected cases. Refer to the cardiologist. Tricuspid regurgitation: Valve replacement a difficult decision depending on the cause. Refer to the cardiologist.

Pulmonic Valve Disease

Causes: Pulmonic stenosis (primarily congenital): Acquired causes include endocarditis and carcinoid. Pulmonic insufficiency: Usually functional secondary to pulmonary hypertension.

Pathophysiology: Pulmonic stenosis: Pressure overload of the right ventricle leading to hypertrophy, dilation, and failure. Pulmonic insufficiency: Volume overload of the right ventricle. Generally well-tolerated.

Symptoms: Pulmonic stenosis: With right heart failure, cardiac output decreases, leading to fatigue, dyspnea, and shortness of breath. Systemic venous hypertension results in right-upper-quadrant tenderness (hepatomegaly), ascites, and peripheral edema. Pulmonic insufficiency: Symptoms generally secondary to pulmonary hypertension and right heart failure.

Diagnosis: Physical examination: Pulmonic stenosis: parasternal heave (right ventricular heave), pulmonic ejection click, systolic murmur at the left base that may radiate to left shoulder, and a delayed and soft P_2. Pulmonic insufficiency: Short, early diastolic murmur associated with a systolic ejection murmur heard in the pulmonic area and increased with inspiration.

Electrocardiography: Pulmonic stenosis: Right atrial and right ventricular hypertrophy. Pulmonic insufficiency: Right ventricular hypertrophy.

Chest radiography: Pulmonic stenosis: Prominent pulmonary artery. Pulmonic insufficiency: Right ventricular enlargement.

Echocardiography: Pulmonic stenosis: Severity of the stenosis and right ventricular size and function. Pulmonic insufficiency: Pulmonic valve structure, severity of the regurgitation, and right ventricular size and function.

Cardiac catheterization: Confirms the echocardiographic data and provides information on coronary anatomy.

Treatment: Asymptomatic: Pulmonic stenosis (mild, gradient < 50 mm Hg).Pulmonic insufficiency: Prophylaxis against subacute bacterial endocarditis and surveillance. Symptomatic: Refer to the cardiologist. Pulmonic stenosis: Generally associated with a gradient greater than 50 mm Hg. Procedure of choice, percutaneous balloon valvuloplasty. Pulmonic insufficiency: Medical therapy for right heart failure (digoxin, diuretics, vasodilators). Need to identify the possible, correctable cause of pulmonary hypertension. If necessary, pulmonic valve replacement with a homograft or xenograft.

SUGGESTED READING

Bonow RO. Management of chronic aortic regurgitation. N Engl J Med 1994;33:736–737.

Bonow RO, Picone AL, Mintose CL. Survival and functional results after valve replacement for aortic regurgitation from 1976 to 1983: influence of preoperative left ventricular function. Circulation 1985;72:1244–1256.

Braunwald E. Valvular heart disease. In: Braunwald E, ed. Heart disease. Philadelphia: WB Saunders, 1992:1007–1077.

Braunwald E. On the natural history of severe aortic stenosis. J Am Cardiol 1990;15:18–20.

Cheitlin M. Valvular heart disease: management and intervention. Circulation 1991;84(Suppl I):259–270.

Leatham A, Bull C, Braimbridge MV, eds. Valve disease and its complications. In: Lecture notes on cardiology. Oxford: Blackwell Scientific Publications, 1991:64–109.

Lund O. Preoperative risk evaluation and stratification of long-term survival after valve replacement for aortic stenosis. Circulation 1990;82:124–129.

Pellikka PA, Nishimura RA, Bailey KR, et al. The natural history of adults with asymptomatic, hemodynamically significant aortic stenosis. J Am Cardiol 1990;15:1012–1017.

Ross J Jr. Afterload mismatch in aortic and mitral valve disease: implications for surgical therapy. J Am Cardiol 1985;5:811–826.

Schick EC. Valvular heart disease. In: Noble J. Textbook of primary care medicine. St. Louis: Mosby, 1996:275–281.

Schlant RC, Alexander RW , eds. Hurst's the heart, arteries, and veins. 8th ed. New York: McGraw-Hill, 1994.

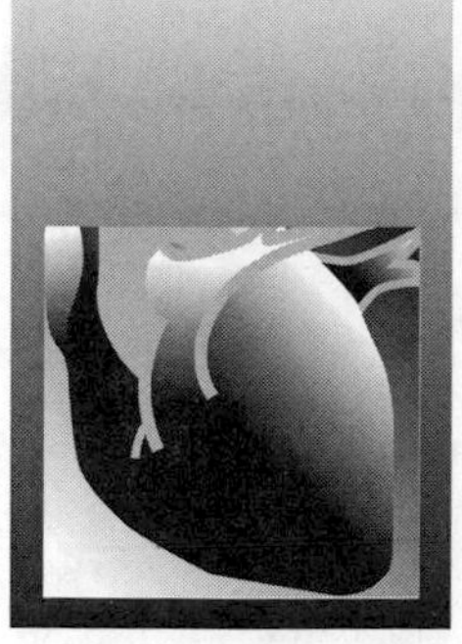

CHAPTER 10

Infective Endocarditis

James A. Arrowood

BACKGROUND

Infective endocarditis results from microbial infection of the endothelial lining of the heart. It characteristically produces vegetations on the valves of the heart but also may involve ventricular septal defects or mural endocardium. Infection of the lining of a large artery is more accurately called infective endarteritis, but it produces a similar clinical syndrome. Infective endocarditis is best classified according to the infecting organism (e.g., *Staphylococcus epidermidis* endocarditis) because the organism determines the disease course as well as therapy.

CAUSES

For ease of description, infective endocarditis may also be classified according to syndrome:

- Native valve endocarditis
- Prosthetic valve endocarditis
- Endocarditis in intravenous drug users

Each of these syndromes involves a different presentation, course, and microorganisms.

Native Valve Endocarditis

Native valve endocarditis occurs on a heart valve that was either previously normal or damaged by congenital or acquired disease. Most patients are older than 50 years of age and have an identifiable predisposing cardiac lesion. Congenital heart disease is present in approximately 10 to 20% of patients with endocarditis. Predisposing lesions include patent ductus arteriosus, ventricular septal defect, and bicuspid aortic valve but do not include uncomplicated atrial septal defect. About 10 to 30% of patients have mitral valve prolapse. Although mitral valve prolapse is common, the risk that anyone with this condition will develop infective endocarditis is low. When prolapse is associated with regurgitation and an audible regurgitant murmur, however, a patient's risk increases. Rheumatic valvular disease is present in about 30% of such patients. Infection is most commonly found in the mitral valve or aortic valve.

Degenerative heart disease also predisposes to endocarditis. Calcific aortic stenosis in older patients has become increasingly important as a cause and has contributed to an observed increase in the median age of patients with endocarditis. Twenty to 40% of patients with infective endocarditis have no recognizable predisposing lesion. Although any organism can produce endocarditis, most cases of native valve endocarditis are caused by the following organisms:

- Streptococci (55%)
- Staphylcocci (30%)
- Enterococci (6%)

Fungi rarely produce native valve endocarditis in patients who do not use intravenous drugs.

Prosthetic Valve Endocarditis

Prosthetic valve infections have become more numerous with increased use of such devices and now account for 10 to 20% of all cases of endocarditis. One to 2% of patients are affected during the first year after surgery, and the rate declines slightly to 1% per year thereafter. Aortic valve prostheses are two to four times more likely to become infected than are mitral prostheses. Prosthetic valve endocarditis occurring within 60 days of surgery (early prosthetic valve endocarditis) usually results from valve contamination at the time of surgery or from perioperative bacteremia. Approximately half of the cases of prosthetic valve endocarditis are caused by staphylococci (*S. epidermidis,* 30%; *S. aureus,* 20%). Gram-negative bacilli account for 15 to 20% of cases, and fungi (usually *Candida* species) cause approximately 10%. The peak time of onset is 3 to 6 weeks after surgery, and the incidence rapidly decreases thereafter. The course of early prosthetic valve endocarditis is fulminant and often associated with valve dehiscence and dysfunction.

Infection occurring 60 days after surgery (late prosthetic valve endocarditis) may be caused by transient bacteremia; it may also result from the same factors causing early endocarditis but has a longer incubation period. About one-third of cases of late prosthetic valve endocarditis are due to streptococci and staphylococci (*S. epidermidis,* 20%; *S. aureus,* 10%). Fungi account for only about 5% of cases of late prosthetic valve endocarditis. The course of the late form may be similar to that of the early form but is more often similar to that of native valve endocarditis, especially when caused by streptococci.

Endocarditis in Intravenous Drug Users

Intravenous drug users are at high risk for endocarditis, and most drug users with endocarditis (80%) do not have predisposing lesions. Most drug users with endocarditis are young men (mean age, 30 years; male-to-female ratio, 3 to 1). Bacteremias in intravenous drug users are most frequently derived from the user's skin or from local infections at injection sites. Direct intravenous injection of bacteria from contaminated drugs or equipment is also possible. *Staphylococcus aureus* causes 50 to 60% of cases, streptococci and enterococci cause 20%, gram-negative bacilli (mostly *Pseudomonas* and *Serratia* species) cause 10%, and fungi (usually *Candida* species) cause 5%. Multiple organisms are isolated from the blood in about 5% of drug users.

Right-sided valvular infection is more common among intravenous drug users. The tricuspid valve is involved in more than 50% of patients, the aortic valve in 25%, the mitral valve in 20%, and the pulmonic valve in 1 to 2%. More than one valve may be infected on either side or both sides of the heart simultaneously. Septic pulmonary infarction or pulmonary emboli from embolization of tricuspid vegetations are common and result in multiple opacities on chest radiographs. Murmurs are frequently absent or not well appreciated with right-sided endocarditis.

PATHOGENESIS

The initial event in the development of infectious endocarditis is the attachment of microorganisms circulating in the bloodstream to an endothelial surface. This is facilitated when thrombi composed of platelets and fibrin have been deposited on previously injured endothelial surfaces. These sterile thrombotic lesions are believed to provide a surface that is more receptive to the attachment of microorganisms during episodes of bacteremia. Endothelial injury is more likely to occur on valves damaged by congenital or rheumatic disease or previous endocarditis or from abnormal flow patterns produced by congenital lesions. The vegetation of infective endocarditis is caused when additional platelets and fibrin are deposited over the attached microorganisms. Microorganisms may then proliferate at a site that is resistant to penetration by phagocytic cells, and the infection continues unchecked by host defense mechanisms. The schema described allows relatively nonpathogenic organisms, such as *S. viridans,* to cause infection, and more virulent organisms, such as *S. aureus,* to infect apparently normal valves. Infection with the more virulent organisms is often more acute and fulminant and may be caused by direct invasion of normal endothelium. Transient bacteremia, which is also required for endocarditis, is thought to result from traumatic procedures involving epithelial surfaces that are usually colonized by bacteria (e.g., dental procedures, urethral surgery, colonoscopy). Thus, antibiotic prophylaxis is recommended for such procedures when a predisposing cardiac lesion is present (see Appendix A).

PATHOPHYSIOLOGY

The clinical features of infectious endocarditis are produced by

- Local infection
- Vegetations
- Constant bacteremia
- Increasing titers of antibodies to the organism

Vegetations may produce valve dysfunction or destruction and result in partial occlusion or insufficiency. Abscesses may develop by direct extension of active infection into adjacent cardiac structures, causing conduction disturbances, fistulous tracts, chordal rupture, or purulent pericardial effusion. Embolization to various organs is also possible and may produce septic infarcts and abscesses. Mycotic aneurysms can develop from septic emboli to the vasa vasorum or direct invasion of the arterial wall. These often develop in the aorta or cerebral arteries and may rupture. High titers of antibodies against the infecting organism lead to the formation of circulating immune complexes, which may cause glomerulonephritis, arthritis, vasculitis, and Osler nodes.

SIGNS AND SYMPTOMS

Symptoms of the subacute form of infectious endocarditis are nonspecific and best described as the general manifestations of an infection.

- Low-grade fever is usually present, but its magnitude and pattern may vary considerably.
- Shaking chills are usually present only in patients with acute infectious endocarditis.
- Fever may be absent in older patients, those previously treated with antibiotics, or those with renal failure or congestive heart failure.

Common symptoms include

- Anorexia
- Fatigue
- Weight loss
- Malaise
- Arthralgias

More specific symptoms are related to the development of complications of the disease from progressive destruction of the valve and embolic and immunologic phenomena. Embolic phenomena are clinically apparent in 15 to 35% of cases of infectious endocarditis. Left-upper-quadrant abdominal pain may signal splenic embolization with subsequent infarction, chest pain, coronary artery embolism, and hematuria from renal embolization.

Neurologic symptoms are present in about one-third of patients because of brain abscess, purulent meningitis, or cerebral artery occlusion. The most common neurologic symptom is headache, which usually improves with supportive care and antimicrobial therapy. Intracranial mycotic aneurysms are strongly suggested by severe, unremitting localized headache; most patients with aneurysms are probably asymptomatic. Aneurysm is typically diagnosed only after the patient presents with a catastrophic hemorrhage.

Endocarditis involving the right side of the heart may present with pulmonary emboli or infarcts. If endocarditis is untreated and valvular destruction occurs, valvular regurgitation can develop and congestive heart failure may dominate the presentation.

Arthritis or vasculitis may occur because of deposition of immune complex in joints and mucocutaneous vessels.

Fever may not be initially present on physical examination, but temperature usually increases during the initial 24 to 48 hours. Heart murmurs are almost always present, except early in the course of acute infections or in patients with right-sided or mural endocarditis. Murmurs are caused by the underlying valvular or congenital heart disease or may be due to dysfunction of the valve from the infectious process. The possibility of endocarditis must always be considered in the febrile patient with a known heart murmur. Splenomegaly and petechiae occur in about 30% of patients with heart murmurs, primarily those with disease of long duration. Petechiae are predominantly found on the conjunctivae, palate, and buccal mucosa but are not specific to endocarditis.

Other peripheral stigmata are found in patients with endocarditis. Fingernails may reveal splinter hemorrhages, represented by linear dark red streaks. These streaks more strongly suggest endocarditis if they are proximally located in the nail bed. Osler nodes are small, tender nodules on the finger or toe pads that occur in 10 to 25% of patients. The nodes are probably due to deposition of immune complex. Janeway lesions are small (1 to 4 mm), nontender, hemorrhagic areas found on the palms and soles. They are more common in acute endocarditis and are due to septic emboli. Roth spots—oval, retinal hemorrhages with a clear pale center—are seen in less than 5% of patients with endocarditis.

LABORATORY TESTING

Blood Cultures

The bacteremia of endocarditis is continuous, and cultures may be obtained at any time regardless of body temperature. In subacute disease and in the absence of previous therapy, three cultures should be obtained at least 1 hour apart. If the patient has previously received antimicrobial therapy is stable and not toxic, antimicrobial therapy may be delayed while further cultures are obtained in an attempt to obtain positive results. When the presentation is acute, three cultures should be obtained at least 30 minutes apart. Only one culture should be obtained from each venipuncture site (at least 10 mL of blood), and both aerobic and anaerobic techniques should be used.

Routine Laboratory Tests

Patients with subacute disease usually have a normochromic, normocytic anemia that may be severe. The leukocyte count in usually normal but may demonstrate the presence of more immature leukocytes. If renal embolization has been extensive or autoimmune glomerulonephritis is present, serum creatinine and blood urea nitrogen levels may be elevated. The erythrocyte sedimentation rate is almost always elevated unless heart or renal failure is present. Urine may be normal in uncomplicated cases but usually reveals proteinuria, microscopic hematuria, or pyuria.

The patient with acute infectious endocarditis usually has a normal hemoglobin level and hematocrit and an elevated leukocyte count. Chest radiography usually reflects the underlying valvular or congenital disease; if the right-sided valves are infected, the lung fields may exhibit multiple foci of infection from emboli. If aortic or mitral regurgitation is present and filling pressures are elevated, pulmonary vascular redistribution will be present with possible edema.

Echocardiography

Echocardiography has become increasingly important in both the diagnosis and management of infectious endocarditis. In the absence of a prosthetic valve, two-dimensional transthoracic studies can identify most vegetations larger than 5 mm in diameter, and transesophageal studies can reliably detect vegetations larger than 3 mm. Reported sensitivities range between 50 and 75% for transthoracic studies and up to 95% by transesophageal technique. Sensitivity of echocardiography is reduced for prosthetic valve endocarditis. Specificity has not been clearly established, but the false-positive rate has been low in patients with proven endocarditis. Thickened valves, thrombi, nodules, tumors, and flail leaflets can be misinterpreted as vegetations. Vegetations may not be visualized during the first 2 weeks of endocarditis; once visualized, however, they usually remain the same size during therapy and for months after successful therapy. As vegetations heal, fibrosis, collagen deposition, and calcification occur, causing the vegetations to appear more echocardiographically dense and smaller. In some cases, this can allow differentiation between active and healed vegetations, especially if serial studies are available. *The absence of a vegetation in someone suspected of having endocarditis does not exclude the diagnosis.* Although the clinical importance of detected vegetations continues to be controversial, most available data suggest that patients with vegetations are at an increased risk for such complications as systemic emboli, congestive heart failure, requirement for surgical intervention, and death. Most complications occur in patients with vegetations larger than 10 mm in diameter.

Doppler echocardiography can also provide important information about the complications produced by endocarditis. This technique allows detection of primary native valve disruption, prosthetic valve dysfunction, and prosthetic valve dehiscence and assessment of the hemodynamic effects of these conditions. Extravalvular complications may also be detected, including perivalvular abscesses, aortic root mycotic aneurysms, intracardiac fistulas, and purulent pericarditis. Sequential echocardiograms can assist in making decisions about the necessity and timing of surgery.

DIAGNOSIS

Infectious endocarditis is diagnosed by clinical presentation or by growing the causative organism from the patient's blood. Infectious endocarditis should be suspected in febrile patients with prosthetic heart valves or new murmurs, especially of the regurgitant type, and in febrile intravenous drug users. Infectious endocarditis should also be considered in patients with heart murmur who have unexplained fever for at least 1 week and in young patients who have had a stroke.

Other diseases producing a clinical picture similar to that of endocarditis include the following:

- Atrial myxoma
- Acute rheumatic fever
- Connective tissue diseases, including systemic lupus erythematosus, thrombotic thrombocytopenic purpura, and sickle cell disease

The aforementioned are distinguished from infectious endocarditis by negative blood cultures.

Summary of Diagnosis

- Blood cultures uncontaminated by antibiotic therapy are the keystone of diagnosis; definitive diagnosis can be made by growing the causative agent from the patient's blood.
- Echocardiography may confirm the presence of vegetations, valvular abnormalities, or intracardiac shunts.
- Chest radiography indicates the presence or absence of congestive heart failure, valvular calcification, and cardiomegaly.
- Fever and a pathologic murmur should prompt a high index of suspicion.
- Presence of native valve abnormality, prosthetic valves, previous "shunt" surgery, or intravenous drug use should also increase the level of suspicion.
- Splenomegaly, Osler nodes, and Roth spots are late manifestations of the disease but are not always present.
- Infectious endocarditis should be strongly suspected in the following patients if they are febrile:
  - Patients with prosthetic heart valves
  - Patients with new heart murmurs, especially of the regurgitant type
  - Intravenous drug users
  - Patients with unexplained fever for at least 1 week and a heart murmur
  - Young person with a stroke
- Other diseases can produce a clinical picture similar to that of endocarditis:
  - Atrial myxoma
  - Acute rheumatic fever
  - Connective tissue diseases
- Negative blood cultures distinguish other conditions from infectious endocarditis

TREATMENT

All patients with endocarditis should be hospitalized for complete diagnostic evaluation, supportive care, and initiation of treatment with intravenous antibiotics. The main goals of treatment are to eradicate all infecting organisms from the vegetation and to monitor and manage complications. For cure, the vegetation must be sterilized. If any organisms are viable after a given course of antimicrobial therapy, relapse is likely. Thus, bactericidial agents must be used rather than bacteriostatic agents, and the agents must be administered in high concentrations and for a long enough period to sterilize the vegetation. Most patients are treated with specific regimens according to accepted guidelines from authoritative sources (see Suggested Readings). For the regimens to be effective, isolation and antimicrobial susceptibility of the infecting organism must be accurately determined. Antimicrobial therapy should be started as soon as possible. For patients suspected of having endocarditis, therapy should be started within 2 to 3 hours after at least three blood cultures are obtained. If antimicrobial agents have been administered within the previous 2 weeks and the course is subacute, therapy may be delayed for 2 to 3 days while additional blood cultures are obtained in an attempt to increase the yield for organism isolation. Intravenous antibiotic therapy usually lasts 4 to 6 weeks. If the response to treatment is good (resolution of fever and negative blood cultures) and the course is uncomplicated (e.g., no significant valvular destruction or heart failure), part of the parenteral course may be administered at home to expedite hospital discharge.

Oral therapy is not recommended. Although it has been used in certain situations, the risks are clearly higher than those with parenteral therapy. If oral therapy is considered, the risks and benefits should be carefully evaluated.

Empirical Therapy before Isolation of an Organism

With the acute onset of endocarditis in a patient who does not use intravenous drugs and has a native valve, therapy should be directed against *S. aureus* and include an antistaphylococcal penicillin. With acute onset in an intravenous drug user, therapy is directed against *S. aureus* and gram-negative bacilli and gentamicin is added to the regimen. If *S. aureus* is likely to be methicillin-resistant, vancomycin should be used instead of an antistaphylococcal penicillin. In patients with a prosthetic valve, therapy should be directed against *S. epidermidis, S. aureus,* and gram-negative bacilli. Vancomycin should be used as well as gentamicin because of the high incidence of methicillin-resistant *S. epidermidis*. If the presentation is subacute in a patient who does not use intravenous drugs, therapy should be directed against enterococci and should consist of ampicillin plus gentamicin. In patients with prosthetic valves, anticoagulation with warfarin is continued through treatment. Anticoagulants are of no value in treating infectious endocarditis and should not be used in patients who do not require them for other reasons.

Treatment should be adjusted when the organism causing endocarditis has been identified. If blood cultures are negative but the clinical response is good, empirical therapy should be continued for the recommended duration of treatment. If blood cultures are negative and the clinical response is poor even after 7 to 10 days of therapy, the possibility of fungal endocarditis should be entertained, especially if large vegetations are present on echocardiography.

After antimicrobial therapy has been initiated, blood cultures should be repeated after 7 to 10 days of therapy (more frequently if the patient is not responding) to assess adequacy of therapy. Most patients become afebrile within 3 to 7 days, but persistent or recurrent fever should raise suspicion of myocardial or metastatic abscess, recurrent emboli, inadequate therapy, or a febrile reaction to the antimicrobial agent. Positive blood cultures may persist for 1 to 2 weeks despite curative therapy, especially if enterococci and *S. aureus* are causing the endocarditis.

Surgical Intervention

Surgical intervention is often required during treatment of patients with endocarditis who are experiencing the following complications:

- Refractory heart failure related to valvular dysfunction
- Prosthetic valve dysfunction or dehiscence
- Myocardial or valve ring abscess
- Uncontrolled infection (persistent bacteremia despite appropriate antimicrobial therapy or when appropriate therapy is not available)
- Repeated relapses

Ideally, patients should be treated with optimal antimicrobial therapy long enough before surgery to sterilize blood cultures. If the patient has a definite indication for surgery, however, the procedure should not be delayed. It is difficult to know when to proceed to valve replacement in patients with emboli; no data are available to indicate the likelihood of additional emboli after the initial event. It has been reported that vegetations 10 mm in diameter or greater are associated with a higher risk for emboli. One approach, therefore, is to consider surgery in patients with two or more emboli

Summary of Treatment

- Confirmation of positive blood cultures
- Consultation with infectious disease specialist for appropriate antibiotics
- Hospitalization for initiation of therapy and to ensure hemodynamic stability and control of the infection
- Duration of therapy usually 4 to 6 weeks
- Home intravenous antibiotics programs possible
- Early referral to cardiologist and surgeon when indicated

or in patients with one embolus and the continued presence of very large vegetations ($\geq$10 mm on two-dimensional echocardiography). The early and long-term mortality and morbidity from valve replacement must be weighed against the unpredictability of further embolic events.

REFERRAL

After endocarditis is diagnosed, the primary care team should obtain two referrals: infectious disease and cardiology. The infectious disease consultant will determine the appropriate choice and duration of antibiotic therapy. The cardiology consultant will follow the hemodynamic stability or instability with the primary care physician, obtain the appropriate echocardiograms, and recommend the timing of cardiac catheterization if surgery is deemed necessary.

PROGNOSIS

Infectious endocarditis is almost universally fatal if left untreated, with cure rates varying according to the infecting organism, the type and position of the cardiac valve involved, and whether complications develop. For native valve endocarditis, cure rates for disease caused by streptococci exceed 90%; rates are 75 to 90% for disease caused by enterococci and 60 to 75% for disease caused by *S. aureus*. Mortality rates are increased if heart failure, renal failure, or a perivalvular abscess develops and with culture-negative disease, gram-negative or fungal infection, involvement of the aortic valve (compared with involvement of the mitral or tricuspid valve), and prosthetic valve infection. A worse prognosis is also seen in elderly and very young patients, patients with emboli or mycotic aneurysm rupture, and patients who need valve replacement.

Early prosthetic valve endocarditis (developing <60 days after surgery) has a higher mortality rate (40 to 80%) than late prosthetic valve endocarditis (developing > 60 days after surgery). This increased mortality rate is the result of infection with antibiotic-resistant staphylococci in the early form of the disease and the result of a higher likelihood of development of valve dysfunction, dehiscence, and intracardiac abscess formation. Early valve replacement in prosthetic valve endocarditis in patients with indications for surgery is associated with a lower mortality rate than is delayed surgery.

PREVENTION

Persons with acquired or congenital heart disease are at increased risk for infective endocarditis. Endocarditis usually follows bacteremia, and certain health care procedures cause bacteremia with organisms that can cause endocarditis. Because these organisms are usually sensitive to antibiotics, endocarditis may be prevented if antibiotics are administered to patients with predisposing heart disease before procedures that may cause bacteremia. Although this has been supported by studies in animals, no prospective study has proven that it is effective in humans. Antibiotic prophylaxis is currently considered the standard of care (see Appendix A).

KEY POINTS

- Search for the cause:
  - Previous dental procedures
  - Surgery
  - Instrumentation
  - Intravenous drug use
- Initiate therapy with a high index of suspicion before blood culture results are available.
- Begin therapy directed against the presumed organism and for the appropriate classification:
  - Native valve
  - Prosthetic valve
  - Intravenous drug use
- The best therapy is prevention.
- Initiate prophylaxis of infective endocarditis in appropriate patients.
- Proper classification of endocarditis by infecting organism allows determination of disease course and treatment.
- Both valvular and congenital heart disease predisposes to endocarditis.
- Staphylococci cause approximately half of the cases of prosthetic valve endocarditis.
- Intravenous drug users are at high risk for endocarditis, primarily caused by *S. aureus*.
- Endothelial surface is more vulnerable to microorganisms when it has been previously damaged (e.g., by congenital or rheumatic disease, previous endocarditis, congenital lesions).
- Infection with more virulent microorganisms may be caused by direct invasion of normal endothelium.
- Common symptoms include anorexia, fatigue, weight loss, malaise, and arthralgias.
- Heart murmurs caused by underlying valvular or congenital heart disease or dysfunction of valve from infectious process are almost always present.
- Blood cultures are critical for diagnosis, and negative blood cultures distinguish other diseases from endocarditis.
- Infective endocarditis is almost universally fatal if left untreated.
- Antibiotics administered prophylactically may prevent endocarditis.

SUGGESTED READING

Datani AS, Taubert KA, Wilson W, et al. Prevention of bacterial endocarditis. Recommendations by American Heart Association. JAMA 1997;227:1794–1801.

Kaye D, ed. Infective endocarditis. 2d ed. New York: Raven Press, 1992.

Marks AR, et al. Identification of high-risk and low-risk subgroups of patients with mitral-valve prolapse. N Engl J Med 1989;320:1031.

Steckelberg JM, et al. Emboli in infective endocarditis: the prognostic value of echocardiography. Ann Intern Med 1991;114:635.

Threlkeld M, Cobbs G. Infections of prosthetic valves and intravascular devices. In: Mandell GL, ed. Principles and practice of infectious diseases. 3d ed. New York, Churchill-Livingstone, 1990.

Wilson WK, Karchmer AU, Datani AS, et al. Antibiotic treatment of adults with infective endocarditis due to streptococci, enterococci, staphlococci and HACEK microorganisms. JAMA 1995;274:1706–1713.

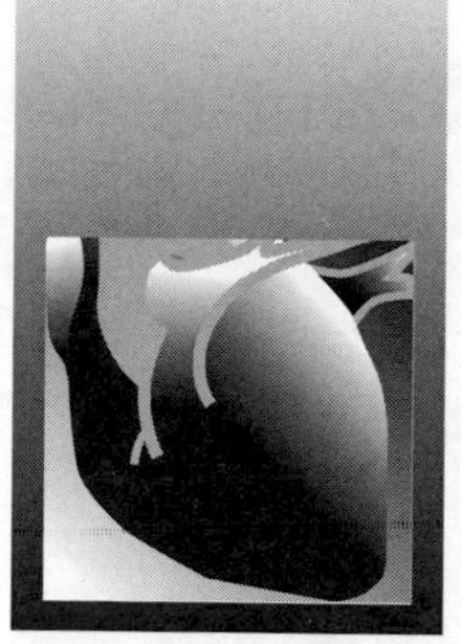

CHAPTER 11

Congenital, Acquired, and Adolescent Cardiovascular Medicine

William B. Moskowitz

BACKGROUND

Cardiovascular disease occurs more often in children than is generally appreciated. More than 600,000 children in the United States have an abnormality of the cardiovascular system: approximately 440,000 have a cardiac defect; an estimated 160,000 have a rhythm or conduction disturbance; and about 40,000 have an acquired disease such as cardiomyopathy, rheumatic heart disease, or Kawasaki disease. In addition, if the current rate of atherosclerosis (a disease that begins in childhood) continues, a substantial portion of the approximately 80 million U.S. children younger than 21 years of age will ultimately die of complications of atherosclerotic disease.

This chapter presents some important issues in pediatric cardiology that will aid the primary care physician in the following:

- Identifying problems
- Raising the level of awareness of potential problems
- Answering some routine office practice questions that come up when dealing with the pediatric patient with heart disease

CONGENITAL HEART DISEASE

Cyanotic Heart Disease

The Neonate

Causes Central cyanosis occurring shortly after birth often reflects hypoventilation, either from the depressant effects of maternal analgesia or from possible unrecognized pneumothorax or diaphragmatic hernia. After the first few minutes of life, central cyanosis often suggests congenital heart disease. Alternatively, right-to-left shunting through a patent foramen ovale or patent ductus arteriosus in the absence of other cardiac defects can lead to marked central cyanosis. This is the case in infants with persistent pulmonary hypertension (persistent fetal circulation), with or without associated pulmonary parenchymal disease. Even in the absence of pulmonary hypertension, central cyanosis secondary to right-to-left shunting through these persistent fetal pathways can occur intermittently, particularly with vigorous crying or straining, through the first several days to week of life.

The physiologic basis of all cases of cyanosis, no matter the disease state, involves at least one of the following five mechanisms:

- Hypoventilation (central or alveolar)
- Right-to-left shunting (intracardiac or extracardiac)
- Ventilation–perfusion mismatch (atelectasis, pulmonary embolism)
- Diffusion impairment (hyaline membrane disease, acute respiratory distress syndrome)
- Inadequate transport of oxygen by hemoglobin (methemoglobinemia)

Cyanosis is clinically evident when the patient has more than 5 g of reduced hemoglobin per dL. Cyanosis due to cardiac lesions must involve right-to-left shunting at some level (atrial, ventricular, or great vessel) and may involve obstruction to pulmonary blood flow. Congenital heart defects leading to cyanosis fall into three general physiologic categories:

- Tetralogy physiology
- Transposition physiology
- Venous admixture physiology

Tetralogy physiology occurs when pulmonary blood flow is obstructed (pulmonary stenosis or atresia) and there is right-to-left shunting through a ventricular septal defect to the aorta. In tetralogy of Fallot with cyanosis, the degree of right ventricular outflow obstruction varies considerably. However, the total resistance through the right ventricular outflow tract exceeds systemic resistance so that right-to-left shunting occurs through the ventricular septal defect. In many patients, the degree of right ventricular outflow obstruction is relatively fixed and determined by the degree of pulmonary valvular stenosis and pulmonary hypoplasia; thus, each month, systemic arterial saturation largely depends on systemic vascular resistance. The degree of hypoxemia increases as systemic arterial pressure and resistance decrease because of hypovolemia, fever, exercise, or drugs that produce vasodilation. Conversely, systemic arterial saturation is elevated by conditions that increase systemic pressure and resistance and thus decrease the amount of intracardiac right-to-left shunting.

Dextroposition of the great arteries is a relatively frequent cardiac defect. The aorta arises entirely from the right ventricle and is anterior and rightward; the pulmonary artery arises from the left ventricle. About half of the hearts with dextroposition of the great arteries have no other abnormality except a persistent patent foramen ovale or a patent ductus arteriosus. The dominant physiologic abnormality is a deficiency of oxygen supply to the tissues. Systemic and pulmonary circulations function in parallel rather than in series; thus, the greatest portion of the output of each ventricle is recirculated to that ventricle. Only a small portion of blood, on which survival depends, is exchanged by intercirculatory shunts to eventually reach the appropriate vascular bed. Systemic and pulmonary artery saturations thus depend on shunting through an atrial septal defect, ventricular septal defect, or patent ductus arteriosus.

The best example of a venous admixture lesion is the single ventricle. Both systemic venous and pulmonary venous atria drain into a common ventricle or mixing chamber. Saturations of the blood leaving the heart by way of the pulmonary artery and the aorta are therefore identical. Many anatomically complicated heart defects (e.g., tricuspid atresia, mitral atresia, double-outlet right ventricle, total anomalous pulmonary venous return, truncus arteriosus) have the same admixture physiology. The degree of cyanosis is directly related to the presence and severity of obstruction to pulmonary blood flow.

Infants with the greatest obstruction to pulmonary blood flow (critical pulmonary stenosis and pulmonary atresia) present the earliest after birth with the greatest cyanosis. These infants have ductal-dependent pulmonary blood flow: the major, if not sole, source of pulmonary blood flow is derived from the aorta through the patent ductus arteriosus. Administration of high concentrations of oxygen (100% inspired oxygen) has little if any effect on increasing systemic SaO_2 in infants with a constricting patent ductus arteriosus. This is also true for infants with dextroposition of the great arteries and most infants with large right-to-left shunts. In contrast, increases in systemic SaO_2 are usually seen in infants with pulmonary parenchymal disease. Infants with persistent pulmonary hypertension and significant right-to-left shunting through a patent foramen ovale or patent ductus arteriosus typically show little or no increase in arterial oxygenation until hyperventilation decreases the PCO_2, which results in pulmonary vascular relaxation.

Diagnosis Clinical evaluation of the cyanotic newborn usually shows tachypnea and hyperpnea, with little or no murmur on auscultation. However, murmurs of pulmonary stenosis, patent ductus arteriosus, or atrioventricular valve regurgitation may be present. Arterial blood gas determination is used to measure PCO_2, which is generally elevated ($>$ 35 to 40 mm Hg) in the presence of lung disease and generally low ($<$ 30 to 35 mm Hg) in the presence of congenital heart disease. Chest radiography is for evaluating the status of pulmonary blood flow, size of the heart, and side of the aortic arch and for ruling out significant pulmonary disease. Electrocardiography (ECG) is of little help in differentiating the cause of cyanosis because most newborns and those with cyanotic congenital heart disease have right ventricular hypertrophy and a rightward axis. Echocardiography with two-dimensional Doppler color imaging is the noninvasive diagnostic procedure of choice for determining the specific anatomic and physiologic derangements when heart disease is present. In addition, this test allows anatomic heart disease to be effectively excluded and physiologic derangements (patent foramen ovale or patent ductus arteriosus; right-to-left shunting) to be measured in persistent pulmonary hypertension. Because of the reliability of two-dimensional color flow echocardiography in experienced hands, diagnostic catheterization of the cyanotic infant is not routinely performed before palliative surgical procedures.

Management The initial stabilization of the cyanotic infant with congenital heart disease includes administration of oxygen, adequate fluids, and glucose; correction of acidosis, if present; and initiation of a prostaglandin E_I infusion. Prostaglandin E_I maintains ductal patency that provides adequate pulmonary blood flow in ductal-dependent defects. Prostaglandin E_I is also useful in dextroposition of the great arteries. Pulmonary blood flow is increased through the patent ductus arteriosus, resulting in increased left-to-right shunting through an adequate atrial septal defect that improves systemic arterial oxygen concentration. Infants with even the most complex cyanotic heart defects can be stabilized during prostaglandin E_I infusion and can be transported to a pediatric cardiac center for treatment.

The treatment strategy for the infant with cyanotic congenital heart disease involves first securing a stable source of pulmonary blood flow with adequate systemic oxygen delivery. Separating the systemic and pulmonary circulations so that all systemic venous blood returns to the lungs and all pulmonary venous blood goes to the body is the ultimate goal. The various procedures performed on the cyanotic infant to attain these goals are listed in Table 11.1. Infants with dextroposition of the great arteries and other cyanotic defects with obligate shunting at the atrial level undergo balloon atrial septostomy in the immediate newborn period. Infants with critical pulmonary valve stenosis and right-to-left atrial shunting may be effectively treated with balloon pulmonary valvuloplasty in the pediatric cardiac catheterization laboratory after they have been stabilized with prostaglandin E_I. Most infants with cyanotic congenital heart disease undergo initial palliation. Several palliative shunts are created in the neonate with obstructed pulmonary blood flow. These shunts improve pulmonary blood flow and allow the pulmonary arteries and child to grow so that definitive surgical therapy may

TABLE 11.1. Palliative and Definitive Procedures for Cyanotic Heart Defects

Procedure	Explanation
Palliative	
Balloon atrial septostomy	Creates atrial septal defect to ensure atrial mixing
Classical Blalock-Taussig Shunt	Subclavian artery end-to-side of pulmonary artery
Gortex interposition graft	Gortex tube graft from side or base of subclavian artery or aorta to pulmonary artery
Classical Glenn shunt	End of superior vena cava (taken off heart) to end of right pulmonary artery (detached from main pulmonary artery)
Bidirectional Glenn shunt	End of superior vena cava (taken off heart) to side of right pulmonary artery, which is left in continuity with main pulmonary artery. Staging to Fontan completion
Definitive repair	
Tetralogy of Fallot	Closure of ventricular septal defect, resection of muscular subpulmonic stenosis, and valvar stenosis. Possible use of outflow tract patch or conduit to enlarge pulmonary artery
Transposition of great arteries, atrial	Baffles systemic venous blood to left ventricle and lungs; baffles pulmonary venous blood to right ventricle and systemic circulation
Transposition of great arteries, Arterial	Switches great arteries to appropriate ventricles; must also translocate coronary arteries
Rastelli repair of transposition of great arteries with ventricular septal defect and pulmonary stenosis	Ventricular septal defect closure to direct left ventricular blood flow to aorta and placement of homograft from right ventricle to pulmonary artery; used also for repair of truncus arteriosus and tetralogy with pulmonary atresia
Fontan procedure	Superior and inferior vena cava returns directed to pulmonary artery by direct right atrial anastomosis, prior bidirectional Glenn shunt, or intra- or extracardiac conduits

be performed later. Infants with severe obstruction to pulmonary blood flow or those with discontinuous pulmonary arteries may have additional sources of pulmonary blood flow from aortopulmonary collateral vessels. These communications may lead to heart failure or pulmonary vascular disease and must be addressed by surgical ligation or coil embolization in the catheterization laboratory before definitive therapy. Few definitive procedures are performed on the neonate.

The Older Infant, Child, and Adolescent

Causes Although most cyanotic children after the neonatal period have known cyanotic heart disease with or without previous palliation, two other groups of children may present with cyanosis at a later age.

The classic presentation in a child 6 to 18 months of age (tetralogy of Fallot) is cyanosis upon crying, exercise, and occasional squatting. This now occurs less frequently because primary care physicians can detect murmurs earlier and make a referral before pulmonary blood flow becomes severely obstructed. These less severely affected children may therefore not require initial palliation but may undergo complete repair as their first and only procedure.

The second group of children presenting with late-onset cyanosis have developed Eisenmenger's syndrome: pulmonary hypertension with right-to-left shunting through a defect that was previously shunting left to right, such as a large ventricular septal defect, patent ductus arteriosus, or complete endocardial cushion defect. Shunting reverses because the pulmonary vascular resistance exceeds systemic vascular resistance. Although uncommon before the age of 2 years in children with a ventricular septal defect, it may occur much earlier in some children, especially those with Down's syndrome.

Diagnosis Clinically, a loud pulmonary component of S_2 is present, and ECG may show right ventricular hypertrophy. Most of these children cannot undergo surgical repair of their defects. Some may be candidates for heart–lung transplantation or lung transplantation with intracardiac repair. A few can undergo repair at increased risk if the pulmonary vascular bed is shown to react to oxygen or to pharmacologic agents.

Before definitive repair of any congenital cyanotic defect, complete catheterization is required to verify the noninvasive diagnoses, exclude associated defects, evaluate the results of previous palliative procedures, and provide the surgeon with the necessary anatomic and physiologic details. Coronary artery patterns must be identified before surgery to avoid injury during arterial-switch procedures and when right ventricular outflow tract reconstruction is being contemplated.

Management The terms "definitive operation" and "total repair" represent entirely different outcomes. With a definitive operative repair, residual defects may persist and late complications may develop that can affect the long-term outcome of the patient. Therefore, an experienced cardiologist, together with the primary care physician, should provide lifelong cardiac follow-up. It is important for the physician to understand the presence, extent, and possible development of postoperative residua or complications (Table 11.2). A child who has undergone palliation with a shunt procedure will eventually outgrow that source of pulmonary blood flow. Increasing polycythemia and cyanosis with decreasing exercise tolerance and endurance are typical. Acute thrombosis of a shunt rarely occurs. Because of persistence of a right-to-left shunt in palliated patients, the risk for systemic embolization, brain abscess, and cerebral embolism is always present.

TABLE 11.2. **Postoperative Residua and Late Complications in Cyanotic Heart Defects**

Defect	Residua and Complications
Shunted lesions	Acute thrombosis
	Progressive cyanosis and polycythemia
	Risk for systemic and cerebral embolization
	Brain abscess
	Deformation of pulmonary artery from shunt
	Endocarditis
Tetralogy of Fallot	Residual ventricular septal defect or pulmonary stenosis
	Branch pulmonary artery stenosis
	Right ventricular dysfunction from pulmonary insufficiency
	Ventricular dysrhythmias
	Heart block
Transposition of great arteries	Atrial repair
	Atrial dysrhythmias and sick sinus syndrome
	Systemic right ventricular dysfunction
	Tricuspid insufficiency
	Superior vena cava or pulmonary venous obstruction
Rastelli repair	Residual ventricular septal defect
	Conduit stenosis and insufficiency
Fontan procedure for univentricular hearts	Atrial dysrhythmias (atrial flutter and sick sinus syndrome)
	Ventricular dysfunction
	Conduit stenosis or branch artery stenosis
	Residual baffle leak (cyanosis)
	Formation of intrapulmonary ateriovenous fistulae (cyanosis)
	Protein-losing enteropathy
	Cirrhosis
	Exercise intolerance

Children who have undergone repair of tetralogy of Fallot may be asymptomatic and lead full lives. However, progressive right ventricle dilation and dysfunction due to volume overload from chronic pulmonary insufficiency may require a pulmonary homograft in the second or third decade of life. Right ventriculotomy, used to repair many complicated defects and some cases of tetralogy of Fallot, may result in conduction defects. Ventricular septal defect closure may also lead to injury to the conduction system with acute complete heart block or incomplete block that may progress to late complete block. The latter may be sudden and associated with Stokes-Adams attacks. Significant ventricular dysrhythmias and ventricular tachycardia are seen in patients with tetralogy of Fallot. Patients usually have significant residual right ventricular outflow tract obstruction or severe pulmonary insufficiency with right ventricular dysfunction.

The arterial-switch operation has become the procedure of choice for dextroposition of the great arteries because of the high incidence of atrial dysrhythmias, conduction abnormalities, and systemic ventricular dysfunction seen on long-term follow-up from atrial-switch procedures. Some complications seen with the atrial-switch operation in the past were probably related to surgical and myocardial preservation techniques that have since been improved. The outcome for children with dextroposition of the great arteries repaired by both methods remains good.

Children with cyanotic heart defects treated by the Fontan procedure do not age in good health. The longer the time since completion of the procedure, the fewer the patients who remain in sinus rhythm. Patients require antidysrhythmia medications for difficult-to-control atrial flutter and other supraventricular tachycardias. A pacemaker is often needed to provide adequate heart rate support so that medications can be used to effectively treat tachydysrhythmias. With time, ventricular dysfunction may follow, requiring therapy with digoxin, diuretics, and afterload-reduction agents. Cirrhosis and protein-losing enteropathy may occur because of chronic elevation of central venous pressure. Some patients develop cyanosis from pulmonary arteriovenous fistulae, which require coil embolization. Although many patients who have had the Fontan procedure continue to do well, many patients find themselves on lists for heart transplantations. It is the role of the primary care physician, along with the cardiologist, to optimize patient outcome and quality of life through attention to details and anticipation of possible long-term problems.

Periodic evaluation for potential rhythm disturbances, residual lesions, conduit or homograft dysfunction, and myocardial dysfunction must be done at intervals commensurate with the patient's clinical status. Medical therapy, interventional catheterization procedures, or surgical therapies are instituted and performed. Prophylaxis against endocarditis is necessary in patients who have had such procedures. If no further interventional or surgical therapies (including heart and heart–lung transplantation) are possible or warranted in a patient, medical management must be carefully monitored. This includes appropriate treatment of congestive heart failure and rhythm disturbances, therapy for severe polycythemia, and prevention of thromboembolism.

Congestive Heart Failure

In pediatrics, most congestive heart failure occurs within the first year of life; half of the patients present within the neonatal period and first few months of life. Excessive workloads imposed on the myocardium because of volume-loading situations (left-to-right shunts, valvular insufficiency, iatrogenic causes) or pressure-loading situations (valvular stenosis, coarctation or interruption of the aorta, hypertension) predominate in infants and children younger than 1 year of age. Rhythm disturbances from tachydysrhythmias (supraventricular or ventricular) or bradydysrhythmias (complete heart block) also occur frequently. Primary myocardial dysfunction from cardiomyopathies, myocarditis, or metabolic aberrations (hypoxemia, sepsis, acidosis, severe anemia, and electrolyte abnormalities) may occur at any age. After the age of 1 year, in addition to complications and residua from previous surgical procedures for congenital heart disease and new onset of dysrhythmias, acquired heart diseases such as rheumatic disease, endocarditis affecting existing heart defects, and myocardial diseases may present with congestive heart failure. Except for newborns with transient myocardial ischemia or depression from perinatal stress, patients with congestive heart failure generally improve only slightly and should be referred immediately for complete evaluation.

The Neonate

Causes The causes and timing of congestive heart failure in infants and children are listed in Table 11.3. Hydrops fetalis is usually due to noncardiac causes but may result from persistent tachydysrhythmias (supraventricular), bradydysrhythmias (complete heart block), severe valvular regurgitation (especially tricuspid valve), cardiac tumors, and large arteriovenous malfor-

TABLE 11.3. Causes and Timing of Heart Failure in Infants and Children

Prenatal	First Days—First Week	First Week—First Months	First Year
Severe anemia	Coarctation of aorta	Coarctation of aorta	Atrial septal defect
Dysrhythmias	Hypoplastic left heart	Patent ductus arteriosus	Other left-to-right shunts
Cardiac tumors	Critical aortic stenosis	Ventricular septal defect	Left ventricular inflow or outflow obstruction
Atrioventricular malformations	Aortic interruption	Complete endocardial cushion defect	Hypertension
Tricuspid regurgitation	Atrioventricular malformations	Transportation of great arteries	Dysrhythmias
Myocardial diseases	Cardiomyopathy	Ventricular septal defect	Iatrogenic
	Coronary anomalies	Truncus arteriosus	
	Perinatal stress	Cardiomyopathy	
		Total anomalous pulmonary venous return	

mations. Heart failure presenting within hours to the first day or so of life is usually due to severe left ventricular outflow tract obstruction, critical coarctation of the aorta, interruption of the aortic arch, critical aortic valvular stenosis, and hypoplastic left heart syndrome. These lesions are ductal-dependent systemic blood flow lesions. Systemic blood flow is derived from the right ventricle by way of the ductus; when the patent ductus arteriosus begins to constrict, systemic blood flow is compromised and congestive heart failure results. Infants with severe myocardial diseases, such as cardiomyopathies or myocarditis from an intrauterine infection, and large arteriovenous malformations (cerebral or hepatic) may also present with congestive heart failure within the first few days of life.

Most term infants with septal defects or patent ductus arteriosus, endocardial cushion defects, unobstructed total anomalous pulmonary venous return, dextroposition of the great arteries with large ventricular septal defect, and truncus arteriosus do not develop congestive heart failure until the second week of life or later. This is due, in part, to the delay in the decrease in pulmonary vascular resistance from prenatal levels. Term infants with less critical coarctation of the aorta and aortic stenosis also present somewhat later. Congenital anomalies of the coronary arteries (origin of the left coronary artery from the pulmonary artery) may result in congestive heart failure. This occurs in association with myocardial ischemia when pulmonary artery pressures decrease and myocardial perfusion is compromised.

Diagnosis In older infants and children, congestive heart failure is readily diagnosed from the clinical manifestations of pulmonary or systemic congestion and impaired myocardial performance with typical murmurs and gallops. The infant, however, usually presents with respiratory distress and, eventually, poor systemic perfusion. Rapid heart rates and noisy, rapid, labored respirations make adequate auscultation of the heart difficult. Accurate determination of liver size is often hampered by hyperaeration from pulmonary hypertension or obstructive pulmonary disease. Before the physical examination, review of the prenatal and birth history may provide evidence of intrauterine problems such as possible infection, dysrhythmia, or fetal distress. A family history of cardiomyopathy, previous births with congenital malformations or fetal death, and maternal illnesses such as diabetes should be obtained. Because growth failure may be a sign of congestive heart failure in the infant, a history of feeding difficulties with easy fatigability, dyspnea, diaphoresis, and tachypnea should be sought.

On initial physical examination, the general state of health or illness is readily discovered and signs of failure to thrive are sometimes apparent. An infant with compromised systemic oxygen delivery from cyanotic congenital heart disease or congestive heart failure has little spontaneous movement. Dysmorphic features may suggest a syndrome associated with congenital heart disease, such as Down's syndrome (endocardial cushion defect, ventricular septal defect) and fetal alcohol syndrome (septal defects and tetralogy of Fallot). Tachycardia (a heart rate of more than 160 beats/min in an infant at rest) suggests increased adrenergic tone in response to diminished cardiac output. Heart rates in excess of 220 beats/min suggest supraventricular tachycardia as the cause of congestive heart failure. Tachypnea is usually present as part of the clinical picture of congestive heart failure. Rapid, shallow respirations with nasal flaring and intercostal retractions with wheezes are characteristic of pulmonary overcirculation in the infant; rales are present in advanced congestive heart failure. Signs of systemic venous congestion such as hepatomegaly and peripheral edema may also accompany congestive heart failure.

Auscultation of the head (occipital area) and liver for continuous bruits diagnostic of arteriovenous malformations should be routinely performed on all infants being evaluated for congestive heart failure. It cannot be overemphasized that blood pressure should be measured in all four extremities in every infant and child being evaluated for congenital heart disease to rule in or out the presence of coarctation of the aorta. In infants, obtaining pulse oximetry and blood pressure measurements in upper and lower extremities effectively rules in or rules out ductal-dependent systemic blood flow lesions. An infant with equal blood pressures in arms and legs and complete SaO_2 (>95%) in the upper and lower extremities cannot have a ductal-dependent systemic blood flow lesion. With the latter lesions, the lower-extremity SaO_2 would be considerably lower than the upper-extremity SaO_2. In these lesions, the patent ductus arteriosus, from the right ventricle and pulmonary artery, is the main source of systemic blood flow. Once the patent ductus arteriosus constricts or closes, the SaO_2 in upper and lower extremities may become similar but perfusion to the body is compromised, with obvious blood pressure alterations.

Further examination of the cardiovascular system may show specific abnormalities. Palpation of the pulses in the upper and lower extremities is mandatory and can reveal coarctation of the aorta or aortic interruption. Generalized low- output states are characterized by diminished pulses throughout. Gallop rhythms may be present, indicating altered ventricular compliance. Murmurs may suggest the cause, but definite diagnosis is made in conjunction with a pediatric cardiologist. Rhythm disturbances detected on auscultation should be documented by ECG. Chest radiography may display cardiomegaly, specific chamber enlargement, and pulmonary overcirculation and may suggest the presence of aortic arch abnormality. Two-dimensional Doppler echocardiography is the diagnostic test of choice to delineate the anatomic and functional alterations in congenital heart disease.

Management Neonates with congestive heart failure requires immediate attention because they are in a tenuous, transitional period in which their condition may rapidly deteriorate. Therefore, when the diagnosis of possible congenital heart disease with congestive heart failure is being entertained, the patient is best served by referral to a pediatric cardiologist. Initial stabilization and therapy for the sick neonate include supplemental oxygen and placement of an intravenous line. If evidence clearly suggests a ductal-dependent systemic blood flow lesion, prostaglandin E_1 infusion may be initiated in consultation with a pediatric cardiologist. This agent may reopen the constricted ductus and restore systemic blood flow, thereby stabilizing the infant. If severe metabolic acidosis (pH < 7.2) is found, bicarbonate therapy should be administered. Pulmonary congestion or low urinary output may improve with diuretics. Respiratory insufficiency or failure responds to positive-pressure mechanical ventilation. In the sick infant, it may be difficult to separate sepsis or pulmonary infection from congestive heart failure; thus, antibiotics may be appropriate after cultures are obtained. Although digoxin remains the mainstay inotropic agent for long-term management of congestive heart failure in infants and children, it is of little use in the sick neonate with poor myocardial function and compromised systemic perfusion. Intravenous infusions of dopamine or dobutamine (5 to 15 μg/kg of body weight per minute) may be required to support cardiovascular function until the congenital heart disease is addressed surgically or the systemic disease causing myocardial dysfunction (sepsis, myocarditis, perinatal stress) is controlled. Surgical and interventional catheterization procedures used to treat congenital heart disease in infants and children are listed in Table 11.4. After stabilization, infants with coarctation of the aorta undergo repair done by using various procedures, depending on the anatomy.

Diagnostic catheterization is usually performed before surgery. The infant with critical aortic valve stenosis may first undergo balloon dilation of the aortic valve to relieve the obstruction; if that is unsuccessful, open valvulotomy is performed. Infants with a hypoplastic left heart may undergo heart transplantation or a Nor-

TABLE 11.4. Surgical and Interventional Catheterization Treatments for Congestive Heart Failure in Infants and Children

Lesion	Procedure
Neonate and infant	
Coarctation of aorta	End-to-end anastomosis Subclavian flap angioplasty Radical shunt anastomosis Dacron/Gortex patch angioplasty Balloon dilation of recurrent coarctation
Interuption of aorta	Primary anastomosis Homograft arch reconstruction Ventricular septal defect closure Balloon dilation Open valvulotomy on bypass
Aortic valve stenosis	Balloon dilation Open valvulotomy on bypass
Hypoplastic left heart syndrome	Norwood operation followed by staged Fontan procedure Transplantation
Patent ductus arteriosus	Surgical ligation Ligation and division
Truncus arteriosus	Removal of pulmonary artery from trunk, attach to right ventricle by homograft, closure of ventricular septal defect
Transposition of great arteries with large ventricular septal defect	Arterial-switch operation with patch closure of ventricular septal defect
Anomalous left coronary artery	Anastomosis of left coronary artery to aorta Pulmonary–aortic tunnel to coronary artery
Arteriovenous malformations	Coil embolization techniques with surgical backup
Older infant and child	
Ventricular septal defect	Pulmonary artery band as palliation Patch closure
Atrial septal defect	Direct suture closure Pericardial patch closure for large defect or sinus venosus defect associated with anomalous pulmonary veins
Partial endocardial cushion defect	Pericardial patch closure of atrial septal defect, suture repair of mitral valve cleft
Complete endocardial cushion defect	Ventricular septal defect and atrial septal defect patch closures, separation of common atrioventricular valve into competent, nonstenotic mitral, and tricuspid valves
Patent ductus arteriosus	Surgical ligation and division Ductal occlusion devices in catheterization laboratory
Aortic insufficiency	Aortic homograft replacement Ross procedure Mechanical valve
Mitral insufficiency	Repair Annuloplasty Homograft replacement Mechanical valve

wood operation, usually without diagnostic cardiac catheterization because echocardiography provides adequate anatomic and hemodynamic information. The Norwood operation includes atrial septectomy, ligation and division of the patent ductus arteriosus, and reconstruction of the aorta from the right ventricle with homograft augmentation of the aortic arch and aortopulmonary shunt placement for a controlled source of pulmonary blood flow.

Between 6 and 12 months of life, the aortopulmonary shunt is replaced by a bidirectional Glenn shunt; the Fontan procedure is then performed. Infants with interruption of the aorta may be able to withstand primary repair of the arch or may require an interposition homograft conduit to restore ascending to descending aortic continuity. Most of these infants have a large ventricular septal defect, which may be closed at the same time as the arch reconstruction; as an alternative, a pulmonary artery band may be placed to prevent pulmonary overcirculation. The infant returns at a later date for pulmonary artery debanding and patch closure of the ventricular septal defect. Truncus arteriosus is repaired by removal of the pulmonary arteries from the common trunk and attaching them to a pulmonary homograft sewn to the right ventricle; the ventricular septal defect is closed to include the aortic trunk from the left ventricle.

Infants with anomalous coronary artery from the pulmonary artery may be critically ill, with low cardiac output from an ischemic, possibly infarcted left ventricle and severe mitral insufficiency. If they can be stabilized, continuity between the anomalous coronary artery and the aorta is surgically restored. This may be done directly in some cases; in others, a tunnel is constructed from the aorta through the pulmonary artery to the anomalous left coronary artery. Despite surgical therapy, some of these infants may still require heart transplantation.

The Older Infant, Child, and Adolescent

Causes Whereas the neonate with congenital heart disease presents with congestive heart failure typically due to a left ventricular obstructive lesion, the older infant with congestive heart failure typically has a significant left-to-right shunt and pulmonary overcirculation, usually caused by septal defects and patent ductus arteriosus. Other causes of volume overload include arteriovenous fistulae, valvular insufficiency, and iatrogenic volume administration. Pressure overload lesions that may have been mildly to moderately severe early in life may progress and become hemodynamically severe as the infant grows. Included in this group are children who have recurrences of their left ventricular obstruction after neonatal procedures. It is important to remember that endocarditis can occur even in infants with congenital heart disease. Therefore, when an infant with a heart defect presents with new onset of congestive heart failure, the diagnosis of endocarditis must be considered. Myocardial dysfunction may be a residual condition from severe neonatal defects. At any age, congestive heart failure may be caused by myocarditis, cardiomyopathy, electrolyte disturbance, endocrine problems, systemic hypertension, or alterations in the chronotropic state of the heart.

Infants and young children with heart failure may appear undernourished as a consequence of decreased systemic perfusion and increased oxygen demands. Chronic nonproductive cough caused by bronchial mucosa congestion, orthopnea, and dyspnea on exertion may also be present. Tachypnea, dyspnea, rales, and other signs of pulmonary congestion, along with signs of systemic venous congestion, are usually present in the older infant and child with congestive heart failure. Evidence of myocardial dysfunction with tachycardia and S_3 gallop on auscultation, cool distal extremities with diffusely diminished pulses, and perfusion are frequent. An S_4 gallop, however, suggests a hypertrophied, noncompliant ventricle, such as that seen with hypertrophic cardiomyopathies, severe left ventricular outflow obstruction, and mitral stenosis.

Diagnosis As in the neonate, blood pressure should be measured in all four extremities of every older child being evaluated for congestive heart failure to rule out coarctation of the aorta. Similarly, all peripheral pulses must be palpated. The heart may be enlarged to palpation or percussion. Typical murmurs of septal defects and patent ductus arteriosus, semilunar valve, and atrioventricular valve stenosis or insufficiency are usually present, leading to definitive diagnosis in consultation with a pediatric cardiologist. It is important to remember that it may be difficult to differentiate respiratory signs of heart failure from primary pulmonary diseases. Infants and children with primary heart disease may have superimposed pulmonary diseases; conversely, severe respiratory disease may compromise myocardial function with signs of heart failure. Comprehensive two-dimensional Doppler echocardiography of the heart is invaluable in such situations to accurately define the cardiopulmonary situation and guide subsequent management.

Management The major goals in the treatment of congestive heart failure include

- Relief of pulmonary and systemic venous congestion
- Improvement of myocardial performance
- Reversal of the underlying disease process
- Repair of the congenital heart defect

Medical management is useful in improving the hemodynamics in preparation for and after surgical or interventional procedures. In selected patients, medical management may be used successfully to postpone interventions that would best be done on a larger child or older child. For the infant in mild to moderate congestive heart failure caused by a moderately sized ventricular septal defect, medical management may allow adequate growth of the infant. The infant may avoid surgical intervention completely because ventricular septal defects frequently diminish in size or close spontaneously.

The timely use of interventional cardiac catheterization procedures has decreased the number of surgical procedures performed in children with congenital heart disease. Specifically, aortic and pulmonary valve stenosis, mitral stenosis, pulmonary artery branch stenosis, and recurrent and native coarctation of the aorta have been successfully repaired in infants and children. Spring coils with nylon fibers used for coil embolization of aortopulmonary collateral vessels and arteriovenous fistulae are now used to close the small patent ductus arteriosus. Large ventricular septal defects, patent ductus arteriosi, and complete endocardial cushion defects are repaired by 1 year of age to prevent the development of pulmonary vascular disease. The repair is done sooner if congestive heart failure is severe, if pulmonary vascular resistance is elevated, or if the child has Down's syndrome (which is associated with earlier progression to pulmonary vascular disease).

The mainstay of medical management of congestive heart failure remains the use of digoxin to improve myocardial function. The digoxin schedule is different in children than in adults and is based on weight. The dose is given intramuscularly or intravenously if the patient is in moderate or severe congestive heart failure. A total digoxin dose is given over 24 hours: half initially, one-fourth 8 hours later, and one-fourth in another 8 hours. The patient is monitored for changes in heart rate and rhythm during this period. A lower total dose is used in the presence of myocarditis or cardiomyopathy because of a possible increased predisposition to dysrhythmias. The total digoxin dose for a full-term infant is 40 μg/kg of body weight. This is reduced to 25 to 30 μg/kg for the premature infant and is increased to 60 μg/kg for infants 1 month to 2 years of age. From ages 2 to 12 years, the total loading dose is 40 to 60 μg/kg. The daily maintenance dose is 10 μg/kg, divided every 12 hours up to a maximum of 0.25 mg/d. The parenteral form of the drug contains 100 μg/mL, and the oral preparation contains 50 μg/mL. After oral administration of digoxin, peak serum levels occur in 1 to 1.5 hours; with intravenous injections, peak levels occur almost immediately. Serum levels become steady-state about 8 hours after a dose is given.

In heart failure, the kidney responds to the relative hypoperfusion by increasing sodium reabsorption, which leads to volume expansion. This produces the clinical problems of systemic and pulmonary congestion, which are improved with the appropriate use of diuretic agents. Diuretics maximize sodium loss by increasing the renal excretion of sodium, water, and other anions. Hypokalemia may therefore accompany diuretic use, and serum potassium levels should be closely monitored, especially if digoxin is also being given. Hypokalemia may be prevented by using dietary potassium supplements or by adding a potassium-sparing agent (spironolactone). Afterload-reducing agents or vasodilators are used to relax vascular smooth muscle and to decrease systemic vascular resistance. Doing so alters loading conditions on the myocardium and improves cardiac performance. Angiotensin-converting enzyme inhibitors are used in infants and children to

- Unload the heart with primary myocardial dysfunction
- Decrease the left-to-right shunt through a large ventricular septal defect
- Decrease the regurgitant fraction (volume overload) from mitral or aortic valve insufficiency
- Afterload the heart in systemic hypertension

Vasodilators have also been used in children with the refractory congestive heart failure seen in cardiomyopathies (including anthracycline cardiotoxicity) and in the management of low-output states after the repair of congenital heart disease.

The two curative procedures among the many possible procedures are division of a patent ductus arteriosus in a patient without pulmonary artery hypertension and closure of a secundum atrial septal defect, which has a low associated risk of conduction and rhythm disturbances. Most heart defects corrected by interventional or surgical procedures may have residua or develop late complications that may alter long-term outcome. Again, long-term cardiac follow-up is appropriate at intervals commensurate with the clinical status of the patient and inherent risk for complications. These patients fall into three identifiable groups:

- Patients who have undergone a definitive operation with no residual disease and no expectation of late complication or future surgery
- Patients who have had successfully repaired defects but develop significant complications with some frequency and may require further intervention
- Patients who have undergone either palliative or limited corrective surgery but who have severe residual disease for which no further surgical therapy is possible, short of transplantation.

In the first group, such defects as atrial septal defect of the secundum type, ventricular septal defect, patent ductus arteriosus, and coarctation of the aorta have been repaired without residua. These patients may have normal exercise tolerance, physical examination, ECG, and chest radiography. Endocarditis prophylaxis is obligatory in all patients for 6 months to 1 year after surgery to allow complete endothelialization of the repair. Patients with coarctation repair continue to require prophylaxis because of the high incidence (approximately 80%) of an associated bicuspid aortic valve. Before stopping prophylaxis after patch closure of the ventricular septal defect and ligation of the patent ductus arteriosus, complete closure should be documented by echocardiography. Only infrequent evaluations are necessary; the patient has no restrictions on regular activity, including participation in sports.

Patients in the second group are prone to residual disease and complications. Valvulotomy, whether balloon or surgical, for aortic stenosis can only be considered palliative because residual or recurrent stenosis, regurgitation, and continued predisposition for endocarditis remain. Prosthetic valves and homograft valves do not grow and will require reoperation, probably more than once, if inserted in young children. Moreover, both mechanical and tissue valves are at risk for thrombus formation and endocarditis, and tissue valves may calcify with earlier deterioration in children. Some patients with repaired coarctation of the aorta will have systemic hypertension and many, especially those who undergo repair during infancy, will have evidence of recoarctation. Previously competent or mildly regurgitant atrial ventricular valves may develop progressive insufficiency and may require repair or replacement. Any residual defect may be the site for endocarditis; thus, prophylaxis is mandatory in these patients. Periodic evaluations for rhythm and conduction disorders, residual lesions, prosthetic valve dysfunction, and myocardial dysfunction are warranted. These patients may participate in sports activities as long as their role is not a competitive one. Children with pacemakers and those requiring anticoagulation for prosthetic valves should not participate in contact-sports activities.

Patients in the final group have end-stage cardiomyopathies, end-stage myocardial failure from several previous operations, severe residual defects, and pulmonary vascular disease. Heart or heart–lung transplantation is now a viable option and may offer some of these patients extended, improved survival. Many patients, however, require continued treatment for progressive congestive heart failure, rhythm disturbances, pulmonary and systemic hypertension, and prophylaxis against endocarditis. Multiple-drug therapies and their interactions, electrolyte imbalance, and worsening symptoms must be monitored.

ACQUIRED HEART DISEASE

Kawasaki Disease

Causes

Mucocutaneous lymph node syndrome or Kawasaki disease is a leading cause of acquired heart disease in the United States and developed world. It is a generalized vasculitis of unknown cause that occurs more often in boys than in girls, with a ratio of about 1.5:1. Eighty percent of cases occur in children younger than 5 years of age; most affected children are younger than 2 years of age. The disease is rare in children after the age of 8 years. Less than 2% of patients have recurrences. The epidemiology of Kawasaki disease indicates that an infectious agent causes the disease. Most cases are observed in the spring and winter, although the disease occurs year-round. Children of all racial backgrounds are affected, but the highest incidence is seen in children of Asian ancestry. Although critical data are lacking, Kawasaki disease may be associated with residence near bodies of water or exposure to house dust mites or recently shampooed carpets. Person-to-person transmission is not thought to occur, even in day care centers, and secondary cases among siblings are rare.

The most serious consequence of Kawasaki disease is the formation of coronary artery aneurysms, which may result in coronary thrombosis, stenosis, and, ultimately, myocardial infarction. Coronary abnormalities such as ectasia or aneurysms occur in 15 to 25% of affected children. Aneurysms usually appear 10 to 28 days after the onset of symptoms. Giant aneurysms (those with an internal dimension $>$ 8 mm) have a substantial risk for thrombosis and possible rupture and usually do not resolve. Smaller aneurysms may decrease in size, resolve with endothelial irregularities, or progress to stenotic lesions.

Diagnosis

Because the cause of Kawasaki disease remains unknown, a specific diagnostic test is not available; the disease is diagnosed on clinical grounds. Clinical criteria have been established to assist the physician in establishing the diagnosis and preventing overdiagnosis. These and other clinical and laboratory findings frequently seen in patients with Kawasaki disease are listed in Table 11.5.

The acute phase of the disease, which lasts 1 to 2 weeks, usually begins with sudden onset of high fever, followed in a short time by a polymorphous skin rash (which may be morbilliform, scarlatiniform, or erythema multiforme), very rarely with bullae or vesicles. Patients frequently have nonpurulent bulbar conjunctivitis, reddening and fissuring of the lips, erythema of the oral mucosa, and prominent strawberry tongue. Nonsuppurative cervical lymphadenitis occurs in the acute phase and is the least prominent of all of the principal clinical findings. The changes in the extremities are most impressive and include erythema and indurative edema of the hands and feet. The child is in constant discomfort and refuses to bear weight on the feet or move his or her swollen, tender hands. During this time, leukocytosis with a shift to the left, anemia, and thrombocytosis are seen.

Cardiovascular manifestations are seen in the acute phase of the disease, and the pericardium, myocardium, endocardium, and coronary arteries may all be involved. Pericardial effusion is present in about one-third of patients but rarely progresses to tamponade. Myocarditis is common and recognized clinically by a tachycardia out of proportion to the degree of fever and a gallop rhythm. Frank heart failure may result from the myocarditis, myocardial infarction, or valvular involvement, primarily mitral regurgitation. The ECG may show decreased R-wave voltage, ST-segment depression, and T-wave flattening or inversion. Prolongation of rate-adjusted P-R and Q-T intervals may result from myocardial inflammation. Dysrhythmias, ventricular more commonly than atrial, may be seen from focal areas of inflammation or ischemia. Acute myocardial in-

TABLE 11.5. Diagnostic Criteria and Frequently Associated Findings in Kawasaki Disease

Diagnostic Criteria	
Fever of at least 5 days' duration[a]	
Presence of 4 of the following features	
Change in extremities	
Polymorphous exanthem	
Bilateral conjunctival injection	
Changes in lips and oral cavity	
Cervical lymphadenopathy	
Other clinical features	
Cardiac	Pancarditis early, coronary abnormalities after 10 days of onset of illness
Gastrointestinal	Hydrops of gallbladder, hepatic dysfunction, abdominal pain, diarrhea, vomiting
Musculoskeletal	Arthritis, arthralgia
Central nervous system	Extreme irritability, aseptic meningitis
Respiratory	Preceding respiratory illness, otitis media, pulmonary infiltrates
Other	Aneurysms of medium-sized noncoronary arteries, peripheral gangrene, testicular swelling
Laborary findings	
Hematologic	Thrombocytosis, neutrophilia with immature forms, elevated erythrocyte sedimentation rate, anemia
Urine	Proteinuria, sterile pyuria
Serum	Hypoalbuminemia, elevated aminotransferase, C-reactive protein, and IgE levels

Reprinted with permission from The Committee on Rheumatic Fever, Endocarditis, and Kawasaki Disease, Council on Cardiovascular Disease in the Young, American Heart Association. Diagnosis and therapy of Kawasaki disease in children. Circulation 1993;87:1777–1790.
[a]In patients with fever and fewer than four principal clinical features, Kawasaki disease can be diagnosed when coronary artery disease is detected by two-dimensional echocardiography or angiography.

farction is usually represented on ECG by marked ST-segment elevation with inversion of T waves and abnormal Q waves over the involved myocardial segment. Coronary aneurysms can be seen as early as 3 days after onset of illness but are most commonly seen 10 days to 4 weeks after the onset. It is uncommon for coronary aneurysms to first present more than 6 weeks after the onset of the disease. Risk factors associated with the development of coronary aneurysms include the following:

- Male sex
- Age younger than 1 year
- Other cardiac involvement, including dysrhythmias
- Prolonged duration of inflammation, including fever for more than 10 days
- Recurrence of fever after defervescence of at least 24 hours

In the second 2 weeks of the disease or during the subacute phase, most patients have desquamation of finger and toe areas that starts in the subungual regions and spreads to palms and soles. The arthritis and arthralgia may persist for many months. If the patient is untreated or treated with aspirin only, fever will last for 1 to 3 weeks and will not respond to antibiotics. Kawasaki disease can be diagnosed in patients with fever and fewer than four principal features if coronary artery disease is detected by two-dimensional echocardiography or coronary angiography. Children with prolonged unexplained febrile illnesses, especially those associated with subsequent peripheral desquamation, should undergo echocardiography 3 to 4 weeks after the onset of the illness to determine whether they are at risk for developing significant coronary abnormalities.

In the presence of classic features, Kawasaki disease can be diagnosed by experienced practitioners before the fifth day of fever. However, many clinical conditions can mimic Kawasaki disease. These include

- Viral or rickettsial exanthems such as measles, Epstein-Barr virus infection, or Rocky Mountain spotted fever
- Bacterial infections such as scarlet fever, staphylococcal scalded skin syndrome, toxic shock syndrome, and leptospirosis drug reactions
- Stevens-Johnson syndrome
- Mercury poisoning
- Juvenile rheumatoid arthritis

A careful history and physical examination with judicious use of laboratory tests will direct the physician to the correct diagnosis. Echocardiography is the primary tool for evaluation and follow-up of the cardiovascular abnormalities, especially the coronary artery abnormalities. Initial echocardiography is done when Kawasaki disease is suspected. This examination establishes the baseline to which all follow-up studies are compared. Attention is focused on coronary artery structure, valve function, myocardial function, and the course of a pericardial effusion (when present). Because early diagnosis and institution of appropriate therapy are particularly important in preventing coronary artery involvement, patients with questionable diagnoses should be referred to a pediatric facility with established expertise in the diagnosis and management of Kawasaki disease.

TABLE 11.6. Recommended Therapy during the Acute Stage of Kawasaki Disease

Intravenous gammaglobulin
- 2 g/kg as single infusion over 12 hours (preferred)

or

- 400 mg/kg per day for 4 days; each dose infused over 2 hours

plus

Aspirin
- 80–100 mg/kg per day orally in 4 equally divided doses until patient is afebrile[a]

then

- 3–5 mg/kg orally once daily for up to 6–8 weeks[b]

Reprinted with permission from The Committee on Rheumatic Fever, Endocarditis, and Kawasaki Disease, Council on Cardiovascular Disease in the Young, American Heart Association. Diagnosis and therapy of Kawasaki disease in children. Circulation 1993;87:1779–1790.

[a]Some clinicians recommend high-dose aspirin until the 14th day of illness.

[b]Discontinue aspirin 6 to 8 weeks after the onset of illness if no coronary arterial abnormalities are observed on echocardiography. Continue indefinitely if there are coronary arterial abnormalities.

Management

Short-term therapy is directed at reducing systemic and cardiac inflammation, whereas long-term therapy is used to prevent coronary thrombosis. Patients with Kawasaki disease are best served by treatment with high-dose aspirin and intravenous gammaglobulin within the first 10 days of the disease (Table 11.6). Early therapy has reduced both the morbidity of Kawasaki disease and the incidence of coronary artery abnormalities from 20% to less than 5% at 6 to 8 weeks after therapy. Therapy should be considered for patients in whom the disease is diagnosed after 10 days since onset, especially if signs of active inflammation or cardiac involvement are present. Children treated with the single-infusion regimen seem to have more rapid defervescence and return of acute-phase reactants to normal than children treated with the 4-day infusion. Intravenous gammaglobulin therapy may not always result in a prompt clinical response. Some patients may have persistent fever for more than 24 hours after infusion completion, and some have recurrence of fever after initial defervescence that lasted at least 24 hours. In both circumstances, retreatment with intravenous gammaglobulin should be considered because prolonged fever and inflammation are associated with an increased risk for coronary artery involvement. Finally, gastrointestinal absorption of aspirin may be impaired in the acute phase of the disease; monitoring of serum concentrations may be helpful in selected cases.

When fever has resolved and acute symptoms are resolving, the aspirin dose should be reduced to 3 to 5 mg/kg and given as a single dose per day for its antithrombotic effect. This regimen is continued for 6 to 8 weeks and then stopped if no coronary artery abnormalities are present on follow-up echocardiography. If coronary abnormalities are present, low-dose aspirin therapy should be continued indefinitely and the patient should be referred to a pediatric cardiologist for long-term follow-up care.

Several issues have arisen from gammaglobulin and aspirin treatment for Kawasaki disease. Because passively acquired antibodies from intravenous gammaglobulin may interfere with effective immunization, it is recommended that the parenteral administration of live-virus vaccines (measles, mumps, and rubella) be delayed for at least 5 months from the time of the last infusion. Risk for Reye's syndrome must be reduced by interrupting aspirin therapy if the patient develops varicella or influenza, although the magnitude of risk from Reye's syndrome is unknown. If a patient is at high risk for myocardial infarction during this interval, dipyridamole may be used to alter platelet activity. To reduce the risk for Reye's syndrome in patients receiving long-term aspirin therapy, influenza vaccine is recommended.

Long-term management of patients with Kawasaki disease depends on the degree of coronary arterial involvement. In all but a few patients, echocardiography should be repeated 6 to 8 weeks after the onset of the disease if there has been no evidence of giant coronary artery aneurysms or thrombus formation and if clinical and laboratory signs of systemic inflammation have resolved. Subsequent echocardiography for patients with no coronary artery disease or with ectasia or a solitary small aneurysm is done 6 to 12 months after the onset of the disease. Stenosis or thrombus formation is most frequently seen in patients with giant aneurysms; such patients require more frequent evaluations. Frequency of follow-up is individualized according to the degree of coronary involvement. Routine follow-up of these higher-risk patients includes echocardiography and ECG. If clinical symptoms or noninvasive tests suggest myocardial ischemia, myocardial perfusion scanning, exercise testing, and possibly cardiac catheterization with coronary angiography may be indicated. Myocardial infarction from coronary thrombosis should be suspected in patients with chest pain, abdominal discomfort, nausea or vomiting, weakness with pallor, diaphoresis, and, in young children, inconsolable crying. Diagnosis is confirmed by ECG changes and elevation of creatine kinase–MB isoenzyme levels.

Patients with no coronary artery changes at any stage of the disease require no therapy after the initial 8 weeks, have no exercise restrictions after that time, and require no follow-up after the first year unless the primary care physician suspects cardiac disease. Patients with transient coronary artery ectasia that disappears during acute illness are treated identically, without follow-up after the first year unless cardiac disease is suspected, although the physician may choose to see the patient at 3- to 5-year intervals. Individual patients with coronary artery aneurysm are maintained on long-term low-dose aspirin therapy with or without additional antiplatelet drugs or warfarin. They are restricted from contact sports (physical activity determined by stress testing) and undergo at least annual evaluations with ECG, echocardiography, and possible pharmacologic or exercise stress testing. In selected cases, coronary angiography may be indicated. The risk level for a given patient with coronary arterial involvement may change over time because of the changes in coronary artery architecture. Coronary angiography may be indicated if a stress test or perfusion imaging study suggests myocardial ischemia or echocardiography suggests significant stenosis. In some patients, coronary artery obstruction may warrant surgical revascularization, which is confounded in the young by technical limitations and low rates of graft patency. Percutaneous transluminal coronary angioplasty has not provided consistent or long-lasting results in this pediatric population. Cardiac transplantation has been performed on a few children with Kawasaki disease after aneurysm rupture, coronary bypass grafting, and end-stage heart failure after myocardial infarction.

Acute Rheumatic Fever

Causes

Rheumatic fever remains the leading cause of cardiac disease throughout the world during the first four decades of life. The epidemiology and microbiology of acute rheumatic fever in the United States have changed over the past 25 years. Although in the United States acute rheumatic fever is predominantly a disease of the poor (the epidemiology of poor neighborhoods mimics the international picture of the disease), recent outbreaks of acute rheumatic fever in this country have occurred in more affluent suburbs. These outbreaks were associated with group A streptococci that had a more mucoid appearance (highly encapsulated serotype strains such as M1, M3, and M18) than did previously encountered strains. The host factors and those associated with the infecting organism that lead to the development of acute rheumatic fever and the explanation for the association with poverty remain incompletely understood. What is clear is that untreated group A streptococcal pharyngitis is the most common antecedent event before an attack of acute rheumatic fever and that appropriate treatment of acute pharyngitis essentially eliminates the risk for acute rheumatic fever. Rheumatic fever does not follow group A streptococcal infection at other sites, such as the skin.

Diagnosis

The clinical manifestations of acute rheumatic fever follow a group A streptococcal infection after an asymptomatic latency period of about 3 weeks. Initial attacks of acute rheumatic fever are seen most commonly in children and adolescents between ages 6 and 11 years and are rare in children younger than 5 years of age. The seasonal incidence of acute rheumatic fever (peak incidence occurs in the spring) is similar to that of streptococcal pharyngitis. Acute rheumatic fever is a postinfectious systemic inflammatory disease that involves many organ systems, such as the central nervous system and joints, in a generally self-limited inflammatory process. However, the cardiac involvement can be severe, acute life-threatening congestive heart failure that may result in long-term disability and cardiac dysfunction. The organ systems initially involved (cardiac, joint, brain, subcutaneous, and cutaneous tissues) and the severity of involvement vary from patient to patient.

Carditis associated with acute rheumatic fever is seen in more than 50% of patients. This percentage has recently increased even further, to as high as 90%, when Doppler echocardiography is added to auscultation in the initial evaluation of the heart. Most deaths associated with acute rheumatic fever are related to carditis, which remains the major cause of acquired mitral insufficiency in children and adolescents. Carditis may be the sole manifestation of acute rheumatic fever but may accompany other manifestations. Cardiac involvement should be evident within 2 weeks of the other manifestations. Initial examination of patients should include a careful physical examination, ECG, and echocardiography. Patients who show no evidence of carditis on the initial examination should be followed closely for evolving carditis during the subsequent weeks.

The ECG may reveal generalized low-voltage, ST-segment changes, and T-wave flattening or inversion. The P-R interval may also be prolonged. Although cardiac involvement in acute rheumatic fever may involve the pericardium, myocardium, and endocardium, pericarditis is rare unless myocarditis is severe. This diagnostic point is helpful in differentiating acute rheumatic fever from other systemic inflammatory diseases (such as systemic lupus erythematosus or juvenile rheumatoid arthritis) in which pericarditis is frequent and usually present without significant myocardial involvement.

Valvulitis, or inflammation of the aortic and mitral valves and the chordae of the mitral valve, is the typical cardiac involvement in acute rheumatic fever. The hallmark of carditis in acute rheumatic fever is mitral insufficiency. Auscultation reveals an apical pansystolic murmur that begins with S_1, is blowing in character, and radiates to the left axilla and back. If the mitral insufficiency is severe, a mid-to-late diastolic rumbling murmur (Carey Coombs murmur) is also heard. Aortic insufficiency occurs in about 20% of cases and, if present, usually accompanies mitral insufficiency. Valvular insufficiency or severe myocarditis may progress to congestive heart failure in about 5% of patients (usually young children). Tachycardia inappropriate for the degree of temperature elevation (an increase $>$ 10 beats/min for each degree of temperature elevation) is an early sign of myocarditis. Heart rate is also an excellent marker of inflammation for monitoring the course of carditis. In addition to tachycardia, dysrhythmias and first- and second-degree heart block may also indicate myocardial involvement. Progressive cardiac enlargement may be a result of worsening mitral or aortic insufficiency, worsening myocarditis, and congestive heart failure or a result of pancarditis with pericarditis and effusion. A friction rub may be heard or palpable, especially when the patient is placed in the upright position.

Other major and minor manifestations of acute rheumatic fever are listed in Table 11.7. Arthritis occurs in about 70% of patients and primarily involves the large joints (knees, ankles, wrists, and elbows) in an asymmetric and migratory distribution. In most patients, arthritic symptoms resolve in approximately 1 week. The involved joints are painful, swollen, warm, and erythematous. A dramatic response to aspirin is characteristic. Syndenham's chorea occurs in less than

TABLE 11.7. Diagnostic Guidelines for Acute Rheumatic Fever[a]

Major Manfestations		Minor Manifestations
Carditis (mitral insufficiency)	50–90%	Clinical Arthralgia Fever
Polyarthritis (migratory, asymmetric)	70%	
Chorea	15%	Laboratory Elevated acute-phase reactants Elevated erythrocyte sedimentation rate Elevated C-reactive protein level Prolonged P-R interval
Erythema marginatum	5%	
Subcutaneous nodules	<5%	

[a]Modified from Dajani AS, Ayoub EM, Bierman FZ, et al. Guidelines for diagnosis of rheumatic fever: Jones criteria, updated 1992. Circulation 1992;87:302–307.
Supporting evidence for antecedent group A streptococcal infection: positive throat culture or rapid streptococcal antigen test; elevated or rising streptococcal antibody titer. If supported by evidence of preceding group A streptococcal infection, the presence of two major or one major and two minor manifestations suggest the diagnosis of acute rheumatic fever.

20% of patients; clinical signs first appear 3 months or more after the initial infection. Involuntary and purposeless movements, muscular incoordination (which affects all muscles but particularly affects those of the face and extremities), and emotional lability are typical. Speech patterns are broken, and, because of difficulties in fine-motor control, handwriting is affected. These bothersome symptoms are usually self-limited, even without therapy, and abate in several weeks; severe cases may persist for many months despite therapy. Erythema marginatum, occurring in about 5% of patients, is characterized as a macular, nonpruritic rash with a serpiginous erythematous border occurring most commonly on the trunk and proximal extremities. An application of warmth, such as a warm bath or shower, has been said to bring out the rash. Subcutaneous nodules (painless, freely mobile 0.5- to 2-cm nodules located on the extensor surfaces of the elbow, knee, ankle, and interphalangeal joints) are uncommon in acute rheumatic fever. They are more typically seen in patients with chronic rheumatic heart disease. The minor manifestations occur with some frequency in acute rheumatic fever but are nonspecific findings shared with other inflammatory and infectious diseases.

Diagnosis

The most recent revision of the Jones criteria are now used to solidify a diagnosis of acute rheumatic fever in lieu of a specific diagnostic test. The diagnosis of acute rheumatic fever requires the presence of two major manifestations or one major and two minor manifestations. Both situations require supporting evidence of recent streptococcal infection. Despite these criteria, other diseases, such as collagen vascular diseases, postinfectious polyarthritis, serum sickness, and infectious arthritis, may need to be considered. Additional laboratory tests may be necessary. If the patient has carditis, especially pericarditis, diseases such as other causes of myopericarditis (viral, bacterial, mycoplasma, rickettsial, or parasitic infections), juvenile rheumatoid arthritis, and lupus should be excluded. Endocarditis on congenital heart defects and Kawasaki disease should also be considered.

Management

Treatment first involves the eradication of group A streptococci from the pharynx; the standard recommended treatment of acute streptococcal pharyngitis is adequate for this. Secondary prophylaxis is critical for the prevention of recurrences of rheumatic fever and, in patients with cardiac involvement, is recommended for at least 5 years after the acute attack and probably for life. Patients without carditis are at lower risk for cardiac involvement with recurrences. Prophylaxis in these patients may be discontinued once they reach their early twenties (provided that the first acute episode had occurred at least 5 years previously). Patients at higher risk for streptococcal pharyngitis should consider extended duration of prophylaxis. Monthly injections of long-acting benzathine penicillin are most reliable, although twice-daily dosing of oral penicillin is also effective. Erythromycin may be used for patients allergic to penicillin. In patients with valvular disease, prophylaxis against bacterial endocarditis and rheumatic fever is important.

Therapy for carditis includes bed rest, anticongestive measures for congestive heart failure, and anti-inflammatory therapy. Salicylate therapy is recommended in patients with mild to moderate carditis; steroids should be reserved for patients with severe carditis, pancarditis, and congestive heart failure. Aspirin is administered at 90 to 100 mg/kg per day, with a serum level goal of 25 mg/dL. Therapy is continued for 4 to 8 weeks; if improvement is noted, therapy is weaned during the next 4 to 6 weeks. Monitoring of heart rate, echocardiography, and acute-phase reactants assist in the weaning process. If steroid therapy is used, it should last no longer than 2 weeks and should be gradually withdrawn over another 2 to 3 weeks. It is important to begin aspirin therapy a week before steroid therapy is discontinued to avoid an inflammatory rebound. Bed rest is important during carditis; after its resolution, increasing levels of activity are permitted. After the first attack of acute rheumatic fever, the residual heart disease frequently disappears or regresses and seldom worsens during the next 10 years if recurrence is prevented by continuous prophylaxis.

Mitral Valve Prolapse

Causes

The hallmarks of mitral valve prolapse on examination include a midsystolic to late systolic click and a systolic murmur. The click occurs when part of a leaflet or both leaflets of the mitral valve extend up into the left atrial cavity during ventricular systole. The murmur represents mitral insufficiency. Although mitral valve prolapse has been found in 1 to 2% of children of all ages, some studies suggest that it may be inherited as an autosomal dominant phenotype. The female-to-male ratio is 2:1. Mitral valve prolapse is associated with several recognizable connective tissue disorders, such as Marfan's syndrome, Ehlers-Danlos syndrome (types I, II, and IV), Stickler's syndrome, and osteogenesis imperfecta syndromes. Many patients with mitral valve prolapse have asthenic habitus, hypomastia, and skeletal abnormalities that do not meet criteria for specific genetic syndromes.

Symptoms in patients with mitral valve prolapse may include palpitations, easy fatigability, exercise intolerance, chest pain, dyspnea, postural phenomena, presyncope or syncope, and neuropsychiatric symptoms. Although these symptoms are usually seen during and after the second decade of life (see Chapter 15), they may also occur in children.

Diagnosis

Cardiac auscultation is the key to the diagnosis. The presence of a nonejection systolic click with or without a late mitral insufficiency murmur constitutes the clinical criteria for the diagnosis of mitral valve prolapse. The findings may vary from day to day. In children, the murmur may be honking or musical or may sound like a seagull; is loudest at the left midsternal border; and radiates toward the apex. Characteristic changes in the timing and intensity of the click and murmur with positional changes are diagnostic (Table 11.8). The systolic click moves toward S_I with upright posture; the systolic murmur becomes longer,

Effect of Postural Changes on Auscultation **TABLE 11.8.**

Variable	Mitral Valve Prolapse	Hypertrophic Cardiomyopathy	Venous Hum
Supine			
Click	Midsystolic	None	None
Murmur	Mitral regurgitation, apical	Systolic ejection murmur, decreased	Absent or decreased
Standing			
Click	Closer to S_1	None	None
Murmur	Earlier, longer, louder	Increased intensity	Increased intensity
Prompt Squatting			
Click	Closer to S_2	None	None
Murmur	Shorter duration	Decreased intensity	Not applicable

S_1, first heart sound, S_2, second heart sound.

may intensify, and may become holosystolic. A murmur may be heard only in the upright position. Prompt squatting from the standing position results in movement of the systolic click and the systolic murmur back toward S_2.

The most impressive changes in continuous auscultation occur after the patient stands from a squatting position, when the click and murmur move back toward S_1. Such postural changes in patients with mitral valve prolapse are related to changes in left ventricular volume, myocardial contractility, and heart rate. Hypertrophic cardiomyopathy with dynamic left ventricular outflow tract obstruction may display similar auscultative variation with postural changes, but nonejection clicks are generally not present.

Evaluation of a child suspected of having mitral valve prolapse should include a family history, general physical examination seeking evidence for connective tissue disease, cardiac examination with auscultation during postural changes, ECG, and echocardiography. Most patients with mitral valve prolapse have normal findings on ECG. Nonspecific ST-segment and T-wave changes and T-wave inversion, especially in the inferior leads, have been described in patients with mitral valve prolapse. Echocardiography does the following:

- Identifies the presence and severity of mitral valve prolapse
- Defines the anatomy of the mitral valve apparatus
- Measures the degree of mitral regurgitation
- Defines additional cardiac abnormalities

The likelihood of finding mitral valve prolapse by using echocardiography in patients with a negative auscultation upon careful physical examination is low. However, typical mitral valve prolapse on echocardiography without auscultatory findings should not be ignored.

In patients who have a history of syncope, palpitations, or other symptoms suggesting dysrhythmias, 24-hour ECG or event recorder and possible exercise stress test may be indicated. Palpitations may be related to dysrhythmias; on 24-hour continuous ECG, however, a discordance is often seen between rhythm abnormalities and symptoms. The causes of chest pain in patients with mitral valve prolapse are incompletely understood. Although syncope or presyncope may have dysrhythmia as a cause, patients with mitral valve prolapse may display orthostatic changes and vasodepressor-vasovagal syncope due to autonomic dysfunction. This dysautonomia may also play a role in the generation of anxiety, panic attacks, and other neuropsychiatric symptoms.

Management

The approach to treatment and follow-up depends on the severity of mitral valve dysfunction, the degree of mitral insufficiency, and the need to prevent or treat complications. Asymptomatic patients with isolated systolic clicks usually have mitral valve prolapse that has limited clinical significance and is generally nonprogressive. Prophylaxis against endocarditis is indicated in patients with mitral valve prolapse and mitral regurgitation. All asymptomatic patients with mitral valve prolapse in the absence of mitral insufficiency or a family history of sudden death associated with mitral valve prolapse may engage in all sports activities. Patients with mitral valve prolapse who are symptomatic (chest pain, palpitations, dysrhythmias, near-syncope, or syncope) or who have mitral insufficiency should have their status further evaluated by a cardiologist before they are cleared for athletic competition. Patients with mitral valve prolapse syndrome may be sensitive to volume depletion; thus, adequate volume should be taken before, during, and after physical activities. Low doses of β-adrenergic blocking drugs have been effective in preventing palpitations, chest pain, and anxiety attacks or panic attacks in patients with mitral valve prolapse, but only after a thorough evaluation to exclude other causes for the symptoms. Despite the reported complications, mitral valve prolapse is benign in most patients. The most important reassurance to give the patient and his or her parents is that mitral valve prolapse rarely has serious consequences.

Hypertrophic Cardiomyopathy

Causes

Several distinct subgroups of children with hypertrophic cardiomyopathy have different pathophysiologic causes of symptoms and, therefore, different prognoses (see Chapter 15 for a discussion of hypertrophic cardiomyopathy in the adult). Infants and young children are first identified with hypertrophic cardiomyopathy because of a murmur, diagnosis of which is confirmed by echocardiography. Symptoms indicating serious disease associated with hypertrophic cardiomyopathy are unusual in patients younger than 10 years of age. The onset of congestive heart failure in the first year of life carries a poor prognosis; few patients survive to the age of 2 years. These patients usually have severe septal hypertrophy with biventricular outflow tract obstruction and unremitting congestive heart failure despite medical and surgical intervention. In older children, adolescents, and young adults, the most common clinical manifestations of hypertrophic cardiomyopathy are dyspnea on exertion, chest pain, presyncope, syncope, palpitations, and sudden death. Chest pain may be typical or atypical ischemic chest discomfort (angina). Exercise intolerance, dyspnea, and orthopnea are often seen in conjunction with clinical signs of congestive heart failure. These signs are due to elevated pulmonary venous and left atrial pressures caused by abnormal left ventricular diastolic function. The severity and type of symptoms may be similar in patients with obstruction to left ventricular outflow and in patients without obstruction. In young adults with hypertrophic cardiomyopathy, the risk for sudden death is increased in patients who have documented nonsustained ventricular tachycardia, evidence of sinus or atrioventricular node disease, or resting sinus bradycardia that does not respond to tachycardic stimuli. The significance of such electrophysiologic abnormalities in children awaits resolution because dysrhythmias are rare in infants and children with hypertrophic cardiomyopathy. Furthermore, the absence of ventricular dysrhythmias during ambulatory ECG monitoring does not indicate a low risk for sudden death.

Sudden death occurs most often in young children and adults aged 12 to 35 years. Sudden death is not limited to symptomatic patients; most patients are asymptomatic or only mildly symptomatic, and sudden death may be the first and only manifestation of hypertrophic cardiomyopathy. In children and adolescents, syncopal episodes and a family history of sudden death indicate high risk. Resting or provocable left ventricular outflow gradients occur in only about 25% of patients with hypertrophic cardiomyopathy. No evidence suggests that the prognosis of such patients differs from that of patients without left ventricular outflow gradients. Most patients die while sedentary or performing mild exertion; about one-third die during or immediately after strenuous physical activity.

Diagnosis

The findings on physical examination in patients with hypertrophic cardiomyopathy vary and are related to the hemodynamic state. Physical findings in patients without left ventricular outflow obstruction may be subtle. The left ventricular impulse is single and not exaggerated, and the systolic murmur may be soft or absent. Performing auscultation with positional changes is critical to the detection of hypertrophic cardiomyopathy (Table 11.8). Even with auscultation, the diagnosis of nonobstructive hypertrophic cardiomyopathy may be difficult to confirm without echocardiography. Classic physical findings include the following:

- Palpable S_4 and a double apical systolic impulse
- Brisk, rapidly collapsing carotid brachial pulses with a distinct bisferious contour
- Harsh, left precordial systolic murmur that decreases in intensity with prompt squatting and increases with standing

Patients with loud systolic murmurs of at least grade 3/6 intensity usually have peak systolic gradients greater than 40 to 50 mm Hg. The murmur is usually most audible along the left lower sternal border or at the apex. Splitting of S_2 is physiologic in most patients but may be paradoxical in patients with severe left ventricular outflow obstruction. When the physical examination yields classic findings, Doppler echocardiography confirms the diagnosis and obviates the need for cardiac catheterization. Catheterization is performed in the following selected situations:

- To evaluate the patient before transplantation
- To obtain myocardial biopsy samples
- To diagnose underlying mitochondrial or metabolic abnormalities
- To evaluate the hemodynamic responses of the left ventricular outflow tract
- To assess pharmacologic treatments before initiating outpatient therapy
- To evaluate the hemodynamic responses to atrial ventricular sequential pacing before pacemaker implantation

Upon referral or discovery of a patient with hypertrophic cardiomyopathy, additional testing other than echocardiography is warranted. The ECG is abnormal in more than 90% of children with hypertrophic cardiomyopathy. Ambulatory 24- to 48-hour ECG monitoring has shown an 80 to 90% incidence of dysrhythmias, including rapid atrial activity and multiform ventricular premature complexes. An incidence of nonsustained ventricular tachycardia is seen in 15 to 30% of patients. Most patients with syncope and those with palpitations have dysrhythmias on 24-hour ECG monitoring. Treadmill exercise testing provokes dysrhythmias in about two-thirds of patients, and about half of these patients have new ST-segment or T-wave abnormalities. Because the findings on ambulatory ECG and exercise testing are not necessarily congruent, both studies are recommended.

Management

The optimum management of hypertrophic cardiomyopathy requires a firm commitment on the part of the physician to impart to each patient the best possible understanding of the disease, its possible complications, potential side effects of therapy, and the need for lifelong follow-up to ensure compliance with therapy. The most important aspect of clinical management is identification and treatment of patients at increased risk for sudden death. Any patient with hypertrophic cardiomyopathy who has survived sudden death must be treated. The following patients also require therapy:

- Patients who are symptomatic with chest pain, dyspnea, presyncope, and syncope or have significant exercise intolerance determined by exercise testing
- Patients with a family history of sudden cardiac death
- Patients with significant left ventricular hypertrophy (wall thickness > 20 mm)
- Patients with potentially life-threatening dysrhythmias, whatever the symptom status

Although the risk for endocarditis appears small in patients with hypertrophic cardiomyopathy, all patients should receive antibiotics before dental or surgical procedures. Because sudden death often occurs during or shortly after severe exertion and because hypertrophic cardiomyopathy appears to be the most common cause of sudden death in young athletes, asymptomatic children with hypertrophic cardiomyopathy should be strongly advised against participation in competitive sports or strenuous physical activities.

β-Adrenergic receptor blocking drugs have been used to relieve symptoms in patients with the obstructive or nonobstructive forms of hypertrophic cardiomyopathy. These drugs may improve symptoms by inhibiting sympathetic stimulation of the heart or decreasing outflow gradients under conditions of increased sympathetic tone, but they do little for resting gradients. They may improve congestive symptoms or chest pain by diminishing myocardial oxygen requirements but have minimal direct benefit on left ventricular diastolic function. After initial improvement, however, symptoms may recur in up to two-thirds of patients receiving β-blockers; this necessitates treatment with higher doses or treatment with calcium-channel blockers. Verapamil, the agent primarily used in children older than 1 year of age, improves left ventricular diastolic function and reduces outlet obstruction in both the short and long term. Many patients with symptoms severe enough to warrant surgical intervention obtain improvement sufficient to postpone surgery. Caution should be taken in initiating therapy in patients with hypertrophic cardiomyopathy who have pulmonary venous congestion, especially in the presence of left ventricular outflow obstruction; these patients may be at increased risk for severe pulmonary edema or sudden death. Disopyramide, an antidysrhythmic agent with potent negative inotropic action, is also an effective agent that benefits some patients with significant left ventricular outflow obstruction.

The treatment of potentially fatal dysrhythmias in hypertrophic cardiomyopathy is essential. The β-blocking agents are often effective in treating supraventricular and ventricular dysrhythmias and are used especially in patients who also have dyspnea or chest pain. No single antidysrhythmic drug, with the possible exception of amiodarone, has been proven to be superior in the prevention of sudden death. Amiodarone, a potent antidysrhythmia drug with many potential side effects, controls several dysrhythmias and has the additional benefit of improving diastolic function. The initiation and evaluation of the efficacy and possible complications of any antidysrhythmic drug or drug combination must be monitored and reassessed carefully in consultation with the pediatric cardiologist.

The therapeutic strategy for the asymptomatic child with hypertrophic cardiomyopathy and no evidence of complex dysrhythmias remains problematic. Many asymptomatic children and young adults have been treated prophylactically in the hope of decreasing the likelihood of sudden death. No available evidence proves that β-blockers or calcium-channel blockers protect against sudden death.

There is widespread enthusiasm for the presurgery use of dual-chambered pacing in patients with obstructive hypertrophic cardiomyopathy and severe drug-refractory symptoms. Atrial ventricular pacing alleviates symptoms and reduces left ventricular outflow gradients in most patients (no benefits have been seen in patients without obstruction). The long-term effects of this therapy in children are still unknown.

The surgical procedures—septal myotomy-myomectomy and mitral valve replacement—are recommended for patients with obstructive hypertrophic cardiomyopathy and severe symptoms that are refractory to medical and electrophysiologic therapies. Although symptoms improve in most patients undergoing surgery, no evidence suggests that surgery decreases the occurrence of potentially lethal dysrhythmias or reduces the risk for sudden death. Hypertrophic cardiomyopathy is one of the most common indications for heart transplantation in children. Indications and timing for the procedure vary according to the patient and include medically refractory or progressive symptoms in patients without obstruction or patients with obstruction who are suboptimal candidates for standard surgical techniques after all other methods have been used.

CONDUCTION AND RHYTHM DISTURBANCES IN CHILDREN

Sudden Death

Causes

Sudden death during childhood is an uncommon but tragic event. The incidence of sudden death in some postoperative patients years after surgery is related to dysrhythmias and conduction abnormalities. The frequency of this problem will probably increase as more patients are followed for longer periods after surgery. Exercise-related sudden death in children is also related to the presence of an aberrant left coronary artery coursing between the aortic and pulmonary artery roots. Myocardial ischemia occurs during exercise as the orifice of the left coronary artery becomes slit-like and the coronary becomes compressed between the great arteries. Syncope during exercise is the usual presentation. A small number of children and young adults with preexcitation also have atrial fibrillation and therefore may be at risk for ventricular fibrillation and sudden death.

An important cause of sudden death in children and young adults is the long Q-T syndrome. A genetic abnormality has been described linking family members. The dysrhythmia associated with the long Q-T syndrome is ventricular tachycardia. It is mediated through adrenergic and central nervous system stimulation, such as startling situations, loud noises, and competitive events. The Q-T interval should be measured and corrected for heart rate. Children who present with syncope or presyncope or have a family history of sudden death or congenital deafness should have ECG to determine the Q-T interval.

Irregular Rhythms

Causes

The most common irregular rhythm is sinus arrhythmia. This is the normal variation in the heart rate with respiration. As the child takes a breath, the heart rate increases. This is most evident in children 5 to 10 years of age. The diagnosis is confirmed by showing the cyclic variation in heart rate on ECG while the P wave and P-R interval do not vary. Sinus arrhythmia virtually rules out the presence of inflammatory or infectious diseases of the heart, such as myocarditis or congestive heart failure.

Premature beats are frequent in children. Atrial premature beats are often seen in newborn infants and usually disappear within the first weeks to first month of life. Premature ventricular contractions are more common in older children and adolescents. These are usually unassociated with any identifiable cause. They may occur in children with congenital heart disease before or, more frequently, after reparative surgery, with myocarditis, electrolyte imbalance, and drug abuse or toxicity. Clinically, children with premature ventricular contractions are asymptomatic or may be aware of their ectopy and report palpitations. Premature ventricular contractions are believed to be of benign origin if they are uniform and single and can be abolished by increases in the intrinsic heart rate by having the child run in place for a short time. Typically, the premature ventricular contractions return as the heart rate declines to a heart rate similar to that at which they were suppressed. Exercise stress testing and 24-hour ECG may be helpful in the evaluation of these children.

Supraventricular Tachycardia (see Chapters 2 and 3)

Diagnosis

The presentation in children depends on the presence or absence of associated congenital heart disease, the state of the myocardium, and the duration and rate of the supraventricular tachycardia. Infants and young children are frequently seriously ill. They may be pale, poorly perfused with cool extremities, restless, and irritable, with signs of congestive heart failure. Heart failure is uncommon when the duration is less than 24 hours and the heart rate is less than 200 beats/min. The heart rate range is 125 to 320 beats/min (average, 240 beats/min). Typically, faster rates are seen in the infant and young child. The QRS complex during supraventricular tachycardia has a normal duration and shape in more than 90% of children. Therefore, if complete bundle-branch block is seen with tachycardia, ventricular tachycardia is strongly suggested. P waves may occur in 50% of patients with supraventricular tachycardia and are most frequently seen to be inverted in leads II, III, and aVF and positive in leads I and aVL. Preexcitation due to Wolff-Parkinson-White syndrome can be found on the sinus ECG in approximately 20% of children who have supraventricular tachycardia; infants show an even higher incidence (25 to 50%). Concealed preexcitation and atrioventricular node reentry tachycardia are also common mechanisms of supraventricular tachycardia in children. Echocardiography is recommended in the initial evaluation after the rhythm has returned to normal in order to exclude intrinsic congenital heart disease, tumors, and cardiomyopathy.

Management

The form of therapy is determined by the urgency of the situation, but the first episode of supraventricular tachycardia in a child should always be treated. If the patient (no matter what the age) is acutely ill with evidence of congestive heart failure or low output, the following should be tried in succession but under appropriate ECG monitoring, with established intravenous access and resuscitation equipment and medications available:

1. Vagal maneuvers (squatting and straining in older children or pressing on the abdomen of infants); ocular pressure is contraindicated because eye damage may result.
2. Ice bag (a bag of ice and water is placed over the face of the patient for 10 seconds)
3. Adenosine given as a bolus followed by a saline bolus will break supraventricular tachycardias that use the atrioventricular node as part of the reentry mechanism (preexcitation and atrioventricular nodal reentry)
4. Cardioversion (1 W/sec per kg)

If supraventricular tachycardia is refractory to the aforementioned interventions, digoxin loading may be initiated in consultation with a cardiologist. Digoxin is not recommended in children older than 1 year of age who have preexcitation because there is a risk for shortening the effective refractory period of the bypass tract; digoxin should also not be given in the presence of atrial fibrillation (about 10% of patients) because it results in one to one conduction to the ventricle producing ventricular fibrillation.

Long-term therapy is continued for 1 year. Supraventricular tachycardia recurs less frequently in treated patients and in patients in whom supraventricular tachycardia developed at 4 months of age or younger. Recurrences are the rule regardless of whether precipitating factors are present. Additional or alternative medications may become necessary. Radiofrequency ablation of refractory supraventricular tachycardia has been successfully performed in even small children and is recommended for medically refractory or life-threatening dysrhythmias and intolerable adverse effects of medications.

Ventricular Tachycardia

Diagnosis

Ventricular tachycardia is rare in children. Only about 25% of affected children have normal hearts. Most patients predisposed to ventricular tachycardia have undergone repair of tetralogy of Fallot or have a prolonged Q-T interval, cardiac tumors, or cardiomyopathy. Children with mitral valve prolapse may have premature ventricular contractions, which have a benign course. Drug toxicity from digoxin and tricyclic antidepressants, as well as severe hypoxemia, hypotension, and hyperkalemia from any cause, may lead to ventricular tachycardia. The concomitant use of erythromycin and theophylline compounds can result in theophylline toxicity and risk for ventricular tachycardia, especially during an acute exacerbation of asthma (when hypoxemia may be present). Patients may have a history of palpitations, chest pain, and syncope or presyncope and a family history of sudden death.

Management

In the treatment of high-grade ventricular ectopy and ventricular tachycardia, possible precipitating events should be determined and treated. Aggressive treatment of the seriously ill child who has an acute onset of premature ventricular contractions and multiform premature ventricular contractions, couplets, and ventricular tachycardia is recommended. In the unstable patient, synchronized direct-current cardioversion (if a pulse is present) or defibrillation (pulseless ventricular tachycardia) is performed with 1.0 to 2.0 W/sec per kg. Successive doubling of the cardioversion charge may be needed. If cardioversion is unsuccessful, hypoxemia, acidosis, hypoglycemia, or other metabolic derangement requiring therapy may be present. The appropriateness and effectiveness of subsequent therapy may be guided by 24-hour ECG monitoring, exercise stress testing, and, in some situations, invasive electrophysiologic testing.

Congenital Complete Heart Block

Causes

The most common cause of persistent bradycardia in newborn infants and children is complete atrioventricular block, defined as complete absence of conduction of atrial impulses to the ventricle. Heart block may be acquired or congenital. Patients with acquired heart block may be further subdivided as having surgical or nonsurgical complete heart block; the latter subgroup has infectious and inflammatory diseases, myopathies, and idiopathies. Infants and children with complex congenital heart disease, including single-ventricle and levotransposition of the great arteries with ventricular inversion, are at risk for spontaneous complete heart block because of intrinsic abnormalities of the atrioventricular node and conduction system. Congenital complete heart block is often diagnosed before birth. Complete heart block unassociated with congenital heart disease is considered a model of passively acquired autoimmunity by which immune abnormalities in the mother lead to production of autoantibodies that cross the placenta and presumably injure the developing fetus. The prevalence of connective tissue disease in mothers of infants with congenital complete heart block ranges from 33 to 64%; half of the mothers are symptomatic, and half have only serologic evidence of disease. Systemic lupus erythematosus is the usual underlying disorder, but Sjögren's syndrome, rheumatoid arthritis, and undifferentiated connective tissue disease have also been reported. Although complete heart block is irreversible, the noncardiac manifestations of neonatal lupus are transient, resolving at about 6 months of age (at the same time that maternal antibodies disappear from the child's serum). Patients should be counseled about the substantial risk for recurrence of heart block, and the fetal heart rate should be monitored. Heart block unassociated with antibodies is usually diagnosed later in life and often starts as incomplete block that progresses to complete heart block. Patients in whom heart block is diagnosed later in life require close follow-up of heart rate and rhythm.

Most deaths from congenital complete heart block occur in the first year of life. Although deaths are uncommon after this time, serious symptoms continue to appear, with syncope, exercise intolerance, and congestive heart failure predominating. Each patient with congenital complete heart block should be thoroughly evaluated for associated congenital heart disease. An ECG and 24-hour ECG should be performed at baseline and should be repeated every 1 to 3 years. Exercise stress tests should be done at 4 to 5 years of age and should be repeated at intervals to evaluate the patient's exercise tolerance and heart rate response and to determine whether ventricular ectopy has developed.

Management

Therapy for symptomatic complete heart block is implantation of a permanent pacemaker. Infants with ventricular rates consistently less than 55 beats/min should be paced because they frequently develop congestive heart failure; infants with significant congestive heart failure usually require pacing at rates of 65 to 70 beats/min to maintain an adequate cardiac output. In older children, ventricular rates of less than 45 beats/min while awake, the presence of frequent or complex ventricular ectopy, syncope, and moderate or severe exercise intolerance are indications for pacing. Viewed in a lifelong perspective, congenital complete heart block may represent a potentially life-threatening disease that is associated with a risk for Stokes-Adams attacks and sudden death at any age, even in the absence of the following high-risk criteria:

- Decreasing ventricular rate
- Low activity rate response
- Frequent ectopy during effort or on 24-hour ECG monitoring
- Mitral insufficiency
- Long corrected Q-T interval and widened QRS interval

Therefore, some centers recommend prophylactic pacing of all adolescents with congenital complete heart block. Sudden death and syncopal episodes may be preventable with pacing, and these operations are associated with low morbidity and mortality. Furthermore, the psychological impact of pacemaker implantation in a child must be considered. Resentment of the pacemaker and problems related to the issue of body image are common in this population.

BACTERIAL ENDOCARDITIS (SEE CHAPTER 10)

Causes

Although endocarditis is more common in older children, it has been reported in children of all ages, including neonates. More than 80% of cases of infective endocarditis in children occur in patients with congenital heart disease and infants and children with indwelling venous catheters. Therefore, bacterial endocarditis must be ruled out in persistently febrile children of any age who have congenital heart disease or indwelling catheters. The incidence of endocarditis varies with the underlying disease state but is highest in patients with prosthetic heart valves, systemic-pulmonary artery shunts, tetralogy of Fallot, unrepaired ventricular septal defect, and aortic valve stenosis. Gram-positive cocci (α-hemolytic streptococci, coagulase-positive and -negative staphylococci) account for about 90% of the recoverable bacteria. Gram-negative bacteria seldom cause endocarditis in children. Fungal endocarditis may occur in intravenous drug addicts, after cardiac surgery, and in neonates with prolonged use of indwelling catheters and those receiving broad-spectrum antimicrobial agents.

Diagnosis

Older children often present with only a history of malaise, headache, arthralgia, or mild anorexia and weight loss and may not have a classic constellation of signs and symptoms. Most of these are related to the hemodynamic alterations brought about by the infection itself, such as valvular insufficiency, congestive heart failure, and conduction abnormalities. However, embolization from vegetations (pulmonary, systemic, or central nervous system) or immunologic reactions (nephritis, splenomegaly, cutaneous manifestations) may bring the patient to medical attention. Changes in the character of cardiac murmurs or the appearance of a new murmur should always raise suspicion. Laboratory evidence may include an elevated erythrocyte sedimentation rate and evidence of anemia and hematuria. Echocardiogram should be done in any patient in whom a diagnosis of endocarditis is being entertained, although small vegetations (< 2 mm) may not be visible. The sine qua non of bacterial endocarditis is a positive blood culture.

The following guidelines have been suggested for obtaining sufficient blood cultures to rule out endocarditis:

- At least 1% of the patient's blood volume cultured over 48 hours

  or
- Three properly drawn blood cultures over 24 hours

The latter should be sufficient to detect 97% of cases of endocarditis; 3 to 5% of cases may have negative blood cultures.

Management

Because complications of endocarditis are often unpredictable, most patients should be monitored carefully in concert with a cardiologist skilled in pediatrics or should be referred to a major pediatric center for at least the initial portion of antibiotic therapy.

Prophylaxis

Any measure that can prevent endocarditis, with its inherent high morbidity and mortality rates, is desirable. Poor dental hygiene, periodontal diseases, and infections may produce bacteremia even in the absence of dental procedures; thus, maintenance of good oral hygiene is important. Antibiotic prophylaxis is recommended for patients at risk for endocarditis when they undergo dental or surgical procedures that may induce bacteremia with organisms likely to cause endocarditis. In patients who are receiving daily penicillin for prophylaxis against splenic dysfunction or rheumatic fever and are about to undergo a dental procedure, antibiotic therapy should be changed to erythromycin because of the development of penicillin-resistant oral flora. En-

TABLE 11.9. Prophylaxis before Surgical and Dental Procedures[a]

Recommended
- Dental procedures known to induce gingival or mucosal bleeding, including professional cleaning
- Tonsillectomy or adenoidectomy; bronchoscopy with rigid bronchoscope
- Esophageal dilation
- Cystoscopy; urethral dilation
- Urinary tract catheterization and surgery, if urinary tract infection is present[b]
- Incision and drainage of infected tissue[b]
- Vaginal delivery in the presence of infection[b]

Not recommended
- Dental precedures not likely to induce gingival bleeding, such as simple adjustment of orthodontic appliances or fillings above the gum line
- Injection of local intraoral anesthetic (except intraligamentary injections)
- Shedding of primary teeth
- Tympanostomy tube insertion
- Bronchoscopy with flexible bronchoscope, with or without biopsy
- Cardiac catheterization
- Endoscopy with or without gastrointestinal biopsy
- Cesarean section
- In the absence of infection for urethral catheterization, dilatation and curettage, uncomplicated vaginal delivery, therapeutic abortion, sterilization procedures, insertion or removal or intrauterine devices

Modified from Datani AS, Bisno AL, Chung KJ, et al. Prevention of bacterial endocarditis. Recommendations by the American Heart Association. JAMA 1990;264:2919–2922.

[a]Selected procedures; table is not meant to be all-inclusive.

[b]In addition to prophylactic regimen for genitourinary procedures, antibiotic therapy should be directed against the most likely bacterial pathogen.

docarditis may still occur despite appropriate antibiotic prophylaxis.

Endocarditis prophylaxis is recommended for most congenital heart disease and acquired heart disease lesions, regardless of whether surgery has been done. The following are the exceptions:

- Isolated secundum atrial septal defect
- Surgical repair without residua after 6 months of secundum atrial septal defect
- Ventricular septal defect
- Patent ductus arteriosus
- Previous coronary artery bypass graft surgery
- Mitral valve prolapse without regurgitation
- Functional or innocent murmurs
- Previous Kawasaki disease or rheumatic fever without valvular dysfunction
- Cardiac pacemakers
- Implanted defibrillators

In general, dental or surgical procedures that induce bleeding from the gingiva or from the mucosal surfaces of the oral, respiratory, gastrointestinal, and genitourinary tracts may cause bacteremia and require prophylaxis. These procedures are listed in Table 11.9. Prophylaxis is most effective when given perioperatively in doses that are sufficient to assure adequate serum concentrations during and after the procedure. The standard prophylaxis regimen is recommended even for high-risk patients, including those with prosthetic valves, conduits, or shunts and patients with a history of endocarditis. Amplified prophylaxis may include ampicillin (50 mg/kg) plus gentamicin (2.0 mg/kg) given intramuscularly or intravenously within 30 minutes before a procedure and repeated 8 hours after the initial dose. High-risk patients who are allergic to penicillin may receive vancomycin (10 mg/kg intravenously over 1 hour starting 1 hour before the procedure).

CHEST PAIN

Causes

Chest pain is a fairly common symptom in pediatric practice, occurring in about 1 in every 300 children seeking medical care. It is often chronic and recurrent, affecting boys and girls equally, at an average age of 12 to 14 years. For most children and adolescents, the cause of the chest pain is undetermined and benign. In the minority of patients, chest pain is caused by the following (in decreasing order of frequency):

- Costochondritis
- Bronchitis
- Other respiratory disease
- Muscular causes (overuse, trauma)
- Gastrointestinal causes (esophagitis, foreign body)

Cardiac causes of chest pain include

- Pericarditis
- Dysrhythmias
- Mitral valve prolapse

Rarely, anginal pain is caused by

- Myocardial ischemia from coronary artery abnormalities
- Hypertrophic cardiomyopathy
- Severe aortic stenosis
- Severe pulmonary hypertension
- Cocaine

Any chest pain has a significant psychological component, and readily identified stress is sometimes associated with the onset of pain. The causes of chest pain in children, unlike in adults, can usually be discovered by a comprehensive history and physical examination, without the need for anxiety-provoking laboratory tests.

Diagnosis

A history of known heart disease (including Kawasaki disease) or lung disease is obviously important because it may suggest exacerbation of a long-standing problem. In evaluating the specific symptom of chest pain, the following are important:

- Severity
- Frequency
- Duration
- Type
- Location

A classic description of sharp, pleuritic chest pain that is intermittent and possibly relieved by sitting up and leaning forward suggests pericarditis. The onset of chest pain around meals or with specific foods may suggest esophagitis, whereas a recent choking episode may indicate foreign-body ingestion. The presence of family turmoil may be temporally related to the onset of pain; teenage girls should be specifically questioned about the likelihood that they are pregnant. In contrast to pain from cardiac causes, benign chest pain often occurs at rest, while reading or watching television, and is not related to exercise.

Exercise-induced anginal chest pain, especially if associated with syncope, should always lead to an extensive cardiac evaluation. Exercise-related nonanginal pain, especially when associated with cough or tightness in the chest, may suggest exercise-induced asthma. Nonanginal chest pain at rest associated with palpitations, syncope, or near-syncope is more likely caused by anxiety, mitral valve prolapse, or dysrhythmia. If the chest pain is chronic, the history should include previous treatments, medications, positions, or other therapeutic methods that seem to relieve the child's pain.

On physical examination, the degree of the patient's agitation or distress may reflect the severity of the chest pain. Additional signs of anxiety, such as excessive hand wringing, muscle tightness, and tics, may suggest an underlying stressful situation at home or school. Heart rate, blood pressure, and respiratory rate and effort should be noted. Inspection of the chest may reveal evidence of trauma or asymmetry due to underlying heart, lung, or skeletal abnormalities. Auscultation may show significant murmurs, tachycardia, or dysrhythmias. Positional changes may be helpful in eliciting the click and murmur of mitral valve prolapse and regurgitation or the murmur associated with hypertrophic cardiomyopathy. A friction rub at the left lower sternal border may suggest pericarditis; distant heart sounds may indicate significant effusion. A narrow pulse pressure, tachycardia, and pulsus paradoxus indicate impending tamponade. Palpation of the chest wall, specifically the costochondral junctions, may reproduce the pain and is characteristic of chostochondritis. Abnormalities on lung-field examination would suggest specific respiratory tract diseases.

For most children with chest pain, laboratory tests are not helpful and are not indicated as part of the evaluation. Chest radiography may be indicated if significant trauma has occurred or if pulmonary abnormality is suspected. An ECG may be helpful if the history or physical examination suggests dysrhythmia or pericarditis. Echocardiography is a rapid, easily performed, sensitive diagnostic tool for the evaluation of the infrequent child whose history or physical findings suggest a possible cardiac cause for the chest pain.

Management

Most children can be followed by their primary care physician. Chest-wall pain syndromes are helped by the following:

- Analgesics
- Rest
- Heat
- Relaxation techniques

A trial of antacids may benefit the child with probable esophagitis, and bronchodilators may dramatically improve symptoms in the child with exercise-induced asthma. The physician should provide counsel and possible further assessment of psychosocial issues. Appropriate reassurance to the patient and family is of utmost importance, especially when the chest pain is idiopathic and likely to persist for many months. Subspecialty referral may be appropriate when specific concerns have been defined.

PREVENTION OF CORONARY ARTERY DISEASE

The cardiovascular risk factors for the development of adult coronary artery disease are already present in many children. Hypertension, various atherogenic blood lipid patterns, smoking, and sedentary lifestyle are commonly listed as major risk factors. Male-pattern obesity, diabetes, male sex, and a positive family history are additional risk factors. Some of these risk factors (smoking, sedentary lifestyle) are behaviors, and some are purely genetic (sex and family history) and therefore unmodifiable; hypertension, dyslipidemia, obesity, and diabetes have both behavioral and genetic antecedents.

Parental and family history may be a useful marker for high-risk patients because the association between parental disease and risk factors in their children probably reflects the impact of behavioral or environmental and genetic factors. In the "family at risk," at least one member has

- Dyslipidemia (high low-density lipoprotein [LDL] cholesterol levels and low high-density lipoprotein cholesterol levels)
- Essential hypertension
- Family history of premature coronary artery disease (before 55 years of age in parents and grandparents)
- Active smoking habit

In addition to allowing the identification of young persons at risk, parental disease is probably a good motivator to enhance compliance in these families for risk factor intervention programs.

Not only does the presence of risk factors independently influence the occurrence of coronary artery disease, but risk factors tend to aggregate in individuals, significantly multiplying that person's risk. Therefore, children who are identified to be at risk on the basis of a single risk factor, such as a screening cholesterol or elevated blood pressure, may have additional risk factors and should be evaluated comprehensively. The practicing physician should assess risk factors in children and encourage changes in lifestyle.

Diet and Cholesterol

The Expert Panel on Cholesterol in Children and Adolescents of the National Cholesterol Education Program has recommended an individual approach to identification and management of children at high risk for developing coronary artery disease and a population approach to lowering the blood cholesterol levels in all American children. The diet recommended by the panel for all children older than 2 years of age (no restrictions on fat intake are recommended below that age) includes no more than 30% of total calories from fat, 15% from protein, and 55% from carbohydrates, preferably complex. Furthermore, 10% of the fat calories or less should come from saturated fats, and less than 300 mg cholesterol should be consumed per day (the Step-One diet). Because food intake varies from day to day, these recommendations are meant to represent an average of nutrient intake over several days.

The panel has recommended that selective cholesterol screening be performed in children and adolescents whose parents or grandparent had documented coronary artery disease, angina pectoris, peripheral vascular disease, or sudden cardiac death at age 55 years or younger. In addition, the offspring of a parent who has been found to have high blood cholesterol levels (≥ 240 mg/dL) should also be screened. Primary care physicians may choose to screen other children who do not have the aforementioned criteria but who are judged to be at increased risk for the development of coronary artery disease. For example, an adolescent who smokes, has high blood pressure, is overweight, or consumes excessive amounts of fat in the diet may benefit from cholesterol testing.

Cholesterol screening of children may be done any time after 2 years of age and should occur routinely in continuing health care. This provides an opportunity for all first-degree family members to have their cardiovascular risk assessed. For children who have at least one parent with a blood cholesterol level of 240 mg/dL higher, the panel recommends that initial screening be measurement of nonfasting total cholesterol level. Children found to have a total cholesterol level of 200 mg/dL or higher should return for a fasting lipoprotein analysis. Children with a total cholesterol level of 170 to 199 mg/dL should have a repeated test; if the average of the two measurements is 170 mg/dL or higher, a lipoprotein analysis should be obtained. For the child with a family history of coronary artery disease, a fasting lipoprotein analysis should be the initial screening test.

A child whose average LDL-cholesterol level is borderline (110 to 129 mg/dL) should receive risk factor advice, begin consuming a Step-One diet, and receive other risk factor intervention. Reevaluation is done in 1 year. A confirmed LDL cholesterol level exceeding 130 mg/dL should lead to a clinical evaluation, which includes a search for secondary and familial causes and aggressive intervention that should include professional dietary counseling and regular follow-up. Referral to a pediatric cardiologist with expertise in dyslipidemia may be warranted in children and adolescents with a family history of premature coronary artery disease, multiple risk factors, or primary or secondary hypercholesterolemia. If, after at least 3 months on the Step-One diet and other modifications (exercise, smoking cessation, and, in obese children, weight loss), cholesterol levels have not been decreased, dietary modification should progress to the Step-Two diet (in which saturated fats are reduced to less than 7% and dietary cholesterol, to less than 200 mg/dL per day) in consultation with a qualified nutrition professional and continuation of positive lifestyle changes.

Drug therapy may be considered in children 10 years of age or older if dietary therapy lasting 6 months to 1 year has not reduced LDL cholesterol levels below those cited previously. Dietary therapy is continued even after drug therapy is instituted. Drug therapy should be considered *a*) if the LDL cholesterol level remains at or above 190 mg/dL, *b*) if the LDL cholesterol level is 160 mg/dL or higher and there is a family history of premature coronary artery disease, or *c*) if there are continued attempts at controlling two or more other risk factors. Children should only rarely be considered for drug therapy because of the known and as-yet-unknown adverse effects of therapy and the expense. The only drugs that are currently used for the routine treatment of hypercholesterolemia in children and adolescents are the bile-acid sequestrants cholestyramine and colestipol. In children, the long-term safety of the other lipid-lowering agents (nicotinic acid, HMG CoA [hydroxymethylglutaryl coenzyme A] reductase inhibitors, probucol, gemfibrozil, and clofibrate) are unknown. Children and adolescents who do not adequately respond to diet plus bile-acid sequestrants may be considered for additional drug therapy in consultation with a lipid specialist.

Hypertension (see also Chapter 5)

Despite the many well-described pathophysiologic causes of secondary hypertension in usually young children (e.g., coarctation of the aorta, renal or renal vascular disease, endocrine disorders, adrenergic tumors, and drugs), hypertension in most older children and adolescents is primary or essential. Early detection, evaluation, and treatment of primary and secondary hypertension in children will improve their long-term health. Hypertensive infants and toddlers require immediate evaluation, diagnostic studies, and treatment directed to the underlying cause of hypertension. Children 3 years of age and older should have their blood pressure measured yearly as part of routine heath care. Accurate blood pressure measurements can be obtained in the office setting with the child at rest, either sitting or lying in a quiet room, using the appropriate- size blood pressure cuff. A larger rather than smaller cuff should be chosen because a small cuff may falsely elevate the measured blood pressure; a larger cuff rarely masks true hypertension. A helpful equation to obtain a "ballpark" blood pressure indicating possible hypertension in children 1 year of age and older is as follows:

$$\text{systolic blood pressure} = 100 + 2.5 \times \text{age (in years)}$$

and

$$\text{diastolic blood pressure} = 70 + 1.5 \times \text{age (in years)}$$

The report of the Second Task Force on Blood Pressure Control in Children included age- and sex-specific percentiles of blood pressure measurements from birth to 18 years. The fourth Korotkoff phase was used to define diastolic blood pressure for children 3 to 12 years of age, and the fifth Korotkoff phase was used for diastolic blood pressure in older children. Three consecutive elevated readings on separate occasions are necessary before diagnosing hypertension.

Children are normotensive if both systolic and diastolic blood pressures are below the 90th percentile for age and sex. Significant hypertension is a systolic or diastolic blood pressure between the 95th and 99th percentiles with severe hypertension, implying a risk for end-organ injury, having measurements exceeding the 99th percentiles for age and sex. An algorithm for the systematic assessment and treatment of elevated blood pressure measurements in children is shown in Figure 11.1. If a child is tall and has weight proportional for age, a blood pressure greater than the 90th percentile for age is probably normal for that child's body size. An obese child is unlikely to have a cause for an elevated blood pressure other than his or her excessive weight. A similar level of blood pressure for age in a child who is tall and lean may be normal for that child's height. If, however, over several visits to the physician a child or adolescent has an average blood pressure greater than the 90th percentile for age but is neither tall nor heavy, there is an increased likelihood that the elevation in blood pressure may be pathologic, especially if the patient has a family history of essential hypertension.

Diagnosis

The most important aspects of the diagnostic evaluation of the hypertensive child or adolescent are the following:

- Detailed family history
- Comprehensive review of systems
- Thorough physical examination
- Urinalysis
- Complete blood cell count
- Measurements of blood urea nitrogen, creatine, uric acid, and electrolyte levels

Additional tests may be indicated on the basis of family history, review of systems, and clinical findings. Assessment of lipoprotein cholesterol levels may also be warranted in selected patients.

Management

After essential hypertension is diagnosed, nonpharmacologic therapies such as dietary intervention, weight control, and physical activity should be instituted first. The use of pharmacologic agents (e.g., β-adrenergic blockers, calcium-channel blockers, angiotensin-converting enzyme inhibitors, and other vasodilators) to control blood pressure should be reserved for patients with severe hypertension or those in whom several months of nonpharmacologic therapies have not controlled the elevated blood pressure. Aggressive pursuit of effective dietary modification, weight control, and physical activity should continue even after drug therapy is begun. Treatment is individualized, and the least amount of intervention required to control blood pressure while maintaining a high degree of compliance is considered optimal. If compliance with a chosen medication is considered good but blood pressure is poorly controlled, a secondary form of hypertension may be present. Essential hypertension usually responds promptly to therapy. The cause of the hypertension should be reassessed in such cases and in patients thought to have essential hypertension who become refractory to combination drug therapy. When blood pressure is well controlled with medications for a time, gradual withdrawal of drug therapy may be considered with careful monitoring of blood pressure, especially if nonpharmacologic therapies have been effective.

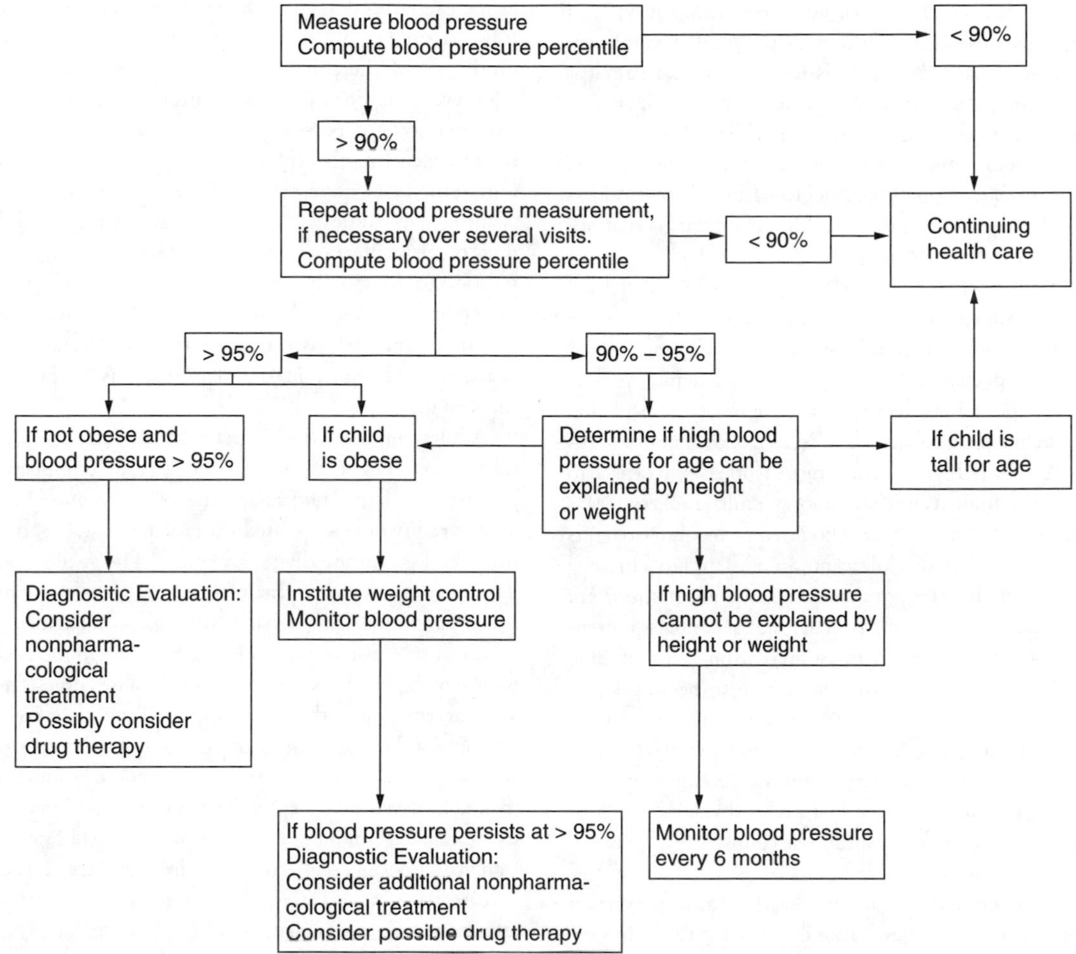

FIGURE 11.1.
Algorithm for identifying children with high blood pressure. Note: Whenever blood pressure measurement is stipulated, the average of at least two measurements should be used. Reprinted with permission fromTask Force on Blood Pressure Control in Children. Report of the Second Task Force on Blood Pressure Control in Children—1996. Pediatrics 1996;98:645–658.

Tobacco Use

Cigarette smoking remains the leading cause of preventable death in the United States, the cause of approximately 20% of deaths annually. Illness and death have also been demonstrated for passive or second-hand smoking. All of the compounds from cigarette smoke implicated as damaging to the cardiovascular system of active smokers have been identified in environmental tobacco smoke or second-hand smoke. Adverse alterations in systemic oxygen transport and lipoprotein profiles have been shown in preadolescent children exposed to long-term passive smoke from their parents. Children passively exposed to long-term cigarette smoke may be at increased risk for coronary artery disease.

Although overall tobacco use in the United States has decreased over the past decade, with about 29% of adult Americans being active smokers, the highest prevalence of smoking is found in teenagers and young adults. Approximately 40% of these children begin experimenting with tobacco in grade school. Initiation of regular daily smoking occurs most commonly in 12- to 14-year-olds; almost 90% of adult smokers began regular use before 21 years of age. Approximately 11% of high school students nationwide use smokeless tobacco because children believe it is less dangerous than cigarettes, despite its direct association with an increased risk for oral cancer. Proatherogenic alterations in lipoprotein composition have also been demonstrated from smokeless tobacco. Nicotine from these products has the same systemic and addictive effects as that absorbed through the lungs.

The onset of tobacco use is primarily a social behavior. Adolescent smoking and other tobacco use are strongly and consistently associated with smoking by parents, peers, and siblings; poor academic performance; poor knowledge of adverse health effects; and the belief that tobacco use is a sign of maturity. Although most high school seniors who smoke expect to stop, the high recidivism among adult smokers (60% failure rate among those who attempt to quit) suggests that many of these adolescents are addicted to a lifelong habit. Primary care physicians can assume an important leadership role in both primary and secondary prevention of tobacco use. Primary prevention helps children and adolescents resist the temptation to begin tobacco use. Secondary prevention emphasizes the reasons to stop smoking and encourages young people to stop. This prevention, however, requires a developmental approach that begins at the first prenatal visit.

Parents who smoke should be counseled to quit. Antitobacco use messages should be part of all routine health maintenance examinations. The most important component in effective smoking cessation is reinforcement. Pregnant women who have stopped smoking during their pregnancy have an extremely high relapse rate after the baby is born. New mothers who can no longer refrain from smoking should be counseled not to smoke in the presence of their children to protect them from tobacco smoke. A behavioral prescription, dependent on the age of the child, has been developed for smoking prevention. For infants, education of parents to the adverse effects of passive smoking on the health of the infant is key. Infants exposed to passive smoke over the long term are at increased risk for sudden infant death syndrome, pneumonia, bronchitis, and asthma. Children of elementary-school and middle-school age will respond to direct education of the harmful and addictive effects of tobacco. Many are already keen on the advertising techniques used to mask the real effects of tobacco use. The goal in this age group is to prevent tobacco use.

Adolescents are at the highest risk for beginning to use tobacco, but they are the most difficult group to influence because even if they understand the long-term morbidity and mortality rates associated with tobacco use, they may deny the risks during their adolescence. The goal in adolescents is to encourage them to continue to not use tobacco or to quit using tobacco through social skills development. Nonsmoking adolescents are taught methods to deal with peer pressures to smoke. Because adolescents are concerned about their body and appearance, the issues of finger and tooth staining, mouth odor, and decreased stamina should be emphasized. Active smoking should be treated by developing a commitment to nonsmoking and using available smoking cessation programs. The physician may also suggest alternatives to improve lifestyle such as regular aerobic activities, which the adolescent may find attractive. As important role models, physicians and their office staff should not smoke or use tobacco products, especially in the presence of their patients. A tobacco-free environment is imperative for the health of children and adolescents.

KEY POINTS

Central Cyanosis in Neonates

Definition: > 5 g of reduced hemoglobin per L

Signs

- Hypoventilation
- Right-to-left shunting
- Ventilation–perfusion defects
- Diffusion impairment
- Inadequate transport of oxygen

Causes

- Tetralogy physiology: right-to-left shunting through a ventricular septal defect
- Transposition of the great arteries. Aorta arises from the right ventricle
- Single ventricle

Diagnosis

- Newborn: tachycardia, hyperpnea
- Refer to pediatric cardiologist for echocardiography

Treatment

- Oxygen, fluids
- Glucose
- Prostaglandin E_1
- Infusion
- Transportation to pediatric cardiac center for catheterization, surgical consideration

Cyanosis in the Infant, Child, and Adolescent

Causes: Late-onset cyanosis, consider Eisenmenger's syndrome (pulmonary hypertension with right-to-left shunting)

Diagnosis

- Loud P_2
- Right ventricular hypertrophy on ECG
- Refer to pediatric cardiologist for echocardiography
- In 16- to 18-month-old children with cyanosis on exertion (crying, exercise), consider tetralogy of Fallot

Treatment

- Refer to pediatric cardiologist for catheterization, surgical consideration
- "Definitive repair" by pediatric cardiologist or surgeon
- Primary physician and pediatric cardiologist consult closely
- Periodic evaluation for rhythm disturbances, residual defects, conduit, or homograft dysfunction at the onset of congestive heart failure

Congestive Heart Failure

Usually occurs within the first year of life

Causes

- Ductal-dependent systemic blood-flow lesions
- Cardiomyopathies
- Myocarditis
- Large atriovenons malformations
- Congenital coronary artery disease

Symptoms: Infants

- Respiratory distress
- Poor perfusion
- Rapid heart rates
- Failure to thrive

Symptoms: Older Children

- Dyspnea on exertion
- Orthopnea
- Paroxysmal nocturnal dyspnea
- Abdominal pain and discomfort
- Tachycardia at rest
- Rales
- Murmurs
- Gallops

Treatment: Neonate

- Refer immediately to pediatric cardiologist

Treatment: Older Infant with Volume Overload, Cardiomyopathy, or Myocarditis

- Refer to pediatric cardiologist
- Medical management

  Digoxin: Infant: 40 μg/kg. Ages 2–12: loading dose 40–60 μg/kg with a maintenance dose of 10 μg/kg divided every 12 hours. Older child: up to 0.25 mg/day.

  Diuretics: monitor for hypokalemia

KEY POINTS

Vasodilator: Angiotensin-converting enzyme inhibitors, angiotensin-1 receptor blockers
Prophylaxis against subacute bacterial endocarditis

- Surgical management
  - Refer to pediatric cardiologist for consideration of definitive therapy and possible surgical correction or palpation
  - Curative: closure of patent ductus arteriosus without pulmonary hypertension and secundum atrial septal defect
- All children should be followed in consultation with pediatric cardiologist

Acquired Heart Disease

Kawasaki Disease (Mucocutaneous Lymph Node Syndrome): Leading cause of acquired heart disease in the United States

Cause

- Generally unknown in most patients
- Generalized vasculitis

Diagnosis

- Occurs more frequently in boys than in girls
- 80% of patients younger than 5 years of age
- Probably infectious
- Formation of coronary artery aneurysms

Symptoms

- Fever
- Rash
- Cervical lymphadenitis
- Erythema
- Edema of hands and feet
- Onset of congestive heart failure
- ECG changes
- Myocardial infarction

Treatment

- Treat early
- Reduce inflammation with high-dose aspirin and intravenous gammaglobulin
- Long-term management depends on degree of coronary artery involvement
- Follow-up in consultation with pediatric cardiologist

Acute Rheumatic Fever: Leading cause of cardiac disease in the first four decades of life

Cause

- Group A streptococci

Symptoms

- Congestive heart failure
- ECG abnormalities
- Pericardial friction rub

Diagnosis

- Seek out antecedent pharyngitis
- 3-week latency period
- Carditis in 50% of patients
- Listen for murmur of mitral regurgitation
- Aortic insufficiency in 20% of patients
- Resting tachycardia
- Cardiac enlargement
- Refer to pediatric cardiologist if acute rheumatic fever is suspected

Treatment

- Treat pharyngitis
- Antibiotic prophylaxis against rheumatic fever
- Prophylaxis against subacute bacterial endocarditis if valvulitis is present
- Bed rest, aspirin, and therapy for congestive heart failure if required

Mitral Valve Prolapse

- 1–2% of children
- Occurs more frequently in girls than in boys
- May be primary or associated with connective tissue disease (e.g., Marfan's and Ehlers-Danlos syndromes)

Cause

- Redundant mitral valve leaflets that extend into the left atrium during ventricular systole

Symptoms

- Palpitations
- Easy fatigability
- Chest pain
- Autonomic dysfunction

KEY POINTS

Diagnosis

- Mid-to-late systolic click heard best at the apex, associated with the murmur of mitral insufficiency
- ECG

Treatment

- Prophylaxis against subacute bacterial endocarditis in patients with mitral regurgitation
- Low-dose β-blockers for palpitations
- Patient may engage in sports activity

Hypertrophic Cardiomyopathy

Hypertrophic cardiomyopathy with heart failure in patients younger than 1 year of age has poor prognosis. Generally, signs and symptoms develop after the age of 10 years.

Symptoms

- Dyspnea on exertion
- Chest pain
- Syncope
- Palpitations associated with congestive heart failure
- Sudden death associated with congestive heart failure; occurs in one-third of patients with hypertrophic cardiomyopathy after strenuous exercise

Diagnosis

- S_4, harsh systolic ejection murmur at the left sternal border that decreases with squatting and increases with standing
- ECG abnormalities in 90% of children with hypertrophic cardiomyopathy
- Echocardiography the gold standard for confirming hypertrophic cardiomyopathy

Treatment

- Refer to pediatric cardiologist
- *No competitive sports*
- β-Blockers and calcium-channel blockers (verapamil) relieve symptoms
- Amiodarone may improve dysrhythmia and ventricular function
- In consultation with pediatric cardiologist, select patients who may benefit from dual-chamber pacing or septal myotomy-myomectomy or mitral valve replacement

Conduction and Rhythm Disturbances: Sudden death possible

Causes

- Hypertrophic cardiomyopathy
- Aberrant left coronary artery
- Preexcitation syndromes
- Long Q-T syndrome (important because it tends to be familial and is treatable)

Benign, irregular rhythms most common

- Sinus arrhythmia
- Atrial premature beats
- Unifocal premature ventricular contractions

Supraventricular Tachycardia

- May progress to congestive heart failure in the infant
- 20% of children with supraventricular tachycardia have Wolff-Parkinson-White syndrome
- With paroxysmal supraventricular tachycardia or atrial flutter, try bedside maneuvers or adenosine
- Refer to pediatric cardiologist for long-term therapy (medical or radiofrequency ablation)

Ventricular Tachycardia

- Uncommon in pediatric population; most commonly seen in patients with repaired tetralogies
- Drug toxicity a major cause
  - Digoxin
  - Tricyclic antidepressants
  - Erythromycin
  - Theophylline
  - Terfenadine (Seldane)

Sustained Ventricular Tachycardia

- Treat with direct-current cardioversion: 1.0 to 2.0 W/sec per kg
- Refer immediately to pediatric cardiologist

Complete Heart Block

- Most common cause of persistent bradycardia in infant and child
- Both congenital and acquired causes
  - Postsurgical

KEY POINTS

- Infectious
- Inflammatory

- Look for lupus in mother and infant with congenital heart block
- Permanent pacing for syncope, easy fatigability, congestive heart failure
- Permanent pacing helps prevent sudden death in child and adolescent

Endocarditis and Chest Pain (see also Chapter 7 and Chapter 10)

- Indwelling venous catheters the cause in 80% of children with congenital heart disease
- Blood cultures required for symptoms of fever plus known congenital heart disease
- Symptoms in older children:
  - Malaise
  - Headache
  - Arthralgia
  - Anorexia and weight loss
  - Fever
  - Hemodynamic alterations
- Use prophylaxis against subacute bacterial endocarditis except in patients who had surgery more than 6 months previously for secundum atrial septal defect, ventricular septal defect, and patent ductus arteriosus
- Secundum atrial septal defects, functional murmurs, and prolapse without regurgitation do not require prophylaxis against subacute bacterial endocarditis

Chest Pain (see also Chapter 7)

- Usually benign in pediatric population
- Typical causes include costochondritis, bronchitis, and musculoskeletal disorders
- Cardiac pain can come from pericarditis, dysrhythmias, and mitral valve prolapse
- Angina is rare, seen only in anomalous coronary arteries and aortic stenosis
- Differentiate cardiac pain from more benign cardiac causes through a careful history
- ECG and chest radiography usually not helpful
- Manage underlying problem

Coronary Artery Disease Prevention

- Search for risk factors
  - Hypertension
  - Hypercholesterolemia
  - Obesity
  - Family history
  - Cigarette smoking: prevent or terminate use
  - Diabetes
  - Sedentary lifestyle
- Screen for cholesterol in children whose parents or grandparents had coronary artery disease at 55 years of age or younger. Test is valid after the age of 2 years

Initial nonfasting cholesterol screening:

- If LDL cholesterol level > 200 mg/dL, fasting lipid profile
  - If LDL cholesterol level 170–190 mg/dL, repeat
  - If LDL cholesterol level 110–128 mg/dL, dietary management
  - If LDL cholesterol level >130 mg/dL, aggressive approach
  - If LDL cholesterol level >160 mg/dL with positive family history, drug therapy
  - If LDL cholesterol level >190 mg/dL, drug therapy
- Screen for hypertension
  - Systolic blood pressure = 100 + 2.5 × age (in years)
  - Diastolic blood pressure = 70 + 1.5 × age (in years)
- Evaluation in hypertensive child should include
  - History
  - Physical examination
  - Electrolyte measurement
  - Measurement of blood urea nitrogen level
  - Measurement of creatinine level
- Treat with lifestyle modifications
  - Weight reduction
  - Exercise
  - Diet
- Pharmacologic treatment only after failure of lifestyle modifications

SUGGESTED READING

Bisset GS, Schwartz DC, Meyer RA, et al. Clinical spectrum and long-term follow-up of isolated mitral valve prolapse in 119 children. Circulation 1980;62:423–429.

Brenner JI, Ringel RE, Berman MA. Cardiologic perspectives of chest pain in childhood: a referral problem? To whom? Pediatr Clin North Am 1984;38:1241–1258.

Dajani AS, Ayoub EM, Bierman FZ, et al. Guidelines for the diagnosis of rheumatic fever: Jones criteria, updated 1992. Circulation 1992;87:302–307.

Dajani AS, Bisno AL, Chung KJ, et al. Prevention of bacterial endocarditis. Recommendations by the American Heart Association. JAMA 1990;264:2919–2922.

Goble MM, Dick M, McCune WJ, et al. Atrioventricular conduction in children of women with systemic lupus erythematosus. Am J Cardiol 1993;71:94–98.

Maron BJ, Spirito P, Wesley Y, et al. Development and progression of left ventricular hypertrophy in children with hypertrophic cardiomyopathy. N Engl J Med 1986;315: 610–614.

Moskowitz WB, Mosteller M, Schieken RM. Lipoprotein and oxygen transport alterations in passive smoking children: the MCV twin study. Circulation 1990;81:586–592.

Perry CL, Silvis GL. Smoking prevention: behavioral prescriptions for the pediatrician. Pediatrics 1987;79:790–799.

Report of the Expert Panel on Blood Cholesterol Levels in Children and Adolescents: National Cholesterol Education Program. Bethesda, MD: U.S. Department of Health and Human Services, 1991. NIH publication no. 91–2732.

Report from the Committee on Rheumatic Fever, Endocarditis, and Kawasaki Disease, Council on Cardiovascular Disease in the Young, American Heart Association. Guidelines for long-term management of patients with Kawasaki disease. Circulation 1994;89:916–922.

Task Force on Blood Pressure Control in Children. Report of the Second Task Force on Blood Pressure Control in Children—1996. Pediatrics 1996;98:645–658.

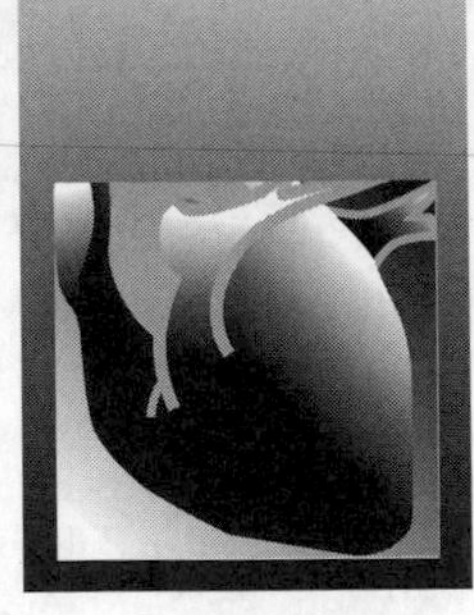

12 CHAPTER

Pericardial Disease

Andrea Hastillo

BACKGROUND

The normal pericardium consists of two thin membranes: the parietal pericardium and visceral pericardium. The latter is the outermost layer of the myocardium. The two layers are separated by about 30 mL of an acellular transudate. Congenital abnormalities are fairly uncommon; acquired disease of the pericardium occurs frequently, however, and accounts for significant morbidity and mortality. Because many diseases involve the pericardium, it is useful to approach pericardial disease by grouping them into the five usual clinical syndromes:

1. Acute pericarditis
2. Pericardial effusion
3. Pericardial constriction
4. Cardiac tamponade
5. Effusive–constrictive pericardial disease

Over the course of disease, one syndrome may blend into another. For example, a patient with tuberculosis may present with a chest pain syndrome characteristic of acute pericarditis that may wane as pericardial effusion develops. Later, despite treatment for tuberculosis, the effusion may disappear, but subsequent fibrosis and calcification may lead to pericardial constriction, with its own set of signs and symptoms. Diagnosis and treatment of the diseases affecting the pericardium depend on the cause, the hemodynamic sequelae of the pericardial disease, and the overall prognosis of the patient. The primary care physician is usually the first to encounter a patient with signs or symptoms related to the pericardial disease. A complete history and physical determine the need for further evaluation, consultation, and testing.

The patient's history, including any of the following conditions, should alert the physician to underlying causes of pericardial disease:

- Lung and breast cancer, which frequently metastasize to the pericardium
- Autoimmune disease, such as systemic lupus erythematosus and rheumatoid arthritis
- Infectious diseases, such as tuberculosis and HIV infection
- Metabolic disorders, including renal failure
- Other common causes, such as transmural myocardial infarction and cardiac surgery

The physical examination may demonstrate alterations in vital signs, pulsus paradoxus, Kussmaul's sign, pericardial rub, or anasarca.

Chest radiography plus 12-lead electrocardiography (ECG) are universally indicated. Echocardiography is usually indicated. Further testing and procedures may require consultation with a cardiologist or cardiothoracic surgeon for tissue or pericardial fluid sampling, cardiac catheterization, or surgery.

ACUTE PERICARDITIS

Acute pericarditis is caused by many different diseases. The diseases that most commonly cause acute pericarditis are listed in Table 12.1. Features of acute pericarditis are listed in Table 12.2.

History/Signs and Symptoms

Classic pericarditis pain is a retrosternal chest pain that is often sharp, worsens in the supine position, and improves while sitting forword. The pain may radiate to the neck and left shoulder and be confused with angina. The positional changes and the sharpness of the pain are helpful in identifying acute pericarditis.

Physical Examination

A fever is expected as a result of acute inflammation. Uncomplicated acute pericarditis should alter neither blood pressure nor respiratory rate. A scratchy three-component pericardial friction rub caused by rubbing of the two inflamed pericardial layers is pathognomonic of acute pericarditis. The rub is best heard with the diaphragm of the stethoscope as the patient sits, leans forward, and holds his or her breath in end exhalation. Although the rub may be heard from the base to the apex, maximum intensity is in the second to fourth intercostal spaces at midsternum or just left of the sternum. Two components occur during diastole and one occurs during systole. Not all three components are always heard, and the rub tends to be of short duration.

TABLE 12.1. Common Causes of Acute Pericarditis

Infection
- Bacterial
- Viral
- Tuberculous
- HIV

Metabolic disorder
- Uremia

Connective tissue disease
- Systemic lupus erythematosus
- Rheumatoid arthritis

Neoplasia
- Breast
- Lung

Other
- Acute transmural myocardial infarction
- Dressler's syndrome
- Post–cardiotomy syndrome
- Radiation therapy

Idiopathic process

Diagnosis and Laboratory Evaluation

Acute pericarditis can be diagnosed by history and physical examination alone. However, chest radiography and 12-lead ECG should be done.

12-Lead Electrocardiography

Acute epicardial inflammation may cause ST-segment elevation in all leads except aVR and V1. In addition, the P-R segment may be depressed (Fig. 12.1). The QRS voltage should be noted because enlarging pericardial effusions may decrease the voltage. The ECG also serves as a baseline with which to observe electrical alternans, a condition that may develop in pericardial tamponade. Differentiation of ST-segment elevation caused by acute myocardial infarction from ST-segment elevation caused by acute pericarditis may be difficult. Table 12.3 suggests some differentiating features.

Chest Radiography

Chest radiography may reveal a normal-sized cardiac silhouette; in the presence of pericardial effusion, however, the silhouette may enlarge. Radiography may also provide a diagnosis if the pericarditis is due to intrathoracic cancer or contiguous infection.

Echocardiography

Echocardiography should be performed to measure small amounts of fluid accumulation because 250 mL must accumulate before the radiographic features of pericardial effusion appear. Echocardiography may provide a more focused diagnosis if metastatic implants are seen or if alterations in pericardial thickness have developed. Cardiac function can also be assessed.

Referral

If there is any question about the diagnosis, a cardiology referral should be obtained. The cardiologist can aid in the decision about the necessity of performing pericardiocentesis, perform the procedure if necessary, and advise the primary care physician about the necessity of open biopsy and drainage by a cardiac surgeon.

Treatment

Hospitalization for de novo pericarditis should be contemplated seriously until the cause is known and hemodynamic status appears stabilized. Pain relief may require aspirin doses similar to those given for arthritis or may require nonsteroidal anti-inflammatory drugs if aspirin fails. Although corticosteroids may relieve pain, they should not be used routinely if the cause of the pericarditis is not clear; they have significant adverse ef-

TABLE 12.2. Features of Acute Pericarditis

History
- Chest pain
- Fever

Physical
- Pericardial rub
- Fever

Special Studies
- Electrocardiography
  - ST-segment elevation
  - P-R depression
- Radiography
  - May be normal

Treatment
- Symptomatic
- Specific for cause

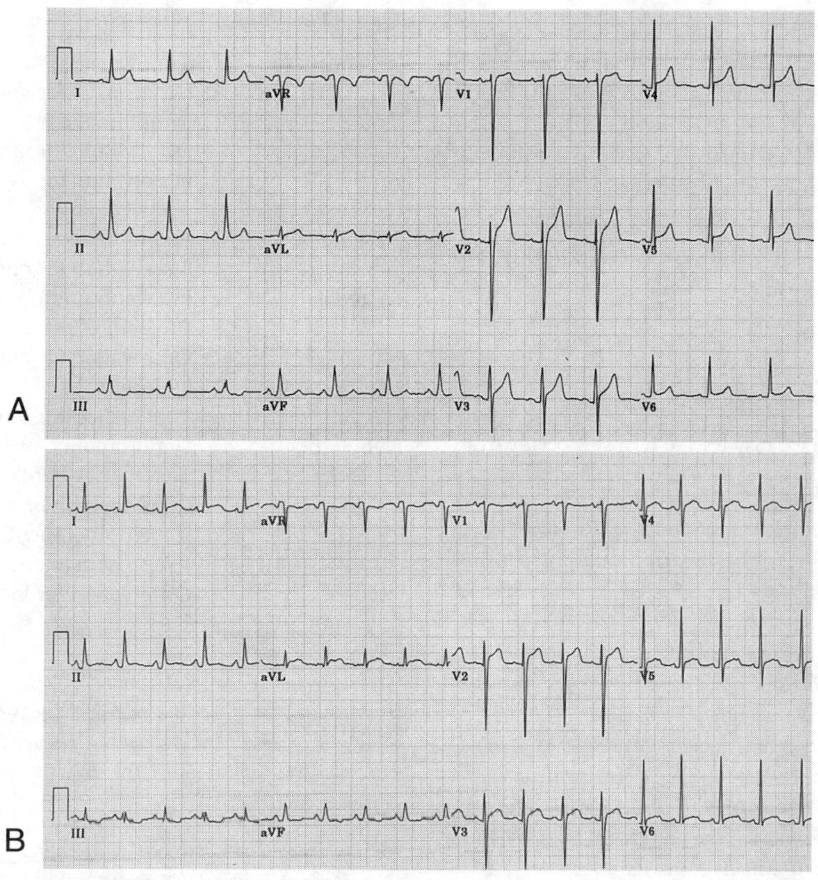

FIGURE. 12.1.

A 34-year-old man with acute pericarditis. **A.,** Baseline electrocardiogram. Early repolarization. **B.,** With acute pericarditis, the electrocardiogram demonstrates diffuse ST-segment elevation in all leads except III, aVF, and V1, a finding compatible with pericarditis. The P-R interval is depressed in leads I and II. Electrical alternans is present in all limb leads and in lead V1.

Differentiation between Acute Myocardial Infarction and Acute Pericarditis **TABLE 12.3.**

Variable	Acute Myocardial Infarction	Acute Pericarditis
Height of ST segment	May be >0.5 mV	Usually <0.5 mV
Location of ST-segment elevation	Often specific to one coronary artery distribution	All leads except V1 and aVR
ST segment configuration	Convex up	Concave up
Terminal QRS complex	Often in ST segment	Separate from ST segment
Q-T interval	Often prolonged	Usually normal

Summary of Diagnosis

- Signs include pericardial friction rub with two or three components.
- It is best heard with patient in the sitting position and the diaphragm of the stethoscope at the left sternal border at end expiration.
- The ECG indicates diffuse ST-segment elevation with no reciprocal changes.
- Acute pericarditis can be diagnosed by history and physical alone, but chest radiography and 12-lead ECG should be done.

fects and withdrawal may lead to relapse. Specific treatments are as follows:

- Uremic pericarditis requires intense dialysis.
- Tuberculous pericarditis requires multidrug therapy and close surveillance to prevent significant constriction.
- Bacterial pericarditis requires specific intravenous antibiotics in addition to drainage of the sac, but even these treatments may not prevent death.
- Neoplastic causes may require intrapericardial instillation of chemotherapeutic or sclerosing drug.
- Common idiopathic or viral acute pericarditis usually requires no specific therapy except for alleviation of symptoms; it usually runs its course in 1 to 3 weeks, although recurrences may develop (Table 12.4).

TABLE 12.4. Specific Treatments for Pericarditis

Type of Pericarditis	Treatment
Idiopathic	Symptomatic Observation for tamponade
Viral	Symptomatic Observation for tamponade Observation for associated myocarditis
Tuberculous	Antituberculous drugs Observation for constriction
Bacterial	Intravenous antibiotics Draining of pericardium Observation for constriction
Uremic	Intense dialysis Observation for tamponade
Neoplastic	Symptomatic Treatment of underlying cancer Consideration of instillation of chemotherapeutic or sclerosing agents Observation for tamponade

Summary of Treatment

- Aggressive treatment of the underlying disorder if it is identified
- Aspirin and nonsteroidal anti-inflammatory agents; steroids only as a last resort

PERICARDIAL EFFUSION

The normal pericardium is distensible and may accommodate up to 2 L of fluid if the effusion develops slowly. Thus, the compliance characteristics of the pericardium and the amount and rate of fluid accumulation determine which signs and symptoms may develop with pericardial effusion. Signs and symptoms may relate to compression of lung or to decreased venous return to the heart as increased intrapericardial pressure increases intracardiac diastolic pressures (Table 12.5). Large pericardial effusions are often due to

- Cancer
- Viral infections
- Radiation therapy
- Collagen vascular disease
- Uremia
- AIDS

The pericardial fluid accumulation seen in these various diseases may be due to

- Inflammation of the pericardium associated with infection
- Hemorrhage after trauma or left ventricular free-wall rupture
- Low oncotic pressure from the nephrotic syndrome
- High hydrostatic pressure due to congestive heart failure
- Increased capillary permeability due to severe hypothyroidism

History/Signs and Symptoms

Some patients are asymptomatic, with no history suggesting pericardial disease. Other patients may have a heavy precordial feeling or report shortness of breath, which may relate to compression of lung tissue or compromised intrathoracic space. Large effusions may even compress the esophagus, thereby leading to dysphagia.

Physical Examination

In the absence of hemodynamic compromise, vital signs may be normal. The respiratory rate may be elevated because of lung compression, and a fever may be present as a result of underlying pericardial disease or even lung compression. Examination of the lungs may reveal Ewart's sign:

- Dullness to percussion
- Increased fremitus
- Egophony
- Bronchial breath sounds at the inferior angle of the left scapula due to the compression of lung by the pericardial effusion

The cardiac apex may be neither visible nor palpable because of the dampening effects of the pericardial fluid. Heart sounds may be distant, and a pericardial rub may still be heard.

Diagnosis and Laboratory Evaluation

Electrocardiography, chest radiography, and echocardiography should be done.

Features of Pericardial Effusion **TABLE 12.5.**

History
  Dyspnea
Physical
  Ewart's sign
  Distant heart sounds
Special studies
Electrocardiography
  Low voltage
  Electrical alternans
Radiography
  Large cardiac silhouette
  Pericardial fat pad
  Displacement
Echocardiography
  Free space that identifies and partially quantitates the pericardial effusion
Treatment
Specific for cause

Electrocardiography

The ECG may demonstrate low voltage or a decrease in voltage compared with baseline. Electrical alternans may be present (Fig. 12.1). In classic electrical alternans, the P wave, QRS complex, and T wave show alternating voltage from beat to beat. Variations are present. For example, only the QRS may vary in voltage, or the voltage may increase and decrease cyclically over many beats. Electrical alternans is not pathognomonic of pericardial effusion and sometimes occurs in persons with marked respiratory distress.

Chest Radiography

Chest radiography should demonstrate an enlarged cardiac silhouette if the effusion exceeds 250 mL in volume (Fig. 12.2). An enlarged cardiac silhouette may also be seen as a result of cardiac dilatation, cardiac hypertrophy, or pericardial thickening without effusion. If the silhouette is due to pericardial fluid, the hilar borders are often obscured because the pericardium reflects onto the great vessels and distorts the usual sharp angle when filled with extra fluid.

Echocardiography

Echocardiography can measure the amount of effusion, reveal alterations in the pericardial thickness, and indicate that hemodynamic compromise has developed because of the effusion. Further tests will depend on the suspected cause of the effusion. Removal of fluid and even tissue biopsy may be necessary for diagnosis and require consultation with a cardiologist or cardiothoracic surgeon. Evaluation of the fluid and tissue should include culture (and sensitivity) for myriad infectious causes, a connective tissue screen, cytology, complete blood counts, and chemistry panels that include measurement of protein and specific gravity.

Summary of Diagnosis

- Signs include distant heart signs and egophony at the left scapula.
- The ECG indicates low voltage and electrical alternans.
- Chest radiography indicates enlarged cardiac silhouette or "globular heart."
- Echocardiography semiquantifies the amount of pericardial effusion.

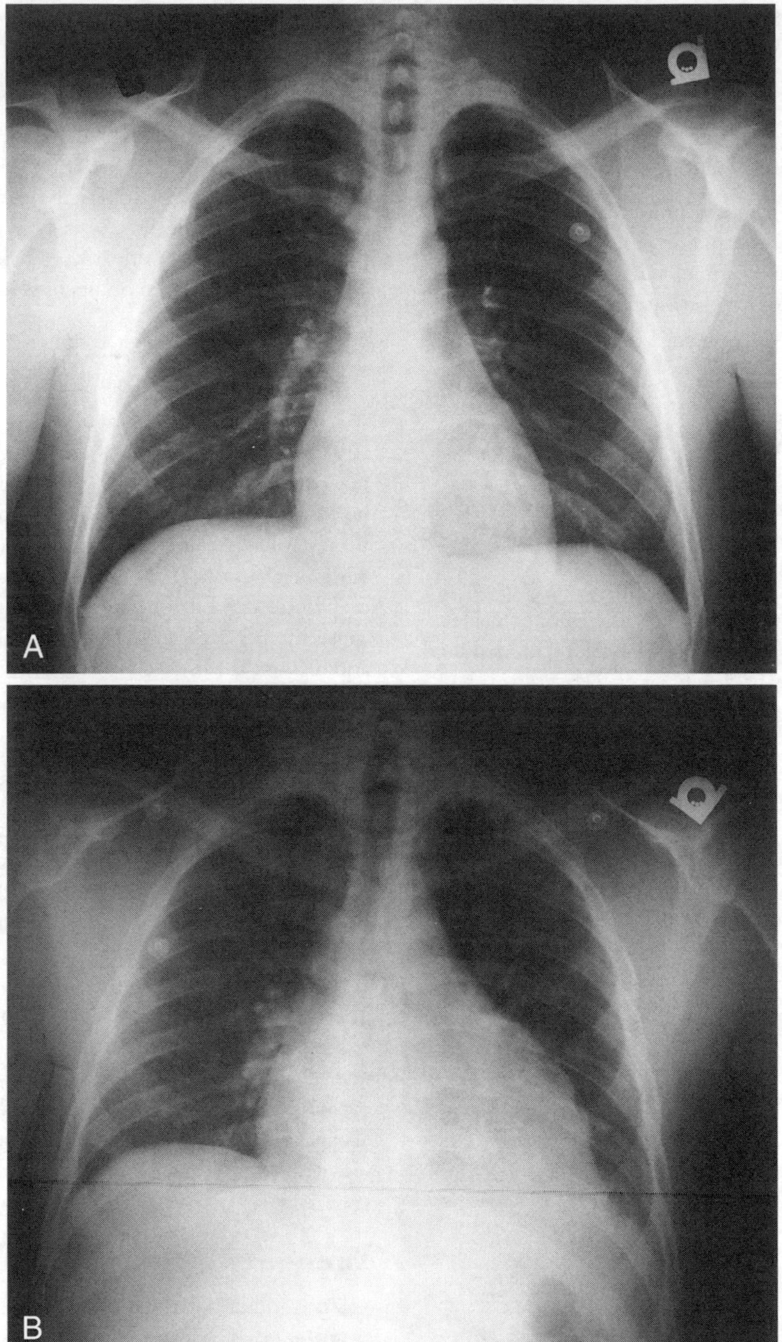

FIGURE 12.2.

Posteroanterior chest radiographs. **A.,** Baseline. **B.,** Diffuse increase in cardiac silhouette. Circumferential pericardial effusion with a volume of about 250 mL is seen on echocardiography. No chamber enlargement.

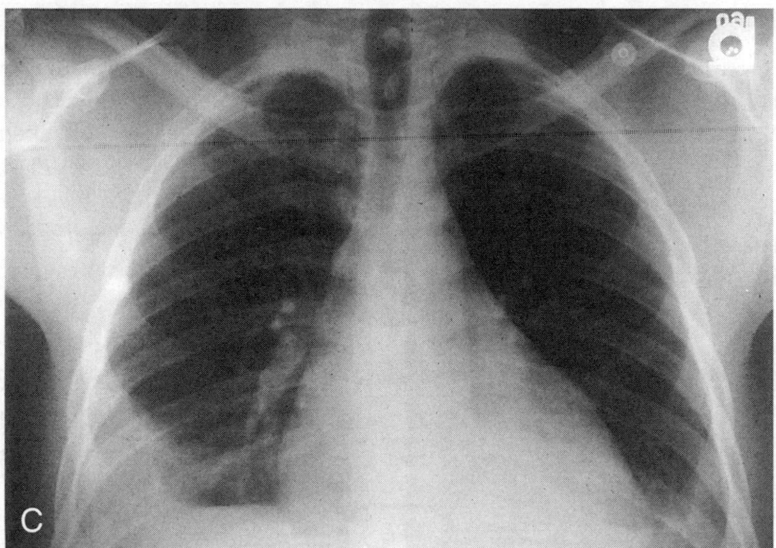

(FIGURE 12.2.—*continued*)
C., Two days later. The cardiac silhouette is diminishing, and pleural effusions are present.

Treatment

Treatment is directed at the underlying cause, if known. Removal of fluid and tissue may be indicated for diagnosis but also for relief of hemodynamic compromise that results from impediment to venous return. Removal of large volumes of fluid may be necessary for compressive symptoms. Careful follow-up of the effusion for development of cardiac tamponade or pericardial constriction is indicated. History, physical examination, and repeated echocardiography are the basic standards for treatment.

Referral is indicated for pericardiocentesis or a pericardial window.

CARDIAC TAMPONADE

When the fluid in the pericardial sac has accumulated rapidly or in such great amounts that the pericardial pressure increases, venous return is impeded. Because the pericardium surrounds the cardiac chambers, this increased pressure causes increased intracardiac pressure, leading to impeded venous return throughout diastole. The decrease in venous return subsequently leads to a reduction in stroke volume and cardiac output. This pathophysiologic process results in the hemodynamic abnormalities of cardiac tamponade. Heart rate increases and vasoconstriction occurs as compensatory mechanisms; if tamponade proceeds slowly, blood volume also increases to maintain cardiac output. If cardiac tamponade occurs acutely or if compensatory mechanisms fail, blood pressure decreases and the patient will die. Common causes of cardiac tamponade are listed in Table 12.6.

History/Signs and Symptoms

The history varies. With acute tamponade, which may occur because of ventricular free-wall rupture with acute myocardial infarction, aortic dissection, or penetrating trauma wound, the patient may be moribund and unable to give any history. If able to speak, the patient usually indicates the presence of dyspnea and chest discomfort (Table 12.7). In less acute tamponade, such as that seen with slowly but progressively enlarging effusions, patients may have generalized weakness, dyspnea, and malaise.

Physical Examination

Acute tamponade is manifest by a very ill-looking patient who is vasoconstricted, often stuporous, tachypneic, tachycardic, and hypotensive and has a narrow pulse pressure (< 30 mm Hg). Neck veins are distended. Pulsus paradoxus, an exaggeration of a normal decrease in systolic blood pressure during inspiration, should be present if blood pressure can be measured. The best way to search for a pulsus paradoxus is to instruct the patient to breathe normally, determine the systolic pressure at which Korotkoff sounds are first heard, and then, over a few respiratory cycles, determine the point at which all systolic Korotkoff sounds are

TABLE 12.6. Common Causes of Cardiac Tamponade

Connective tissue disorder
Hyperalimentation with central line
Metabolic disorder: uremia
Neoplasia
Post–cardiac surgery
Post–myocardial infarction, and especially if patients have received anticoagulation, post–thrombolytic treatment
Trauma

TABLE 12.7. Features of Cardiac Tamponade

- History
  - Dyspnea
  - Chest pain
  - Weakness
- Physical
  - Venous hypertension
  - Arterial hypotension
  - Tachycardia
  - Pulsus paradoxus
  - Quiet apical impulse
- Special studies
  - Electrocardiography
    - Electrical alternans
  - Radiography
    - May be normal
  - Echocardiography
    - Free space that identifies the effusion or blood
  - Catheterization
    - Equalization of diastolic pressure
- Treatment
  - Pericardiocentesis
  - Specific for etiology

heard. The difference in these two systolic pressures is normally 10 mm Hg or less. If the difference is greater, a pulsus paradoxus is present. Determining this difference may be very difficult if the patient is critically ill with tamponade. Furthermore, the most common cause of pulsus paradoxus is respiratory disease with exaggerated respirations, not pericardial disease. The cardiac examination may reveal a quiet apical impulse with normal or distant heart sounds. A pericardial rub may be present. If tamponade developed gradually, hepatomegaly and edema may be present.

Summary of Diagnosis

- Signs include venous hypertension, pulsus paradoxus, hypotension, and tachycardia at rest.
- The ECG indicates electrical alternans.
- Echocardiography indicates diastolic collapse of right atrium or right ventricle.

Diagnosis and Laboratory Evaluation

Chest radiography, ECG, and echocardiography should be performed. The ECG discloses a decrease in voltage and electrical alternans. Echocardiography displays diastolic collapse of the right atrium and right ventricle, a graphic example of the compressive features of the high pericardial pressure. Right heart cardiac catheterization may be necessary in complicated cases. Diagnosis and treatment may proceed concomitantly, with emergency pericardiocentesis.

Treatment

Acute pericardial tamponade may require emergency removal of fluid. As equipment is being readied, volume infusion may augment intravascular volume sufficiently to maintain a cardiac output adequate for survival. A cardiologist or cardiothoracic surgeon should review the case and proceed with therapy and diagnosis as indicated. Evaluation of the cause of the pericardial effusion with tamponade proceeds similarly to that done for acute pericarditis and pericardial effusion. Open or closed pericardiocentesis is required for medical or surgical emergencies.

PERICARDIAL CONSTRICTION

Acute pericarditis, even if treated properly, may be complicated by the development of pericardial constriction. This is particularly true for tuberculosis and undrained purulent pericarditis. Common causes of constrictive pericarditis are

- Previous cardiac surgery
- Tuberculosis
- Radiation therapy
- Viral infection

Mediastinal irradiation in excess of 4000 rads may be associated with constrictive pericarditis, which may develop over only a few months. In constriction, the pericardium thickens, the layers fuse with fibrous scar, and, approximately half of the time, the layers calcify. These pathologic processes result in a decrease in pericardial compliance and an increased resistance to myocardial expansion during diastole. Calcification may extend into the myocardium itself, and prolonged constriction may even lead to atrophy of the myocardium. Isolated calcification of the pericardium does not necessarily cause or indicate constrictive pericardial disease. During early ventricular diastole, resistance to venous return is normal; as venous flow continues and the ventricle expands, however, distention of the ventricle will be constrained by the less than normally distensible pericardium. This leads to a rapid increase in intracardiac pressure and sudden elevation in resistance to venous return. As venous return decreases, stroke volume and cardiac output are reduced. To compensate, the heart rate increases to maintain cardiac output; blood volume will likewise increase. The symptoms and signs of pericardial constriction relate to decreased cardiac output and increased extravascular fluid (e.g., fatigue, lethargy, dyspnea, ascites, and peripheral edema).

History/Signs and Symptoms

Symptoms of pericardial constriction are often insidious because the disease tends to progress slowly and temporizing compensatory mechanisms prevent sudden changes in symptoms. The patient may report decreased exercise tolerance, an increase in abdominal girth due to hepatomegaly or anasarca, peripheral edema, palpitations, or a generalized run-down feeling (Table 12.8). The patient may have a history of cardiac surgery, radiation therapy to the chest, tuberculosis, or anterior chest trauma. Certain tumors may also cause pericardial constriction.

Physical Examination

The patient may be extremely cachectic with severe anasarca. Sinus tachycardia is expected. Atrial dysrhythmia is common because of infiltrative epicardial disease or atrial distention. Blood pressure may be normal or low. The neck veins may be distended and display Kussmaul's sign (venous engorgement on inspiration). The jugular venous pressure normally decreases during inspiration. Lung examination may be normal, but pleural effusions are common. The cardiac apex is usually not displaced but may be difficult to palpate. Heart sounds may display a rhythm irregularity. An S_3 called a pericardial knock may be heard soon after S_2. The patient may have an enlarged liver, peripheral edema, and anasarca.

TABLE 12.8. Features of Constrictive Pericarditis

- History
  - Dyspnea
  - Abdominal swelling
  - Edema
  - Fatigue
- Physical
  - Kussmaul's sign
  - Pericardial knock
  - Ascites
  - Hepatomegaly
  - Edema
- Special studies
  - Electrocardiography
    - Atrial arrhythmias
    - ST-T changes
  - Radiography
    - Normal-size heart
    - Pericardial calcification
  - MRI, CT, Echocardiography
    - Thickened pericardium
  - Catheterization
    - Equalization
    - Dip-plateau or square root sign
- Treatment
  - Pericardial stripping

CT, computed tomography; MRI, magnetic resonance imaging.

Diagnosis and Laboratory Evaluation

In addition to ECG and chest radiography, cardiac catheterization is indicated for suspected pericardial constriction.

Electrocardiography

The ECG may demonstrate low voltage and various atrial dysrhythmias in addition to nonspecific ST-segment and T-wave abnormalities.

Chest Radiography

Chest radiography may reveal a normal-sized cardiac silhouette; pericardial calcification may be absent or may be extensive. Pleural effusions, evidence of old tuberculosis, or active tumor may be present.

Echocardiography, Computed Tomography, and Magnetic Resonance Imaging

Echocardiography may reveal thickened pericardium, but computed tomography may be better for this purpose. Determining the extent and location of the constriction is important in determining surgical approaches to pericardial removal, if indicated. Magnetic resonance imaging is important to determine whether myocardial atrophy and fibrosis are present because these abnormalities usually herald an extremely high postoperative mortality rate as a result of acute cardiac dilatation and failure.

Differential Diagnosis

The signs and symptoms of pericardial constriction may be confused with those of restrictive cardiomyopathy; only data from magnetic resonance imaging and cardiac catheterization may differentiate the two. Cardiac catheterization should reveal the presence of equalization of right and left heart pressures during late diastole. Signs of constriction depend on the volume status of the patient, and diagnosis may require volume manipulation with intracardiac catheters in place.

Treatment

Treatment must be initiated as early as possible. Patients who are prone to progress from acute pericarditis to constrictive physiology (e.g., tuberculosis, bacterial pericarditis) should be carefully followed in anticipation of development of constrictive pericarditis. Treatment of constriction consists of careful and methodical surgical removal of the offending pericardium. With advanced stages, it may be impossible to effectively remove adequate amounts of pericardium because of invasion of the myocardium by the fibrotic or calcific process. In addition, atrophy and fibrosis of the myocardium may be so profound that, at best, improvement is delayed and follows an uneven postoperative course; at worst, death may occur because of acute myocardial dilatation and failure after pericardiectomy. Surgery may be impossible because of evidence of myocardial atrophy and fibrosis.

EFFUSIVE–CONSTRICTIVE PERICARDIAL DISEASE

History/Signs and Symptoms

Effusive–constrictive pericardial disease is characterized by varying signs and symptoms of constriction and tamponade (Table 12.9). Common causes include

- Idiopathic pericarditis
- Neoplastic disease
- Radiation therapy
- Tuberculosis

TABLE 12.9. Features of Effusive–Constrictive Pericarditis

History
- Fatigue
- Chest discomfort
- Dyspnea

Physical
- Venous hypertension
- Prominent jugular venous X-wave changes to prominent Y after fluid removal
- Pericardial knock may appear after fluid removal

Special studies
- Radiography
- Enlarged cardiac silhouette
- Echocardiography
- Catheterization
  - After fluid removal, development of square root sign

Treatment
- Pericardial stripping
- Specific for cause

Summary of Diagnosis

- Signs include Kussmaul's sign, venous hypertension pericardial knock (rare), ascites, hepatomegaly, and peripheral edema.
- The ECG indicates atrial arrhythmias.
- Chest radiography should be checked for pericardial calcification.
- Echocardiography or magnetic resonance imaging indicates a thickened pericardium.
- Cardiac catheterization equalization of pressures: right atrial pressure = right ventricular end-diastolic pressure = pulmonary artery diastolic pressure = pulmonary capillary wedge pressure. All of these are elevated.

Physical Examination

The patient may report chest pain and weakness in addition to dyspnea. Venous hypertension is present. Neck veins demonstrate prominent X waves before the effusion is removed. After removal of pericardial fluid, the prominent Y descent characteristic of pericardial constriction and a pericardial knock may appear.

Diagnosis and Laboratory Evaluation

Diagnosis of effusive–constrictive pericardial disease depends on a high index of suspicion and invasive studies; thus, early consultation is indicated.

Chest radiography demonstrates an enlarged cardiac silhouette. Echocardiography should demonstrate fluid and perhaps a thickened pericardium. Magnetic resonance imaging or computed tomography of the chest may be beneficial. Right heart catheterization should confirm the emergence of constrictive hemodynamic characteristics after removal of pericardial fluid.

Treatment

Surgical removal of the offending pericardium is necessary. Refer to cardiac surgeon.

KEY POINTS

Acute Pericarditis

Causes: Virus, bacteria, uremia, systemic lupus erythematosus, rheumatoid arthritis, metastatic disease, radiation therapy.

Symptoms: Chest pain that is worse in the supine position; relieved by sitting upward; and aggravated by breathing, coughing, and sneezing.

Signs: Pericardial friction rub with three components. Best heard in the sitting position with the diaphragm of the stethoscope at the left sternal border at end expiration.

ECG: Diffuse ST-segment elevation. Symptomatic treatment with aspirin and nonsteroidal anti-inflammatory drugs. Steroids used only as a last resort.

Progression: Can progress to effusion, tamponade, or constriction.

Pericardial Effusion

Cause: Identical to causes of acute pericarditis.

Symptoms: Patients are initially asymptomatic and progress to dyspnea.

Signs: Distant heart signs; egophony at the left scapula.

ECG: Low-voltage electrical alternans.

Chest radiography: Enlarged cardiac silhouette; "globular heart."

Echocardiography: Semiquantifies amount of pericardial effusion.

Treatment: Specific for cause. If patient is symptomatic, referral for pericardiocentesis or pericardial window.

Cardiac Tamponade

Causes: Hyperalimentation with a central line, previous cardiac surgery, post–myocardial infarction, blunt trauma, closed chest trauma and penetrating wounds.

Symptoms: Dyspnea, chest pain, and weakness.

Signs: Venous hypertension, pulse paradoxus, hypotension, tachycardia at rest.

ECG: Electrical alternans.

Echocardiography: Diastolic collapse of right atrium or right ventricle.

Treatment: Medical or surgical emergency, opened or closed pericardiocentesis.

Effusive–Constrictive Pericardial Disease

Causes: Tuberculosis, previous cardiac surgery, radiation therapy, infection.

Symptoms: Dyspnea, abdominal swelling, edema, and fatigue.

Pericardial Constriction

Causes: Tuberculosis, previous cardiac surgery, radiation therapy, infection.

Symptoms: Dyspnea, abdominal swelling, edema, fatigue.

Signs: Kussmaul's sign, venous hypertension, pericardial knock, ascites, hepatomegaly, and peripheral edema.

ECG: Atrial arrhythmias.

Chest radiography: Search for pericardial calcification.

Echocardiography and magnetic resonance imaging: Search for pericardial calcification.

Cardiac catheterization: Equalization of pressures: (right atrial pressure = right ventricular end-diastolic pressure = pulmonary artery diastolic pressure = pulmonary capillary wedge pressure; all of these are elevated).

Treatment: Refer to cardiac surgery for pericardial stripping.

SUGGESTED READINGS

Arsenian MA. Cardiovascular sequelae of therapeutic thoracic radiation. Prog Cardiovasc Dis 1991;33:299–301.

Braunwald E. Pericardial disease. In: Isselbacher KJ, Braunwald E, Wilson JD, et al, eds. Harrison's principles of internal medicine. 13th ed. New York: McGraw-Hill, 1994:1094–1101.

Corey GR, Campbell PT, Van Trigt P, et al. Etiology of large pericardial effusions. Am J Med 1993;95:209–213.

Dasco CC. Pericarditis in AIDS. Cardiol Clin 1990;8:697.

Reynolds MM, Hecht SR, Berger M, et al. Large pericardial effusions in the acquired immunodeficient syndrome. Chest 1992;102:1746–1747.

Rienmüller R, Gürgan M, Erdmann E, et al. CT and MR evaluation of pericardial constriction: a new diagnostic and therapeutic concept. J Thorac Imaging. 1993;8:108–121.

Shabetai R. Diseases of the pericardium. In: Wyngaarden JB, Smith LH Jr, Bennett J, eds. Cecil's textbook of medicine. 19th ed. Philadelphia: W.B. Saunders, 1992:343–348.

Zakowski MF, Ianuale-Shanerman A. Cytology for pericardial effusions in AIDS patients. Diagn Cytopathol 1993;9: 266–269.

Ziskind AA, Pearce AC, Lemmon AA, et al. Percutaneous balloon pericardiotomy for the treatment of cardiac tamponade and large pericardial effusions: description of technique and report of the first 50 cases. J Am Coll Cardiol 1993;21:1–5.

13 CHAPTER

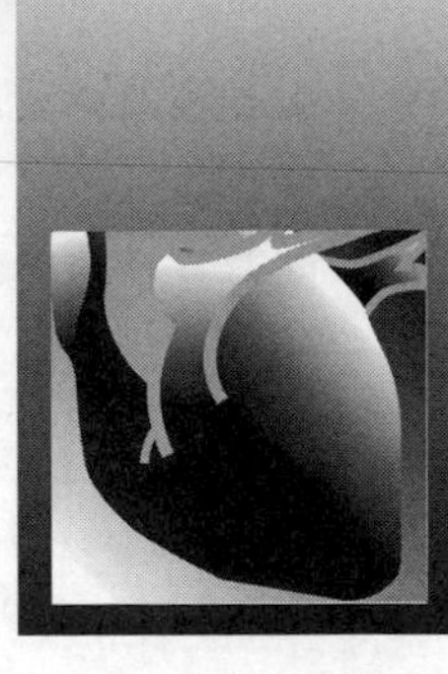

Pulmonary Hypertension

R. Paul Fairman

BACKGROUND

Chronic pulmonary arterial hypertension is an uncommon cardiovascular problem, but it may complicate the management of many disorders or develop without apparent cause. Primary care physicians should be familiar with signs and symptoms that herald the presence of pulmonary hypertension and should be able to initiate an evaluation. Although specialist consultation is usually required to confirm the diagnosis and begin treatment, primary care physicians should be prepared to manage some (but not all) stable pulmonary hypertensive conditions.

The normal pulmonary vascular bed differs from the systemic circuit—it accommodates the entire cardiac output, but its vessels contain minimal smooth muscle and no precapillary muscle and are subject to little nervous or humoral control. The pulmonary vascular tree is highly compliant; the pressures and resistance within it are about one-fifth of those in the systemic circulation and are primarily determined by the dynamic activities of the right and left ventricles. Even when pulmonary blood flow increases several-fold with exercise, pulmonary artery pressure remains low. Because of its low resistance and high capacitance nature, high pressure affects the pulmonary circuit significantly less than it affects the systemic circuit. The clinical significance of elevated pressures is also distinctly different. Systemic hypertension leads to end-organ damage in the kidneys and brain and to left ventricular dysfunction and failure. The clinical significance of pulmonary hypertension is limited to the condition's effects on right ventricular function.

Arterial Hypertension Versus Venous Hypertension

In this chapter, as in most clinical settings, the term "pulmonary hypertension" is used as shorthand for pulmonary *arterial* hypertension. Pulmonary *venous* hypertension rarely causes sustained pulmonary arterial hypertension. Pulmonary venous hypertension is usually a result of left ventricular failure or mitral stenosis. Whenever pulmonary venous and capillary pressures increase, an obligatory increase in pulmonary artery pressure occurs. If venous pressure is sufficient to increase pulmonary capillary pressure (pulmonary artery wedge pressure) above 21 mm Hg, interstitial edema begins to form. In most patients, alveolar flooding develops when the pressure exceeds 25 mm Hg. Pulmonary arterial hypertension caused by venous hypertension is treated by correcting the underlying cardiac problem. Occasionally (most often in patients with mitral stenosis), chronic elevation of pulmonary venous and capillary pressures leads to a disproportionate increase in pulmonary artery pressure. Despite the structural changes in the configuration of pulmonary arterioles, this form of pulmonary hypertension is improved, if not corrected, when valvular obstruction is surgically relieved.

Chronic Hypertension Versus Acute Hypertension

The term "pulmonary hypertension" generally refers to a chronic condition. Pulmonary pressures progress from normal to elevated over many months, if not several years or decades. Most cases of pulmonary hypertension that present acutely are exacerbations of a persistent and long-standing condition; a careful history reveals evidence for the chronic nature. True acute pulmonary hypertension is generally a result of acute pulmonary embolism or the acute respiratory distress syndrome. Acute pulmonary hypertension is not discussed in this chapter.

CHRONIC PULMONARY ARTERIAL HYPERTENSION

Pulmonary hypertension is defined by an elevated pulmonary artery pressure, but pulmonary hypertension does not indicate the cause of the altered physiology. Numerous conditions may elevate pulmonary artery

TABLE 13.1. Common Causes of Pulmonary Arterial Hypertension

Primary
- Primary pulmonary hypertension

Secondary
- Parenchymal lung disease
  - Chronic obstructive pulmonary disease
  - Cystic fibrosis
  - Pulmonary fibrosis (from any cause)
- Chest-wall abnormalities
  - Obesity hypoventilation (usually coexists with sleep apnea)
  - Severe kyphoscoliosis
- Pleural fibrosis
- Neuromuscular disease
  - Sleep apnea
  - Muscular dystrophy
- Obliterative vascular disease
  - Persistent or recurrent pulmonary emboli
  - Scleroderma
  - Sickle cell disease
- Congenital heart disease
  - Atrial septal defect
  - Ventricular septal defect
  - Patent ductus arteriosus

pressures, and most cases of pulmonary hypertension are secondary to cardiac or pulmonary disease. Only a small percentage of cases are primary (Table 13.1).

Chronic pulmonary hypertension inevitably causes hypertrophy of the normally thin-walled right ventricle. When the pressure elevations are sufficiently severe and prolonged, right heart failure occurs. When elevated pulmonary artery pressures are caused by abnormalities in the pulmonary system (lungs, chest wall, neuromuscular apparatus), the changes in right ventricular form or function are known as cor pulmonale. Diagnosis of cor pulmonale does not require right heart failure.

Like systemic hypertension, pulmonary hypertension is defined by elevated vascular pressures that are arbitrary. Normal pulmonary artery pressures in adults at rest and residing at sea level are 25 mm Hg systolic and 10 mm Hg diastolic (mean value for both, 15 mm Hg). At higher elevations and a lower ambient Po_2, pulmonary artery pressures are much higher. In healthy Andean natives living at 12,000 to 14,000 feet above sea level (where the Po_2 is only about 80 mm Hg [compared with 150 mm Hg at sea level]), mean pulmonary artery pressure is 28 mm Hg; with exercise, it increases to 60 mm Hg. Although these pressures are abnormal for most populations, they cause no untoward effects in the native inhabitants.

Despite this exception, it is fairly standard to define pulmonary artery hypertension by the pressures within the pulmonary artery. A mean pulmonary artery pressure greater than 20 mm Hg or a systolic pressure greater than 35 mm Hg constitutes pulmonary hypertension. Mild (systolic pressure, 35 to 45 mm Hg) elevations in pulmonary artery pressure are likely to generate few, if any, symptoms and only minor physiologic adaptations, making the condition nearly impossible to diagnose. The only clinical impact of mild to moderate forms of pulmonary hypertension is the risk for progression over time if it is not identified and treated and the likelihood of markedly higher levels of pulmonary hypertension developing with exercise or hypoxemia. Moderate pulmonary hypertension (systolic pressure, 45 to 60 mm Hg) may cause sufficient clinical abnormalities to permit identification of the condition, even in patients with symptoms or signs of pulmonary or cardiac disease. Higher levels of pulmonary arterial pressure may lead to right ventricular failure or, under conditions of acute stress, may be associated with chest pain, syncope, hemoptysis, and sudden death.

Pathophysiology

Of the factors that contribute to pulmonary hypertension (Table 13.2), hypoxemia is most important because it is the most common and most treatable. Alveolar hypoxia causes vasoconstriction of the pulmonary vasculature. Under normal circumstances, this response allows the lung to decrease blood flow to poorly ventilated lung units, maintaining normal ventilation or perfusion relationships and satisfactory arterial oxygen tensions. When much of the lung is affected by disease, however, alveolar hypoxia and the resulting widespread vasoconstriction elevate pulmonary artery pressures. When pro-

TABLE 13.2. Mechanisms Responsible for Chronic Pulmonary Hypertension

- Pulmonary vasoconstriction (hypoxia, acidosis)
- Loss of vascular bed by scarring or destruction of alveolar walls
- Thickening of arterial walls (remodeling)
- Increased pulmonary vascular flow (left-to-right shunts)
- Vascular occlusion (blood clots, sickle cell, schistosomiasis)

longed, pulmonary vasoconstriction induces anatomic changes in pulmonary arterioles that perpetuate the hypertensive response. Similarly, acidosis, either respiratory or metabolic, also causes pulmonary vasoconstriction, although the response is less severe. The combination of hypoxia and acidosis is synergistic. The contribution of these two factors to long-standing pulmonary hypertension is treatable.

Loss of the pulmonary vascular bed contributes to many cases of pulmonary hypertension. This mechanism alone rarely causes resting pulmonary hypertension; half of the pulmonary vascular bed may be lost (pneumonectomy) without significant increases in resting pulmonary artery pressures, although exercise may increase pressures substantially. Nevertheless, many pulmonary diseases destroy pulmonary blood vessels. Emphysema destroys entire alveolar walls and their capillaries; interstitial diseases are characterized by selective fibrosis of components of the alveolar wall, and vascular diseases occlude vessels.

The pulmonary vascular cross-sectional area may also be decreased by direct thickening of arterial and arteriolar walls. Such changes are most prominent in primary pulmonary hypertension and scleroderma but are seen to lesser degrees in other types of pulmonary hypertension.

Augmented pulmonary artery blood flow may also lead to pulmonary hypertension. Patients with congenital left-to-right intracardiac shunts develop pulmonary hypertension over many years. Initially, the pulmonary circulation can accept the augmented blood flow without anatomic changes in blood vessels. Eventually, pulmonary vessels become thickened (remodeled) and pulmonary artery pressure begins to increase. Pressures in the pulmonary circuit may approach systemic values; eventually, right-sided intracardiac pressure may exceed pressure on the left side and reverse the shunt direction, a condition commonly known as the Eisenmenger syndrome.

Acute embolic obstruction of pulmonary arteries increases pulmonary artery pressure transiently but does not exceed a mean pressure of 30 to 40 mm Hg unless the patient has preexisting heart or lung disease. However, chronic thromboembolic disease does not have the defining characteristics of acute embolic obstruction. Small-vessel occlusion of the pulmonary vasculature can lead to elevated pulmonary artery pressures. This is confirmed by two other diseases that occlude vessels: a) sickle cell disease and combination hemoglobinopathies and b) schistosomiasis.

In most patients with chronic pulmonary hypertension, more than one mechanism contributes to the pressure elevation. Indeed, elevated pulmonary artery pressure from any cause seems to lead to anatomic changes in the pulmonary vasculature that further elevate pressure. The longer the pressure remains elevated, the more severe and less reversible the anatomic changes become.

TABLE 13.3. **Symptoms of Chronic Pulmonary Arterial Hypertension**

Dyspnea
Fatigue
Chest pain
Syncope
Hemoptysis

Signs and Symptoms

Symptoms directly attributable to elevated pulmonary artery pressures (Table 13.3) are best identified in patients with primary pulmonary hypertension. In patients with secondary forms of pulmonary hypertension, symptoms are usually dominated by the cardiac or pulmonary problem that is responsible for the elevated pulmonary artery pressures. In these patients, it may be difficult to identify the onset of significant pulmonary hypertension because symptoms of pulmonary hypertension overlap with those of the initiating cardiac or pulmonary process. Chronic pulmonary hypertension may generate few symptoms until pulmonary artery pressures are already extreme. Slow progression allows the right ventricle sufficient time to become enlarged, sustaining higher workloads and maintaining normal oxygen delivery except at high levels of exertion.

Dyspnea is a common symptom. It begins insidiously, limiting vigorous activities first and eventually interfering with routine activities. In patients with secondary forms of pulmonary hypertension, the dyspnea of the underlying heart or lung disease may be indistinguishable from that due to pulmonary hypertension. Exertional fatigue is similarly common. Both dyspnea and fatigue may result from the heart's inability to increase its output in the face of elevated pulmonary vascular resistance.

Chest pain resulting from pulmonary hypertension may have features similar to those of classic angina, including substernal location; pattern of radiation; and heavy, crushing, or constricting qualities. The pain of chronic pulmonary hypertension is probably caused by an imbalance of oxygen requirement and supply in the pressure-overloaded right ventricle. The pain of acute pulmonary hypertension results from a different mechanism, sudden distention of the main pulmonary arteries.

Syncope, an uncommon symptom of pulmonary hypertension, indicates severe disease. It usually occurs with, or just after, exertion and results from an inability to increase cardiac output with exercise.

Similarly, **hemoptysis** is uncommon in patients with mild to moderate chronic pulmonary hypertension and therefore suggests severe disease.

Raynaud's phenomenon is common in pulmonary hypertension associated with connective tissue disorders; it is uncommon in patients with primary pulmonary hypertension.

For many patients (especially those with neuromuscular diseases, sleep apnea, and obesity/hypoventilation syndrome), pulmonary hypertension remains undetected until the process becomes severe enough to exhaust all compensatory mechanisms. The right ventricle fails and the patient presents with symptoms and signs of edema, right-upper-quadrant pain, distended jugular veins, and, sometimes, ascites.

Physical Examination

In patients with pulmonary hypertension, lung examination shows no abnormalities. All of the physical examination signs of pulmonary hypertension are found in examination of the heart; they are manifestations of cardiovascular adaptations to elevated pressures in the pulmonary circulation. As the right ventricle becomes enlarged and dilates, its pulsations become palpable just to the left of the sternum as a lift or heave. Closure of the pulmonic valve becomes accentuated by high pressures in the pulmonary artery, and the intensity of the pulmonary component of the second heart sound (P_2) eventually exceeds that of the aortic component (A_2). Fixed splitting of S_2 should suggest the diagnosis of an atrial septal defect. Dilatation of the right ventricle may eventually lead to tricuspid insufficiency and a right parasternal systolic murmur that increases with inspiration. Right ventricular gallops are common with moderate to severe pulmonary hypertension. They are heard best in the parasternal area. The presystolic S_4 originates from right atrial emptying into the poorly compliant right ventricle, and the mid-diastolic S_3 is a sign of a failing right ventricle. When right ventricular failure develops, right atrial pressures increase and distended jugular veins may be identified. A hepatojugular reflux may be present, and peripheral edema or even ascites may develop. Peripheral cyanosis suggests severely reduced cardiac output, and central cyanosis suggests a right-to-left shunt. Clubbing of the fingers is most commonly identified in patients with congenital heart disease, cystic fibrosis, or interstitial lung disease. It does not occur in patients with primary pulmonary hypertension.

Laboratory Evaluation

Long-standing heart or lung disease precedes the diagnosis of pulmonary hypertension in 80 to 90% of all cases. Evaluation to confirm the presence of pulmonary hypertension may require only one or two tests beyond information already known about the patient. For patients who do not have known heart or lung disease and who report dyspnea, fatigue, or right heart failure, the diagnostic process may be long.

Chest radiography may identify disease of the pulmonary parenchyma that had been unappreciated (pulmonary fibrosis or emphysema):

- Cardiac silhouette may be enlarged.
- On the lateral view, the right ventricle may fill the anterior clear space behind the sternum.
- Prominent pulmonary arteries and "pruning" of the vasculature are common with advanced disease.
- Enlargement of the right descending (interlobar) pulmonary artery is a specific sign of pulmonary hypertension but, like other radiographic signs, is not sensitive.

Pulmonary function should always be measured in a patient with possible pulmonary hypertension. As **spirometry values** decline, the risk for pulmonary hypertension increases. In chronic obstructive pulmonary disease (COPD), a forced expired volume in 1 second (FEV_1) less than 800 mL should suggest the possibility of pulmonary hypertension; in restrictive diseases, a forced vital capacity less than 50% of the patient's predicted value should suggest this possibility. **Arterial blood gases** should be measured. Hypoxemia (or, in patients with known heart or lung disease, worsening hypoxemia) is the most common finding associated with pulmonary hypertension. Acidosis may also be present and a secondary cause of elevated pulmonary artery pressures.

The **electrocardiogram** may provide indirect evidence of pulmonary hypertension because of hypertrophy or dilation of the right ventricle. As right ventricular muscle mass increases, the QRS axis shifts to the right. The right ventricular electrical signal becomes a more dominant force, leading to more prominent rightward forces. A QRS axis greater than 110°, an RSR′ complex in leads V1 and V2, and incomplete right bundle-branch block denote right ventricular hypertrophy. These abnormalities are found less often in patients with COPD because the position of the heart in such patients is extensively altered by air trapping. Large P waves in the inferior leads (P pulmonale) are identified more frequently in acute pulmonary hypertension and are unreliable signs of chronic pulmonary hypertension.

Other testing may be ordered in select cases to identify specific disorders that may cause pulmonary hypertension:

- Right heart catheterization is the gold-standard diagnostic test for pulmonary hypertension. Although it is not required in patients with obvious causes of pulmonary hypertension (COPD, sleep apnea, neuromuscular disorders, pulmonary fibrosis), it is often necessary for patients whose disease process is less clear (primary pulmonary hypertension, intracardiac shunts, chronic thromboembolic disease).
- Echocardiography is required in any patient in whom the diagnosis of pulmonary hypertension is being seriously considered. Hypertrophy or dilation of the right ventricle is evident in all patients with symptomatic pulmonary hypertension.
- Doppler evaluation of the flow signals is the best noninvasive technique for estimating pulmonary artery pressures.
- Lung scanning may identify chronic thromboembolic lung disease or significant right-to-left shunting. In primary pulmonary hypertension, the lung scan is normal or shows only a "salt and pepper" nonhomogeneous pattern.
- High-resolution computed tomography may be useful for identifying occult pulmonary fibrosis.
- Magnetic resonance imaging of the thorax may document mediastinal fibrosis.
- Polysomnography identifies sleep apnea.
- Laboratory evaluation for liver disease or connective tissue disorders is helpful in some patients.
- Lung biopsy as a diagnostic technique in pulmonary hypertension is controversial. Transbronchoscopic biopsy does not provide suitable tissue for diagnosis, and open-lung biopsy engenders substantial risks for patients. Nearly all cases of pulmonary hypertension can be adequately evaluated without biopsy.

PRIMARY PULMONARY HYPERTENSION

Primary pulmonary hypertension is very rare. Contrary to statements in most textbooks, the disease is not limited to young women. Data in the National Institute of Health Registry indicate that just over 40% of patients are men and that ages range from the teens to older than 60 years.

Signs and Symptoms

Patients with primary pulmonary hypertension usually present with unexplained dyspnea or fatigue. A small percentage of patients may have chest pains or Raynaud's phenomenon, but other symptoms (syncope, right heart failure, or hemoptysis) are absent early in the disease. Physical examination of the lungs yields normal findings, and cardiac abnormalities may be limited and subtle (increased P_2). The diagnostic possibilities in such a patient are extensive:

- Cardiac or pulmonary conditions
- Chronic liver disease
- Connective tissue disorders
- Chronic fatigue syndrome
- Psychiatric problems

Routine evaluation identifies a cause for most patients with unexplained dyspnea or fatigue. Hemoglobin concentrations and results of pulmonary function testing, lung scanning, and pulse oximetry evaluation of oxygenation are normal in most patients with primary pulmonary hypertension. The electrocardiogram may suggest the diagnosis because of findings of right atrial enlargement and right ventricular hypertrophy. Echocardiography confirms the presence of right ventricular hypertrophy and may be able to estimate pulmonary artery pressure. At this point (if not earlier), the patient should be referred to a specialist who can complete the evaluation and initiate treatment.

Laboratory Evaluation

Diagnosis is suspected on the basis of clinical, radiographic, and echocardiographic outcomes. Confirmation requires cardiac catheterization after diverse causes of secondary pulmonary hypertension from heart, mediastinal, lung, and systemic disease and abnormal respiratory control mechanisms are excluded.

Treatment

Therapy for primary pulmonary hypertension remains unsettled but generally consists of anticoagulation with warfarin, vasodilation with high-dose calcium-channel blockers or intravenous prostacyclin, and consideration for lung transplantation.

Prognosis

Although recent multicenter studies have documented some heterogeneity in the course of primary pulmonary hypertension, the overall prognosis is poor. The mean survival after diagnosis is just under 3 years. Some patients respond to treatment and have an improved prognosis, and a small subgroup seems to progress only slowly; any well-informed patient, however, will find the prognostic view bleak. The primary care physician may have a difficult time conveying to the patient an accurate picture of the severity of a disease that is so rarely encountered, so poorly understood by most physicians, and so unknown by the public. The physician must carefully educate the patient so that she or he may plan for the changes in physical capacity, earning power, and lifespan that accompany such a diagnosis. The need to provide support for the entire family in such a turbulent situation cannot be ignored.

Referral

The diagnosis of primary pulmonary hypertension requires the concentrated attention of several specialists; a primary care physician should not feel compelled to manage such a complicated diagnostic process. However, he or she should be prepared to identify patients who may have the disease and initiate an evaluation that can advance the diagnostic process.

No primary care physician should attempt to treat primary pulmonary hypertension. The intricacies and risks of vasodilator therapy and the timing of possible lung transplantation should be delegated to a specialist accustomed to dealing with such issues. Indeed, a diagnosis of primary pulmonary hypertension should prompt referral to a transplantation center.

SECONDARY PULMONARY HYPERTENSION

Chronic Obstructive Pulmonary Disease

Chronic obstructive pulmonary disease is a common cause of pulmonary hypertension, but most patients with chronic obstructive lung disease do not develop clinically significant pulmonary hypertension.

Signs and Symptoms

Elevated pulmonary artery pressures are universal in patients with disabling COPD, but most will not develop right ventricular failure. Emphysema and chronic bronchitis coexist in every patient with chronic obstructive pulmonary disease, but it is the patient whose disease is dominated by the features of chronic bronchitis who most often develops pulmonary hypertension. Several other features should make a physician particularly suspicious about pulmonary hypertension. Severe airflow obstruction ($FEV_1 < 800$ mL) is commonly present, and hypoxemia is an almost universal finding. Spirometry need not be done frequently, but every patient with symptoms of obstructive lung disease should be tested at least once. Repeated testing is not required except when the patient's usual level of functioning changes substantially. Conversely, oxygenation should be tested regularly. Pulse oximetry allows frequent, noninvasive, and inexpensive testing. Significant oxygen desaturation (<88%) should always be treated with supplemental oxygen. Oxygen saturations greater than 88% at rest, although insufficient to be recognized by third-party payers as reimbursable for supplemental oxygen, should not exclude a diagnosis of pulmonary hypertension by the physician. Patients with marginal oxygenation (SaO_2, 89 to 92%) at rest may develop significant hypoxemia with exercise when oxygen requirements are greater and ventilation perfusion matching is poorer, or during sleep when respiratory efforts are weaker. Oxygenation should be evaluated with exercise or overnight if the patient has worsening exercise tolerance, polycythemia, electrocardiographic manifestations of right ventricular hypertrophy, or peripheral edema that cannot be explained by resting oxygen saturations and other features of the case.

Treatment

Pulmonary hypertension associated with COPD rarely becomes severe, but it contributes to reduced exercise tolerance and early death. Thus, pulmonary hypertension should be treated; management is no different from that in all patients with clinically significant obstructive lung disease.

Smoking Cessation

Smoking cessation is the foundation of treatment for chronic obstructive pulmonary disease and for COPD-related pulmonary hypertension. Consistent and repeated efforts should be made to help smokers end their habit. Bronchodilators partially relieve symptoms, although pulmonary function testing may reveal little reversibility. Ipratopium bromide is the best bronchodilator for patients with chronic bronchitis and emphysema. β-Adrenergic agents and theophylline preparations may be added to ipratopium and may help some patients, although not much scientific evidence supports the use of these preparations.

Pneumococcal vaccine should be administered every 6 to 10 years, and annual influenza vaccinations should be encouraged. Long-term steroid therapy has little proven benefit in COPD (unless asthma is a major part of the patient's disease) and should be avoided because of adverse effects. Inhaled steroids are effective in asthma but have not been adequately tested in chronic bronchitis and emphysema to recommend their use.

Correcting Hypoxemia

Hypoxemia must be corrected whenever it is identified. Patients with resting hypoxemia should receive sufficient oxygen (usually 1 to 2 L/min by nasal canulae) to increase the PO_2 to greater than 60 to 65 mm Hg or SaO_2 to greater than 90%; patients should use the oxygen as close to 24 hours per day as possible.

Correction of hypoxemia is the one treatment for COPD that has been shown to improve survival. Survival is improved when hypoxemia is corrected for just 12 hours each day but is greatest when satisfactory oxygen levels are maintained throughout the day. Controlled supplemental oxygen therapy rarely results in significant worsening of alveolar ventilation, but clinicians should evaluate the PCO_2 if a patient develops symptoms suggesting hypercapnia. Finally, every effort should be made to optimize management for patients requiring oxygen; up to half of all patients who initially require oxygen improve sufficiently with standard treatment that long-term oxygen use is no longer required. Other measures that may help some patients include exercise rehabilitation and physical therapy.

Episodes of Right Ventricular Failure

During acute exacerbations of COPD, gas exchange worsens and patients with pulmonary hypertension may develop frank right ventricular failure. The primary treatment goal during such an episode is to ensure adequate arterial oxygenation with low-flow oxygen. Intravenous diuretic treatment of the severe edema associated with this condition should be withheld until satisfactory oxygenation has been achieved. Correction of hypoxemia is often sufficient to induce diuresis. If diuretics are also administered, the ensuing diuresis may be extremely large and the enhanced loss of hydrogen ions and chloride results in metabolic alkalosis that can suppress respiratory drive.

Lung Reduction Surgery and Lung Transplantation

Two newer forms of treatment may improve the outlook for selected patients with COPD: lung reduction surgery and lung transplantation. The effects of lung reduction surgery on pulmonary artery pressures are unknown (severe pulmonary hypertension is a contraindication to the procedure), and lung transplantation improves the condition. These surgical approaches should be considered for patients who are disabled, those whose lives are moderately to severely restricted, and those who require constant oxygen supplementation.

Treatment Alternatives

Treatment alternatives in acute exacerbations of chronic obstructive pulmonary disease are controversial.

Digoxin

Administration usually increases cardiac output and pulmonary artery pressures. The benefits of digoxin are questionable unless there are signs of coexistent left heart dysfunction.

Vasodilator administration has also been attempted under the assumption that afterload reduction benefits the right ventricle. Although many agents have been tried, none is specific for the pulmonary vascular circuit and the side effects of nonspecific vasodilation (worsening hypoxemia and systemic hypotension) have limited their use. More recently, inhaled nitric oxide has been used as a specific vasodilator for the pulmonary circulation. Given by continuous inhalation, it dilates vessels only where ventilation delivers it and therefore does not worsen ventilation-perfusion relationships. Furthermore, the nearly immediate metabolism of nitric oxide limits any systemic effect. Whether this gas will have any clinically significant advantage in acute exacerbations of COPD has not been tested.

Interstitial Lung Disease

Signs and Symptoms

Interstitial lung diseases are a heterogeneous group of disorders that include sarcoidosis, connective tissue diseases, occupational pneumoconioses, radiation- and drug-associated fibrosis, and idiopathic pulmonary fibrosis. Dyspnea and exercise limitation are the dominant symptoms in all interstitial lung diseases. Irritating, dry cough may be troubling late in the course. Restrictive pulmonary functions and chest radiographs demonstrating widespread fibrosis and infiltration are classic findings of interstitial lung disease. Pulmonary hypertension in such patients results from loss of the pulmonary vascular bed and hypoxemia. Physicians should suspect pulmonary hypertension when a patient's forced vital capacity decreases to less than 50% of his or her predicted value. Significant hypoxemia can be missed in these patients if oxygenation is evaluated only at rest. Oxygen saturations in the mid-90% range at rest may decrease to extraordinarily low values with minimal exertion. Similar desaturation probably occurs at night (although this is not as well documented for patients with interstitial lung disease as for those with

COPD). It is more difficult to prevent exercise desaturation with low levels of supplementary oxygen in patients with interstitial lung disease than in patients with COPD, and pulmonary hypertension often progresses despite oxygen therapy.

Scleroderma presents a special situation. It may produce interstitial fibrosis and honeycombing of the lung or may affect the pulmonary vasculature, producing a clinical picture much like primary pulmonary hypertension. Although no serologic tests are diagnostic for scleroderma or the various forms of pulmonary disease associated with it, two serum antibodies are helpful. Half of the patients with the hypertensive form of lung disease have a circulating anticentromere antibody, and the anti-SCL70 antibody is associated with the fibrotic form of lung disease.

Treatment

The prognosis for patients with interstitial lung disease is generally poor, and the disease may progress to death over months to a few years. Some forms are particularly rapid. Treatment with steroids and immunosuppressive agents is helpful for a few patients, and lung transplantation should be considered in every patient with progressive disease.

Referral

Referral to a specialist is indicated for any patient with a new diagnosis of a restrictive lung disease (especially if it has developed over a period of several months) and for any patient whose disease has progressed while he or she has received standard therapy.

Sleep Apnea/Obesity Hypoventilation

Signs and Symptoms

The fundamental cause of the sleep apnea syndrome is unknown, but the syndrome presumably represents a disorder of respiratory control revealed during sleep. However, anatomic features also play a substantial role: most patients are obese, and the diameter of the upper airway is smaller in patients with sleep apnea than in those who do not experience sleep apnea. In addition, hormonal influences seem important; men are affected much more often than women, and the incidence among women increases after menopause.

Whatever the pathogenesis, patients with the sleep apnea syndrome typically stop breathing for 20 to 40 seconds several hundred times per night. During these episodes, SaO_2 decreases and CO_2 levels increase. Hypoxemia and acidosis stimulate pulmonary pressor responses, and it has been postulated that, after years of intermittent pressure elevations, patients develop permanent pulmonary hypertension. However, this has not been confirmed in patients with uncomplicated sleep apnea. In fact, most patients with sleep apnea have normal blood gases and pulmonary artery pressures during their waking hours. Some patients present to their physician with all of the signs and symptoms of right heart failure, severe daytime hypersomnolence, and severely deranged blood gases. More often than not, these patients are morbidly obese or have an intrinsic pulmonary disease, such as asthma or COPD, in addition to sleep apnea. The colorful appellation of Pickwickian syndrome is memorable but does not define the several processes that may be responsible for the clinical picture. It is more useful to identify each of a patient's disorders so that each can be treated appropriately. Most often, these include the sleep apnea/obesity hypoventilation syndromes. Although sleep apnea can be treated with nocturnal positive airway pressure or various surgical techniques, treatment of obesity-related hypoventilation invariably requires weight loss.

Treatment

When patients with sleep apnea develop right ventricular failure, the highest priority is the restoration of satisfactory oxygenation. If this can be achieved, pulmonary artery pressures can be reduced and the overburdened right ventricle relieved. Oxygen supplementation may be sufficient in some patients, but others may require ventilatory assistance with intubation or noninvasive techniques to achieve satisfactory blood gases. Diuretics and cardiotonics offer little benefit and some risk in such patients. Progesterone may be a useful adjunct because it stimulates ventilation and improves alveolar ventilation and oxygenation. Vasodilator therapy aimed at the pulmonary circuit should be avoided because it is more likely to precipitate problems than to correct right ventricular failure.

Kyphoscoliosis

Kyphoscoliosis progresses to cor pulmonale only when the deformity of the spine is far advanced and is located high in the thoracic vertebral column. An angle of kyphosis exceeding 100° or scoliosis exceeding 120° compresses the lung and limits respiratory muscle function so severely that hypoventilation and hypoxemia develop. Although dyspnea is the most frequent symptom in these patients, many affected persons lead such limited lives that dyspnea is avoided and hypoventilation and pulmonary hypertension develop unnoticed until right heart failure appears.

Alveolar hypoventilation can result from generalized disease of muscles (muscular dystrophy) or, more commonly, from such neurologic disorders as amyotrophic lateral sclerosis, myasthenia gravis, or poliomyelitis. The lungs and airways remain normal unless aspiration, retained secretions, and repetitive bouts of pneumonia intervene. Acute respiratory failure may be the presenting problem, but chronic hypoxemia and hypercarbia are necessary for progression to pulmonary hypertension. The only satisfactory treatment is assisted mechanical ventilation. This treatment once usually required tracheostomy and a volume ventilator; in the past 5 years, however, substantial strides have been made in noninvasive mechanical ventilation techniques. One of these techniques is now favored as the first form of treatment.

Eisenmenger's Physiology

Signs and Symptoms

A large defect in the atria, ventricles, or great vessels with left-to-right shunting may lead to injury of the pulmonary vasculature with anatomic remodeling of pulmonary arteries and arterioles. Pulmonary artery pressure increases over time, and the changes in the pulmonary vasculature become permanent. Eventually, right ventricular or right atrial pressures increase in response to the pulmonary hypertension and the shunt becomes reversed, a condition known as Eisenmenger's physiology. In patients with isolated ventricular septal defects, the clinical syndrome of Eisenmenger's physiology is evident at a mean age of 14 years; in patients with atrial septal defects, the syndrome is usually identified late in the third decade of life. The usual symptoms for such patients are dyspnea that initially appears with exertion and eventually even at rest. Oxygen saturations may be low, and cyanosis generally worsens with exertion. Exercise limitation is a significant problem. Syncope and hemoptysis are late symptoms. Polycythemia is almost universal. Given the protracted nature of the process (2 to 4 decades), the right ventricle has sufficient time to become enlarged; thus, pressures may be almost equal to systemic pressures in the pulmonary circuit. Right ventricular failure is a late manifestation of the process and is often accompanied or precipitated by supraventricular arrhythmia (atrial fibrillation most often).

Treatment

Ultimately, lung transplantation with surgical correction of the heart defect or heart and lung transplantation is the only treatment. However, patients may live for many years even with severe pulmonary hypertension. Vasodilators and diuretic therapy usually provide little benefit and may precipitate major complications. Management of the patient with Eisenmenger's physiology is often difficult and should be provided by an experienced specialist.

Summary of Treatment

Primary Pulmonary Hypertension

- Anticoagulation
- High-dose calcium-channel blocker therapy
- Intravenous prostacyclin therapy
- Consideration of lung transplantation

Secondary Pulmonary Hypertension

Chronic Obstructive Pulmonary Disease

- Chronic bronchitis especially; $SaO_2 < 88\%$: supplemental oxygen
- Evaluation of nocturnal and exercise SaO_2
- Standard management of COPD
- Smoking cessation
- Cornerstone of therapy: bronchodilator, pneumococcal vaccine, and annual influenza shots
- Consideration of rehabilitation and physical therapy
- Lung reduction surgery and lung transplantation
- Treatment of right heart failure
- Digoxin and vasodilators used only with caution.

KEY POINTS

Primary and Secondary Pulmonary Hypertension

- High index of suspicion should be engaged, especially in patients with primary COPD.
- Follow Sao_2: Measurement of this variable is a rapid, safe, and effective way to monitor these patients.
- Perform pulmonary function studies on all patients suspected of having pulmonary hypertension.
- Rule out sleep apnea in appropriately identified patients; the condition may be treatable and correctable.
- All patients suspected of having pulmonary hypertension should have echocardiography to rule out shunt physiology.
- Diagnosis of restrictive lung disease deserves a referral to a pulmonary specialist, especially if a lung biopsy is being considered.

SUGGESTED READING

Barst RJ, Rubin LJ, McGoon MD, et al. Survival in primary pulmonary hypertension with long-term continuous intravenous prostacyclin. Ann Intern Med 1994;121:409–415.

Bergofsky EH, Riedel M, Stanek V. Cardiorespiratory failure in kypho-scoliosis. Medicine (Baltimore) 1959;38:263–317.

Cooper JD, Patterson GA, Pohl MS. Current status of lung transplantaion: report of the St. Lous International Lung Transplant Registry. Clin Transplant 1992;5:77–81.

Cooper JD, Trulock EP, Triantafillou A, et al. Bilateral pneumectomy (volume reduction) for chronic obstructive pulmonary disease. J Thorac Cardiovasc Surg 1995;109: 106–119.

D'Alonzo GE, Barst RJ, Ayres SM, et al. Survival in patients with primary pulmonary hypertension. Ann Intern Med 1991;115:343–349.

Flenley DC, Muir AL. Cardiovascular effects of oxygen therapy for pulmonary arterial hypertension. Clin Chest Med 1983;4:297–308.

Goldstein RS, Gort EH, Stubbing D, et al. Randomised controlled trial of respiratory rehabilitation. Lancet 1994; 344:1394–1397.

Meyer TJ, Hill NS. Noninvasive positive pressure ventilation to treat respiratory failure. Ann Intern Med 1944;120: 760–770.

Nocturnal Oxygen Therapy Trial Group. Continuous or nocturnal oxygen therapy in hypoxemic chronic obstructive lung disease: a clinical trial. Ann Intern Med 1980;93:391–398.

Palevsky HI, Fishman AP. The management of primary pulmonary hypertension. JAMA 1991;265:1014–1020.

Pearl RG. Inhaled nitric oxide. The past, present, and future. Anesthesiology 1993;78:413–416.

Penaloza D, Sime F, Banchero N, et al. Pulmonary hypertension in healthy men born and living at high altitudes. Am J Cardiol 1963;11:150–157.

Powars D, Weidman JA, Odom-Maryon T, et al. Sickle cell chronic lung disease: prior morbidity and the risk of pulmonary failure. Medicine (Baltimore) 1988;67:66–76.

Raghu G. Idiopathic pulmonary fibrosis: a rational clinical approach. Chest 1987;92:148–154.

Rich S, Brundage BH. High-dose calcium channel-blocking therapy for primary pulmonary hypertension: evidence for long-term reduction in pulmonary arterial pressure and regression of right ventricular hypertrophy. Circulation 1987;76:135–141.

Rounds S, Hill NS. Pulmonary hypertensive diseases. Chest 1984;85:397–405.

Sorour AH. Schistosomal cor pulmonale. In: Shaper AG, Hutt MSR, Fejfar Z, eds. Cardiovascular disease in the tropics. London: British Medical Association, 1974.

Strohl KP, Cherniack NS, Gothe B. Physiologic basis of therapy for sleep apnea. Am Rev Respir Dis 1986;134:791–802.

Sugerman HJ, Fairman RP, Sood RK, et al. Long-term effects of gastric surgery for treating respiratory insufficiency of obesity. Am J Clin Nutr 1992;55:597S–601S.

Wood P. The Eisenmenger syndrome: or pulmonary hypertension with reversed central shunt. Br Med J 1958;2:755–762.

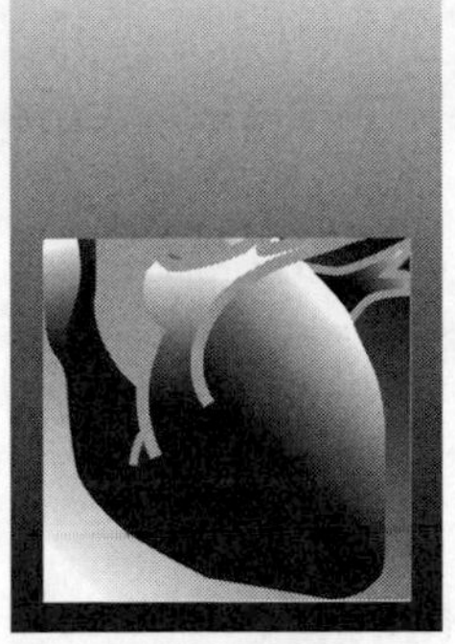

CHAPTER 14

Pregnancy and Heart Disease

Andrea Hastillo

BACKGROUND

Pregnancy causes a variety of physiologic changes. In some women with preexisting cardiac disease, these changes may not be tolerable, and pregnancy may be contraindicated. In other women, cardiac status may not be normal but pregnancy may be associated with an acceptable risk. This chapter is designed to help the primary care physician determine which women are at extreme risk with pregnancy, what risks pregnancy presents in women who do not have clear-cut contraindications to pregnancy, and how the mother's cardiac disease may affect the fetus or neonate.

CAUSES

During pregnancy, the maternal plasma volume increases about 20% by week 20 and 40% by week 40. Also by week 40, the erythrocyte volume increases by about 30% over the prepregnancy state, resulting in the physiologic anemia of pregnancy. Increased renal tubular absorption of sodium also increases total-body sodium and water. Cardiac output peaks by 20 to 24 weeks and plateaus at about 50% above the prepregnancy state. The greater cardiac output is maintained by an increase in heart rate, possibly to 150% of baseline. During pregnancy, pulmonary artery pressures remain at the baseline level, whereas systemic vascular resistance decreases.

As the uterus grows, it becomes an important factor in altering venous return and impedance simply by its compressive effect on the inferior vena cava or aorta. This effect is magnified when the woman is in the supine position, and it may result in syncope and bradycardia. Hemodynamic changes around delivery occur rapidly and are multifactorial because cardiac output increases with delivery and soon after. Cardiac output returns to near-predelivery levels hours after delivery; heart rate also decreases. Cardiac output reaches prepregnancy levels about 2 to 6 weeks after delivery.

The problems of pregnancy relate to the inability of the diseased heart to tolerate the hemodynamic alterations that occur with pregnancy (e.g., fixed valve stenosis with increasing intravascular volume), the risk to the mother of the development of new diseases associated with pregnancy (e.g., endocarditis, peripartum cardiomyopathy), the effects of lowered maternal cardiac output on the fetus (decreased uterine blood flow), and the risk to the fetus of medications or procedures necessary to treat the mother (e.g., teratogenicity or fetal growth retardation). Women with cardiac disease arising from congenital, rheumatic, and hypertensive causes, among others, may now survive pregnancy with a viable fetus if they are screened properly and followed carefully.

Despite its decreasing etiologic role in cardiac disease among women of childbearing potential, rheumatic heart disease remains the most common cause. Its occurrence has been bolstered by the influx of immigrants from countries where rheumatic fever remains active.

PREGNANCY OUTCOMES IN HEART DISEASE

New York Heart Association Functional Classification

The prepregnancy New York Heart Association (NYHA) functional classification of congestive heart failure helps to assess the maternal risks of pregnancy.

Women who are in NYHA class I or II have a mortality rate of less than 1% with pregnancy. Patients in class III or IV face a 5 to 15% mortality rate (Table 14.1). Fetal mortality rates parallel the maternal rates: a fetal mortality rate of 20 to 30% is associated with functional class III or class IV in the mother.

Exceptions to the NYHA classes may include patients with significant pulmonary hypertension, cyanotic lesions without surgical repair, or Marfan's syndrome (especially when accompanied by a dilated aortic root); in these patients, pregnancy may be strongly contraindicated.

TABLE 14.1. Mortality Risks in the Pregnant Cardiac Patient

Mortality < 1%
New York Heart Association class I or class II
- Atrial septal defect
- Ventricular septal defect
- Patent ductus arteriosis
- Pulmonic or tricuspid disease
- Corrected tetralogy of Fallot
- Mitral stenosis
- Porcine cardiac valve

Mortality 5–15%
New York Heart Association class III or class IV
- Mitral stenosis with atrial fibrillation
- Aortic stenosis
- Metallic prosthetic valve
- Coarctation of aorta
- Uncorrected tetralogy of Fallot
- Marfan's syndrome with normal aorta on echocardiography

Previous myocardial infarction

In addition, factors such as previous cardiac or vascular disorders (coarctation of the aorta, patent ductus arteriosus, valve replacement), dysrhythmias, or coronary disease may affect the risks of pregnancy. Therefore, if a patient with known cardiac disease wishes to become pregnant or is already pregnant, a team health care approach is warranted.

Because maternal and fetal survival are so intertwined, a full database that includes the following information is imperative:

- Past surgical procedures
- Current functional status
- Oxygenation

A woman with acyanotic heart disease in NYHA class I or II should be able to tolerate pregnancy. However, pregnancy is usually contraindicated if

- Pulmonary hypertension has developed.
- Unrelieved cyanotic congenital heart disease is present.
- Class III or IV functional status persists despite medication.

Outcomes of Specific Conditions

Congenital Heart Disease

Live birth occurs in about 80% of pregnancies in acyanotic mothers compared with 45 to 55% of pregnancies in hypoxemic mothers. About 72% of pregnancies in women with cyanotic congenital heart disease who have undergone palliative surgery have live births compared with 42% of pregnancies in women with uncorrected cyanotic lesions. Infants of cyanotic mothers are also smaller and more premature. The specifics of genetic counseling are best left to geneticists; however, the incidence of congenital heart disease is about 5 to 8 per 1000 births in the general population and about 2 to 8 per 100 in children of women with congenital heart defects.

Rheumatic Heart Disease

Rheumatic fever prophylaxis should be continued throughout pregnancy. The regurgitant lesions of aortic and mitral insufficiency are better tolerated by pregnant women who do not have heart failure.

Marfan's Syndrome

Marfan's syndrome poses a risk for aortic dissection and rupture for the pregnant woman, especially with the remodeling of the aorta and the associated hyperdynamic state of pregnancy. Genetic counseling is indicated because the syndrome is autosomal dominant. Although patients with aortic roots less than 40 mm do better with pregnancy than do women with larger aortic roots, death still occurs in women with smaller root size.

Hypertension

Preexisting chronic essential hypertension increases the risk for preeclampsia, although it is important to inform the potential gravida that in most instances (>85%) pregnancy will be uncomplicated. Nonetheless, the incidence of premature delivery, fetal growth retardation, abruptio placentae, acute renal failure, and even fetal hypertensive crises is more common in this group. These increases are related to superimposed preeclampsia, duration of hypertension, and age older than 30 years.

The hypertensive patient contemplating pregnancy needs to be informed of the following:

- Mild to moderate essential hypertension is usually associated with a favorable outcome.
- Potential for adverse outcomes is related to the antihypertensive drugs, the hypertension itself, and the possibility and risks of preeclampsia.
- The patient's lifestyle should be altered during pregnancy.
  - Restriction of activity
  - Continuation of sodium restriction if hypertension is salt sensitive
  - Avoidance of alcohol and tobacco

Dilated Cardiomyopathy

Women with dilated cardiomyopathy who remain in class III or IV functional status should reconsider their desire to become pregnant. Even without a superimposed pregnancy, their own survival is poor. The additional burden of a 40% increased blood volume portends a poor maternal outcome even with excellent multispecialty care. Fetal loss is increased and the risk for thromboembolic disease is increased.

Peripartum Cardiomyopathy

Of special note is the management of women who have survived peripartum cardiomyopathy, are not in class III or class IV heart failure, and are contemplating pregnancy or are already pregnant. The cause of this cardiomyopathy, which is associated with the development of signs and symptoms of heart failure in the peripartum period, is unknown. Affected women may quickly have complete recovery, may remain debilitated because of the cardiac disease, or may progressively deteriorate and die. Should survivors become pregnant again? Those who remain in functional class III or class IV should not. Some data indicate that survivors are more prone to redevelopment of peripartum cardiomyopathy with subsequent pregnancies even if they had returned to a normal cardiac status after the initial episode. The subsequent bout may be fatal or irreversible.

Patient Evaluation

A full patient history (with attention to functional status) and physical examination should be performed. In addition to the usual laboratory studies, electrocardiography and echocardiography are indicated. Depending on the results, consultation with a cardiologist, maternal–fetal specialist, anesthesiologist, and neonatologist may be warranted. Medications may need to be altered immediately to prevent teratogenic effects; especially important is the discontinuation of therapy with angiotensin-converting enzyme inhibitors.

Physical Examination

A good physical examination should predate pregnancy because the pregnancy not only alters abnormal physical findings but may also lead to new physical findings caused by pregnancy-induced hemodynamic changes. These latter findings may be misconstrued as indicating cardiac disease and may lead to unnecessary testing and even inappropriate counseling.

The cardiac apex is displaced laterally and superiorly as the uterus grows. An S_3 develops in about 95% of pregnancies, whereas a new S_4 occurs in only 10 to 15%. A venous hum is commonly heard in pregnancy and is diminished or stopped when the patient lies supine or when the jugular vein is compressed. The mammary souffle is a continuous murmur heard at the base of the heart, presumably caused by increased mammary flow. It should disappear with strong compression of the stethoscope over the chest.

Both systolic and diastolic murmurs may develop during pregnancy. A systolic ejection murmur may be heard over the pulmonic area because of increased blood volume. The benign systolic Still's murmur may be heard in the third to sixth intercostal space between the sternum and apex and may be confused with mitral insufficiency or a ventricular septal defect. A high-pitched diastolic murmur caused by pulmonic insufficiency may be heard with pregnancy but resolves quickly after delivery. A murmur reminiscent of tricuspid stenosis may also appear during pregnancy. Both systolic and diastolic murmurs may develop concomitantly.

During pregnancy, the diaphragm is elevated and the respiratory rate is higher. Coupled with basilar rales associated with compression that is indirectly related to the enlarged uterus, heart failure may be suspected even in normal women. The common occurrence of peripheral edema in pregnancy further complicates the picture.

Mitral stenosis, the most common lesion in rheumatic heart disease, may be first diagnosed during pregnancy, when the new changes in hemodynamics lead to symptoms or intensify the diastolic murmur. Atrial arrhythmias, especially atrial fibrillation, may develop during pregnancy and result in severe, life-threatening deterioration.

Both mitral and aortic regurgitant murmurs may become significantly less audible or even disappear during pregnancy, presumably because of deceased peripheral resistance. Recurrence or increasing intensity after delivery should alert the health care practitioner to the possibility of endocarditis, but this may be the result of peripheral resistance increasing to prepregnancy levels.

Referral

All pregnant patients with rheumatic heart disease should be referred to an obstetrician specializing in high-risk patients and to a cardiologist. Discussions of the risks and benefits of pregnancy, as well as participation in the patient's care, are necessary should pregnancy be desired and achieved. The patient should be counseled about the risks that pregnancy presents to herself and to the fetus; genetic counseling may be indicated. The patient should be warned about the potential physical limitations she may need to endure with pregnancy and, if appropriate, should be reminded of her own shortened life span.

Hypertrophic Cardiomyopathy

Genetically transmitted hypertrophic cardiomyopathy is the most common form of hypertrophic cardiomyopathy in pregnant women. It is transmitted as an autosomal dominant disorder with variable penetrance. Successful pregnancy is possible, but sudden unexpected death may occur in patients with this disease. Avoidance of venous pooling or other causes of reduction of venous return is important. Any suspicion of dysrhythmias must be carefully evaluated. Women with hypertrophic cardiomyopathy should be counseled about genetic transmission of their disease, the risks of pregnancy, the potential drugs they may need, and the risks to the fetus.

Coronary Artery Disease

Women suspected of having coronary artery disease are best evaluated and counseled before, not during, pregnancy. The risks associated with radiation and coronary surgery are primarily directed toward the fetus. In the pregnant patient, coronary artery angioplasty is more dangerous because of the pregnant woman's predisposition to coronary artery dissection. Pregnancy complicated by myocardial infarction is very risky for the mother during late pregnancy or delivery, and thrombolytic therapy is contraindicated in pregnancy. Thus, women of childbearing age who have known coronary disease or strong risk factors for premature coronary disease should be counseled early about pregnancy, alteration of risk factors, and their own prognosis.

Treatment

Mitral Stenosis

Digoxin may be used prophylactically in pregnant women with mitral stenosis and sinus rhythm to prevent rapid atrioventricular conduction if atrial fibrillation develops. Balloon angioplasty of the mitral valve has been successfully used to relieve the stenotic lesion during pregnancy. However, both aortic stenosis and mitral stenosis can be difficult to treat during pregnancy.

Anticoagulation during Pregnancy

Indications for anticoagulation during pregnancy include deep venous thrombosis, pulmonary emboli, implantation of certain prosthetic valves, and atrial fibrillation. Women with these disorders are at high risk for severe adverse events (e.g., thrombosis of the valve, pulmonary embolization, and stroke) if anticoagulation is stopped.

The U.S. Food and Drug Administration has placed warfarin in the "contraindicated" pregnancy risk category (Table 14.2). Warfarin is contraindicated during pregnancy as a result of its teratogenic effects and hemorrhage-induced abnormalities.

Barbour and Pickard's review of anticoagulant use in pregnant women stresses the lack of good studies in this complex area. Although heparin is the anticoagulant of choice, the route of administration, the dosage, and even the frequency and duration of use are controversial. Metabolic changes induced by pregnancy further muddle the dosing issue. Because heparin does not cross the placenta, this drug is often used instead of warfarin. Long-term heparin use may lead to maternal osteopenia, which is seldom symptomatic and appears to be reversible. Early (<1 week after initiation of heparin therapy) transient thrombocytopenia due to reversible agglutination and aggregation often develops. Antiplatelet antibody thrombocytopenia occurs less frequently (in < 0.2% of patients) and usually develops 6 to 14 days after heparin therapy begins. Thrombocytopenia requires termination of heparin therapy.

Prosthetic valves often necessitate anticoagulation. Many different approaches to maintaining anticoagulation during pregnancy in a woman with a prosthetic valve are available, including the following:

- Continuous heparin infusion
- Twice-daily subcutaneous heparin therapy, with the activated partial thromboplastin time at 1.5 times the control value obtained 6 hours after a dose is administered
- Early heparin use, warfarin therapy during the second and third trimesters, and resumption of heparin therapy (and discontinuation of warfarin use) around the time of delivery

The incidence of anticipated fetal problems with warfarin vary. The problem with heparin includes sudden, even massive, valve thrombosis and varied incidences of embolization.

In 1992, the American College of Chest Physicians issued its options for prophylaxis in pregnant women with mechanical prosthetic valves:

- Heparin every 12 hours to prolong the activated partial thromboplastin time to 1.5 to 2.5 times the control value (drawn 6 hours after a dose is administered)
- Adjusted-dose heparin until week 13, warfarin until the middle of the third trimester, and a switch back to heparin until delivery.

If the latter option is selected, the clinician should recall the medicolegal implications of prescribing a contraindicated drug during pregnancy and should clearly inform the patient of the risks. With optimal administration of heparin, the last dose is given 24 hours before induction of labor to decrease the risk for maternal bleeding during delivery. As pregnancy progresses, the heparin dose may need to be increased until about week 34 to avoid thrombotic complications.

Although prosthetic valve implantation allows many women to safely and successfully undergo pregnancy, the dangers of anticoagulation, emboli, and thrombi and the rate of valve deterioration accelerated by pregnancy must be discussed with the patient. Metallic valves generally require continuous anticoagulation, whereas bioprosthetic valves less frequently require anticoagulation. This benefit, however, must be weighed against the accelerated deterioration of bioprosthetic valves induced by pregnancy. Pregnancy may hasten calcification of the bioprosthetic valves, which, in turn, requires earlier replacement. In one study, 35% of pregnant women with bioprosthetic valves required replacement soon after delivery (two during pregnancy). The woman should be aware that the second valve replacement will be more difficult than the first and that the next replacement will theoretically be even more difficult.

TABLE 14.2. U.S. Food and Drug Administration Pregnancy Risk Category

Drug Group	Category	Fetal Adverse Effects
Adenosine	C	
Amiodarone	D	Hypothyroidism Hyperthyroidism Bradycardia Q-T prolongation
Angiotensin-converting enzyme inhibitors	C—Trimester 1 D—Trimester 2 and 3	Neonatal renal failure Oligohydramnios Skeletal abnormalities Death
Certain β-Blockers		
Propranolol	C	Fetal growth retardation
Metoprolol	C	Bradycardia Neonatal apnea Hypoglycemia Low birthweight
Atenolol	D	
Certain calcium-channel blockers		
Verapamil	C	
Diltiazem	C	
Digoxin	C	
Dobutamine	B	
Epinephrine	C	Fetal tachycardia Fetal anoxia Uterine relaxation
Heparin	C	
Lidocaine	B	Fetal bradycardia Neonatal hypotonia Cardiac and central nervous system toxicity increased with fetal acidosis
Methyldopa	B	
Nitrates: patch, ointment, spray	C	
Phosphodiesterase inhibitors	C	
Procainamide	C	
Quinidine	C	Possible eighth-nerve damage Possesses oxytocic properties
Warfarin	X	Teratogenic Fetal hemorrhage

Category A: No controlled studies in women show a risk to the fetus in the first trimester of a risk in later trimesters. The possibility of fetal harm seems remote.
Category B: Studies of animal reproduction have not demonstrated a fetal risk or have shown an adverse effect (other than a decrease in fertility). However, controlled studies in pregnant women in the first trimester have been done to confirm these findings, and there is no evidence of a risk in later trimesters.
Category C: Either studies in animals have revealed adverse effects on the fetus (teratogenic or embryocidal effects, or other) but there are no confirmatory controlled studies in women, or studies in both women and animals are not available. Because of the potential risk to the fetus, drugs should be given only if use is justified by a greater potential benefit.
Category D: Positive evidence of human fetal risk exists. Despite the risk, benefits from use in pregnant women may be acceptable in select circumstances (e.g., if the drug is needed in a life-threatening situation, or for treating a serious disease for which safer drugs cannot be used or are ineffective). An appropriate statement appears in the "warnings" section of the labeling.
Category X: Studies in animals or human beings have demonstrated fetal abnormalities, or there is evidence of fetal risk based on human experience. Thus, the risk of using the drug in pregnant women clearly outweighs any possible benefit, and the drug is contraindicated in women who are pregnant or who may become pregnant. An appropriate statement appears in the "contraindications" section of the labeling.
Pregnancy categories obtained from 1998 *Physicians' Desk Reference.*

Marfan's Syndrome

Treatment with β-blockers is helpful in theory and should be combined with blood pressure control and exercise limitation to maximize maternal survival.

Hypertension

Chronic essential hypertension of a mild degree may not have been treated before pregnancy, but the timing of treatment of diastolic hypertension during pregnancy is crucial. The Working Group on High Blood Pressure in Pregnancy recommends that treatment be initiated for a diastolic blood pressure of 100 mm Hg. For pressures of 90 to 99 mm Hg, therapy may be considered if evidence suggests end-organ damage or renal disease. Therapy for mild to moderate hypertension is instituted to prevent hypertensive vascular damage, but no evidence supports or refutes the notion that treatment of chronic hypertension in the first half of pregnancy prevents superimposed preeclampsia.

Many drugs have been used to treat hypertension during pregnancy. The Working Group recommends methyldopa as the drug of choice because it is effective and appears to be safe. β-Blockers are often used, are relatively safe, and are efficacious during late pregnancy, but there are concerns about fetal growth retardation if therapy with these drugs is started at mid-gestation. Nifedipine has been used safely in pregnant women, although data on initiation of therapy during early pregnancy (<26 weeks gestation) are lacking. The drug is teratogenic in rats when used at high doses. Hydralazine has been used for long-term treatment of hypertension in pregnancy but may cause fetal thrombocytopenia. Thus, methyldopa remains the drug of choice for long-term treatment of hypertension during pregnancy. Although use of diuretics in pregnancy is discouraged, the Working Group endorses continuation of diuretic therapy in women who received this treatment before pregnancy. For salt-sensitive hypertension, diuretic therapy may even be initiated during pregnancy.

Dilated Cardiomyopathy

The standard drug therapy for dilated congestive heart failure includes digoxin, angiotensin-converting enzyme inhibitors, and diuretics. Digoxin is considered a safe drug in pregnant women. Angiotensin-converting enzyme inhibitors and angiotensin-receptor blockers are contraindicated after the first trimester of pregnancy because of such adverse fetal effects as neonatal renal failure and death. Interruption of a stable, standard heart failure regimen in a mother whose NYHA class is III or IV could still result in a poor outcome. Second-line drugs, such as hydralazine, may also be associated with adverse effects. With diuretic therapy, careful attention must be paid to electrolyte stability. The phosphodiesterase inhibitors milrinone and amrinone or dobutamine infusion could become necessary for maternal viability. Use of these drugs in pregnant women has been limited.

Coronary Artery Disease

Antianginal medications used in these women to treat coronary artery diseases may increase the risk for adverse affects to the fetus. Therapeutic regimens should be designed to maximize maternal benefit while minimizing fetal harm. Aspirin is considered an essential drug in anginal therapy. Aspirin for other diseases is given at a low dose during pregnancy.

Endocarditis Prophylaxis

Patients with a variety of cardiac lesions, most commonly congenital and valvular, should be considered for endocarditis prophylaxis (see Appendix A). Genitourinary manipulation may lead to bacteremia and, most commonly, endocarditis due to *Enterococcus faecalis* (enterococci). The most recent recommendations of the American Heart Association are that the usual uncomplicated cesarean section does not require endocarditis prophylaxis. For the uncomplicated vaginal delivery, endocarditis prophylaxis is not indicated. Endocarditis prophylaxis is indicated if the patient has a prosthetic valve, a surgically constructed systemic-to-pulmonary shunt or conduit, or a history of endocarditis. If manual removal of the placenta becomes necessary, prophylaxis should be administered.

Cardiac Dysrhythmias

Pregnant women with and those without preexisting cardiac disease may develop many cardiac rhythm abnormalities during pregnancy. Supraventricular dysrhythmias are more common than ventricular dysrhythmias. Neither may require intervention, depending on associated cardiac disease and symptoms. Removal of potential precipitating factors such as caffeine, emotional stress, or substance abuse, coupled with reassurance, may suffice. Maternal risk for the ongoing dysrhythmia is usually obvious, whereas the result of a decreased uterine blood flow may be recognized only at the time of birth. Any drug or active intervention used to treat cardiac dysrhythmias during pregnancy presents some risk to the fetus. Such use should be guided by symptoms and the potential risk to the mother as well as fetus.

Because of variation in cardiac output, gastrointestinal absorption of drugs, renal blood flow, hepatic enzymatic activity, and protein binding and other changed variables during pregnancy, metabolism of drugs varies and usual blood drug concentrations may be inaccurate. Placental transfer varies depending on several variables. Despite widespread use of most antiarrhythmic agents, little information is available on fetal risk and placental transfer. Long-term follow-up of children born after fetal exposure to various drugs may be limited or basically nonexistent.

Use of antiarrhythmic agents is therefore often guided by the known risk that the drugs present to the fetus, the clinical stability of the situation, and the risk to the mother or fetus if the rhythm abnormality is not treated. In the case of cardiovascular collapse, emergency treatment is imperative for survival of the mother, fetus, or both. The Food and Drug Administration has developed a risk classification for drugs used during pregnancy (Table 14.2). If a patient is planning pregnancy or is pregnant and requires antiarrhythmic agents, appropriate consultation with an obstetrician specializing in high-risk patients and with a cardiologist should be undertaken.

Digoxin Digoxin is used to control the ventricular rate in atrial fibrillation and atrial flutter; it is often used for short-term treatment of paroxysmal supraventricular tachycardia as well as for prophylaxis.

Although a category C drug, digoxin is considered "safe," with no significant reported adverse effects in fetuses and neonates. Digoxin clearly crosses the placenta and has been given orally to the mother to treat fetal tachycardia. It is found in breast milk but, according to the American Academy of Pediatrics' Committee on Drugs, is compatible with breast feeding.

Antiarrhythmic Agents

CLASS I **Quinidine** has not been documented as teratogenic, but transient neonatal thrombocytopenia, eighth-nerve damage in the fetus, and premature labor have been reported. Quinidine is considered relatively safe during pregnancy and is used for certain dysrhythmias associated with the Wolff-Parkinson-White syndrome, ventricular dysrhythmias, and maintenance of sinus rhythm after cardioversion of supraventricular tachycardia.

Procainamide is similarly used. It also crosses the placenta and is used to control fetal atrial fibrillation and atrial flutter (after rate control with other medications). Procainamide is not teratogenic in the first trimester. Because it is so slowly eliminated, as is its active metabolite, and because of the danger of inducing antinuclear antibodies and a lupus-like syndrome with long-term use, the drug is usually not given unless the patient's heart fails or the patient cannot tolerate quinidine.

Lidocaine is indicated to treat acute ventricular dysrhythmias. It is not known to be teratogenic. Because the fetal-blood pH is lower than the maternal pH, the lidocaine concentration will be higher in the fetus. This difference assumes importance when the fetus is in distress and the fetal pH may decrease even more. Cardiac and central nervous system toxicity may result, and low initial Apgar scores may reflect this toxicity. As with nonpregnant patients, pregnant women with decreased hepatic blood flow or congestive heart failure should receive lower loading and maintenance dose of lidocaine. The smallest amount possible should be used for the shortest period to avoid fetal toxicity.

CLASS II: β-ADRENERGIC ANTAGONISTS Despite evidence of embryotoxicity in animal studies, no β-blocker has been shown to cause fetal abnormalities. Extensive experience with the use of β-blockers in the pregnant hypertensive population and in pregnant women with other indications for β-blockers indicates some differences in risk to the neonate. β-Blockers have been used in pregnant women for the following:

- Hypertension
- Thyrotoxicosis
- Fetal tachycardia
- Atrial and ventricular premature contraction
- Supraventricular and ventricular tachycardia
- Atrioventricular block in atrial fibrillation and flutter

Propranolol has been used extensively in pregnancy, and a variety of adverse fetal effects are known, including

- Fetal bradycardia
- Hyperbilirubinemia
- Hypoglycemia
- Prolonged labor
- Birth apnea requiring intubation
- Intrauterine growth retardation (a controversial effect)

Metoprolol does not appear to share propranolol's effect in causing fetal bradycardia, hypoglycemia, or growth retardation.

Atenolol may decrease birthweight but does not appear to cause respiratory difficulties, hyperbilirubinemia, or hypoglycemia.

β-Blockers with intrinsic sympathomimetic activity have variable effects on birthweight, heart rate, and glycemic status.

CLASS III **Amiodarone** is used to treat both ventricular and supraventricular rhythm abnormalities. It contains large concentrations of iodine and has been associated with severe neonatal hypothyroidism. Furthermore, significant amounts of the drug are secreted into breast milk. Transient fetal bradycardia and neonatal Q-T prolongation have been described, although no teratogenicity has been reported. Use of this drug should be limited to treatment of refractory dysrhythmias that have not responded to safer antiarrhythmic intervention.

CLASS IV: CALCIUM-CHANNEL BLOCKERS **Verapamil** and **diltiazem** are used for both supraventricular and ventricular dysrhythmias. Diltiazem is increasingly administered through a continuous infusion to control the ventricular response rate in atrial fibrillation and to convert the dysrhythmia. Verapamil may affect fetal atrioventricular node conduction and vascular tone. The affect of ver-apamil on the fetus has led to administering the drug to the mother to treat fetal supraventricular tachycardia. Both the mother and fetus have incurred side effects, including bradycardia, heart block, decreased contractility, and hypotension. Maternal hypotension may lead to fetal distress; thus, intravenous therapy should be used with caution. Despite these effects, verapamil remains an important drug for the treatment of narrow QRS paroxysmal supraventricular tachycardia and for treatment of fetal supraventricular tachycardia resistant to digoxin. Diltiazem has been teratogenic in animal studies and has caused stillbirths and decreased fetal weight. Its use in pregnant women is limited.

OTHER DRUGS **Adenosine** is used to terminate many supraventricular tachycardias. It is given intravenously; unlike verapamil, however, its half-life lasts only seconds and adverse effects should reverse quickly. In one study, the full 12 mg was administered to a woman 41 weeks pregnant; no effect on heart rate was seen in the fetus, which was being continuously monitored by Doppler ultrasonography. During pregnancy, adenosine's degrading enzyme is reduced; because of an increase in intravascular volume, however, the usual 6-mg or the higher 12-mg dose may be needed. Data on use of this drug in pregnant women are limited.

Cardiopulmonary Resuscitation Treatment of this catastrophic event in the pregnant woman is altered by the need to position the woman differently, by difficulties with effective closed-cardiac compression, and by the need to consider early emergency cesarean section if the resuscitation is proceeding poorly and fetal viability is compromised.

Current Advanced Cardiac Life Support (ACLS) Guidelines generated by the American Heart Association stress that cardiopulmonary resuscitation is performed differently in pregnant women. The enlarged uterus may compress the aorta and inferior vena cava, impairing cardiac output and venous return. The woman needs to be rolled toward her left side to displace the uterus to the left and help minimize caval and aortic compression. This may require that a rescuer kneel on the right side of the woman, using his or her thighs to support the woman's shoulders and flank. As an alternative, the rescuer can insert another type of wedge, such as a pillow, to keep the uterus displaced leftward.

Otherwise, standard resuscitative measures and procedures are followed by standard pharmacologic therapy. Early consideration of the fetus should take place. Emergency delivery should be considered for any potentially viable fetus. Thus, at the onset of the resuscitation, a cardiothoracic surgeon should be summoned, as should the obstetrician and neonatologist, to participate in this complex decision. Early delivery (within 5 minutes of the woman's cardiac arrest) is suggested by some authors if the woman continues to lack a pulse.

Summary

- Drugs used for various rhythm abnormalities in the mother (or, as is often the case, for such problems as hypertension or hypertrophic cardiomyopathy) should be used with great caution and only after all reasonable nonpharmacologic interventions fail.
- Limited data on the effects of many of these drugs in pregnant women should temper physicians' use of them.
- The manner in which these drugs may affect the safety of breast feeding is important.
- The primary care physician should expect to discuss the chances of fetal abnormalities or adverse affects of medications with the woman who wishes to become or is already pregnant. Such discussions may result in avoidance or termination of pregnancy.
- Elective use of any cardiac medication in a pregnant patient should begin only after a thorough investigation of potential adverse effects of these drugs, risk–benefit assessment, and thorough discussion with the patient.
- The primary care physician may also be responsible for resuscitative efforts in a pregnant woman and must be aware of the current ACLS guidelines to maximize survival for both the pregnant woman and the fetus.

KEY POINTS

Hemodynamic Changes with Pregnancy

- Increase in plasma volume
- Increase in cardiac output
- Increase in uterus size with compressive effects on the inferior vena cava
- Increase in erythrocyte mass, but not in proportion to the increase in plasma volume; this produces "dilutional" anemia

Physical Findings Altered by Pregnancy

- Cardiac apex displacement laterally and superiorly
- Development of S_3
- Venous hum, which decreases in the supine position or with compression of the jugular vein
- Mammary souffle: continuous murmur heard at the base of the heart
- Development of murmurs (systolic ejection murmur at the left sternal border)

Pregnancy Outcome

- NYHA classes I and II are associated with 1% maternal mortality rate; classes II and IV, with 5 to 15% maternal mortality rate.
- Pulmonary hypertension is considered a contraindication to pregnancy.
- Cyanotic lesions that are not surgically repaired lead to increase in fetal mortality rate.
- Marfan's syndrome leads to maternal risk for aortic dissection.
- Prosthetic valve requires a switch from warfarin to heparin.
- Women with a history of coronary heart disease or with multiple risk factors should be counseled about the increased risk for maternal morbidity and possibly death.

SPECIAL CONCERNS

Infective Endocarditis Prophylaxis Not indicated in uncomplicated cesarean and vaginal deliveries. Indicated with native prosthetic valves, diseased native valve shunts, conduits, or a history of endocarditis.

Anticoagulation Initially, stop warfarin therapy. Switch to heparin, then warfarin beginning at week 13. Two weeks before delivery, switch back to heparin.

Prosthetic Valves Bioprosthetic valves may rapidly deteriorate during pregnancy.

Hypertension Methyldopa still drug of choice; β-blockers acceptable.

Medications Antiarrhythmic drugs quinidine, procainamide, and lidocaine are not teratogenic but should be used with caution. β-Blockers safe, but cause many maternal and fetal effects. Amiodarone not teratogenic, but watch for fetal hypothyroidism and prolonged Q-T interval. Digoxin safe and effective. Verapamil indicated for fetal atrioventricular block. Adenosine safe; 12-mg bolus required.

Cardiopulmonary Resuscitation Pregnant woman must be positioned to her left side. Standard cardiopulmonary resuscitation protocols. Consider emergency cesarean section if cardiopulmonary resuscitation is not effective.

SUGGESTED READINGS

Barbour LA, Pickard J. Controversies in thromboembolic disease during pregnancy: a critical review. Obstet Gynecol 1995;86:621–633.

Cox JL, Gardner MJ. Treatment of cardiac arrhythmias during pregnancy. Prog Cardiovasc Dis 1993;36:137–178.

Dajani AS, Bisno AL, Chung KJ, et al. Prevention of bacterial endocarditis: recommendations by the American Heart Association. JAMA 1990;264:2919–2922.

Elkayam U, Gleicher N. Congenital heart disease. Heart Failure 1993;9:46–58.

Ginsberg JS, Hirsh J. Use of antithrombotic agents during pregnancy. Chest 1992;102:385S–390S, 1992.

Ginsberg JS, Kowalchuk J, Hirsh J, Brill-Edwards P, et al. Heparin therapy during pregnancy. Arch Intern Med 1989; 149:2233–2236.

Hess DB, Hess L, Wayne M. Management of cardiovascular disease in pregnancy, and medical complications during pregnancy. Obstet Gynecol Clin North Am. 1992;19: 679–695.

Lee RV, Rodgers BD, White LM, et al. Cardiopulmonary resuscitation of pregnant women. Am J Med 1986;81: 311–318.

Leffler S, Johnson DR. Adenosine use in pregnancy: lack of effect on fetal heart rate. Am J Emerg Med 1992;10: 548–549.

Lindheimer MD, Cunningham FG. Hypertension and pregnancy: impact of the Working Group Report. Am J Kidney Dis. 1993;21(Suppl 2):29–36.

National High Blood Pressure Education Program Working Group on High Blood Pressure in Pregnancy: a consensus report from the group convened by the National High

Blood Pressure Education Program, National Heart, Lung, and Blood Institute. Am J Obstet Gynecol 1990; 163:1689–1712.

Rotmensch HH, Elkayam U, Frishman W. Antiarrhythmic drug therapy during pregnancy. Ann Intern Med 1983; 98:487–497.

Sbarouni E, Oakley CM. Outcome of pregnancy in women with valve prosthesis. Br Heart J 1994;71:196–201.

15 CHAPTER

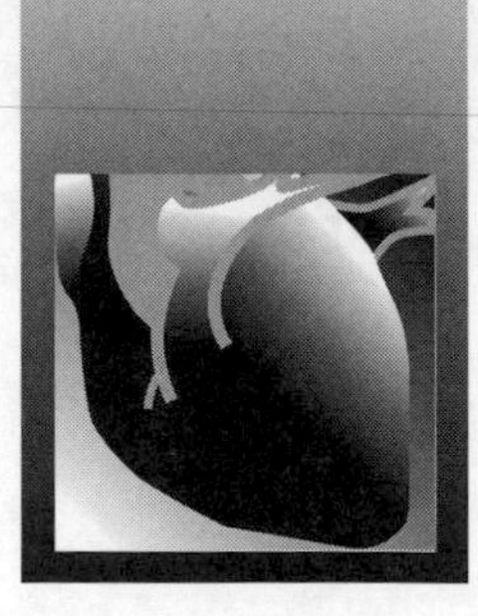

Hypertrophic Cardiomyopathy, Mitral Valve Prolapse, and Cocaine Heart Disease

Andrea Hastillo

HYPERTROPHIC CARDIOMYOPATHY

Background

Hypertrophic cardiomyopathy encompasses a wide variety of morphologic and clinical syndromes characterized by the development of left ventricular hypertrophy in the absence of a systemic or other cardiac disease that could cause this degree of ventricular hypertrophy. Although idiopathic hypertrophic subaortic stenosis is an example of hypertrophic cardiomyopathy, only about one-fourth of patients with hypertrophic cardiomyopathy actually demonstrate outflow tract obstruction.

Histologic examination reveals that the myofibrils are entangled as a result of varying degrees of hypertrophy. The intramural coronary arteries are usually narrowed because of medial and intimal thickening related to abnormal amounts of smooth-muscle cells, collagen, elastin, or connective tissue deposition. Diffuse myocardial fibrosis is present. The mitral valve is usually abnormal and often demonstrates exaggerated systolic anterior mitral leaflet excursion, which may cause the mitral leaflet to touch the intraventricular septum or form a dynamic outflow tract obstruction. Mitral insufficiency is common as a result of this systolic anterior excursion.

Signs and Symptoms

The hypertrophy of the ventricle is usually asymmetric; the septum is normally the most hypertrophied area. Hypertrophic cardiomyopathy may display an autosomal dominant genetic transmission; however, morphologic expression in both sporadic and heritable hypertrophic cardiomyopathy is not complete until early adulthood. The type and degree of hypertrophy may vary among first-degree relatives.

Hypertrophy of the base of the septum associated with abnormal systolic motion of the anterior mitral leaflet may lead to a subaortic outflow tract obstruction. As the blood is ejected though this narrowed outflow tract, an increase in its velocity may cause a Venturi effect that pulls the mitral leaflet even further toward the septum, worsening the outflow obstruction. This may also lead to new or worsening mitral insufficiency.

Ventricular diastolic compliance and relaxation are decreased in hypertrophic cardiomyopathy and may result in a diminished end-diastolic volume. Combined with the smaller than normal left ventricular cavity caused by cardiac muscle hypertrophy encroaching on the chamber, stroke volume may be severely decreased. Thus, maintaining active diastolic filling (atrial contraction) is important in these patients. Symptoms relating to a decrease in ventricular diastolic compliance include congestive failure and low-output left ventricular failure.

Ischemia is characteristic of hypertrophic cardiomyopathy and is partly caused by increases in oxygen demand relating to the increased muscle mass and higher ventricular tension not met because of abnormal coronary arteries and decreased coronary flow gradient. In about 10 to 15% of patients with hypertrophic cardiomyopathy, the ischemia-induced necrosis and fibrosis may cause end-stage dilated cardiomyopathy similar to the dilated cardiomyopathy of systolic dysfunction. Fibrosis and ischemia form the substrate for dysrhythmias, another clinical feature of hypertrophic cardiomyopathy. About 10% of patients develop atrial fibrillation, which may be associated with hemodynamic deterioration and emboli. Ventricular dysrhythmias may occur, and even asymptomatic, nonsustained ventricular tachycardia is associated with an increased risk for sudden death.

Physical Examination

Physical findings vary and may relate to the presence of a dynamic outflow tract obstruction. The carotid pulse may demonstrate a rapid upstroke that is suddenly interrupted because of subvalvular obstruction. The cardiac impulse may be normal, sustained, diffuse, or displaced, but specific features may be a double apical impulse, a palpable S_4, or a systolic thrill caused by mitral insufficiency. On auscultation, the presence of an S_4, preserved A_2 (aortic component of S_2), and absence of an ejection click are expected. Murmurs of mitral insufficiency and subvalvular aortic stenosis may be present. The systolic murmur of outflow obstruction often varies and is expected to develop or become louder with maneuvers that increase contractility, decrease ventricular volume, or decrease aortic impedance. These result in an overall decrease or more rapid decrease in intraventricular volume during systole and allow obstruction to worsen. Simple maneuvers may be used in an attempt to determine the cause of the murmur:

Standing:	Decrease ventricular volume, intensifying the murmur
Squatting:	Slow ventricular ejection, softening the murmur
Valsalva maneuver (prerelease):	Intensifies the murmur

It is important to perform these maneuvers in patients in whom outflow obstruction is suspected and to remember that certain physical activities and medications may worsen or lessen the obstruction (Table 15.1).

TABLE 15.1. Variation in the Intensity of the Systolic Murmur of Left Ventricular Outflow Tract Obstruction

Variable	Bedside or Office Maneuvers	Systolic Outflow Murmur Intensity
Increase preload	Squatting	Decrease
Increase afterload	Squatting	Decrease
Decrease contractility with β-blocker therapy		Decrease
Decrease preload with diuretics and nitrates	Standing Valsalva maneuver	Increase
Decrease afterload	Standing	Increase
Increase contractility		Increase

Laboratory Tests

Electrocardiography (ECG) is nondiagnostic, but huge lateral Q waves or septal R waves associated with evidence of left ventricular and septal hypertrophy may be found. Echocardiography may be diagnostic; in uncomplicated cases, cardiac catheterization may not be indicated.

Clinical Course

Symptoms commonly appear in early life (20 to 40 years of age). One echocardiogram, especially in the patient with a family history of hypertrophic cardiomyopathy, should not be misinterpreted as indicating that the patient is free of the disease. Hypertrophy may develop rapidly during young adulthood, even tripling the rate at which hypertrophic cardiomyopathy develops in a matter of a few years. Therefore, surveillance echocardiography is indicated in certain patients. The presence of a suspicious murmur, chest pain, or palpitations in a young person should provoke concern. Symptoms include those related not only to ischemia, dysrhythmia, and congestive heart failure but also to infective endocarditis and sudden death. The annual rate of death from hypertrophic cardiomyopathy in an in-hospital population is about 2 to 4%.

Athletic Activity

Hypertrophic cardiomyopathy is the most common cause of sudden cardiac death in young, competitive athletes. Risk factors for sudden death include

- Young age (more commonly seen in persons aged 15 to 35 years)
- Nonsustained ventricular tachycardia
- Previous cardiac arrest
- Severe hypertrophy
- Presence of left ventricular outflow tract obstruction (degree of gradient does not relate to risk)
- Family history of malignant hypertrophic cardiomyopathy (two or more first-degree relatives died suddenly of hypertrophic cardiomyopathy before 50 years of age)
- History of syncope

The 26th Bethesda Conference has made specific recommendations regarding athletic activities for patients with hypertrophic cardiomyopathy. Competitive sports are to be avoided altogether, although some distinction among patients' tolerance for activity may be possible.

Diagnosis

Evaluation for a new diagnosis of hypertrophic cardiomyopathy should include a thorough history and physical examination (emphasize family history; maneuver patient), ECG, echocardiography, and 24-hour ambulatory ECG.

Treatment

Prophylaxis against infective endocarditis is indicated (see Appendix A). Endocarditis may involve the abnormal mitral valve and the mural plaque, which may develop on the septum where the anterior mitral leaflet makes contact. Otherwise, treatment in asymptomatic persons is usually not indicated. However, treatment of asymptomatic, nonsustained ventricular tachycardia is controversial and should be discussed with the cardiology consultant.

Mild to moderate symptoms usually require treatment. β-Blockers have been helpful for relieving palpitations and symptoms of angina, heart failure, and cerebral hypoperfusion. These drugs have also helped relieve angina, palpitations, and the symptoms of heart failure and cerebral hypoperfusion as a result of their ability to increase ventricular volume and decrease oxygen demand.

Verapamil may alleviate symptoms, even when propranolol has failed, because it may markedly reverse some of the diastolic compliance problems.

If symptoms worsen or are refractory to these usual medications, the use of disopyramide may be considered. Cautious use of diuretics may be tried in patients with severe congestive symptoms and no obstructive symptoms. With such treatment, the clinician walks the fence between overdiuresis and continued congestion. The dosage of drugs used to treat hypertropic cardiomyopathy often becomes very high; following are typical maximum levels:

β-Blocker, propranolol:	320 mg/d
β-Blocker, atenolol:	100 mg/d
Calcium-channel blocker, verapamil:	640 mg/d
Disopyramide:	600 mg/d

In patients who do not exhibit outflow tract obstruction but do not respond to medical therapy, little remains but to consider cardiac transplantation. Patients who develop fibrosis and progress to the dilated phase are treated as having a dilated cardiomyopathy; possible treatments include transplantation.

In patients who demonstrate left ventricular outflow tract obstruction, dual-chamber pacing and surgical intervention should be considered. Partial removal of the offending hypertrophied septum with possible mitral valve replacement should be analyzed before transplantation alternatives are considered.

Dual-chamber pacing is being developed for treating hypertrophic cardiomyopathy with left ventricular outflow tract obstruction. Data indicate that by prematurely depolarizing the right ventricle (electronic ventricular pacing), the sequence and rate of left ventricular contraction will be abnormal and lessen the outflow tract gradient, possibly even interrupting the Venturi effect. An atrial pacing wire is used to assure atrial–ventricular synchrony to maximize ventricular filling. Evidence suggests that the gradient may lessen over long-term pacing.

The surgical procedure is usually successful in reducing the resting gradient, although a provokable gradient may remain. The septum does not tend to regrow. Major adverse effects of the surgery include a perioperative mortality rate of 5%, iatrogenic ventricular septal defect, and conduction abnormalities requiring permanent electronic pacing. The algorithm for managing hypertrophic cardiomyopathy is presented in Figure 15.1.

Finally, early research is progressing on a new method to treat recalcitrant outflow tract obstruction: intentional controlled infarction of the offending septum. Controlled infarction is accomplished by instillation of absolute alcohol into the artery. That provides arterial blood supply to the septum, usually the first septal perforator. Initial data have been promising.

Referral

Referral to a cardiac surgeon with expertise in septal surgery for hypertrophic cardiomyopathy is indicated when

- Dual-chamber pacing fails or is not indicated
- Patient with outflow tract obstruction remains in class III or class IV failure or angina

MITRAL VALVE PROLAPSE

Background

Mitral valve prolapse occurs in about 3 to 5% of the general population. The condition may involve an autosomal dominant genetic transmission, with a more thorough expression in women. Mitral valve prolapse is characterized by abnormal mitral valve leaflets that are positioned superior to the mitral annular plane during systole. One or both of the mitral leaflets will therefore prolapse into the left atrium during ventricular systole. Prolapse may relate to structural abnormalities of the mitral valve, such as those occurring with myxomatous degeneration of the mitral valve, causing elongated chordae and redundant leaflets, ruptured chordae tendinae, Marfan's syndrome, or even rheumatic fever.

Physiologic prolapse may occur in the absence of structural mitral leaflet abnormalities in some conditions in which the left ventricular cavity becomes smaller, such as with dehydration, the Valsalva maneuver, or atrial septal defect.

It is important to differentiate between prolapse due to structural causes and prolapse due to physiologic causes; the former is associated with more complications.

Signs and Symptoms

Clinical syndromes associated with mitral valve prolapse include the following:

- Mitral insufficiency
- Chest pain, which may be typical or atypical for angina
- Dysrhythmias
- Embolic stroke
- Autonomic dysfunction

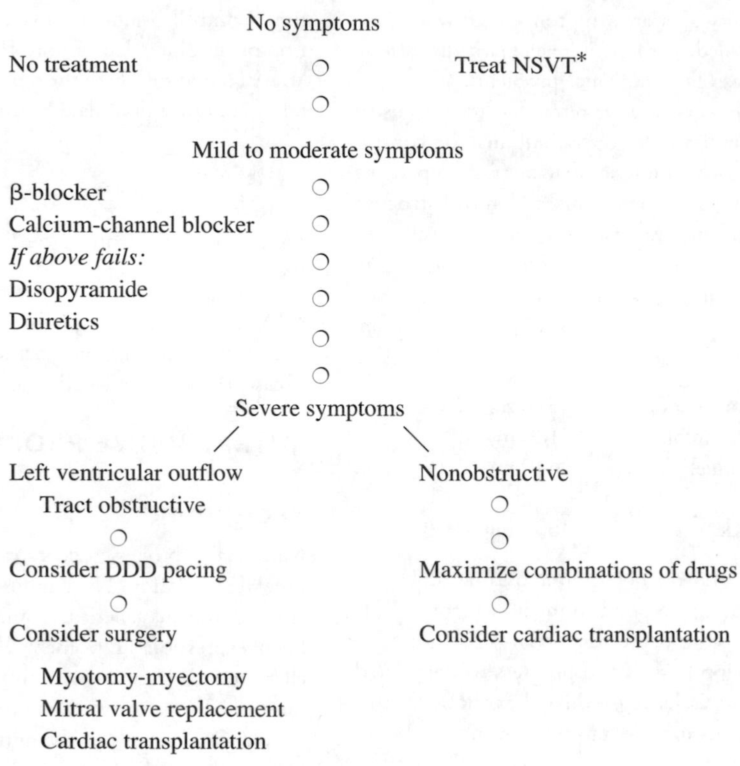

FIGURE 15.1.
Algorithm for treatment of hypertrophic cardiomyopathy. *NSVT,* nonsustained ventricular tachycardia.

Chest pain is often atypical for angina pectoris, although occasional thallium scans suggest that areas of the heart may be ischemic in the absence of angiographic epicardial coronary artery disease. Lightheadedness, postural syncope, fatigue, and palpitations may be multifactorial in origin because of ischemia, dysrhythmias, dynamic changes of mitral insufficiency, and autonomic dysfunction. In addition, these patients are at an increased risk for endocarditis and platelet thrombi, both of which may be associated with emboli manifest by stroke or transient ischemic attacks.

Physical Examination

Physical findings vary and are often transient. Midsystolic clicks may result from sudden tension on the chordae at the time the mitral leaflets prolapse maximally into the left atrium. If mitral insufficiency results from the mitral prolapse, the murmur is usually midsystolic and located at the apex and may vary greatly with ventricular volume changes. The murmur often possesses unusual qualities, such as a honking or whooping sound.

The position of the click or onset of the murmur vary with changes in myocardial contractility, systemic vascular resistance, and ventricular volume. Increasing the left ventricular volume by increasing preload and slowing ejection of blood from the left ventricle by increasing afterload or decreasing contractility tend to delay the onset of prolapse. This delay or increase in left ventricular volume leads to a later occurrence of the click and onset of the murmur. One or both may, in fact, disappear. The opposite occurs if the ventricular volume is decreased or if blood is ejected more rapidly: the click and onset of the murmur will occur earlier or will appear if not previously present. Therefore, simple maneuvers such as standing (which acutely decreases afterload and preload) or squatting (which acutely increases afterload and preload) help diagnose this entity.

Laboratory Tests

The ECG is nondiagnostic. Chest radiography is normal in 80% of patients. Echocardiography is used to confirm the clinical diagnosis and often reveals the diagnosis in the "absence" of clinical features. Cardiac catheterization is not necessary unless the question of other cardiac disease, such as coronary disease, is present or if mitral valve replacement or repair is being contemplated.

Clinical Course

The natural history of mitral valve prolapse is strongly influenced by whether the prolapse is physiologic or structural in origin. Structural prolapse, such as that characterized by redundant, thickened leaflets, is associated with the following additional complications:

- Chest pain
- Development of severe mitral regurgitation
- Stroke
- Significant dysrhythmias
- Infective endocarditis
- Sudden death

The incidence of these complications varies widely.

Mitral valve prolapse is the most common underlying factor associated with infective endocarditis in persons who are not drug addicts. It occurs more frequently in the presence of a murmur and in patients with structural abnormalities. One study indicated that the annual risk for developing infective endocarditis in the presence of prolapse associated with a murmur is about 1 in 1400. Another study found an incidence of 6% over a 6-year follow-up.

In one study, severe mitral insufficiency requiring surgery developed in 9% of patients during a 6-year period. Another study indicated that only 4% of patients required surgery for this complication during a 14-year follow-up. Thus, 4 to 9% of patients with severe mitral regurgitation due to prolapse will eventually require surgery.

Stroke may occur in up to 7.5% of patients and may occur in patients who have prolapse only. In one study, mitral valve prolapse was found in 40% of persons younger than 45 years of age with cerebral strokes or transient ischemic attacks.

The possibility of an increased risk for serious dysrhythmias due to mitral valve prolapse not associated with severe mitral regurgitation is controversial. The increased risk for sudden death in patients with mitral valve prolapse appears small.

Treatment

Prophylaxis against infective endocarditis is indicated for patients with mitral valve prolapse associated with a murmur. In the absence of a murmur, however, the decision for prophylaxis must weigh the risk associated with the antibiotics against the risk associated with the procedure being contemplated in the context of the structural properties of the mitral valve.

A wide variety of β-blockers are available to treat the various atrial and ventricular dysrhythmias, as well as chest pain syndromes associated with mitral valve prolapse.

In an attempt to decrease the risk for emboli, use of aspirin in certain patients with mitral valve prolapse appears effective. Consultation with a neurologist may be necessary to help guide therapy in patients with documented stroke or transient ischemic attacks.

Patients with mitral insufficiency should be carefully followed clinically and with echocardiography. Mitral valve prolapse associated with severe mitral insufficiency requiring surgical intervention may necessitate only mitral valve repair instead of valve replacement.

Restriction of physical activity depends on the degree of mitral insufficiency plus the presence of syncope, dysrhythmias, history of embolic events, and family history of sudden death. The 26th Bethesda Conference addressed restriction of physical activity.

COCAINE HEART DISEASE

Background

Cocaine use is protean, the abuser fits no stereotype, and the toxic effects of the drug are multiple. Cardiovascular complications are common, resulting from all three major routes of cocaine use: smoking, nasal sufflation, and intravenous injection.

Cocaine blocks the peripheral and central reuptake of catecholamines and releases catecholamines from central and peripheral stores. Central nervous system effects result in increased sympathetic activity and perpetuate a positive feedback loop of central nervous system agitation and further heightened peripheral sympathetic activity. Central nervous system effects include seizures and hyperthermia.

α-Stimulation may increase blood pressure and myocardial oxygen demand. It may concurrently decrease oxygen supply by increasing coronary vascular resistance and increasing the risk for in situ thrombi formation by causing coronary artery vasoconstriction. β-Stimulation may increase heart rate and automaticity, increase contractility, and therefore increase oxygen demand.

The local anesthetic effect of cocaine may lengthen myocardial depolarization and depress contractility. Effects on calcium and potassium flux may lengthen the P-R and Q-T intervals and even result in torsades de pointes. Other important effects include hypersensitivity reactions and increased platelet aggregation. Cocaine use is associated with an increased incidence of the following:

- Left ventricular hypertrophy
- Myocarditis
- Accelerated coronary atherosclerosis
- Abnormal intramural coronary arteries
- Infective endocarditis
- Ischemia

Ischemia is probably caused by an increase in oxygen demand not met because of a limited blood supply mediated by coronary artery vasoconstriction, platelet aggregation and thrombus formation in coronary arteries, narrowed intramural coronary arteries, and accelerated coronary atherosclerosis. One-third of persons with infarction ascribed to cocaine have normal coronary arteries; another one-third have thrombus formation but not the high incidence of plaque fissuring and hemorrhage noted in typical atherosclerotic infarctions not associated with cocaine.

Coronary vasoconstriction may occur in vessels without typical atherosclerotic plaque, although constriction is more marked in areas with atherosclerotic disease. Similarly, in situ thrombi may develop in vessels without preexisting disease. Long-term cocaine use is a risk factor for development of premature coronary artery disease.

Signs and Symptoms

Presumably, patients may have silent cardiac disease, including silent episodes of ischemia. A large problem, however, is that many persons do develop symptoms; one of these is often chest pain, which brings the patient to medical attention.

Clinical features of ischemia are based on a limited number of retrospective studies and even fewer prospective studies of ischemic syndromes in the cocaine user. The typical person with cocaine-associated chest pain is in the late-20-year to mid-30-year age group, a cigarette smoker, and not a first-time user. The chest pain syndrome may be typical or atypical angina: it is often dull and retrosternal, with an unexplained pleuritic component; it may radiate to the arms or neck. If associated with infarction, it is more like typical angina. Concurrent cigarette smoking hastens the onset of time from cocaine use to onset of chest pain. Individually, both cigarette and cocaine use cause coronary artery vasospasm. Used together, their effects are additive, especially in the coronary artery segments with preexisting atherosclerotic disease.

Chest pain may occur during cocaine use but may also develop hours later. With most infarctions, pain develops within 3 hours after cocaine use. However, cocaine withdrawal is also associated with repetitive episodes of both symptomatic and silent ST-segment elevations on ECG, presumably because of coronary artery vasoconstriction. Therefore, pain and even infarction may be significantly delayed. A significant frequency of intermittent ST-segment elevations may occur for more than 3 weeks after cessation of cocaine before tapering.

Chest pain is associated with ECG abnormalities in up to as 80% of patients. Nearly half of patients with cocaine-associated chest pain demonstrate ECG criteria for thrombolytic intervention. In this group of young patients, ST-T changes may be difficult to interpret because they may represent early repolarization or left ventricular hypertrophy.

The incidence of myocardial infarction in cocaine users is unknown, but prospective studies indicate an incidence of only about 6%; in contrast, retrospective studies have reported an incidence of 0 to 31%.

Laboratory Tests

Diagnosis of myocardial infarction or even myocardial ischemia in this population is difficult. ST-segment changes on ECG are not specific because the chest pain may be highly suggestive of ischemia in a nonischemic state or blatantly nonsuggestive in an ischemic state.

Dependency on enzymatic markers for infarction is heightened. Cocaine-induced sympathetic hyperactivity may be associated with seizures, skeletal-muscle injury, and rhabdomyolysis and may result not only in elevation of total creatine kinase levels but also increased creatine kinase–MB levels. Clinical evaluation of the data, including evaluation of creatine kinase patterns in relation to the time of pain onset and offset may help in interpretation. Use of the assay for cardiac troponin I may help resolve this issue because cardiac troponin I levels should not increase as a result of skeletal-muscle injury.

Emergency department triage becomes very important because of the many patients with cocaine-associated chest pain coming to the emergency department. Persons with obvious infarction and changing ST segments or documented new ST-segment elevations or Q waves are immediately placed in the intensive care unit. The less straightforward situation of chest pain with nonspecific ST-segment abnormalities on ECG or a history indicating disease or drug use without ECG changes still requires evaluation. The ability to obtain "fast track" enzyme or nuclear studies in observation areas designed for equivocal chest pain syndromes can safely and efficiently triage these patients in less than 24 hours.

Treatment

Therapy for presumed cocaine-induced myocardial ischemia or infarction differs from that for typical atherosclerotic disease. Diagnosis requires a high index of suspicion, and questioning about drugs of abuse should be part of any history of chest pain. Careful consideration to the clinical situation and searching for changing ECG patterns may be necessary. Even echocardiography may be performed to guide therapy for cocaine-associated myocardial ischemia.

Because no prospective clinical studies have examined alterations in treatment of presumed cocaine-induced ischemic syndromes, the following deviations from standard care are only suggestions:

- Oxygen use is standard.
- Aspirin is usually given, although there is a concern about intracerebral bleeding if the patient has cocaine-induced systolic hypertension.
- Consider the early use of benzodiazepines to decrease stimulation of the central nervous system and to decrease anxiety, tachycardia, and hypertension.
- Nitroglycerin can decrease cocaine-induced vasoconstriction. It is a first-line drug in cocaine-associated myocardial ischemia.
- If pain persists or if infarction is probable, treatment choices become more problematic.
- Calcium-channel blockers should theoretically be beneficial. Evidence suggests that verapamil reverses cocaine-induced coronary artery vasoconstriction, but there is concern that central nervous system toxicity may increase. Therefore, calcium-channel blockers may be administered as a second-line therapy if nitroglycerin, aspirin, and benzodiazepines do not control ischemic pain. Benzodiazepines must be given first to decrease the risk for central nervous system toxicity.
- α-Blockers are considered to be potentially helpful but are seldom used.
- β-Blockers are not recommended and should be avoided in patients with recent cocaine use and myocardial ischemia. Unopposed α-effects may result in further coronary vasoconstriction and may increase systemic hypertension. β-Blockers may result in paradoxical hypotension and even death by worsening the negative inotropic effect caused by severe cocaine toxicity.

Theoretically, thrombolytic therapy for patients with cocaine-induced myocardial infarction is indicated, but concerns about cocaine-associated systemic hypertension and intracerebral hemorrhage temper the use of this therapy. Furthermore, the high incidence of confusing electrocardiographic ST-segment changes noted in cocaine-associated chest pain may make the use of thrombolytic agents less attractive. Changing ST-segment elevations indicating myocardial injury and early use of echocardiography showing myocardial wall-motion abnormalities in the ECG matching area may help in management decisions. It is reasonable to use thrombolytic agents in patients with unequivocal evidence of acute myocardial infarction who have no usual contraindication to this treatment. In equivocal cases or situations in which emergency cardiac catheterization is readily available, catheterization followed by intracoronary thrombolysis or primary angioplasty is an appropriate consideration.

Use of the usual antiarrhythmic agent, lidocaine, must proceed with caution in the patient with recent cocaine use. Lidocaine and cocaine may both cause seizures and dysrhythmias. Data on this issue in humans are limited, and lidocaine should be avoided in the first 2 to 4 hours after cocaine use. Lidocaine therapy 4 to 5 hours after cocaine use appears safe.

The short-term prognosis of cocaine-associated ischemia and even infarction is good. Therefore, cocaine-induced ischemia without infarction may be treated with only a brief hospitalization, but the key to prognosis involves defining patients who have associated coronary atherosclerosis and preventing further cocaine and cigarette use. Selection of one of the many variations of stress testing may help identify patients with fixed atherosclerotic disease. If this disease is found, its treatment is similar to that of routine atherosclerotic disease; a few changes are made if the patient plans to continue cocaine use.

Further evaluation of the patient with cocaine-associated myocardial infarction should follow evaluation used in patients with myocardial infarction not associated with cocaine.

All patients should be cautioned to stop cocaine use; further use may, even with no evidence of fixed disease, result in further chest pain, possible ischemia, infarction, and even death. Continued use may result in premature coronary atherosclerosis. Again, use of β-blockers in persons who use cocaine should be avoided.

KEY POINTS

Hypertrophic Cardiomyopathy

- Genetic disease is characterized by abnormal ventricular hypertrophy.
- Only 25% of patients have hypertrophic cardiomyopathy with obstruction (idiopathic hypertrophic subaortic stenosis).
- Mitral insufficiency is common because of septal hypertrophy and abnormal systolic motion of the anterior mitral valve.
- Ventricular diastolic compliance and relaxation are abnormal. Maintenance of normal sinus rhythm is important.
- Thickened muscle can become ischemic resulting in chest pain.

Symptoms: Begin as a young adult: chest pain (angina-like), palpitations, congestive heart failure, syncope, and sudden death. Common cause of sudden death in the young athlete. The diagnosis of hypertrophic cardiomyopathy should exclude the patient from competitive and/or isometric sports for medical and legal reasons.

Diagnosis

Physical examination: Systolic ejection murmur at the left sternal border that increases with standing, decreases with squatting, and intensifies with the Valsalva maneuver

ECG: Nondiagnostic, but large lateral and septal Q waves in the young may be found

Echocardiography: Gold standard; should be ordered for all suspected cases

Therapy: Refer to a cardiologist.

Medical: β-Blockers, verapamil, disopyramide, prophylaxis against bacterial endocarditis.

Surgical: Transplantation for hypertrophic cardiomyopathy without obstruction in refractory cases. Septal myotomy with possible mitral valve replacement.

Electrical: Dual-chamber pacemaker in hypertrophic cardiomyopathy with obstruction.

Mitral Valve Prolapse

- Affects 4 to 5% of the general population; autosomal dominant; more common in women.
- Abnormal mitral valve leaflets prolapsing into the left atrium during systole.

Symptoms: Chest pain (typical or atypical for angina), dysrhythmia, stroke, or autonomic dysfunction.

Diagnosis

Physical examination: Midsystolic clicks with the apical, holosystolic murmur of mitral regurgitation.

ECG: Nondiagnostic.

Chest radiography: Normal in 80% of patients.

Echocardiography: Gold standard; should be ordered on all patients with suspected prolapse to confirm the diagnosis.

Therapy: Prophylaxis against bacterial endocarditis in all patients with the murmur and echocardiographic confirmation.

Medical: β-Blockers, aspirin to prevent emboli.

Surgical: Indicated for severe, refractory cases with congestive heart failure (4 to 9% of cases); mitral valve replacement or repair.

Cocaine and Heart Disease

- Cocaine is protean in society. Any young person, regardless of socioeconomic status, presenting with a chest pain syndrome should be screened for cocaine.
- Cocaine heart disease can present with three major manifestations of heart disease:
  - Sudden death
  - Congestive heart failure (i.e., cocaine-related cardiomyopathy)
  - Coronary artery disease
- Cocaine induced coronary artery disease

Symptoms: Angina-like chest pain or the pain of myocardial infarction. May be associated with confusion, disorientation, seizures, or hyperthermia because of the central nervous system effects of cocaine.

Diagnosis

Physical examination: Tachycardia, S_4 gallop.

ECG: Findings of angina (ST-segment depression); findings of myocardial infarction (ST-segment elevation); may develop hours after cocaine use.

Treatment: For suspected cocaine-induced myocardial infarction.

- Oxygen
- Benzodiazepines
- Aspirin, 325 mg
- Nitroglycerin, both sublingual and cutaneous
- Calcium-channel blockers (verapamil)
- Thrombolytic therapy (*if no contraindications*)
- β-Blockers—*not recommended*

SUGGESTED READINGS

Maron BJ, Mitchell JH. 26th Bethesda Conference. Recommendations for Determining Eligibility for Competition in Athletes with Cardiovascular Abnormalities, January 6–7, 1994. J Am Coll Cardiol 1994;24:845–899.

Hypertrophic Cardiomyopathy

Maron BJ, Barry J. Hypertrophic cardiomyopathy. Curr Probl Cardiol 1993;18:637–704.

Maron BJ, Isner JM, McKenna WJ. Task Force 3: Hypertrophic cardiomyopathy, myocarditis and other myopericardial disease and mitral valve prolapse. J Am Coll Cardiol 1994;24:880–885.

Mitral Valve Prolapse

Carabello BA: Mitral valve disease. Curr Probl Cardiol 1993;18:421–480.

Düren DR, Becker AE, Dunning AJ. Long-term follow-up of idiopathic mitral valve prolapse in 300 patients: a prospective study. J Am Coll Cardiol 1988;11:42–47.

MacMahon SW , Hickey AJ, Wilcken DEL, et al. Risk of infective endocarditis in mitral valve prolapse with and without precordial systolic murmurs. Am J Cardiol 1987;59: 105–108.

Marks AR, Choong CY, Sanfilippo AJ, et al. Identification of high-risk and low-risk subgroups of patients with mitral valve prolapse. Circulation 1989;320:1031–1036.

Cocaine Heart Disease

Chakka S, Myerburg RJ. Cardiac complications of cocaine abuse. Clin Cardiol. 1995;18:67–72.

Hollander JE. The management of cocaine-associated myocardial ischemia. N Engl J Med 1995;333:1267–1272.

Hollander JE, Burstein JL, Hoffman RS, et al. Cocaine-associated myocardial infarction, clinical safety of thrombolyic therapy. Chest 1995;107:1237–1241.

Kloner RA, Hale S, Alker K, et al. The effects of acute and chronic cocaine use on the heart. Circulation 1992; 85: 407–419.

Nadamanee K, Gorelick DA, Josephson MA, et al. Myocardial ischemia during cocaine withdrawal. Ann Intern Med 1989;111:876–880.

Nelson L, Hoffman RS. How to manage acute MI when cocaine is the cause. J Crit Illness. 1995;10:39–43.

16 CHAPTER

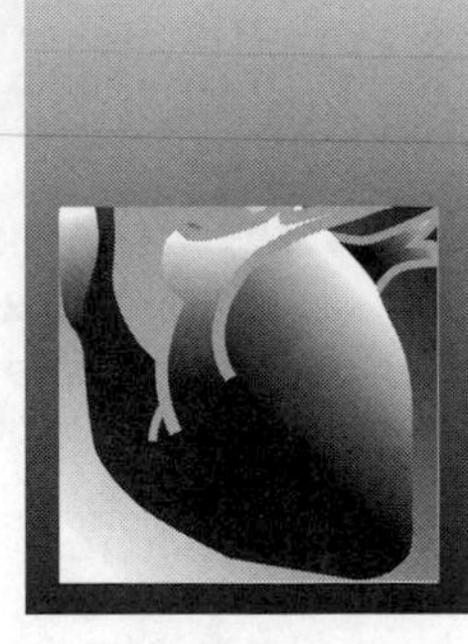

Diagnostic Evaluation and Management of Syncope

Carlos A. Morillo

INTRODUCTION

Syncope, defined as a transient loss of consciousness and posture with spontaneous recovery, is a common medical problem that accounts for approximately 1% of hospital admissions and 3% of emergency department visits. Recurrent, unexplained syncope is a challenging clinical problem, and the cause remains elusive in up to 50% of patients despite many costly investigations. This cost approaches $5000 per patient; an estimated $750 million is spent each year to evaluate patients with syncope.

The incidence of syncope varies with different age groups. In the Framingham study of 2336 men and 2873 women (30 to 62 years of age at study entry) followed for 13 biannual examinations, 3% of men and 3.5% of women experienced syncope. The prevalence of syncope increased with age, from 0.7% in men 35 to 44 years of age to 5.6% in men 75 years of age or older. In a study of elderly institutionalized patients (older than 75 years of age), Lipsitz and coworkers reported an annual incidence of syncope of 6%, with a recurrence rate of 30%. The risk for death among patients with syncope is 1.5 times that of age- and sex-matched controls. In patients older than 65 years of age who have syncope of cardiovascular origin, the risk for death is 33%; in contrast, the risk is 6 to 12% in patients with a noncardiac cause of syncope.

CAUSES

The cause of syncope may be classified as cardiac and noncardiac. Cardiac causes are attributed to 8 to 39% of patients. Despite the use of multiple noninvasive and invasive diagnostic tests, the cause of syncope remains unknown in 30 to 50% of patients. Table 16.1 summarizes the most frequent cardiac and neurovascular causes of syncope. Metabolic and cerebrovascular causes of syncope are infrequent and are not discussed in this chapter.

TABLE 16.1. Causes of Syncope

Type of Syncope	Cause
Cardiac	
Mechanical	Aortic stenosis
	Hypertrophic obstructive cardiomyopathy
	Pulmonary embolism
	Pulmonary hypertension
	Myxoma (left atrium)
	Cardiac tamponade
Electrical	Bradyarrhythmias
	Sinus node disease
	Atrioventricular Node Block
	Tachyarrhythmias
	Paroxysmal supraventricular tachycardia
	Atrial flutter or fibrillation
	Ventricular tachycardia or ventricular fibrillation
Neurovascular	Autonomic dysfunction (orthostatic hypotension)
	Carotid sinus hypersensitivity
	Neurocardiogenic (vasovagal) syncope
	Postprandial syncope
	Long Q–T syndrome

Cardiac Syncope

Cardiac causes of syncope are mechanical or electrical.

Mechanical

Mechanical causes of syncope are due to marked and abrupt reduction in cardiac output that leads to cerebral ischemia, dizziness, and syncope. Reduced cardiac output is associated with the following:

- Aortic stenosis and hypertrophic obstructive cardiomyopathy triggered by exercise due to increased obstruction (dynamic or functional)
- Pulmonary embolism causing cerebral ischemia
- Pericardial constriction
- Myxomas in the left atrium causing intermittent obstruction of the mitral valve or embolization to the brain stem
- Infrequent myxomas that cause intermittent or persistent obstruction of the ventricular outflow tract, simulating aortic or pulmonary stenosis

Electrical

Electrical causes of syncope include bradyarrhythmias and tachyarrhythmias. Syncope is caused by a reduction in cardiac output that leads to global cerebral underperfusion. Dizziness or syncope generally occurs when the patient is in an upright position. However, a large decrease in cerebral blood flow, particularly in patients with compromised left ventricular function, may also lead to syncope while the patient is supine.

Syncope may result from electrical causes depending on the following:

- Rate of bradyarrhythmia or tachyarrhythmia
- Presence of cerebrovascular obstruction
- Integrity of compensatory mechanisms that maintain peripheral vasoconstriction

Syncope due to bradyarrhythmia can be caused by sinus node dysfunction or atrioventricular (AV) node block (see Chapter 3 for a detailed discussion of the following electrocardiographic diagnoses).

Sinus node dysfunction is characterized by marked sinus bradycardia or prolonged pauses. In patients with sick sinus syndrome, bradyarrhythmias may alternate with episodes of atrial fibrillation (Fig. 16.1) and long pauses, and syncope may occur after sudden termination of atrial fibrillation.

Atrioventricular **node block** that leads to syncope is usually due to infranodal or high-degree AV node block, which is associated with an unstable, slow idioventricular escape rhythm. Conversely, AV node block is usually associated with a stable junctional escape rhythm at a rate of 50 to 60 beats/min, sufficient to maintain hemodynamic stability.

During electrophysiology evaluation, ventricular tachycardia is noted in 15% of patients with syncope. When the rate of ventricular tachycardia exceeds 200 beats/min, the incidence of syncope is 36%; in contrast, only 5% of patients with a ventricular tachycardia rate less than 200 beats/min experience syncope. Patients with underlying congestive heart failure have a higher incidence of syncope, indicating that the rate of ventricular tachycardia and the status of left ventricular function may determine whether the patient will develop syncope.

Supraventricular tachycardia is rarely associated with syncope. However, when extremely rapid rates (>250 beats/min) are associated with underlying heart disease, syncope can occur. In some cases, syncope may be due to impaired vasomotor control rather than to the rapid heart rate. Supraventricular tachycardia fast enough to induce syncope is generally seen in patients with an accessory AV connection (Wolff-Parkinson-White syndrome) and episodes of atrial fibrillation. In this setting, the ventricular rate may exceed 300 beats/min and may degenerate into ventricular fibrillation and cardiac arrest. Paroxysmal atrial flutter or fibrillation (Fig. 16.1) may be associated with dizzy spells or presyncope, particularly in patients with compromised left ventricular function.

Neurovascular Syncope

The **neurovascular causes of syncope** are the most common. Autonomic dysfunction, either primary or secondary, is generally manifested by orthostatic hypotension associated with inappropriate chronotropic response that may lead to dizziness and syncope. Elderly patients are at a higher risk for orthostatic hypotension because of decreased postural cardioacceleration. Among the many causes of autonomic dysfunction are the following:

- Diabetes mellitus
- Alcoholic neuropathy
- Parkinsonism
- Other idiopathic disorders, such as the Shy-Drager syndrome
- Pharmacologic therapies

Drug-induced orthostatic hypotension causes recurrent dizzy spells or syncope in 12 to 15% of elderly patients and should always be suspected. Diuretics, calcium antagonists, angiotensin-converting enzyme inhibitors, and nitrates are frequently prescribed in elderly patients for the management of hypertension, congestive heart failure, and ischemic heart disease (Table 16.2). With age, reduced postural cardioacceleration and decreased baroreceptor gain increase the risk for orthostatic hypotension. Other pharmacologic agents frequently associated with orthostatic hypotension include phenothiazines, antidepressants, sedatives, and narcotics.

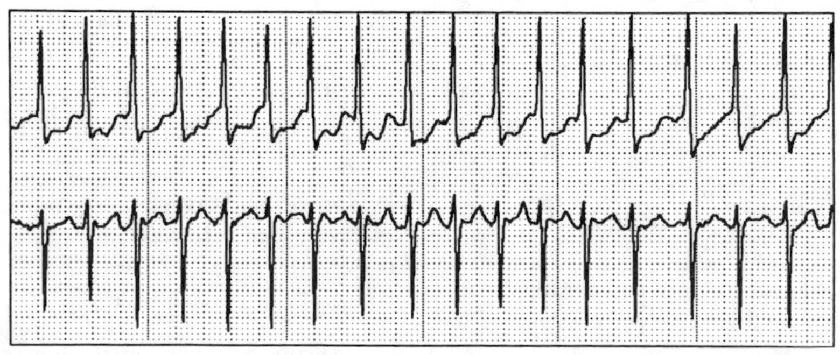

FIGURE 16.1.
Two-channel Holter electrocardiographic recording in a patient with recurrent, unexplained near syncope. Baseline rhythm was sinus bradycardia. Recording shows an asymptomatic episode of atrial fibrillation with rapid ventricular response.

Carotid sinus hypersensitivity infrequently causes syncope and is characterized by severe vasodepression (> 50 mm Hg decrease in systolic blood pressure), marked cardioinhibition bradycardia with heart rate of 40 beats/min or less, or asystole lasting more than 3 seconds (Fig. 16.2). Syncope is most frequently seen in elderly patients with underlying ischemic heart disease, hypertension, and systemic atherosclerotic disease. Of elderly patients admitted acutely with a fractured hip, 36% were found to have experienced syncope and to have carotid sinus hypersensitivity. This observation suggests that carotid sinus hypersensitivity may identify elderly patients at risk for falls and hip fractures and may be a more frequent cause of syncope than previously recognized.

TABLE 16.2. **Drug-Induced Orthostatic Hypotension**

Cardiovascular drugs
Diuretics
Calcium-channel blockers
β-adrenergic blockers
Angiotensin-converting enzyme inhibitors
Nitrates
Other antihypertensive drugs (guanethedine, prazocin, clonidine)
Anti-Parkinsonian drugs
Levodopa plus decarboxylase inhibitors
Bromocriptine
Selegiline (deprenyl)
Anticholinergics
Antidepressants
Tricyclic antidepressants (amitriptyline, imipramine)
Azolopyridines (trazodone)
Monoamine oxidase inhibitors (phenelzine, nialamide)
Antipsychotic agents
Phenothiazines
Butyrophenones

Neurocardiogenic (vasovagal) syncope, one of the most frequent causes of syncope, generally, but not exclusively, occurs in patients with no evidence of structural heart disease. Prodromal symptoms such as dizziness, blurred vision, nausea, and diaphoresis precede the hypotension and bradycardia that lead to syncope. Reflex activation of ventricular mechanoreceptors and impaired arterial baroreceptor response to orthostatic stress have been postulated as potential mechanisms.

Postprandial syncope is almost invariably seen in elderly patients and is related to increased blood flow to the splanchnic bed that triggers a vasodepressor reaction. Affected patients have severe diaphoresis, dizziness, and syncope 10 to 30 minutes after ingesting a large meal. Patients sometimes also report orthostatic hypotension.

Congenital or acquired prolongation of the Q-T interval may present as rapid ventricular polymorphic tachycardia (torsades de pointes) associated with severe hemodynamic collapse and syncope. Congenital long Q-T syndrome may initially manifest as seizures, usually triggered by unexpected or startling stimulus. A family history of unexpected sudden death is usually found in patients with the congenital long Q-T syndrome. Acquired long Q-T syndrome should be suspected in patients with unexplained syncope who are receiving type I antiarrhythmic agents, such as quinidine and procainamide. Similarly, phenothiazines, tricyclic antidepressant agents, and electrolyte disturbances, es-

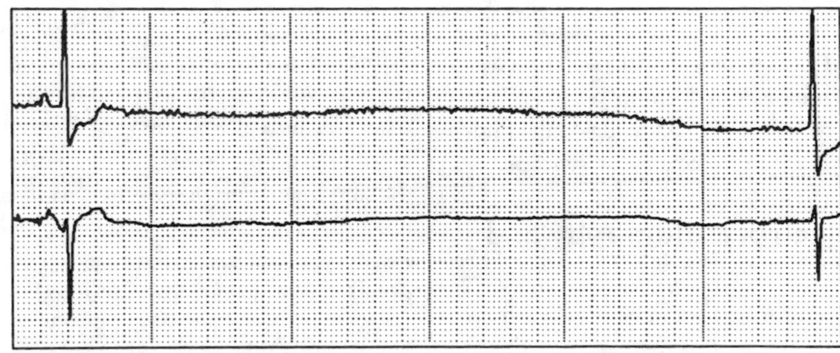

FIGURE 16.2.
Recording shows a sinus pause lasting 5 seconds that was associated with syncope. The cause of syncope was sick sinus syndrome, which was treated with permanent pacing.

pecially hypokalemia, have been associated with prolonged Q-T interval.

DIAGNOSIS: OFFICE EVALUATION

History and Physical Examination

A complete history and physical examination remain the cornerstone of the diagnostic evaluation of syncope. The history and physical examination produce a diagnosis in approximately half of the patients who experience syncope.

A thorough interview with the patient about the circumstances that precipitated the syncopal episode and an interview with witnesses are essential. Family history of recurrent syncope or sudden death suggests the possibility of hypertrophic cardiomyopathy or congenital long Q-T syndrome. A complete drug history should be obtained to determine the potential for iatrogenic syncope.

Physical examination should include the following:

- Measurement of blood pressure in supine and upright positions
- Identification of signs of
  - Aortic stenosis
  - Hypertrophic cardiomyopathy
  - Atrial myxoma
  - Pulmonary hypertension

Electrocardiography

Electrocardiography (ECG) findings that may be helpful in identifying a potential cause of syncope include

- Evidence of previous myocardial infarction
- Prolongation of the Q-T interval
- Short P-R interval and delta waves indicating the Wolff-Parkinson-White syndrome
- High-degree AV block

Other abnormalities that may be found on ECG are ventricular hypertrophy, bundle-branch block, first-degree AV block, and premature ventricular or atrial complexes. These findings have been documented in 75% of patients with syncope but are generally incidental findings not necessarily related to the cause of syncope.

Ambulatory Electrocardiography and Loop Monitors

Continuous ECG monitoring should be performed for at least 24 hours in an attempt to discover an arrhythmic cause of syncope. Because syncope is often sporadic and infrequent, ambulatory ECG is rarely diagnostic. Only in 1 to 3% of patients has syncope been documented during 24 to 48 hours of ambulatory monitoring. Unless arrhythmia is associated with syncope or severe presyncope, arrhythmia should not be attributed as the cause of syncope. Such abnormalities as atrial fibrillation with a rapid ventricular response, sinus pauses lasting less than 3 seconds, AV Wenckebach block, or a burst of nonsustained ventricular tachycardia are more frequently observed in elderly patients; unless they are associated with syncope or presyncope, these abnormalities should be considered incidental.

Loop monitors have recently been introduced to assess patients with recurrent unexplained syncope. These long-term, patient-activated devices record 1 to 5 minutes of the patient's ECG during the syncopal episode. The major limitation of this device is the need for self-activation; this is especially problematic in patients with short prodromes or no warning symptoms. Nonetheless, the diagnostic yield with loop monitors has been reported to be 25%.

Exercise Treadmill Testing

Exercise treadmill testing should be performed in patients with syncope provoked during or after exercise or in association with chest pain, unless evidence clearly shows aortic stenosis or hypertrophic cardiomyopathy. Catecholamine-mediated ventricular tachycardia is sometimes associated with syncope provoked during exercise in young patients with no evidence of structural heart disease. This tachycardia is characterized by a left bundle-branch block and inferior axis during the tachycardia.

Carotid Sinus Massage

Carotid sinus massage should be performed routinely in both the supine and upright positions, especially in elderly patients. The incidence of neurologic complications in elderly patients has recently been revised to 0.14%. Pressure over the carotid sinus should be applied for 5 seconds, and at least 1 minute should be allowed to pass before the contralateral side is massaged. Carotid sinus hypersensitivity is characterized by asystole lasting longer than 3 seconds or a 50–mm Hg decrease in systolic blood pressure. Routine evaluation of carotid sinus massage in the supine and upright positions has identified carotid sinus hypersensitivity as the cause of syncope in 45% of elderly patients with recurrent syncope. Contraindications to carotid sinus massage include

- Carotid bruits
- History of ventricular tachyarrhythmia
- Recent myocardial infarction
- Recent cerebral infarction

DIAGNOSIS: NONINVASIVE HOSPITAL TESTING

Head-up Tilt-Table Testing

The mechanism that leads to the development of neurocardiogenic syncope provoked by upright tilt remains unclear. Essentially, two tilt-table test protocols have been proposed:

- Drug-free prolonged tilt protocol lasting 45 to 60 minutes
- Upright tilt with graded isoproterenol infusions lasting 10 to 30 minutes

The advantages of the former protocol include a sensitivity ranging from 40 to 75%, excellent specificity (93%), and acceptable short-term reproducibility (80%). A minor disadvantage of this protocol is the prolonged time required for the test. The infusion of isoproterenol significantly shortens the protocol and increases sensitivity to about 70% (specificity, 70 to 92%).

A positive tilt-table test result is defined as the induction of presyncope or syncope associated with a systolic blood pressure of 70 mm Hg or less or bradycardia with a heart rate of 50 beats/min or less. Most important, the reproduction of symptoms that resemble the clinical presentation is necessary to correctly diagnose neurally mediated syncope. Although no definite indications for tilt-table testing have been recommended, some basic guidelines are summarized in Table 16.3.

TABLE 16.3. Who Should Undergo Tilt-Table Testing?

Patients with recurrent, unexplained syncope
. . . Preceded by prodromal symptoms such as
Dizziness
Diaphoresis
Nausea
Blurred vision
Headache
Weakness
. . . With no evidence of structural heart disease
. . . With evidence of structural heart disease
Coronary artery disease
Myocardial infarction
Dilated cardiomyopathy
. . . With negative findings on signal-averaged electrocardiography or electrophysiologic study
. . . With hypertrophic obstructive cardiomyopathy
. . . Developing after exercise

Signal-Averaged Electrocardiography

Signal-averaged ECG is a relatively new noninvasive technique that increases the amplitude of the QRS complex several thousand times. This computer-based technique allows the detection of low- amplitude signals buried in the terminal portion of the QRS complex. These signals represent late potentials that are due to slow conduction arising from electrically abnormal ventricular myocytes secondary to an old myocardial infarction. The presence of late potentials is highly correlated with inducibility of ventricular tachycardia during electrophysiologic assessment. Signal-averaged ECG is useful for determining the need for further electrophysiologic testing in patients with unexplained syncope and a history of myocardial infarction associated with an ejection fraction less than 40%. Sensitivity and specificity in this setting range from 50 to 89% and 55 to 100%, respectively. A positive result on signal-averaged ECG predicts the induction of ventricular tachycardia by programmed electrical stimulation in approximately 72% of patients with unexplained syncope. A negative result on signal-averaged ECG (no evidence of late potentials) has a negative predictive value of 93%, indicating that ventricular tachycardia is unlikely to be the cause of the syncopal episode. In summary, signal-averaged ECG may help to stratify patients with unexplained syncope associated with a previous myocardial infarction and ejection fraction less than 40%. A positive result on signal-averaged ECG in this setting should prompt further invasive electrophysiologic testing.

DIAGNOSIS: INVASIVE HOSPITAL TESTING

Electrophysiologic Studies

Invasive electrophysiologic testing is indicated in patients with recurrent unexplained syncope in which noninvasive assessment has not indicated a potential cause. The diagnostic yield of electrophysiologic testing is higher in patients with organic heart disease, particularly those with previous myocardial infarction and left ventricular ejection fraction less than 40%. An arrhythmic cause of syncope may be identified in up to 50% of these patients. In a recent study, however, invasive electrophysiologic testing identified a potential cause for syncope in 68% of elderly patients (older than 75 years of age) with recurrent unexplained syncope. Abnormal findings included sinus node dysfunction in 55% of patients, abnormal His-bundle conduction in 39%, and ventricular tachycardia in another 14%. Several patients had multiple abnormalities.

Figure 16.3 summarizes the incidence and abnormal electrophysiologic findings in patients with recurrent unexplained syncope in the presence or absence of organic heart disease. Overall, a potential cause for syncope was identified in 44% of patients: ventricular tachycardia in 20%, supraventricular tachycardia in 9%, AV node dysfunction in 8%, and sinus node dysfunction in 7%. Dizziness and syncope occur frequently in elderly patients with sinus bradycardia. Although indications for electrophysiologic study in patients with recurrent syncope and sinus bradycardia remain controversial, some general guidelines are summarized in Table 16.4. If sinus node recovery time is abnormal, permanent pacing is indicated. Elderly patients have a higher incidence of sinus node and AV node abnormalities that can be easily treated by permanent cardiac pacing. In addition, the coexistence of multiple electrophysiologic abnormalities is higher in patients older than 75 years of age.

TREATMENT

Treatment of the patient with recurrent syncope is determined by establishing the potential cause of syncope and guiding therapy toward prevention of recurrent episodes. Correction of mechanical causes of syncope, such as aortic stenosis or hypertrophic cardiomyopathy, may be enough to prevent recurrence of syncope.

Bradyarrhythmic causes of syncope are usually managed by implanting a permanent pacemaker. See Table 16.4 for suggested guidelines on the management of patients with syncope and sinus bradycardia. Simi-

Summary of Diagnosis

- Electrical causes are bradyarrhythmias and tachyarrhythmias.
- Mechanical causes are aortic stenosis, pulmonary embolism, and hypertension.
- Neurovascular causes are orthostatic hypotension, carotid sinus hypersensitivity, vasovagal syndrome, and long Q-T syndrome.
- Drug-induced causes are common cardiovascular drugs, anti-Parkinsonian agents, antidepressant agents, antipsychotic drugs.
- History and physical examination remain the cornerstone of the diagnostic evaluation.
- Perform ECG in all patients and ambulatory ECG and loop monitoring when indicated.
- Conduct exercise treadmill testing in patients with an exertional component in the absence of aortic stenosis and hypertrophic cardiomyopathy with obstruction.
- Perform carotid sinus massage, especially in elderly patients. Listen carefully for carotid bruits.
- For the patient with difficult-to-diagnose syncope, refer to the cardiologist for tilt-table testing, signal-averaged ECG, or electrophysiologic studies.

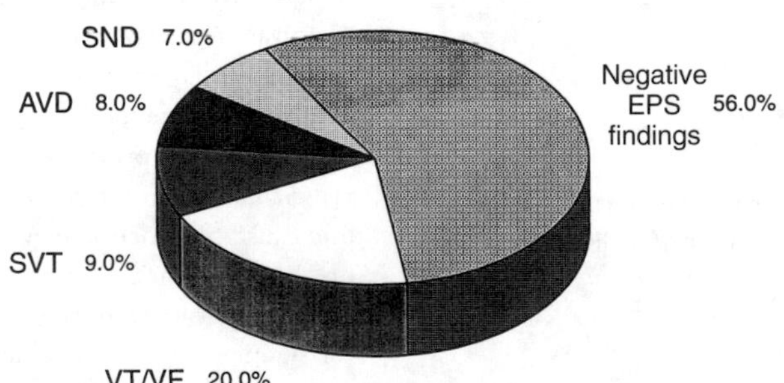

FIGURE 16.3.

Causes of syncope identified by electrophysiologic study in 1146 patients. *AVD,* atrioventricular node dysfunction; *EPS,* electrophysiologic study; *SND,* sinus node dysfunction; *SUO,* syncope of unexplained origin; *SVT,* supraventricular tachycardia; *VT/VF,* ventricular tachycardia/fibrillation.

Guidelines for Patients with Syncope and Sinus Bradycardia **TABLE 16.4.**

Type of Syncope	Measurements	Treatment
Asymptomatic sinus bradycardia	Heart rate ≤ 40 beats/min	Observation
Persistent sinus bradycardia	Heart rate ≤ 40 beats/min	Electrophysiologic study recommended Permanent pacemaker may be implanted if bradycardia persists
Symptomatic sinus bradycardia	heart rate ≤ 40 beats/min	Electrophysiologic study indicated
Abnormal sinus node recovery time	> 1500 ms	Permanent pacemaker indicated

larly, **tachyarrhythmic causes of syncope** may be managed with pharmacologic therapy or by eliminating the arrhythmic substrate with radiofrequency catheter ablation. Therapy for ventricular tachycardia or fibrillation may be selected during electrophysiologic evaluation or with such devices as implantable defibrillators.

Syncope related to **orthostatic hypotension** may result from many factors, particularly impaired neurovascular regulation or depleted intravascular volume. Orthostatic hypotension is usually potentiated by several drugs frequently prescribed in elderly patients, such as nitrates, diuretics, angiotensin-converting enzyme inhibitors, guanethidine, prazosin, methyldopa, and phenothiazines. Dose adjustments or discontinuation of therapy may be necessary. **Orthostatic hypotension of idiopathic origin** may be treated by correcting associated blood volume depletion and instructing the patient to use elastic stockings and to sleep with the bed elevated to at least 20°. If these measures fail, administration of fludrocortisone in doses ranging from 0.1 mg/d to 1.0 mg/d is often useful. Other pharmacologic measures that may be used in addition to fludrocortisone include α-agonists, prostaglandin inhibitors, and β-blockers.

Neurocardiogenic syncope usually occurs in clusters and courses and has a benign prognosis. In patients with frequent incapacitating symptoms, however, therapy with β-blockers, disopyramide, fludrocortisone, or theophylline may be justified. Neurocardiogenic syncope can manifest with prolonged asystole, and the patient may be at a higher risk for injury and recurrent syncope. In such cases, dual-chamber pacemakers have been implanted with relative success.

The management of syncope is particularly challenging in the elderly patient, who may have several comorbid conditions and may require therapy for many potential causes of syncope. Thorough investigation of syncope may identify the cause in 50 to 80% of patients. In patients in whom the cause of syncope remains elusive, the prognosis depends on the concurrent presence of structural heart disease. Recurrence of syncope is generally low during prolonged follow-up in patients without an identified cause of syncope.

Summary of Treatment

- Treatment is guided by an accurate diagnosis.
  - Aortic stenosis: valve replacement or annuloplasty
  - Bradyarrhythmias: pacemakers
  - Tachyarrhythmias: drug therapy or radiofrequency ablation
  - Orthostatic hypotension: discontinuation of therapy with offending drugs
  - Primary orthostatic hypotension: maintain volume; elevate bed to 20°; prescribe use of elastic stockings; administer fludrocortisone, α-agonists, or prostaglandin inhibitors
- Noncardiac syncope is usually associated with a benign prognosis.
- Suspicion of cardiac cause merits a referral to the cardiologist.

GUIDELINES FOR THE PRIMARY CARE TEAM

The diagnostic evaluation of the patient with recurrent dizzy spells and unexplained syncope is challenging and complex. Orthostatic hypotension is a frequent, preventable, and generally overlooked cause of dizziness and syncope. A stepwise approach is recommended by starting the workup with noninvasive testing, such as head-up tilt-table testing, particularly in patients with

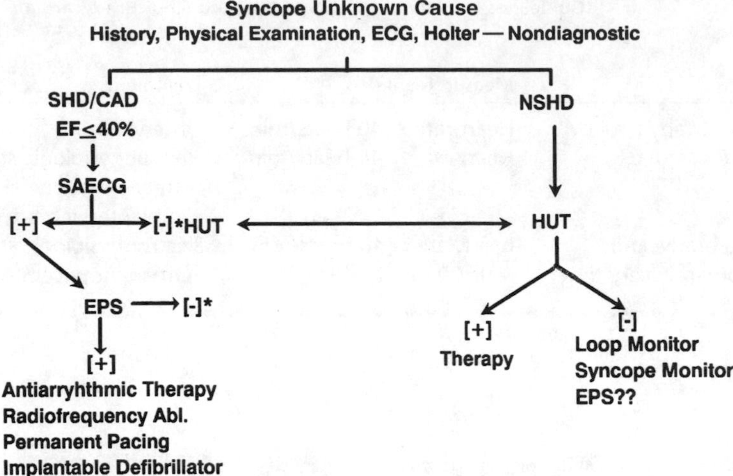

FIGURE 16.4.
Algorithm proposed for the evaluation of unexplained syncope.

no evidence of structural heart disease (Fig.16.4). Invasive assessment should be reserved for patients with symptomatic bradycardia and patients with structural heart disease and depressed ejection fraction. In elderly patients, the incidence of cardiac and neurovascular causes of recurrent syncope is high and multiple causes frequently coexist. Therapy depends on the identification of the potential cause of syncope.

KEY POINTS

- A careful history and physical examination is essential.
- Cardiac causes of syncope can be associated with significant morbidity and mortality. A rapid and accurate diagnosis is required.
- Noncardiac syncope is generally benign.
- A careful drug history is required, especially in elderly patients.
- When considering the diagnosis of carotid sinus hypersensitivity in elderly patients, do not perform carotid sinus massage in the presence of carotid bruits, a history of ventricular tachyarrhythmias, or recent myocardial or cerebral infarction.

SUGGESTED READINGS

Brooks R, Ruskin JN. Evaluation of the patient with unexplained syncope. In Cardiac electrophysiology: from cell to bedside. 2nd edition. Zipes DJ, Jalife J (eds). Philadelphia: WB Saunders. 1996:1247–1264.

Kapoor W. Evaluation and management of the patient with syncope. JAMA 1992;268:2553–2560.

Klein GJ, Gersh BJ, Yee R. Electrophysiological testing: the final court of appeal for diagnosis of syncope? Circulation 1995;92:1332–1335.

Kosinski D, Grubb BP, Temesy-Armos P. Pathophysiological aspects of neurocardiogenic syncope: current concepts and new perspectives. PACE 1995;18:716–724.

McIntosh SJ, Lawson J, Kenny RA. Clinical characteristics of vasodepressor, cardioinhibitory, and mixed carotid sinus syndrome in the elderly. Am J Med 1993;95: 203–208.

Morley CA, Sutton R, Kenny RA. Incidence of complications after carotid sinus massage in older patients with syncope. J Am Geriatr Soc 1994;42:1248–1251.

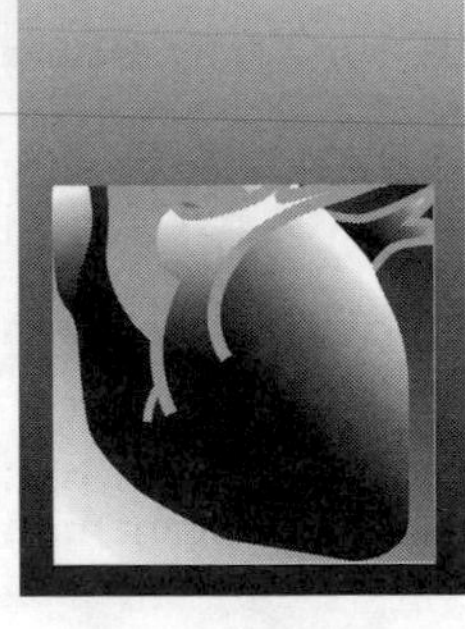

17

CHAPTER

Aortic Dissection

Henry F. Clemo

INTRODUCTION

Intimal dissection is the most common fatal disease involving the aorta. At least 9000 cases of aortic dissection are diagnosed each year in the United States. If untreated, approximately 75% of patients presenting with new aortic dissection die within 2 weeks of onset of symptoms. Aortic dissection is diagnosed before death in only 50% of cases. This syndrome is a medical and surgical emergency and must be included in differential diagnoses of all patients presenting with sudden, cataclysmic onset of chest or back pain.

In aortic dissection, the intimal layer of the aorta suddenly tears away. Arterial blood then enters the space between the intimal and medial layers of the aorta, creating a false lumen. The shearing force of blood in this false lumen separates the intima from the media for variable distances and causes destruction of the medial layer so that only the adventitia contains arterial blood flow. Separation of the intima from the media and adventitia can cause disruption of the aortic valve, arterial bleeding into the pericardium or pleural space, occlusion of coronary artery ostia, and disruption of blood flow into the great vessels. The intima is usually torn secondary to the shearing forces of the intraaortic flow of blood. In older, hypertensive patients, the vasa vasorum of the intimal layer may rupture, thereby causing a hematoma between the intima and media. This hematoma may enlarge and subsequently tear the intima.

CLASSIFICATION

Aortic dissection is classified as proximal (or ascending) and distal (or descending) types. The division of aortic dissection into proximal and distal types is based on the prognosis and treatment of each type.

Proximal Aortic Dissection

Proximal aortic dissections start in the ascending thoracic aorta and may end either in the aortic arch or descending aorta. Proximal dissections account for 60 to 70% of all aortic dissections. Proximal aortic dissection has a poor outcome and is usually treated with surgical intervention.

Distal Aortic Dissection

Distal aortic dissections are limited to the aortic arch and descending aorta. Distal aortic dissection has a somewhat better outcome and can often be managed medically.

Acute Versus Chronic Dissection

Aortic dissection may also be classified as **acute** or **chronic.** Aortic dissection is defined as acute if the patient presents within 2 weeks after the onset of symptoms and as chronic if presentation occurs more than 2 weeks after symptoms develop. Approximately 75% of patients with untreated aortic dissection who present with the acute form die within 2 weeks of onset of symptoms.

CAUSES

The various identified risk factors for aortic dissection are listed in Table 17.1. Aortic dissection more often affects men than women (ratio, 3:1). Most patients present later in life, typically in the sixth and seventh decades. Hypertension is present in 70 to 90% of patients. Although arterial atherosclerosis is common in patients presenting with aortic dissection, the causal relationship of atherosclerosis to aortic dissection has not been well defined. Several reports have documented perforation of intimal, atherosclerotic plaques allowing flow of blood into the medial layer of the aorta.

Various congenital connective tissue disorders predispose an individual to aortic dissection. The most important congenital connective tissue disorder is **Marfan's syndrome,** an autosomal dominant syndrome characterized by skeletal, ocular, and cardiovascular abnormalities. Cystic medial degeneration is the intrinsic defect of Marfan's syndrome. The most common cardiovascular

Risk Factors for Aortic Dissection **TABLE 17.1.**

Hypertension
Congenital conditions
- Marfan's syndrome
- Ehlers-Danlos syndrome
- Turner's syndrome
- Noonan's syndrome
- Bicuspid or unicuspid aortic valve
- Coarctation of the aorta

Connective tissue diseases
- Systemic lupus
- Giant-cell aortitis
- Relapsing polychondritis

Iatrogenic
- Venous coronary artery bypass grafting
- Cross-clamping of the aorta
- Aortic valve replacement or repair
- Cardiac catheterization
- Interventional coronary angioplasty
- Diagnostic arteriography
- Interventional arteriography

complications include aneurysm and subsequent dissection of the ascending thoracic aorta. The patient with Marfan's syndrome is also at risk for aortic and mitral valvular regurgitation. Although aneurysms in other locations are rare in patients with Marfan's syndrome, they occasionally occur in the descending aorta, internal carotid arteries, and pulmonary arteries. Marfan's syndrome is the most common associated condition in patients who present with aortic dissection before the age of 40 years.

Other, more rare conditions have been reported in association with aortic dissection. Of note is that approximately 50% of aortic dissections occurring in women younger than 40 years of age develop during pregnancy, especially in the third trimester. Other risk factors are usually coexistent. Patients with congenital bicuspid aortic valves have an incidence of aortic dissection that is 50 times the incidence in patients with tricuspid aortic valves. Trauma is not usually associated with aortic dissection unless other risk factors coexist. Aortic dissection is a rare but serious complication of cardiac surgery (secondary to cross-clamping, aortotomies made for venous bypass grafts to coronary arteries, intraoperative perfusion of coronary arteries with cardioplegia solution or blood, or the period after aortic valve replacement) and of procedures such as cardiac catheterization, coronary angioplasty, and diagnostic and interventional arteriography.

SIGNS AND SYMPTOMS

The patient with aortic dissection typically presents with sudden, cataclysmic pain. The pain may be described as tearing, ripping, or searing. The pain of aortic dissection is maximal on inception; in contrast, the pain of cardiac ischemia builds up to a crescendo.

The location of the pain may provide a clue to the location of the dissection. Often, anterior chest pain is associated with proximal dissection, whereas back and abdominal pain are associated with distal dissection. The pain may be migratory, following the progression of the dissection of the intima. In up to 15% of cases, however, the presentation of aortic dissection may be painless. The major sites of pain and correlation with location of aortic dissection are summarized in Table 17.2. Other symptoms, such as shock or syncope, are clues to impending cardiovascular collapse. Patients with proximal dissection often present with hemodynamic shock (50%), cardiac tamponade (30%), and aortic regurgitation (60%). The patient may also report various neurologic and gastrointestinal symptoms that may indicate impaired blood flow to the brain, spinal cord, or gastrointestinal system.

TABLE 17.2. Major Site of Pain and Location of Dissection

Type of Pain	Proximal Dissection	Distal Dissection
Anterior chest only	54%	8%
Posterior chest only	12%	52%
Anterior and posterior chest	5%	21%
Face, ear, neck, throat, or jaw	23%	2%
Abdomen	4%	15%

Modified from Spittell PC, Spittell JA, Joyce JW, et al. Clinical features and differential diagnosis of aortic dissection: experience with 236 cases (1980 through 1990). Mayo Clin Proc 1993; 68:642–651.

PHYSICAL EXAMINATION

Physical examination is usually unrevealing in patients with aortic dissection. The most common finding is the diastolic murmur of aortic regurgitation, which has been found in up to 70% of patients with proximal aortic dissection. A pulse deficit is found in only 6% of patients. The deficit is usually in either the right or left carotid or femoral artery or in the left subclavian artery. Neurologic deficits are found in 6% of patients; spinal ischemia is the most common finding.

DIAGNOSTIC TESTING

The definitive diagnosis of aortic dissection requires a diagnostic imaging study, which must be performed immediately after a patient presents with a suspicion of aortic dissection. The diagnostic imaging study should

- Confirm the diagnosis of dissection
- Ascertain whether the ascending aorta is involved
- Demonstrate whether other abnormal anatomic features, such as aortic regurgitation or pericardial effusion, exist

The diagnostic test of choice depends on

- Imaging equipment available
- Speed with which a particular imaging study can be done
- Experience of the imaging physician at the institution to which the patient presents
- Stability and other coexistent health problems of the patient

Diagnostic imaging studies now available include

- Chest radiography in anterior and posterior views
- Electrocardiography (ECG)
- Aortography
- Computed tomography (CT)
- Magnetic resonance imaging (MRI)
- Echocardiography: transesophageal (TEE) and transthoracic (TTE)
- Coronary angiography

Chest Radiography and Electrocardiography

Chest radiography is the most revealing routine clinical test in patients suspected of having aortic dissection. Up to 80% of patients may have an increase in aortic diameter, and 20% may have mediastinal widening. On the other hand, ECG often demonstrates only left ventricular hypertrophy. Less than 2% of patients presenting with aortic dissection have evidence of acute myocardial infarction on ECG. The clinician should immediately consider aortic dissection in the patient who presents with cataclysmic chest or back pain and ECG findings unrevealing for ongoing cardiac ischemia. Rapid diagnosis of aortic dissection is paramount. When the initial history, physical, chest radiography, and ECG are considered, acute aortic dissection is diagnosed only 58% and 72% of the time in patients with proximal and distal aortic dissection, respectively. Other common initial diagnoses include myocardial infarction or ischemia, aortic stenosis, congestive heart failure, or aortic aneurysm. These diagnoses are described in Table 17.3.

Aortography

Aortography has been the traditional diagnostic test of choice; in recent years, however, CT, MRI, and TEE have supplanted its use. The sensitivity and specificity of aortography are 90 to 95% for diagnosis of aortic dissection. False-negative results can occur, especially when the false lumen has thrombosed or when the false and true lumens are simultaneously opacified with radiopaque dye. The intimal flap may not be visualized if the catheter tip is not properly placed. Aortography does provide information on perfusion of peripheral arteries. If the aortic root is visualized, aortic regurgitation may be diagnosed. The main drawback of aortography is that it is invasive and relatively time-consuming to perform. Risk may be added when the unstable patient must be transported to the angiography suite or if large amounts of radiopaque dye are used in a patient with renal compromise.

Computed Tomography

Computed tomography has become more popular for diagnosis of aortic dissection. Its sensitivity varies between 82 and 100% and specificity ranges from 80 to 100%, depending on the quality of diagnostic equipment available. Recently, the advent of helical (spiral) CT allows the rapid acquisition of images during the period when peak intravascular concentrations of radiopaque dye are obtained; this improves the quality of images obtained. In addition, reconstruction of overlapping images assists in the delineation of small abnormalities, such as intimal flaps and site of entry into the false lumen. The sensitivity and specificity of helical CT in diagnosing aortic dissection approach 100%.

TABLE 17.3. **Initial Clinical Impression after History, Physical Examination, Chest Radiography, and Electrocardiography**

Impression	Proximal Dissection	Distal Dissection
Aortic dissection	58%	72%
Aortic aneurysm	6%	13%
Atypical chest pain	2%	2%
Myocardial infarction	6%	0%
Congestive heart failure	6%	0%
Sudden death	6%	0%
Unstable angina	4%	0%
Aortic stenosis	4%	0%
Pulmonary embolus	2%	0%

Modified from Spittell PC, Spittell JA, Joyce JW, et al. Clinical features and differential diagnosis of aortic dissection: experience with 236 cases (1980 through 1990). Mayo Clin Proc 1993;68:642–651.

Helical CT is available at many hospitals in the United States. An example of an aortic dissection diagnosed with helical CT is shown in Figure 17.1. The main advantages of CT include

- Its noninvasive nature
- Speed with which the study can be done (especially with helical CT)
- No contraindication to its use in patients with metal devices, such as joint replacements, stents, or pacemakers

The drawbacks to CT include

- Inability to reliably visualize branch vessels
- Inability to assess aortic regurgitation
- Use of radiopaque dye in the patient with renal compromise

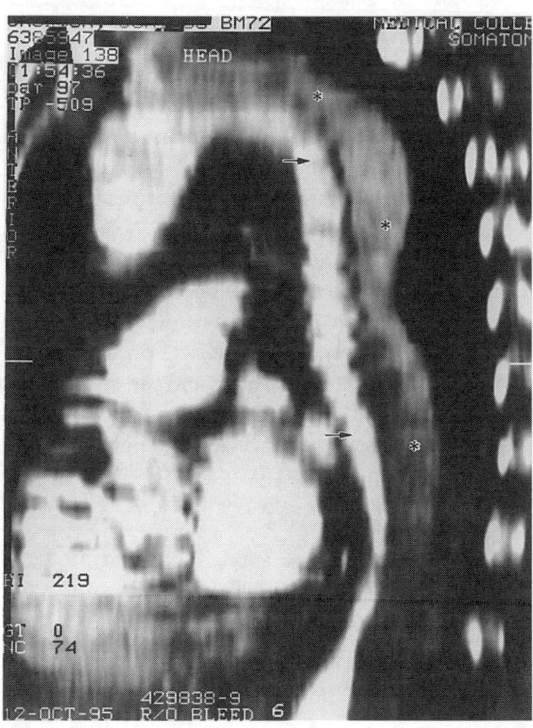

FIGURE 17.1.

Helical computed tomographic scan of chronic aortic dissection involving the arch and descending aorta. A sagittal reconstruction is shown. Imaging and reconstruction were performed in approximately 15 minutes. The arrow and asterisk denote the true and false lumens, respectively. The same patient is shown in Figure 17.2. (Courtesy of T.J. Cole, MD, Department of Radiology, Medical College of Virginia.)

Magnetic Resonance Imaging

Of the diagnostic imaging tests available, MRI has the best sensitivity and specificity (100%). Magnetic resonance imaging accurately delineates the aorta and site of entry into the false lumen. Cine-MRI, which gates the MRI image to ECG, allows some quantitation of aortic regurgitation.

Scanning with MRI has the following advantages:

- Its noninvasive nature
- No radiopaque dye required
- Accurate visualization of pericardial effusion

Although MRI appears to be ideally suited to the diagnosis of aortic dissection, several drawbacks limit its use in the unstable patient:

- Length of time of the study
- Inability to image patients who are intubated and those on mechanically controlled intravenous infusions
- Inability to image patients with metal prostheses (e.g., pacemakers, stents, joint replacements)

Figure 17.2 demonstrates aortic dissection as imaged with MRI.

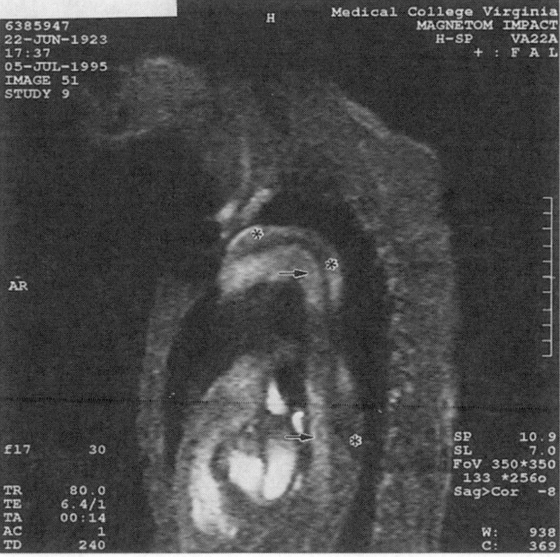

FIGURE 17.2.

Magnetic resonance image of acute dissection involving the arch and descending aorta. A sagittal reconstruction is shown. The arrow and asterisk denote the true and false lumens, respectively. The same patient is shown in Figure 17.1. (Courtesy of T.J. Cole, MD, Department of Radiology, Medical College of Virginia.)

Echocardiography

The most useful imaging technique in the unstable patient is echocardiography. Echocardiography is truly portable and may be done at the bedside in a matter of minutes. The unstable patient does not need to be transported to the radiology suite for a possibly time-consuming study.

Two methods of echocardiography are currently in use: TTE and TEE. Comparison of both methods follows:

	TTE	TEE
Sensitivity	59–85%	95–100%
Specificity	63–96%	77–100%
Diagnostic capabilities	Aortic regurgitation (with flow Doppler) Pericardial effusion Regional wall-motion abnormalities Ejection fraction Cardiac chamber size Reliable information about aortic root	Aortic regurgitation (with flow Doppler) Pericardial effusion Regional wall-motion abnormalities Ejection fraction Cardiac chamber size Reliable information about aortic root, aortic arch, descending thoracic aorta, coronary artery roots
Drawbacks	Poor quality images in patients who are obese or who have chronic obstructive pulmonary disease (up to 10 % of patients)	Semi-invasive: requires esophageal intubation

With older, single-plane TEE probes, the upper portion of the ascending aorta and proximal aortic arch may not be fully imaged because of interference from the trachea. Biplane and omniplane TEE probes have partially overcome this problem. Transesophageal echocardiography requires esophageal intubation, which may be contraindicated in patients with such esophageal disease as cancer, varices, and stricture. Figure 17.3a and 17.3b depict a proximal dissection as imaged by TEE.

If a large pericardial effusion is diagnosed with TTE in the unstable patient suspected of having aortic dissection, the patient should be taken directly to surgery. Time should not be wasted on obtaining other diagnostic imaging studies.

Coronary Angiography

Coronary artery disease occurs in 8 to 33% of patients presenting with proximal aortic dissection. Coronary artery bypass grafting may be done concurrently in up to 38% of patients undergoing repair of proximal aortic dissection. Because of these findings, controversy exists as to whether the older patient with aortic dissection should undergo coronary angiography before surgical repair of the dissection. The willingness to perform coronary angiography, especially in the unstable patient, should be tempered by several considerations:

- Coronary angiography may delay life-saving surgery by at least 1 hour or more.
- Performing coronary angiography in the patient with proximal aortic dissection may be technically difficult.
- Ostial atherosclerotic coronary disease or dissection involving the coronary cusps may be directly visualized by the surgeon in the operating room.
- Most postsurgical deaths in the aortic dissection patient are not due to myocardial infarction.
- In the unstable patient who is presenting with proximal aortic dissection, coronary angiography should not be routinely obtained because of the risk associated with delaying surgery.
- In the stable patient, coronary angiography may be indicated if coronary artery bypass grafting has been done previously, if cardiac risk factors exist, or if ECG suggests cardiac ischemia.

Selection of Imaging Method

The selection of imaging method depends in part on the available imaging techniques and expertise at the hospital to which the patient with suspected aortic dissection presents. Preference of the consulting surgeon should also be considered. A suggested decision tree for choosing an imaging method is presented in Figure 17.4. If helical CT is available, it may be a reasonable alternative to MRI.

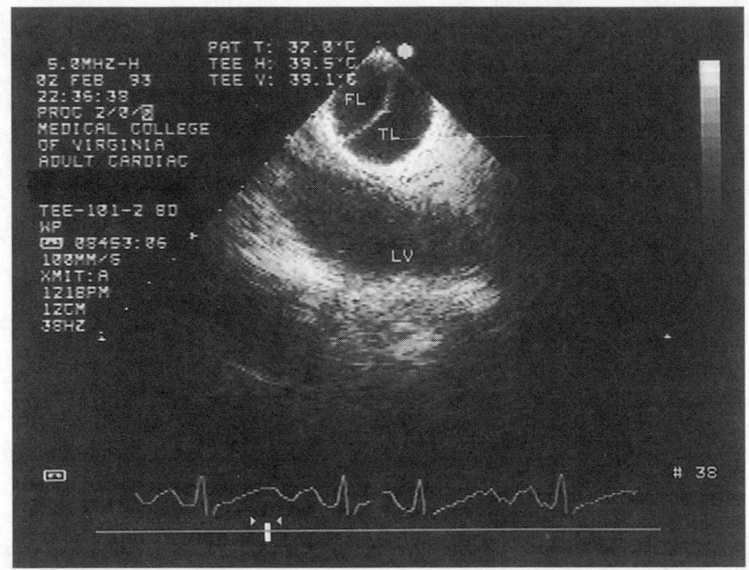

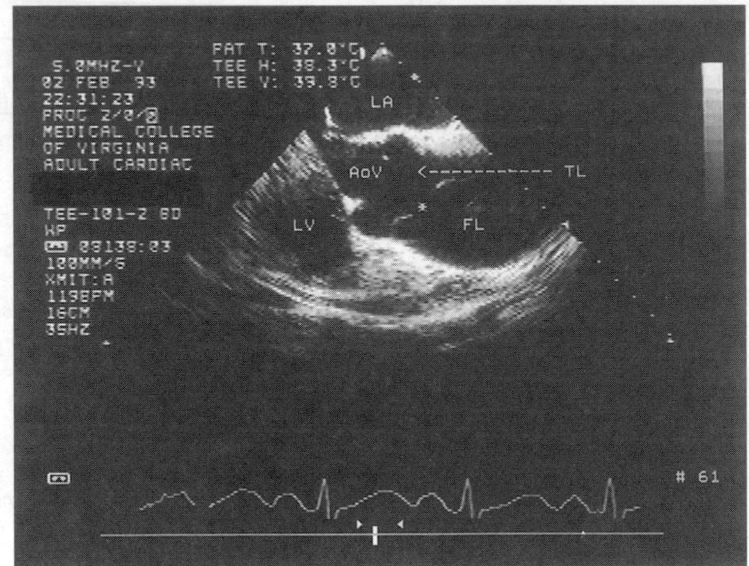

FIGURE 17.3.

Proximal aortic dissection as imaged by transesophageal echocardiography. **A.,** Cross-sectional view of the descending aorta. **B.,** Longitudinal view of the aortic valve and proximal aorta. Asterisk in panel B denotes the proximal site of entry into the false lumen. *AoV,* aortic valve; *Fl,* false lumen; *LA,* left atrium; *LV,* left ventricle; *TL,* true lumen. (Courtesy of W. Paulsen, MD, Division of Cardiology, Medical College of Virginia.)

TREATMENT

Short-term Medical Management

In the patient in whom aortic dissection is suspected, medical treatment should be initiated even before definitive diagnosis has been made. The goals should be to

- Eliminate pain
- Reduce systolic blood pressure to 100 to 120 mm Hg (i.e., the lowest pressure commensurate with perfusion of the cerebral, cardiac, and renal vasculature)
- Reduce heart rate and the velocity of ventricular ejection

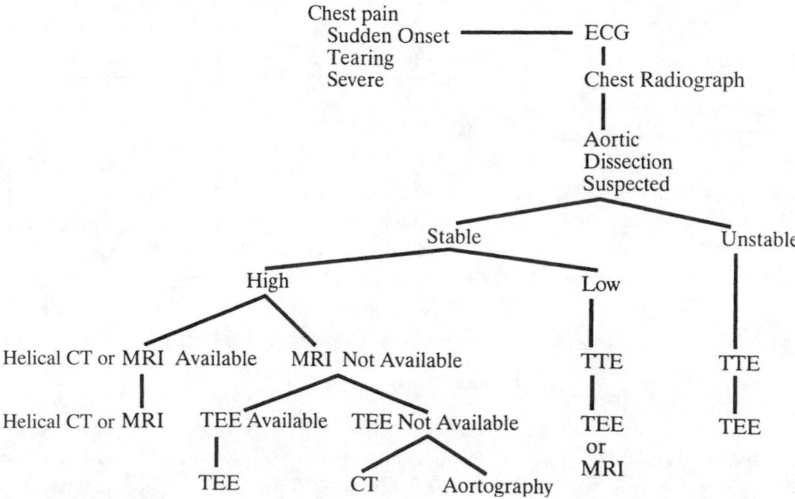

FIGURE 17.4.
Decision tree for imaging of thoracic aortic dissection. Helical computed tomography (*CT*) may be substituted for magnetic resonance imaging (*MRI*), if available. *ECG,* electrocardiography; *TEE,* transesophageal echocardiography; *TTE,* transthoracic echocardiography. (Reprinted with permission from the American College of Cardiology, ACC Educational Highlights. Vol. 11, Number 1. Fall 1995:16.)

Summary of Diagnosis

- Occurs more frequently in men than in women and in elderly persons with history of hypertension
- Sudden onset of severe, ripping chest pain that is maximal at onset
- Anterior chest pain = proximal dissection
- Back and abdominal pain = distal dissection
- Physical examination may be unrevealing
- New onset of diastolic murmur of aortic insufficiency, 70% of proximal dissection, which occurs in pericardial friction rub
- Pulse and neurologic deficits in only 6% of patients with aortic dissection
- Chest radiography: mediastinal widening or increase in aortic diameter (80% of patients)
- Diagnosis confirmed with TEE and, if indicated, followed by cardiac catheterization, aortography, or CT

When systolic blood pressure is being reduced, the patient's cardiac rhythm and arterial blood pressure must be continuously monitored. A pulmonary artery catheter should be placed so that cardiac output and pulmonary capillary wedge pressure may also be monitored. Only intravenous medications should be administered to ensure rapid control of heart rate and blood pressure (see Table 17.4).

To reduce heart rate and velocity of ventricular ejection, a β-blocker should be administered. **Esmolol,** an intravenous β-blocker with a short half-life (minutes) and cardioselective properties, is a reasonable agent to use in the patient with acute aortic dissection because the dose can be quickly titrated. Other agents that may be used in the acute setting include **intermittent, intravenous propranolol or metoprolol. Labetalol** is an intravenous agent with mixed α- and β-blocking properties and may be used as a single agent for decreasing heart rate and blood pressure. In the patient with reactive airway disease, **intravenous diltiazem** may be used as a continuous infusion to control heart rate and, to a lesser extent, blood pressure. **Verapamil** as an intermittent intravenous injection may be used also. Digoxin is contraindicated because of its positive inotropic effects.

If the patient with acute aortic dissection is still hypertensive despite reduction of heart rate and contractility, a vasodilator should be added. The vasodilator agent of choice is **sodium nitroprusside** because it has a short half-life and its dose may be titrated quickly. Sodium nitroprusside should be used with an agent to reduce heart rate because, when used alone, it may

TABLE 17.4. Intravenous Medications Commonly Used To Treat Acute Aortic Dissection

Agent	Loading Dosage	Maintenance Dosage	Adverse Effects
Diltiazem	10–20 mg over 5 minutes May repeat in 5–10 minutes	10–20 mg/h	Hypotension Bradycardia Congestive heart failure
Esmolol	500 μg/kg over 1 minute	50–200 μg/kg per minute, increase in increments of 50 μg/kg per minute (preceded by 500 μg/kg reloading dose)	Hypotension Bradycardia Congestive heart failure Shortness of breath at higher doses
Enalapril		0.625–1.25 mg every 6 hours	Renal failure Angioedema Hypotension Hyperkalemia
Labetalol	20 mg over 5 minutes	40–80 mg every 10 minutes for total of 300 mg After this, may give 40–80 mg every 12 hours	Hypotension Bradycardia Congestive heart failure Shortness of breath at higher doses Halothane effect
Metoprolol	5 mg as bolus Repeat every 5 minutes, total of 3 repetitions	10–20 mg intravenous piggyback every 6 hours	Hypotension Bradycardia Congestive heart failure Shortness of breath at higher doses
Nitroprusside		0.1–10 μg/kg per minute	Hypotension Central nervous system effects Gastrointestinal effects Cyanate toxicity
Propranolol	0.5–3 mg over 5 minutes	1–3 mg/h or 0.05–0.15 mg/kg every 4–6 hours	Hypotension Bradycardia Congestive heart failure Shortness of breath
Verapamil	5–10 mg over 5 minutes Repeat once in 15 minutes	10–20 mg intravenous piggyback every 8 hours	Hypotension Bradycardia Congestive heart failure

increase heart rate and the velocity of left ventricular contraction. After infusion of sodium nitroprusside lasting 48 hours or more, cyanate toxicity may develop, manifested by nausea, restlessness, hypotension, or somnolence. Intravenous hydralazine should be avoided because the drug is incorporated into medial-layer mucopolysaccharides and thus may cause weakening of the aortic wall. Intravenous medications and their major adverse effects in the acute medical management of aortic dissection are summarized in Table 17.4.

Surgical Management

A skilled cardiovascular surgeon should be consulted immediately if aortic dissection is suspected. Consultation should not be deferred until definitive imaging studies have been performed. The surgeon may provide invaluable assistance in the preoperative diagnosis and care of the patient suspected of having aortic dissection. The operating room may also be readied; this avoids delay, which may be catastrophic for the unstable patient.

Several types of aortic dissection demand immediate surgical attention:

1. Proximal aortic dissection
2. Distal aortic dissection if complicated by
   - Rupture or impending rupture (i.e., saccular aneurysm)
   - Progression with compromise of vital organs (i.e., kidneys, GI system)
   - Retrograde extension to the ascending aorta
   - Dissection in patients with Marfan's syndrome

Other patients with distal dissection may warrant surgical intervention if they continue to experience pain despite maximal medical management or if the resultant aneurysm is 5 cm or larger in diameter. Typically, the treatment of choice for stable distal aortic dissection is medical.

The surgical repair of aortic dissection requires excision of the intimal tear, obliteration of the false channel, and reconstitution of the true lumen of the aorta (often with a synthetic graft). If patency of other vessels (coronary and renal vessels, great vessels) is compromised, flow must be reestablished with synthetic grafts or repair of the dissection. If the aortic valve is involved in the dissection, it may be resuspended or replaced.

The overall operative mortality rate for aortic dissection is 5 to 27%. The most common causes of death are hemorrhage and congestive heart failure. Factors that predict operative death include

- Age
- Atherosclerotic heart disease
- Diabetes mellitus
- Cardiac tamponade
- Compromise of blood flow to the brain, kidneys, and viscera
- Pulmonary disease

The survival rate for patients who undergo surgical repair and survive to discharge is 90 to 93% at 1 year and 40 to 60% at 10 years.

Some patients who have had previous surgical repair of aortic dissection may present again with aortic dissection. Patients at particular risk are those with connective tissue disease, such as Marfan's syndrome, or those with poorly controlled hypertension.

Management of Aortic Arch Dissection

The treatment of aortic arch dissection is controversial. The arch is the least common site of involvement in aortic dissection but is the most lethal. Surgical repair of the aortic arch is associated with a 21 to 55% operative mortality rate. The 4-year survival rate is 45% with surgical treatment and 43% with medical treatment. Four-year survival rates may be higher in patients with concomitant proximal and arch aortic dissection who undergo repair of both dissections than in patients who undergo repair of the proximal dissection only. The recent use of hypothermic circulatory arrest may reduce the operative mortality rate of aortic arch repair.

Long-term Medical Management

Uncomplicated distal aortic dissection should be managed medically, in consultation with the cardiologist. A β-blocker should be used to reduce heart rate and ventricular ejection shear even if the patient is normotensive. If a β-blocker is contraindicated because of reactive airway disease, a **calcium-channel blocker** such as verapamil or diltiazem should be used. If hypertension continues despite the use of these agents, a **vasodilator,** such as a long-acting calcium-channel blocker (e.g., felodipine, amlodipine, and extended-release nifedipine) or **an angiotensin-converting enzyme inhibitor** (e.g., captopril, enalapril, and lisinopril) should be added. Hydralazine should not be used. A target systolic blood pressure of 100 to 120 mm Hg should be reached.

Surgical consultation should be obtained if the patient with uncomplicated distal dissection develops any of the following:

- Recurrent pain
- Signs of vital-organ compromise
- Extension of the dissection to the ascending aorta
- Aneurysmal dissection with a diameter of 6 cm or greater
- Inability to control hypertension medically

Intermittent imaging studies should be obtained as described in the following section on follow-up screening.

The patient who has undergone surgical repair of an aortic dissection should be treated with a β-blocker (or diltiazem or verapamil if β-blockers are contraindicated). Hypertension should also be treated aggressively.

Follow-up Screening

Surveillance is essential in the patient who has an aortic dissection which has either been stabilized medically or corrected surgically. False lumens may exist distal to the repaired portion of aorta in most patients undergoing surgical repair. Aneurysm may occur in up to 50% of patients with aortic dissection and poorly controlled hypertension and in up to 10% of patients who are receiving antihypertensive therapy. The patient with

Marfan's syndrome may develop new dissections in other sites in the aorta. At least 20% of patients who undergo surgical repair may later need repeated surgery. For these reasons, follow-up imaging should be performed regularly to assess for aneurysm formation. The timing of imaging studies should be guided by the existence of aneurysm, as well as evidence of recurrence of hypertension. If an aneurysm is detected or if hypertension is present, imaging studies should be performed every 3 months. In the stable patient, however, biannual or annual examinations may be sufficient.

Magnetic resonance imaging is probably the imaging test of choice for follow-up given the noninvasive nature of the test and the avoidance of contrast dye. In patients who cannot undergo MRI, helical CT is a reasonable alternative. Both of these methods allow evaluation of the entire aorta, the point of insertion of the great vessels, and prosthetic grafts. Both methods also allow easy comparison to results of previous studies.

Summary of Treatment

- Short-term treatment: eliminate pain and reduce systolic blood pressure to 100 to 120 mm Hg. Administer intravenous esmolol, propranolol, or metoprolol and then sodium nitroprusside for vasodilatation (watch for cyanide toxicity).
- Consultation or referral: cardiologist (for TEE and intravenous drug management), cardiovascular surgeon.
- Immediate surgical attention: proximal aortic dissection and chronic aortic dissection with complications (e.g., rupture renal compromise, retrograde extension, Marfan's syndrome)
- Long-term medical management for uncomplicated distal dissection: β-blockers, calcium-channel blockers. Do not use hydralazine.

CONCLUSION

Aortic dissection is a life-threatening condition that should be considered a medical and surgical emergency. Aortic dissection should always be considered in the differential diagnosis of the patient presenting with sudden, cataclysmic chest or back pain. Immediate medical management is initiated to decrease blood pressure and ventricular ejection velocity. Surgical consultation must be obtained as soon as possible. The diagnosis of aortic dissection should be confirmed with definitive imaging such as TEE, MRI, or helical CT. Aortic dissection should be categorized as proximal or distal. Most proximal dissections should be surgically repaired, whereas most distal dissections may be managed medically. All patients with aortic dissection should receive long-term therapy to reduce heart rate, contractility, and blood pressure. Follow-up imaging should be obtained regularly to screen for aneurysm formation.

KEY POINTS

- Aortic dissection is associated with significant morbidity and mortality rates.
- High index of suspicion is necessary to differentiate between aortic dissection and angina or myocardial infarction.
- Rapid, complete diagnosis is essential.
- Consultation or referral: both cardiologist and cardiovascular surgeon when considering diagnosis of aortic dissection
- Intravenous drug administration is required.
- Antihypertensive medications (i.e., β-blockers), administered intravenously, are effective drugs.
- Physical examination should focus on root involvement.
- Physical examination often reveals new onset of the murmur of aortic insufficiency or pericardial friction rub.
- In elderly men with history of hypertension presenting with excruciating chest pain radiating to the back, consider aortic dissection.
- If the dissection involves the coronary ostia, myocardial infarction may occur. ECG will show myocardial infarction. Treat patient for aortic dissection, not myocardial infarction.

ACKNOWLEDGMENTS

T.J. Cole, MD, Department of Radiology, and W. Paulsen, MD, Division of Cardiology, Department of Medicine, Medical College of Virginia for images of aortic dissection. Dr. Clemo is the recipient of a Clinician-Investigator Development Award (HL 02798) from the National Heart, Lung, and Blood Institute.

SUGGESTED READINGS

Cigarroa JE, Isselbacher EM, DeSanctis RW , et al. Diagnostic imaging in the evaluation of suspected aortic dissection. N Engl J Med 1993;328:35–43. Objective discussion of the pros and cons of various imaging methods and their use in the diagnosis of aortic dissection.

DeBakey ME, McCollum CH, Crawford ES, et al. Dissection and dissecting aneurysms of the aorta: 20 year follow up of 527 patients treated surgically. Surgery 1982;92:1118–1134. DeBakey, the pioneer of surgical repair of aortic dissection, reviews his experience in managing this condition.

Fann JI, Miller DC. Aortic dissection. Ann Vasc Surg 1995; 9:311–323. Well-organized tables summarizing basic data underlying clinical decision-making in aortic dissection.

Finkbohner R, Johnston D, Crawford S, et al. Marfan syndrome. Long-term survival and complications after aortic aneurysm repair. Circulation 1995;91:728–733.

Glower DD, Fann JI, Speier RH, et al. Comparison of medical and surgical therapy for uncomplicated descending aortic dissection. Circulation 1989;82(suppl 5):IV39–IV46. Provides evidence that medical therapy is superior to surgery in uncomplicated distal aortic dissection.

Nienaber CA, von Kodolitsch Y, Nicolas V, et al. The diagnosis of thoracic aortic dissection by noninvasive imaging procedures. N Engl J Med 1993;328:1–9. Review of sensitivity and specificity of various imaging methods in the diagnosis of aortic dissection.

Roberts WC. Aortic dissection: anatomy, consequences, causes. Am Heart J 1981;102:195–214. Anatomic description of aortic dissection and its complications based on autopsy specimens.

Slater EE, De Sanctis RW. The clinical recognition of dissecting aortic aneurysm. Am J Med 1976;60:625–633. Review of clinical symptoms and signs in aortic dissection.

Spittell PC, Spittell JA, Joyce JW , et al. Clinical features and differential diagnosis of aortic dissection: experience with 236 cases (1980 through 1990). Mayo Clin Proc 1993; 68:642–651. Critical analysis of clinical features of aortic dissection from the Mayo Clinic experience.

Spittell PC. Diseases of the aorta. In: Textbook of cardiovascular medicine. EJ Topol, ed. Philadelphia: Lippincott-Raven; Philadelphia; 1998:2519–2536.

18 CHAPTER

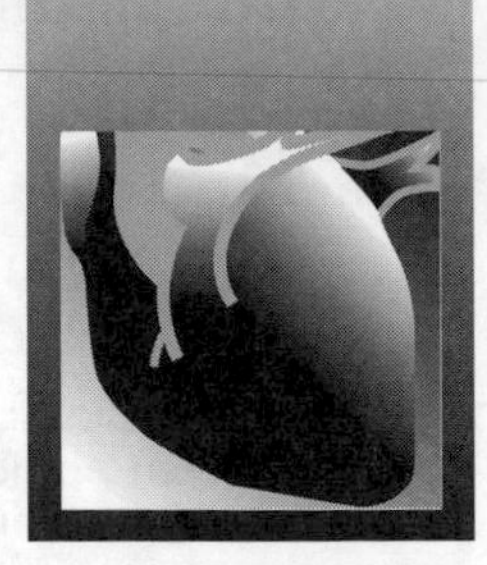

Peripheral Vascular Disease: Arterial and Venous

Jeffery B. Dattilo
Raymond G. Makhoul

ARTERIAL DISEASE: ANEURYSMS

An aneurysm is a localized dilatation of an artery to one and one-half to twice the normal diameter of the artery.

Abdominal Aortic Aneurysms

Aneurysms of the abdominal aorta are common and are increasing in frequency. The major risks of these aneurysms are rupture and sudden death. Approximately 15,000 deaths per year in the United States are due to aneurysm rupture, making it the 13th leading cause of death.

Abdominal aneurysms may be fusiform or saccular; fusiform aneurysms are the most common. Men are more likely to have aneurysms than women (ratio, 4:1). The location of abdominal aortic aneurysms is infrarenal in 90 to 95% of patients; thus, most are amenable to surgical resection. About 40% of patients have an associated aneurysm of the common or internal iliac artery.

Causes and Pathogenesis

Aortic aneurysms were traditionally thought to be caused by atherosclerosis because of the high incidence of atherosclerosis in these patients. More recently, however, several alternative hypotheses on the causes of abdominal aneurysms have emerged. These include

- Genetic predisposition for aneurysms
- Increased proteolytic enzyme activity in the aortic wall
- Hemodynamic influences
- Cystic medial necrosis
- Dissection
- Ehlers-Danlos syndrome
- Syphilis

The accepted physical principle to explain expansion of an aneurysm is the law of LaPlace. Simply stated, the radius is directly proportional to the tension applied to the vessel wall. (Fig. 18.1) Experimental evidence in animal models exists for all of these causes, but the cause in human aneurysms remains unclear.

Clinical Manifestations

Most infrarenal abdominal aortic aneurysms (70 to 75%) are asymptomatic at the time of discovery. They may be discovered at the time of routine physical examination or during radiologic studies such as intravenous pyelography, lumbosacral spinal radiography, computed tomography of the abdomen, and abdominal ultrasonography. An aneurysm may be discovered at laparotomy for other abdominal abnormalities.

The causes of symptoms due to abdominal aortic aneurysms include

- Rupture
- Expansion
- Pressure on adjacent structures
- Embolization
- Dissection
- Thrombosis

By far, the most common presenting symptoms are abdominal, back, or flank pain. The classic triad of a palpable, pulsatile abdominal mass; excruciating abdominal or back pain; and hypotension is said to be pathognomonic of a ruptured aneurysm. In one retrospective series of patients with aneurysm rupture, 83% of patients had a palpable pulsatile mass, 72% had abdominal and back pain, and 45% had hypotension. Fewer than half of patients had all three symptoms. Misdiagnosis of ruptured abdominal aortic aneurysm is common and results in high mortality. About 10% of patients may have pain

$$\textbf{Tension} = \textbf{Pressure} \times \textbf{Radius}$$

FIGURE 18.1.
Law of LaPlace.

that mimics renal stones (e.g., flank pain radiating to the hip, genitalia, or thigh). Patients sometimes experience an acute, unilateral, painful neuropathy secondary to compression of the femoral or obturator nerves by the aneurysm. An aneurysm infrequently ruptures into the inferior vena cava, resulting in an acute aortocaval fistula manifested by lower-extremity edema and high-output congestive heart failure. Rupture of an aneurysm into the gastrointestinal tract with massive gastrointestinal bleeding has been reported.

Most aneurysms are lined with mural thrombi, which may dislodge, embolize to the lower extremities, and result in acute ischemia. The aneurysm sometimes acutely thromboses above the iliac bifurcation, causing acute ischemic symptoms.

Diagnosis

An infrarenal abdominal aortic aneurysm greater than 5 cm in size can usually be diagnosed on physical examination, except in obese patients. Typically, the aneurysm is palpated as a prominent lateral pulsation located midway between the xiphoid and the umbilicus. Palpation below the umbilicus is too low to detect the abdominal aorta because the abdominal aorta has already given rise to the common iliac arteries at this level. The differential diagnosis of a pulsatile abdominal mass also includes a normal but ectatic aorta and a retroperitoneal mass overlying a normal aorta.

The oldest method of objectively diagnosing an abdominal aneurysm is plain abdominal radiography in the anterior-posterior and lateral projections. In 50 to 70% of patients, enough calcium is present in the aortic wall to make the diagnosis, but an accurate estimate of the size of the aneurysm is possible in only 75% of these patients. Therefore, negative findings on plain radiography of the abdomen cannot reliably rule out the presence of an aneurysm.

The most commonly used imaging methods to detect an abdominal aortic aneurysm and to accurately document its size are B-mode ultrasonography and computed tomography. **Ultrasonography** should be the method of choice for the following:

- Initial evaluation of a pulsatile abdominal mass
- Subsequent studies to follow the size of the aneurysm
- Use in aneurysm screening programs

The following are the advantages of ultrasonography:

- Wide availability
- Quick performance
- Relatively low cost
- No known harmful side effects

Studies comparing the accuracy of ultrasonographic measurement of aneurysms to the actual size of the aneurysm have shown the technique to be accurate to within 2 to 3 mm.

For patients with symptomatic aneurysms in whom rupture is suspected, ultrasonography is not accurate; another test, such as computed tomography, should be used. **Computed tomography** uses ionizing radiation to obtain cross-sectional images of the aorta and other intraabdominal structures. The following are the advantages of computed tomography:

- It is highly accurate in predicting aneurysm size.
- It allows evaluation of the aneurysm in relation to the renal arteries.
- It can delineate retroperitoneal hematoma (in cases of aneurysm rupture) or periaortic thickening (in cases of inflammatory aneurysm).

Thus, it is the preferred method of preoperative aneurysm evaluation.

Although **magnetic resonance imaging** can be used to evaluate aneurysms, this method has many disadvantages, including cost, slow imaging speed. and contraindications to scanning.

Arteriography is not a good diagnostic study for abdominal aneurysms and should be used only in selective cases as a preoperative test before surgical resection.

Treatment

As mentioned previously, the major risk of an abdominal aortic aneurysm is rupture and the high mortality rate. When rupture occurs, the postoperative mortality rate is about 50%; if the patients who die before arriving at the hospital are considered, the mortality rate approaches 80%. To select the best treatment for these aneurysms, the natural history must be understood.

A 1977 autopsy study of 265 patients with nonresected aneurysms less than 5 cm in diameter showed that aneurysms ruptured in 34 (12.8%). Almost one in four aneurysms in the 4- to 5-cm range had ruptured. The major flaw of this study is that the measurement of aneurysm size in the postmortem state probably underestimates the size of these aneurysms. More recent population-based studies suggest that the risk for aneurysm rupture begins to rapidly increase at aneurysm diameters of 5 cm, with a 5-year rupture rate ranging from 25 to 41%. Given that the approximate yearly expansion rate of abdominal aortic aneurysm is 0.5 cm , the natural history of large abdominal aneurysms is ominous (Table 18.1). Thus, surgical resection and grafting of aneurysms that are at least 5 cm in diameter in good-risk patients is reasonable.

TABLE 18.1. Natural History of Abdominal Aortic Aneurysms

Diameter (cm)	Annual Rupture Rate (%)
5.0	4.0
5–7	6.6
≥7	19.0

Note: Annual growth rate is 0.5 cm/y.

TABLE 18.2. Perioperative Mortality Rate for Resection and Grafting of Abdominal Aortic Aneurysm

Operation	Mortality Rate (%)
Elective	3–5
Symptomatic (nonruptured) aneurysm	20
Ruptured aneurysm	50

A more controversial issue involves aneurysms between 4 and 5 cm in diameter, the so-called small abdominal aortic aneurysms. In these patients, the options are twofold: surgical resection or close observation with serial ultrasonography every 6 months. The decision to operate may be influenced by many factors, including the patient's age; the presence of such comorbid conditions as cardiac, pulmonary, and renal function; and the documented rate of growth of the aneurysm. No published randomized trials have compared surgical and nonsurgical management of small aneurysms, although some are currently in progress. Until the results of these studies are available, a reasonable approach would be to refer patients with aneurysms of 4 cm or greater in diameter to an experienced surgeon for evaluation and consideration for resection.

The results of standard, elective operative repair of nonruptured abdominal aortic aneurysms are excellent, with a mortality rate of 3 to 5% in most modern series (Table 18.2). The most common cause of perioperative death is myocardial infarction. Surgery for symptomatic but nonruptured aneurysms carries a mortality rate of about 20%, whereas the perioperative mortality rate for ruptured aneurysms is about 50%. Likewise, the long-term survival of patients undergoing elective aneurysm repair is excellent, matching that of age-matched persons without aneurysms. A new development in the treatment of aneurysms is endovascular grafting via a transfemoral approach. This technique should be considered investigational; only clinical trials with adequate long-term follow-up will determine the eventual usefulness of this approach.

Iliac Artery Aneurysms

Common iliac artery aneurysms occur most frequently in association with abdominal aortic aneurysms. Isolated iliac aneurysms are rare, accounting for less than 1% of atherosclerotic aneurysms. They usually involve the common or internal iliac arteries; the external iliac artery is usually spared. Because of their location in the pelvis, isolated iliac aneurysms may be difficult to detect on abdominal examination until they become very large or symptomatic. In many instances, they may be palpated on rectal or pelvic examination, especially if the internal iliac artery is involved. Symptoms commonly consist of lower abdominal, flank, or pelvic pain.

Iliac aneurysms may be diagnosed by plain radiography, ultrasonography, or computed tomography. Most iliac aneurysms tend to be large when discovered and have a relatively high rate of rupture. Because of this, patients with iliac aneurysms 3 cm or greater in diameter should be considered for surgical resection.

Femoral Artery Aneurysm

Femoral artery aneurysms are the second most common of the peripheral aneurysms. True aneurysms involve all three layers of the arterial wall and are largely secondary to atherosclerotic degeneration. They are strongly associated with abdominal aortic and popliteal aneurysms and occur bilaterally about 50% of the time. Femoral artery aneurysms limited to the common femoral artery are called type I, and those involving the orifice of the deep femoral artery are termed type II.

Clinical Manifestations

Approximately 25% of atherosclerotic femoral aneurysms are asymptomatic; the remainder present with such symptoms as arterial ischemia, local compression of the femoral nerve, and artery or groin pain. The ischemic symptoms may be secondary to embolism or thrombosis of the aneurysm. Rupture is rare, occurring in less than 2% of patients.

Diagnosis

Femoral artery aneurysms are usually diagnosed by physical examination of a pulsatile groin mass; ultrasonography is the most useful confirmatory test.

Treatment

Surgical repair is indicated for all symptomatic atherosclerotic femoral aneurysms and those that are asymptomatic and greater than 2.5 cm in diameter. Small asymptomatic aneurysms can be monitored with serial **ultrasonography.** The surgical technique involves replacement of the aneurysm with a graft, usually synthetic. For aneurysms involving the deep femoral artery (type II), **reimplantation** of that vessel may be necessary. The results of femoral artery aneurysm resection are excellent, with very low morbidity and mortality rates.

Popliteal Aneurysms

The popliteal region is the most common site of peripheral arterial aneurysms. The cause of popliteal aneurysms is **atherosclerosis** in 95% of patients. Rare causes include popliteal artery entrapment by the gastrocnemius muscle, bacterial infection, collagen disorders, and trauma. These aneurysms typically present in the seventh decade of life, and the male-to-female ratio is approximately 30:1.

Popliteal aneurysms occur bilaterally in about half of patients. These patients have an increased incidence of associated abdominal aortic, iliac, and femoral aneurysms. Conversely, the incidence of popliteal aneurysm in patients presenting with abdominal aortic aneurysm is about 6%.

Clinical Manifestations

Most patients with popliteal aneurysms present with symptoms. Leg ischemia ranging from claudication to limb-threatening gangrene is the most common manifestation of popliteal aneurysms. Symptoms are due to

- Thrombosis of the aneurysm
- Embolization to the tibial vessels
- A combination of the aforementioned

Less commonly, large popliteal aneurysms may cause local compressive symptoms, such as venous obstruction or nerve impingement with pain and tenderness. Unlike abdominal aortic aneurysms, rupture is rare, occurring less than 5% of the time.

Diagnosis

The diagnosis of popliteal aneurysm is principally clinical and requires a high degree of suspicion. Particular attention should be paid to patients with a contralateral popliteal aneurysm or a strong family history of aneurysmal disease. Most popliteal aneurysms present as pulsatile popliteal masses or as firm, nonpulsatile masses if they are thrombosed. Some may be diagnosed by plain **radiography** if the wall contains vascular calcifications. The diagnosis is best confirmed by **ultrasonography,** which documents the size of the aneurysm and the presence or absence of mural thrombus. **Arteriography** is indicated before operative repair of these aneurysms.

Treatment

Treatment for all symptomatic aneurysms is **surgical.** For asymptomatic aneurysms, treatment is controversial. A reasonable approach is that operative therapy should be considered when aneurysms reach 2 cm in size in a patient who is a good candidate for surgery. The aim of surgery for popliteal aneurysm is to eliminate the aneurysm from the circulation while restoring blood flow to the leg. The surgical procedure of choice is **ligation** above and below the aneurysm with bypass, preferably using autogenous saphenous vein. With large aneurysms causing local compressive symptoms, **resection** of the aneurysm with grafting may be necessary. This operation, however, is associated with a higher morbidity rate because of the associated dissection in the popliteal space.

In patients with acute thrombosis of a popliteal aneurysm and limb-threatening ischemia, **intra-arterial thrombolytic therapy** in addition to **operative repair** may be an option. This therapy, usually consisting of urokinase infusion, is aimed at clearing the tibial and pedal vessels of thrombus and may be administered either preoperatively or intraoperatively.

The long-term results of surgery for popliteal aneurysm depend on the nature of the aneurysm (symptomatic versus asymptomatic), the quality of the distal runoff vessels, and the type of graft used.

Carotid Artery Disease

Approximately 500,000 persons sustain a stroke each year in the United States; 200,000 of these persons die. The patients who do not die of stroke are often left disabled, and the resulting cost to the patient and society is immense. About one-third of ischemic strokes are caused by atherosclerotic disease of the major extracranial vessels, most commonly the carotid artery bifurcation. The appropriate treatment of carotid bifurcation stenosis has been controversial, in part because of a lack of randomized trials. Recently, however, the results of studies dealing with both symptomatic and asymptomatic lesions have become available. This information allows more definitive guidelines in the management of these lesions.

Pathology and Pathophysiology

The most common lesion in patients with carotid disease is an atherosclerotic plaque at the carotid bifurcation. This location seems to be particularly susceptible to lesion formation. The exact reasons for this are not clear but are probably related to the unique hemodynamic characteristics of the carotid bifurcation. One popular theory is that carotid atherosclerotic lesions localize to areas of low-flow velocity and low shear, such as the carotid sinus opposite the flow divider.

The earliest stage of the atherosclerotic lesion is the fatty streak, which appears as yellow-white discolorations on the intimal surface of the arterial wall. The fatty streak progresses to early atherosclerotic plaque and finally complicated plaque. Complicated plaque is responsible for the symptoms associated with carotid bifurcation disease and is characterized by calcification, hemorrhage, and infarction. Most symptoms from carotid artery disease are caused by emboli from the surface of a plaque; these emboli consist of cholesterol, platelets, or thrombin. Less commonly, symptoms may be secondary to carotid stenosis or occlusion and hypoperfusion secondary to inadequate collateral circulation. Other lesions that may be encountered in the carotid artery, but with much less frequency, include carotid kinks and coils, carotid aneurysms, fibromuscular dysplasia, carotid body tumors, radiation injury, and vasculitis.

Clinical Manifestations

From a clinical perspective, patients with carotid artery stenosis may be asymptomatic or symptomatic. Symptomatic patients may experience one of many neurologic events, including

- Transient ischemic attacks
- Reversible ischemic neurologic deficit
- Amaurosis fugax
- Evolving stroke
- Frank stroke
- Nonfocal symptoms

Diagnosis

A careful history and physical examination with emphasis on the **neurologic examination** and the **vascular examination** are essential. A thorough history for the presence of coronary and peripheral vascular occlusive disease and such stroke risk factors as hypertension, cigarette abuse, use of oral contraceptives, hyperlipidemia, and diabetes mellitus is taken. The presence or absence of carotid bruits should be noted.

If symptoms suggest carotid disease or if a carotid bruit is heard, further investigation with duplex scanning may be warranted. The duplex scanner combines real-time, B-mode ultrasonography with pulsed Doppler flow measurements. By measurement of the peak systolic frequencies and spectral broadening, the degree of stenosis can be estimated. Improvements in technology and familiarity with duplex scanning has enabled some surgeons to rely on duplex scanning rather than angiography in performing carotid endarterectomy.

Duplex scanning has three major limitations:

- It is highly operator dependent.
- It does not sample the entire carotid artery (the arch vessels, proximal common carotid artery, and intracranial carotid artery cannot be seen).
- Nonstenotic but clinically important lesions, such as ulcers, may be difficult to evaluate.

Angiography remains the best method for assessing the cerebral circulation. It has the advantages of delineating the entire vascular tree from the aortic arch to the intracranial circulation. In addition, the collateral circulation in the brain can be evaluated and a clear picture of carotid bifurcation plaques and ulcers can be obtained. Drawbacks include the following:

- Contrast nephrotoxicity and allergy
- Puncture-site hematomas
- Potential for precipitating neurologic events

Magnetic resonance angiography is an emerging, promising technology for visualization of the cerebral vascular system that has limited application.

Management

For years, the optimal management of patients with carotid stenosis has been controversial. Part of this controversy was due to the lack of sufficient data on the natural history of the disease and the relative efficacy of medical and surgical treatment in reducing the rate of stroke and death. Recently, the results of many multicenter, randomized studies comparing medical management and surgery (carotid endarterectomy) have become available.

Asymptomatic Carotid Stenosis

Asymptomatic carotid lesions are often found when a bruit is noted in the neck on physical examination. On duplex scanning, most carotid bruits are shown to be associated with some degree of carotid disease, but only one-third are hemodynamically significant (>50% diameter stenosis). Conversely, the absence of a bruit does not rule out the presence of significant carotid bifurcation disease.

The rationale for carotid endarterectomy for asymptomatic carotid bifurcation lesions is to reduce the long-term risk for stroke in the distribution of that carotid artery. Five randomized trials were designed to study the efficacy of prophylactic carotid endarterectomy for the treatment of patients with asymptomatic carotid stenosis. The largest of these trials, the Asymptomatic Carotid Atherosclerosis Study (ACAS), recently concluded that there was a clear benefit in favor of surgery (Fig. 18.2). For patients with stenosis greater than 60% diameter reduction, the relative reduction in risk for stroke was 55% in the surgical group compared with the patients who did not undergo surgery.

It is reasonable to refer patients with asymptomatic carotid stenosis of at least 60 to 80% diameter reduction for evaluation by an experienced surgeon for consideration for endarterectomy. The results of this and other studies are applicable only if the combined stroke and mortality rate with surgery is low. With carotid endarterectomy for asymptomatic stenosis, this rate should be less than 3%.

Symptomatic Carotid Stenosis

The symptoms related to symptomatic carotid artery lesions have already been discussed, as have patient evaluation and diagnostic studies. The options for treatment are medical management versus surgical management. The risk factors known to be associated with an increased risk for stroke in patients with carotid artery disease include

- Age
- Hypertension
- Ischemic heart disease
- Diabetes mellitus
- Cigarette smoking

Elimination or treatment of some of these risk factors, such as hypertension and cigarette smoking, may reduce the risk for stroke. The use of drugs to reduce the risk for stroke has focused primarily on antiplatelet agents, including aspirin, ticlopidine, dipyridamole, and, most recently, clopidogrel. Meta-analysis of several randomized studies has shown a 2% absolute reduction in nonfatal stroke with the use of antiplatelet agents.

Three randomized trials compared surgical management with medical management for symptomatic carotid disease. The best known of these studies is the North American Symptomatic Carotid Endarterectomy Trial (NASCET). Surgery was clearly beneficial in patients with single or multiple transient ischemic attacks or a mild stroke within a 6-month interval and 70% or greater stenosis (Fig. 18.2). The best strategy for symptomatic lesions with stenosis between 30% and 69% is uncertain. Surgery should be performed only by an experienced surgeon who has documented good results for carotid endarterectomy.

PERIPHERAL ARTERY OCCLUSIVE DISEASE

Acute Arterial Occlusion: Thrombosis and Embolus

Causes

Thrombosis and embolism are considered medical and surgical emergencies. Rapid differentiation between

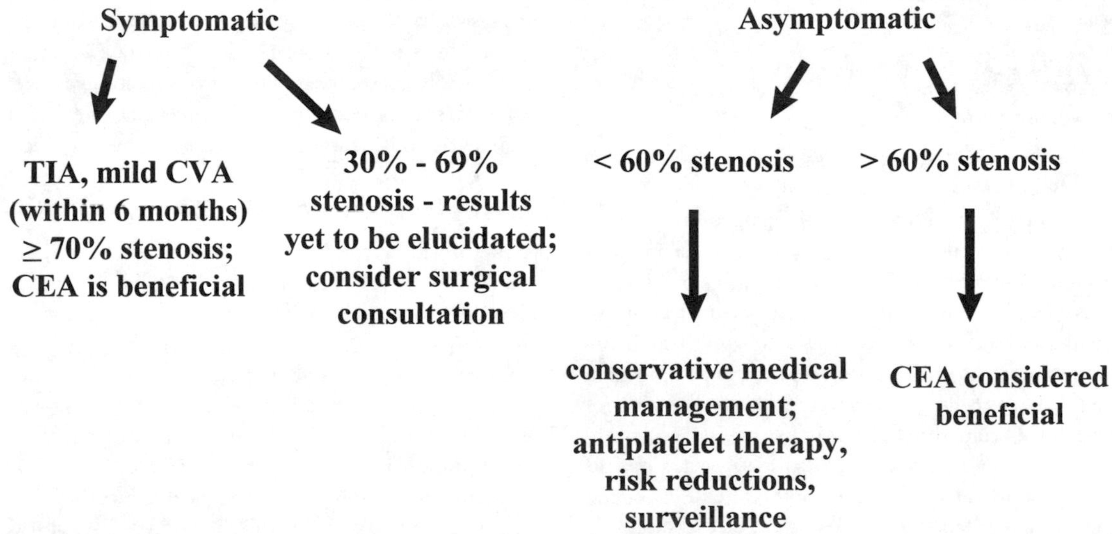

FIGURE 18.2.
Management of carotid stenosis. CEA, carotid endarterectomy; CVA, cerebrovascular accident; TIA, transient ischemic attack.

thrombosis and embolism is critical because the treatment of these two problems differs and morbidity depends on the timely restoration of blood flow to the extremity.

The most common cause of acute arterial occlusion is embolus from the heart. Causes of embolism originating in the heart include

- Arrythmias
- Mitral stenosis
- Mural thrombus from a ventricular aneurysm

Emboli from sources other than the heart include

- Abdominal aortic aneurysms
- Iliac, femoral, and popliteal aneurysms
- Ulcerated plaques in the upstream vascular tree

Seventy percent of emboli from the heart lodge in the arteries below the inguinal ligament; the most common site is the superficial femoral artery.

By far, the most common cause of acute thrombosis is disruption of a preexisting atherosclerotic plaque with subsequent exposure of the prothrombotic core of the plaque. In the absence of preexisting arterial occlusive disease, arterial injury is the usual cause of acute thrombosis. Injuries most commonly seen with thrombosis are the following:

- Posterior knee dislocations
- Fractures
- Repeated trauma (cervical rib)
- Iatrogenic vascular injuries

Diagnosis

The "five Ps" are classic hallmarks of acute arterial ischemia:

- Pain
- Pallor
- Pulselessness
- Paresthesia
- Paralysis

A sixth "P" often included is poikilothermia.

A careful history should be taken, with specific notation of the presence or absence of previous symptoms, such as claudication. In addition, a history of atrial fibrillation may be elicited in some patients, suggesting the diagnosis of embolism. On physical examination, signs of chronic ischemia such as loss of hair and atrophic nails suggest previous underlying atherosclerosis. Examination for pulses in the opposite extremity is essential because a normal vascular examination in the unaffected limb suggests embolism rather than thrombosis. Chest radiography, electrocardiography, and echocardiography may also be useful in these patients.

Treatment

The cornerstone of treatment for acute arterial ischemia is **heparinization** and **referral** to a surgeon. The patient should be given a bolus of 5000 to 10,000 U of heparin intravenously and an infusion of 1000 U/h. Depending on the diagnosis and the degree of ischemia, the options for treatment include

- Surgical embolectomy
- Surgical bypass
- Arteriography with urokinase infusion

Good long-term results may be achieved with prompt diagnosis and treatment.

Chronic Arterial Insufficiency

Pathology and Pathophysiology

Atherosclerosis is the most common cause of the degenerative pathologic changes seen within arteries. Risk factors for atherosclerosis include tobacco use, diabetes, hypertension, hyperlipidemia, and genetic factors. Hypotheses on the cause of atherosclerosis abound. One of the most popular is that atherosclerosis results from a continuing repair process of the arterial wall in response to repeated endothelial-cell damage. According to this theory, the cells are damaged by such factors as hyperlipidemia, increased shear stress of hypertension, and hormone dysfunction. With the accumulation of blood-borne monocytes and platelets in the vessel wall, mitogens are released. The mitogens stimulate smooth-muscle cell proliferation and migration, leading to plaque formation. Lesions may eventually become more complex, containing a necrotic core covered by a fibrous cap; they may then ulcerate or develop hemorrhage or calcification.

The common sites of atherosclerotic lesions are near areas of the arterial tree exposed to high shear, such as at arterial branch bifurcations and posteriorly fixed sites. Younger patients generally have aortoiliac lesions, whereas the elderly present with disease involving the superficial femoral and tibial arteries. Below the inguinal ligament, the distal superficial femoral artery is the most common site for atherosclerotic occlusive disease in nondiabetic persons. In diabetic patients, the distal popliteal and tibial vessels are commonly diseased; the more proximal arteries are often spared (Fig. 18.3).

Clinical Manifestations

The spectrum of symptoms in the patient with atherosclerotic occlusive lesions ranges from no symptoms

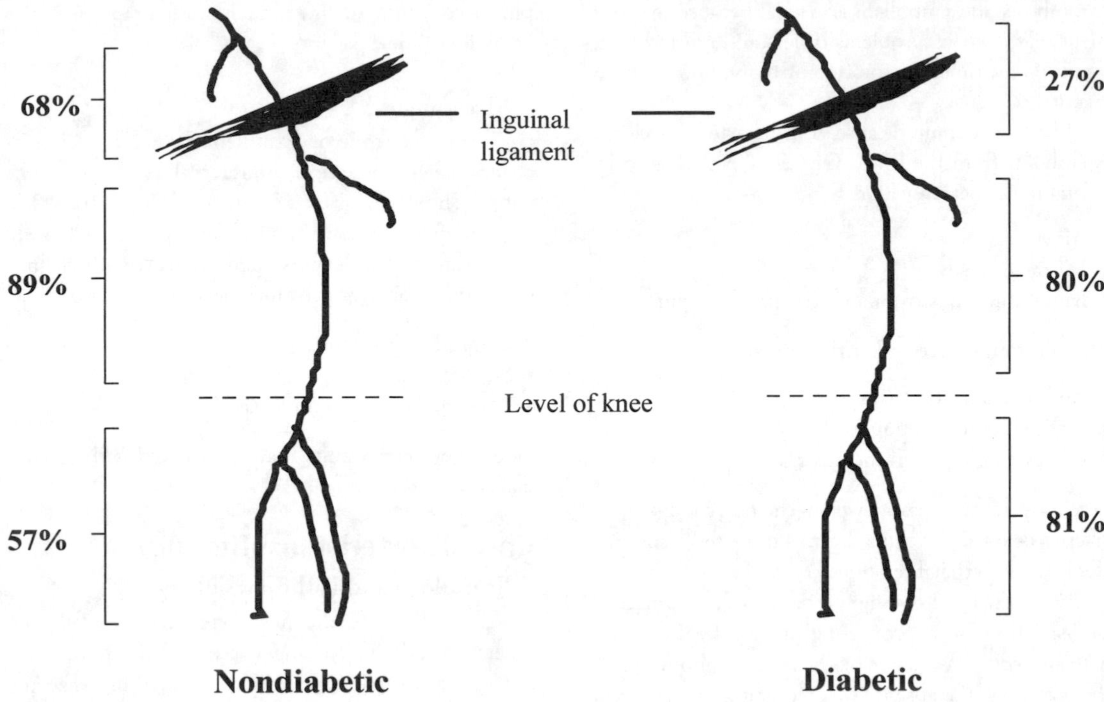

FIGURE 18.3.
Frequency of atherosclerotic lesions in the lower limb. (Adapted from Ernst CB, Stanley J. Current therapy in vascular surgery. St. Louis: Mosby; 1995.)

to painful ischemic tissue loss and depends on the degree of disease present. Symptoms include

- Intermittent arterial claudication
- Ischemic rest pain
- Tissue loss

Spinal stenosis may mimic arterial claudication.

Intermittent arterial claudication is the most commonly encountered symptom in these patients. Claudication can be defined as limb pain brought on by exertion and relieved by periods of rest, often in a reproducible manner. This symptom is based on an oxygen supply-and-demand phenomenon. With exercise, the muscles distal to the areas of stenosis or occlusion undergo an ischemic period and the patient experiences pain. With rest, the demand lessens and the limited blood supply can again adequately perfuse the tissue. Conditions that may mimic arterial claudication include spinal stenosis and venous claudication.

Ischemic rest pain, or pain at rest, is seen in more advanced atherosclerotic disease, usually involving multiple segmental occlusions. Unlike claudication, rest pain does not involve muscle groups but rather the foot, especially the toes and metatarsal heads. Early on, it may present as dysesthesias in the foot with elevation. This is typically relieved when the patient hangs the foot down or ambulates. Rest pain may be difficult to differentiate from diabetic neuropathy and in many cases may coexist with this condition. If left untreated, ischemic rest pain almost always progresses to tissue loss.

Tissue loss from arterial ischemia is typically painful and is commonly associated with other manifestations of ischemia. The ulcer usually has a necrotic base and is often located in areas prone to chronic pressure or trauma. In addition, patients may present with gangrenous (black) or pregangrenous, cyanotic (blue) toes.

Diagnosis

A thorough examination, including a careful history with attention to smoking, related disease states (hypertension, diabetes, coronary artery disease, hyperlipidemia), and time course of symptoms is the most important diagnostic tool. A comprehensive vascular examination comprises inspection, palpation, and auscultation. It is important to look for signs of chronic arterial insufficiency, including skin color changes and compromised skin integrity. A simple maneuver to detect an ischemic leg is to place the lower extremity in a dependent position and observe for increased redness (dependent rubor). In addition, loss of hair and nail thickening are signs indicating chronic ischemia. The upper- and lower-extremity arteries should be palpated for the presence and intensity and are graded as follows:

0 = absent
1+ = diminished
2+ = normal
3+ = enlarged
4+ = aneurysmal

If pulses cannot be palpated, determination of blood flow must be confirmed with hand-held Doppler examination. Auscultation of the carotid, abdominal aorta, and femoral arteries for bruit is an important aspect of the vascular examination. Segmental arterial pressures

- Provide an objective and quantitative method of assessing the circulation
- Confirm the diagnosis
- Localize the occlusive lesions providing a baseline against which to measure future studies
- May predict the chances of healing an ulcer or wound with conservative measures

A quick test that can be done in the office or at the bedside is the ankle/brachial index. This is performed by measuring the systolic blood pressure of the brachial artery and the systolic blood pressure at the ankle. The ratio of the ankle pressure to the brachial pressure is then calculated. A normal ankle/brachial index is 1.2 to 1.0. Patients with claudications have indexes ranging from 0.9 to 0.6. Patients with rest pain or tissue loss typically have indexes less than 0.5 (Fig. 18.4). In patients with calcified noncompressible vessels, such as diabetic patients, the ankle/brachial index is not useful. In diabetic patients, the blood pressure cuff cannot easily collapse the vessel; thus, the index is artificially elevated. In these patients, the toe pressure, which is not subject to this problem, is a more reliable indicator of the actual perfusion. Normally, the toe pressure is 20 to 30 mm Hg less than the ankle pressure.

Arteriography has little use in the diagnosis of chronic arterial insufficiency and should be reserved only for patients requiring intervention with angioplasty or surgery (Table 18.3).

Treatment

The presence of mild to moderate claudication is a relatively benign condition that rarely poses a threat of limb loss to the nondiabetic patient. In general, 75% of these patients remain stable or improve over a 5-year period. Only 5 to 7% must have amputation eventually. Two subsets of patients with claudication who exhibit a more accelerated course of symptoms are diabetic patients and patients who continue to smoke. The treatment of patients with mild to moderate claudication involves the following:

- Patient education and reassurance
- Modification of risk factors
- Exercise
- Pharmacologic therapy

The patient should initially be told the natural history of claudication. Most patients with claudication smoke cigarettes, and a major effort should be made to break this addiction. Daily exercise increases walking distance in about two-thirds of patients. Two theories for this effect exist: 1) an increase in collateral channels of circulation and 2) a conditioning of the muscle beds that increases their efficiency in dealing with a limited blood supply. Drug treatment usually includes aspirin (325 mg/d) and pentoxifylline at 400 mg three times daily. Randomized studies have documented a modest increase in patients' walking distance with the use of pentoxifylline. Only in patients with severe, disabling claudica-

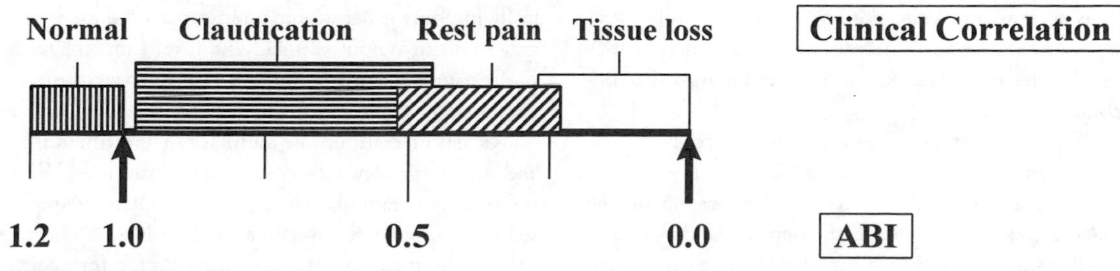

FIGURE 18.4.
Ankle/brachial index and clinical correlation.

TABLE 18.3. Indications for Invasive Diagnostic and Therapeutic Interventions for Occlusive Disease

Clinical Presentation	Invasive Diagnostic and Therapeutic Intervention
Intermittent claudication (walk > 1 block)	Not indicated
Severe claudication (walk < ½ block)	Indicated if it limits lifestyle
Rest pain	Indicated but may be done electively
Tissue loss, with nonhealing ischemic ulcer	Indicated; assess aggressively

tion should surgery be considered. Balloon angioplasty may be an option when aortoiliac stenosis is suspected, because the results in these cases are often good.

In patients with ischemic rest pain, tissue loss, or gangrene, surgical referral is clearly indicated. Advances in surgical techniques and anesthetic management allow bypass surgery to be performed safely and effectively. Five-year patency rates exceed 80% for aortoiliac reconstructive procedures and are approximately 70% for infrainguinal bypasses. In some patients with severe comorbid conditions, primary amputation may be the best option.

VENOUS DISEASE

To better understand the pathophysiology of venous disease, knowledge of the normal anatomy and physiology of the venous system is essential. In humans, the veins of the lower extremity can be separated into three systems:

- Superficial
- Deep
- Perforator

The **superficial venous system** consists of the greater saphenous vein, the lesser saphenous vein. and the tributaries of these two veins. Blood from the foot and medial aspect of the knee drain into the greater saphenous vein. The greater saphenous vein then empties into the common femoral vein, and the lesser saphenous terminates in the popliteal vein. The superficial veins are involved in varicose vein problems, and it is usually the secondary and tertiary tributaries that become varicose.

The **deep system of veins** follows the course of the major arteries of the leg and shares their names. These veins form the major venous drainage system of the lower extremity. In the calf, the perineal and posterior tibial veins are the deep veins that drain most of the blood of the musculature of the calf and then join at the knee to form the popliteal vein. This continues in the thigh as the superficial femoral vein, which is joined by the deep femoral vein to form the common femoral vein.

The **perforator veins** connect the deep and superficial veins in the lower extremity. These veins, which are more numerous below the knee, typically penetrate the fascia of the leg to connect the superficial and deep systems. Valves of the perforator veins direct blood from the superficial to deep venous system. The major driving force for venous return in the lower extremity is the pumping action of the muscles of the calf and thigh. During exercise, the calf muscle pump reduces venous pressure in the deep veins by emptying them; when the muscles relax, the superficial veins rapidly drain into the deep system.

Venous Stasis

About 50% of patients with acute deep venous thrombosis develop the post-thrombotic syndrome as a result of chronic venous insufficiency. The pathophysiology of venous thrombosis involves recanalization of the deep veins with resultant deformity and incompetence of the venous valves. The deep venous system then effectively transmits the gravitational pressure of the blood column unimpeded from the level of the heart to the ankles. This, coupled with incompetent perforating veins, results in transmission of the high venous pressure to the superficial tissues of the leg. The perforator veins in the lower leg near the medial malleolus are clinically important because incompetence of these vessels may result in venous stasis ulcers. Over time, the result is often stasis dermatitis (brawny skin changes caused by hemosiderin from the stagnant blood) or eventual venous stasis ulceration. The **hallmark of treatment** is leg and foot elevation with compression stockings. While the patient is ambulating, an Unna boot impregnated stocking applied for weeks at a time is also effective therapy. Surgical therapy, including perforator vein ligation and venous reconstruction, is not often used and offers variable results.

Varicose Veins

The anatomic distribution of varices is determined by inspection of the legs in the recumbent and standing positions. Patients with primary varicose veins report heaviness, aching, burning, fatigue, throbbing, or pain that may be relieved by walking, leg elevation, or external compression. Hand-held Doppler and duplex ultrasonography are essential in defining the extent of the disease and evaluating the patency of the deep system. Treatment options for varicose veins include elastic compression support, surgical removal of the varices and vein stripping, and sclerotherapy.

Deep Venous Thrombosis

The pathophysiology of venous thrombosis involves disruption of the endothelium, platelet deposition, and the formation of a hemostatic plug. In 1856, Virchow introduced the term "thrombosis" and the three potential mechanisms responsible for this condition (Virchow's triad):

1. Stasis
2. Endothelial damage
3. Hypercoagulability

The usual location for the formation of a nidus of thrombus is the venous valvular sinuses. A propagating thrombus may become attached to the opposite wall, causing interrupted flow, retrograde thrombosis, and signs of venous stasis in the extremity. Alternatively, the thrombus may propagate without occluding flow and develop a long, floating tail that may embolize to the lungs, causing pulmonary embolism.

TABLE 18.4. Clinical Aspects of Deep Venous Thrombosis

Event	Incidence (%)
Patients presenting with signs and symptoms of DVT who actually have DVT	30–50
Calf DVTs that are clinically demonstrable	5
Above the knee DVTs that present with clinically demonstrable signs and symptoms	40–50

DVT, deep venous thrombosis.

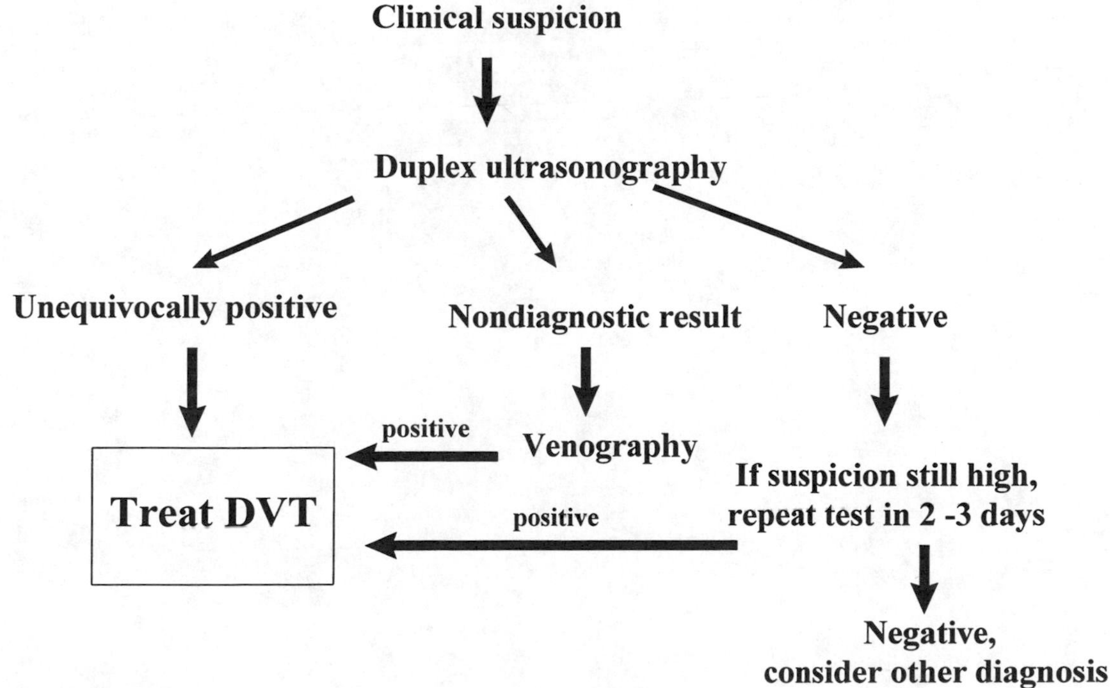

FIGURE 18.5.
Diagnostic evaluation of deep venous thrombosis.

Diagnosis

Deep venous thrombosis is diagnosed according to clinical observations and results of confirmatory tests. Clinical suspicion should always compel the practitioner to pursue further diagnostic workup of these patients, although only 30 to 50% of patients who appear with signs and symptoms of deep venous thrombosis actually have the condition. In addition, 5% of patients with calf deep venous thrombosis show clinical evidence of the disease state (Table 18.4). The severity of the clinical presentation is determined by the following:

- Location and extent of the thrombosis
- Degree of resulting occlusion
- Presence or absence of collaterals

Venous obstruction and hypertension are greater in patients with thrombosis of the proximal ileofemoral and femoral veins than in those with thrombosis of the calf veins. The most reliable confirmatory tests for deep venous thrombosis are duplex ultrasonography and contrast venography (Fig. 18.5). When performed properly, these tests are equivalent in making the diagnosis.

Treatment

The mainstay of treatment of deep venous thrombosis is anticoagulation, first with heparin and then with warfarin. In some instances, lytic therapy with urokinase or its equivalent plus placement of a vena caval filter may be useful. In rare instances of limb-threatening ileofemoral thrombosis, surgical thrombectomy may be needed.

KEY POINTS

Peripheral Vascular Disease

- Characterization: Common (occurs more frequently in men than in women); danger of rupture and sudden death; 90% infrarenal.
- Cause: Usually atherosclerosis.
- Diagnosis: Usually asymptomatic. Triad of palpable abdominal mass, abdominal or back pain, and hypotension = rupture. Aneurysm greater than 5 cm is usually associated with calcium in the aorta. Definitive diagnosis: B-mode ultrasonography or computed tomography.
- Management: Refer to vascular surgeon without delay. Mortality rate with elective surgery for nonruptured aneurysm, 3 to 5%.

Iliac, Femoral, and Popliteal Aneurysms

- Iliac aneurysms: Occur with abdominal aortic aneurysms. Difficult to detect on abdominal examination; easier on rectal or pelvic examination. Lower abdominal, flank, or pelvic pain. Ultrasonography or computed tomography: diameter greater than 3 cm, refer to vascular surgery.
- Femoral aneurysm: Common, bilateral in 50% of patients. Three-quarters of patients are symptomatic: arterial ischemia, local compression, pain. Rupture is rare. Treatment: diameter greater than 2.5 cm, refer to vascular surgeon.
- Popliteal aneurysms. Disease of the elderly. Occurs more frequently in men than in women. Half of cases are associated with other aneurysms. Symptoms of leg ischemia. Rupture is rare. Treatment is symptomatic, surgical.

Carotid Artery Disease

- Cause: Atherosclerotic plaque at the carotid bifurcation. Symptoms due to emboli (transient ischemic attacks, amaurosis fugax, stroke).
- Diagnosis: Search for risk factors; carotid bruits, duplex scanning. Definitive diagnosis: angiography.
- Management: Asymptomatic: stenosis greater than 50 to 80%, refer to vascular surgeon. Symptomatic: medical therapy; aggressively treat risk factors; antiplatelet agents (aspirin, ticlopidine, dipyridamole). Surgical therapy: with stenosis greater than 70%, surgery is clearly beneficial. With stenosis of 30 to 70%, surgery is controversial.

Arterial Occlusion: Thrombosis and Embolism

- Medical and surgical emergencies. Rapid differentiation a must.
- Cause: Acute arterial occlusion, embolus from the heart. Acute thrombosis, rupture of a preexisting atherosclerosis plaque.
- Diagnosis: "5 Ps" (pain, pallor, pulselessness, paresthesia, and paralysis). Careful examination of the pulses.
- Treatment: Intravenous heparin (bolus of 5000 to 10,000 U and infusion of 1000 U/h).
- Presentation of chronic arterial insufficiency: asymptomatic, claudication; symptomatic, pain at rest. Diagnosis: Segmented arterial pressure. Management: Mild to moderate claudication; medical management (insufficiency progresses in smokers and diabetic patients): exercise program, risk factor modification. Ischemic rest pain, refer to the vascular surgeon.

Venous Disease

- Venous stasis: 50% of patients with deep venous thrombosis, edema, and stasis dermatitis. Treatment: Leg and foot exercise and compression stockings.
- Varicose veins: Evaluate with handheld Doppler scanner and duplex ultrasonography. Treatment: Elastic compression support, surgical removal, sclerotherapy.
- Deep venous thrombosis: High index of suspicion. Venous obstruction and hypertension are greater in patients with thrombosis of the proximal iliofemoral and femoral veins.
- Diagnosis: Duplex ultrasonography and contrast venography.
- Treatment: Heparin and warfarin remain the mainstay. Refer to vascular surgeon when considering the possibility of lytic therapy or vena caval filter.

SUGGESTED READINGS

Aneurysms

ADAM VA Cooperative Study Group. Variability in measurement of abdominal aortic aneurysms. J Vasc Surg 1995; 21:945.

Bicherstaff LK, Hollier LH, Van Peenan HJV, et al. Abdominal aortic aneursym: the changing natural history. J Vasc Surg 1984;1:6–12.

Cronenwett JL, Murphy TF, Zelenock GB, et al. Actuarial analysis of variables associated with rupture of small abdomial aortic aneursms. Surgery 1985;98:472–483.

Ernst CB. Abdominal aortic aneurysm. N Engl J Med 1993;328:1167–1173.

Hollier LH, Taylor LM, Ochsner J. Recommended indications for operative treatment of abdominal aortic aneurysms. J Vasc Surg 1992;15:1046–1056.

Nevitt MP, Ballard DJ, Hallett JW Jr. Prognosis of abdominal aortic aneurysms: a population-based study. N Engl J Med 1989;321:1011.

Carotid Artery

Executive Committee for the Asymptomatic Carotid Atherosclerosis Study (ACAS). Endarterectomy for aymptomatic carotid artery stenosis. JAMA. 1995;273: 1421–1428.

Moore WS, Barnett HJ, Beebe HG, et al. Guidelines for carotid endaterectomy. A multidisciplinary consensus statement from the ad hoc committee, American Heart Association. Stroke 1995;26:188–201.

North American Symptomatic Carotid Endarterectomy Trial Collaborators. Beneficial effect of carotid endarterectomy in symptomatic patients with high grade carotid stenosis. N Engl J Med 1991;325:445–453.

Arterial Insufficiency/Venous Disease

Clagett GP, Krupski WC. Antithrombotic therapy in peripheral arterial occlusive disease. Chest 1995;108 (Suppl):431S.

Ernst CB, Stanley J. Current Therapy in Vascular Surgery. St. Louis: Mosby, 1995.

Imparato AM, Kim GE: Intermittent claudication: its natural course. Surgery 1975;78:795–799.

Kempczinski R. The Ischemic Leg. Chicago: Year Book; 1985.

Moore WS. Vascular surgery: a comprehensive review. Philadelphia: WB Saunders; 1991.

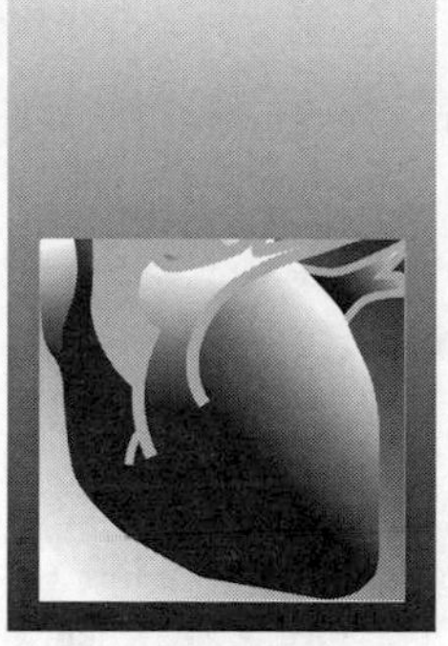

CHAPTER 19

Congestive Heart Failure

Michael L. Hess
David E. Tolman

BACKGROUND

Congestive heart failure represents the end stage of many of the causes of heart disease. A good working definition of congestive heart failure, formulated by Eugene Braunwald, states that "Congestive heart failure is a pathophysiologic state in which cardiac output is inadequate to meet the metabolic needs of the body." This is obviously an all-encompassing statement that includes both systolic dysfunction of the myocardium (which commonly produces the congestive heart failure syndrome) and diastolic dysfunction. Ninety percent of patients who are seen by the primary care physician present with systolic dysfunction.

In this context, congestive heart failure is defined as a systemic syndrome produced as a result of a failing myocardium or a significant increase in left ventricular end-diastolic pressure despite normal cardiac function. For example, a cardiomyopathic process is defined as a left ventricular ejection fraction less than 40%. The resultant decrease in cardiac output sets into motion a series of pathophysiologic sequences that produces the congestive heart failure syndrome. An example of congestive heart failure with normal ventricular function is moderate to severe mitral or aortic regurgitation, which, in turn, can elevate left ventricular and left atrial pressure and produce the congestive heart failure syndrome despite a left ventricular ejection fraction greater than 50%. Cardiomyopathy is treated medically, and the mitral or aortic insufficiency is treated first medically and then with appropriate valve repair or replacement. This distinction is important. If the primary care provider is faced with this dilemma, referral to a cardiologist is recommended.

Two basic, underappreciated problems occur with patients who have congestive heart failure:

1. Frequency of the disease
2. Fatality of the disease

Congestive heart failure is a common disease. In 1994, 454,000 patients with new occurrences of symptomatic heart failure were discharged from hospitals in the United States. Congestive heart failure represents the most common diagnosis-related group (DRG) classification for Medicare. In 1995, approximately 702,000 patients were in this category.

Congestive heart failure is a fatal disease. The Framingham data show that about 50% of men and 34% of women die within 4 years of disease onset. If a primary care physician elects to refer a patient to a cardiologist or to a center with expertise in heart failure, this selected patient population can carry up to a 20 to 40% 1-year mortality rate. Indeed, these patients are at an extremely high risk.

CAUSES

The causes of congestive heart failure are listed in Table 19.1. The leading cause of congestive heart failure remains coronary artery disease presenting as ischemic cardiomyopathy. The reason for this is twofold:

First, a large proportion of patients with myocardial infarction develop ischemic cardiomyopathy. Second, the U.S. population is aging. The fastest-growing segment of the U.S. population consists of persons older than 80 years of age. Medical science has yet to dissect out the aging process from coronary artery disease.

The second most common presentation, especially in younger patients, is primary, dilated cardiomyopathy (Fig. 19.1). The causes of dilated cardiomyopathies are many. The most common causes of primary, dilated cardiomyopathies in the United States include:

- Alcohol
- Familial cardiomyopathies
- Molecular defects in the genetic sequence
- Adriamycin and radiation, especially in women
- Numerous viral causes

Congestive heart failure caused by hypertension is decreasing significantly in the United States. This decrease

TABLE 19.1. Causes of Congestive Heart Failure

Coronary artery disease
- Greater than 50% of all patients with congestive heart failure have coronary artery disease; this percentage is increasing
- Better care after acute myocardial infarction
- Aging population

Cardiomyopathy
- Multiple causes: alcohol-related, sarcoid, genetic, familiar
- Occurs more frequently in men than in women

Hypertension
- Incidence is decreasing

Valvular heart disease
- Calcific aortic stenosis in the elderly
- Mitral valve syndrome in younger patients
- Rheumatic heart disease in the "medically underserved" parts of the world

Congenital heart disease

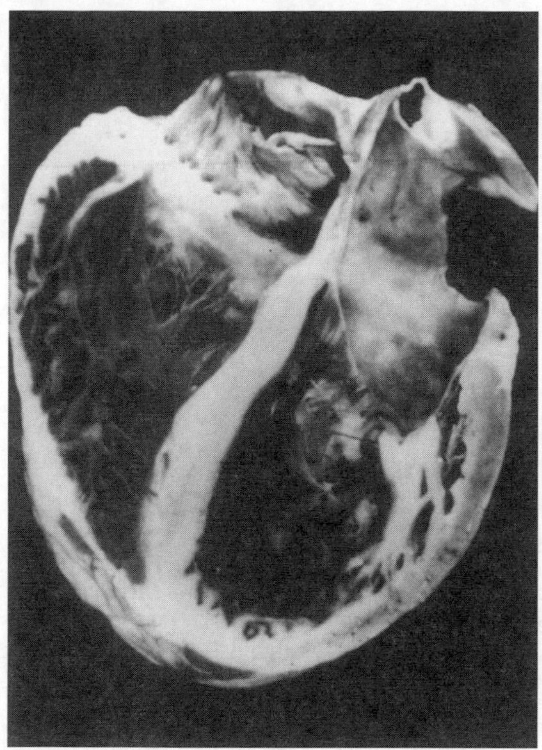

FIGURE 19.1.
Gross pathology of a case of dilated cardiomyopathy. Four-chamber enlargement and dilatation of both atria and ventricles are present. Note the marked thinning of the free walls of both the right and left ventricle and the intraventricular septum. This pathologic process results in a significant increase in biventricular volumes.

is due to extensive work by the entire medical community. However, the number of patients with congestive heart failure due to hypertension is still high. Valvular heart disease is limited to calcific aortic stenosis in the elderly and the mitral valve syndromes in younger patients in the United States.

Rheumatic heart disease has declined significantly in North America and Europe but is still a major problem in underdeveloped countries. Cases of rheumatic fever still occur in the United States. Whether these occurrences will translate into a reemergence of rheumatic heart disease is unknown but is worth considering.

The frequency of congenital heart disease is stable. With treatment, children who have complex, congenital heart disease remain healthy throughout childhood, adolescence, and early adulthood. Dilated, congestive cardiomyopathy becomes a problem in the third and fourth decades of life.

PATHOPHYSIOLOGY

Cardiomyopathy, which is defined as a left ventricular ejection fraction less than 40%, causes a decrease in contractility of the heart. As can be seen from Figure 19.2, this decrease in contractility produces a decrease in cardiac output. The decrease in cardiac output then activates a "neurohumoral storm." This storm is responsible for the original theory that the patient undergoes a series of compensatory mechanisms. These mechanisms, however, are not compensatory but rather pathophysiologic.

The principle reason for this pathophysiologic sequence is that the major sensor mechanisms—the **baroreceptor system** and the **kidney**—cannot perceive a decrease in cardiac output from hypovolemia. The decrease in cardiac output activates a series of mechanisms aimed at increasing total peripheral resistance and increasing intravascular volume. This pathophysiologic sequence includes activation of the sympathetic nervous system in patients with congestive heart failure; this is responsible for

- Resting tachycardia
- Cold clammy skin
- Diaphoresis
- Narrow pulse pressure

Plasma catecholamine levels markedly increase, and the norepinephrine level directly correlates with the prognosis—the higher the norepinephrine level, the worse the prognosis. The renin-angiotensin system is activated as part of this renally mediated sequence. Angiotensin I is cleaved by converting enzyme to angiotensin II. Angiotensin II, like norepinephrine, is a potent vasoconstrictor but is also a ubiquitous neurohormone. Angiotensin II stimulates the hypothalamus and, as a result, drives the thirst mechanism.

The patient who presents to the primary care physician with heart failure and hyponatremia is compelled to drink large quantities of water because of the effect of angiotensin II on the hypothalamus. Angiotensin II stimulates the posterior pituitary to increase the generation of antidiuretic hormone. This, in turn, increases intravascular volume. The older name for antidiuretic hormone is vasopressin, another potent vasoconstrictor. Angiotensin feeds to the adrenal cortex and increases the generation of aldosterone, which, in turn, increases intravascular volume. Thus, this "neurohumoral storm" (composed of norepinephrine, angiotensin II, antidiuretic hormone, and recently identified endothelin) bombards the periphery, increasing intravascular volume and increasing systemic vascular resistance. This increase in systemic vascular resistance increases the im-

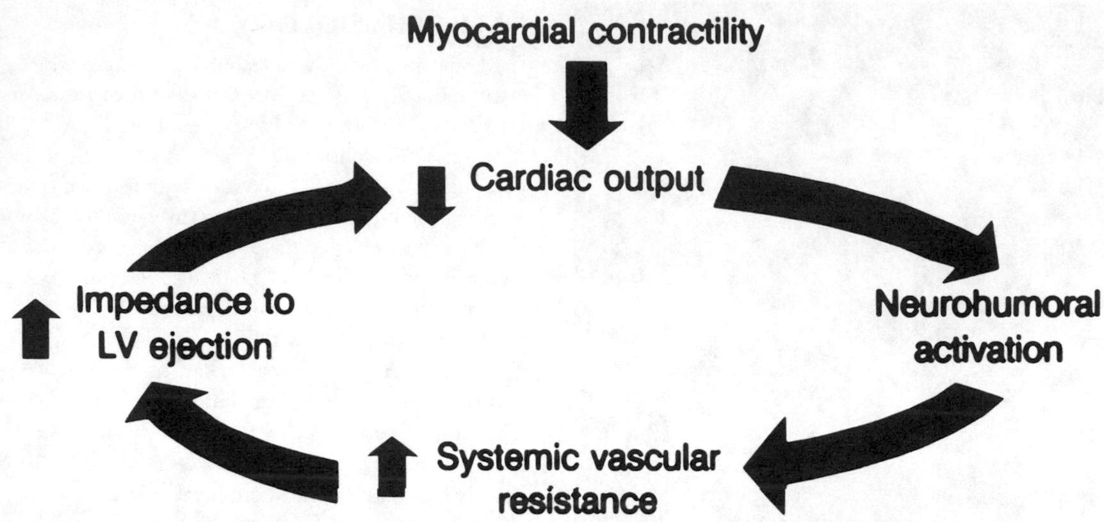

FIGURE 19.2.
The positive feedback loop of the pathophysiology of decompensated congestive heart failure. Each of the various causes of congestive heart failure produces a decrease in myocardial contractility, which then causes a decrease in cardiac output and activates the "neurohumoral storm": norepinephrine angiotensin, antidiuretic hormone, and endothelin, which cause a significant increase in systemic vascular resistance. This increase in resistance increases the impedance to left ventricular (*LV*) ejection, which results in a further decrease in stroke volume and cardiac output, which further activates the neurohumoral storm. Thus, the patient is caught in a progressive vicious cycle of positive feedback that can result in decompensated heart failure.

pedance to left ventricular ejection, which is the resistance the heart must overcome in order to eject its normal stroke volume. This further decreases stroke volume and cardiac output; the patient with congestive heart failure is then caught in a vicious circle of positive feedback, with a progressive decrease in cardiac output and an increase in systemic vascular resistance at the expense of a decrease in left ventricular ejection. All of these steps lead to the downhill spiral of decompensated congestive heart failure.

CLINICAL MANIFESTATIONS

Congestive heart failure has no predilection for any specific age group. However, the peak incidence is between the ages of 35 to 74 years, with a preponderance of men over women with both coronary artery disease and dilated cardiomyopathies. Congestive heart failure has a wide spectrum of clinical presentations. Patients can be asymptomatic for months to years, with incidental findings of cardiomegaly seen on routine chest radiography. At the other extreme, the initial clinical presentation can be acute pulmonary edema manifested by ventricular failure, malignant arrhythmias, or even cardiac arrest. The clinical symptoms of congestive failure are usually reflected as a combination of "forward failure"—reduced cardiac output with the symptoms of fatigue, weakness, and decreased exercise tolerance—and "backward failure"—pulmonary congestion without systemic congestion. Often, the initial symptoms are symptoms of left ventricular failure:

- Dyspnea
- Dyspnea on exertion
- Orthopnea
- Paroxysmal nocturnal dyspnea

Symptoms occurring later in the disease often reflect right ventricular failure and usually indicate a poor prognosis:

- Peripheral edema
- Hepatomegaly
- Ascites

Anginal chest pain as a presenting symptoms at the time of diagnosis occurs in 20 to 40% of patients. The anginal symptoms in these patients may be related to subendocardial ischemia resulting from decreased perfusion associated with increased left ventricular end-diastolic pressure. Exercise tolerance and symptoms often do not correlate with the severity of left ventricular failure. Many patients with severe left ventricular dysfunction (ejection fractions < 20%) are minimally symptomatic and have good exercise reserve.

Physical signs vary depending on the stage of congestive heart failure. Findings on physical examination may also vary; patients may appear to be normal or may show classic signs of decompensated left ventricular failure. Patients with **left ventricular failure** may develop the following signs and symptoms:

- Tachypnea
- Wheezing
- Pulmonary rales
- Decreased breath sounds during auscultation
- Dullness to percussion (suggesting pleural effusion)

In the **final stage of severely reduced cardiac output,** the following physical signs and symptoms are present:

- Hypotension with a narrow pulse pressure and a resting tachycardia caused by the sympathetic overdrive
- Weak peripheral pulses due to the decrease in stroke volume with poor capillary refill
- Cold and cyanotic extremities, signifying poor perfusion due to significant peripheral vasoconstriction and decreased stroke volume
- Hypokinetic and laterally displaced left ventricular impulse on palpation
- Possible right ventricular impulse, best identified in the subxiphoid area

Auscultation may reveal the following:

- Regurgitant murmurs from mitral and tricuspid regurgitation due to dilatation of the base of the heart and abnormal closure of the valves
- An S_4 gallop, signifying decreased compliance of the ventricle
- Development of the S_3 gallop, a hallmark on physical examination of the failing left ventricle
- Both S_3 and S_4 gallop sounds combined into a summation gallop

The physical signs of **concomitant right ventricular failure** (jugular venous distention, hepatomegaly, and peripheral edema) and of left ventricular failure (an S_3 gallop) are present in less than one-third of patients at the time of diagnosis. These signs of biventricular failure usually imply a poor prognosis.

LABORATORY STUDIES

In addition to the history and physical examination, the clinical diagnosis of congestive heart failure depends on a **noninvasive evaluation.** The importance of laboratory information relies mainly on the exclusion of preexisting or coexisting cardiac disease.

Initial evaluation of all patients who present with congestive heart failure should include resting electrocardiog-raphy for the determination of the presence or absence of myocardial ischemia and lateral and posterior-anterior chest radiography. The most common presenting finding on chest radiography is left ventricular enlargement resulting in a cardiothoracic ratio exceeding 0.5 (a typical chest radiography is shown in Fig. 19.3). As left ventricular function deteriorates below a critical level (ejection fraction < 30%), several conditions develop:

- Pulmonary venous congestion
- Interstitial edema
- Alveolar edema
- Pleural effusions (in heart failure, the right pleural effusion may be greater than the left)

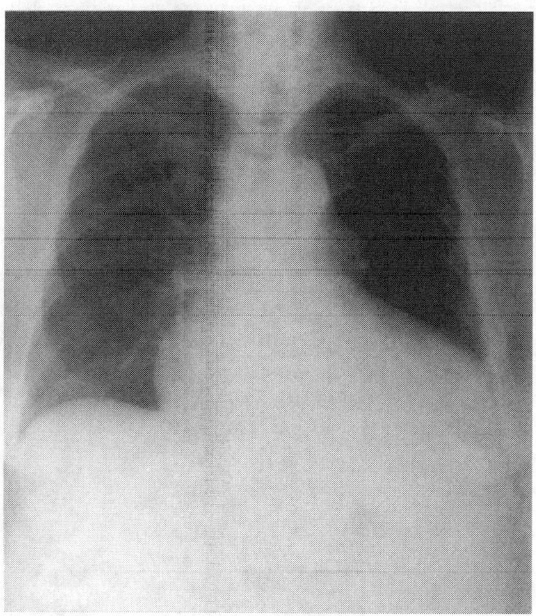

FIGURE 19.3.

Chest radiograph in the posterior-anterior view of a 54-year-old man with documented primary cardiomyopathy and an ejection fraction of 20%. The radiograph demonstrates both the pathology and pathophysiology of this patient with decompensated congestive heart failure. There are left ventricular enlargement and dilatation (cardiothoracic ratio > 0.5) together with a left pleural effusion and residual pulmonary venous hypertension as a result of the increase in left ventricular end-diastolic pressure and left atrial pressure.

Electrocardiography

Common electrocardiographic abnormalities include nonspecific S-T and T-wave changes with or without left ventricular hypertrophy and intraventricular conduction delays. Left bundle-branch block is more common than right bundle-branch block and is often the presenting feature in asymptomatic patients. T-wave inversion in the absence of discrete myocardial infarction may be present depending on the extent of myocardial fibrosis, especially in primary cardiomyopathies. Abnormal P waves suggestive of right or left atrial enlargement are seen in the latter stages of the disease. Atrial flutter or atrial fibrillation have been observed in about 20% of patients at the time of diagnosis. Ventricular dysrhythmias are frequently recorded on ambulatory Holter monitors, and up to 90% of patients with New York Heart Association class III and class IV congestive heart failure show multiform premature contractions or nonsustained ventricular tachycardia. Patients with complex ventricular dysrhythmia carry a significantly higher mortality rate. Some patients with complex ventricular dysrhythmia and reduced left ventricular ejection fraction appear to be at high risk for sudden death.

Echocardiography

Echocardiography is a cornerstone of the noninvasive diagnostic evaluation of patients with congestive heart failure. In addition to its role in assessing the morphologic changes (this can be seen from Fig. 19.4), echocardiography provides valuable information on chamber size, wall thickness, atrial enlargement, regurgitant flow, and pulmonary artery pressures. Echocardiography also identifies important physiologic aspects of the heart. Global hypokinesis with ejection fractions less than 30% and a left ventricular end-diastolic dimension of 5.0 cm or greater marks a symptomatic stage of congestive heart failure. Although global hypokinesis is the rule, regional wall-motion abnormalities have been described as a secondary phenomenon in dilated congestive cardiomyopathies. In addition to examining ventricular size and function, echocardiography is also helpful in assessing the anatomy and function of the valves, visualizing thrombi, and identifying pericardial involvement. All patients presenting with the signs and symptoms of congestive heart failure should undergo echocardiography.

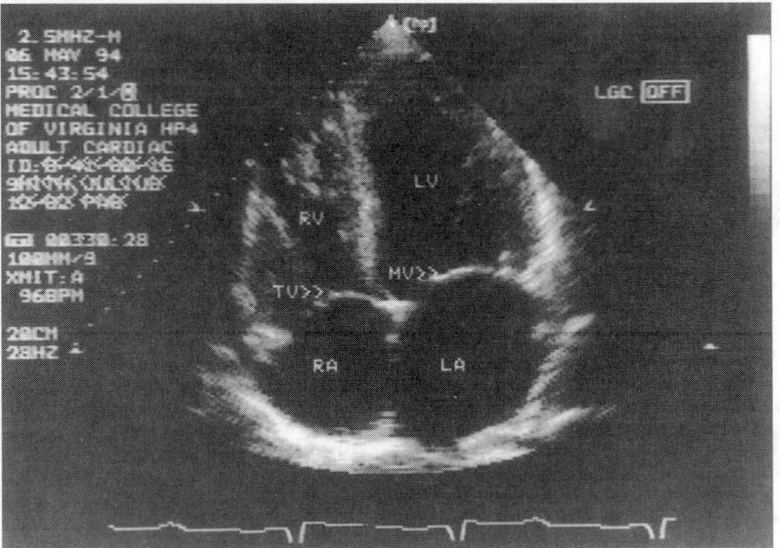

FIGURE 19.4.

Two-dimensional echocardiogram in the apical view in a patient with decompensated congestive heart failure. The left ventricular internal diameter (*LV*) is enlarged to 7.0 cm (normal, 3.3 to 6.1 cm), and the left atrium (*LA*) is significantly dilated to 7.0 cm (normal, 2.8 to 4.3 cm). The right ventricle and right atrium are also dilated, with internal diameters of 5 cm (normal, 2.2 cm to 4.4 cm) and 6 cm (normal, 2.5 to 4.9 cm), respectively. Thus, the echocardiogram demonstrates excellent correlation with the gross pathology (see Fig. 19.1). (Courtesy of Dr. J.V. Nixon, Echocardiographic Laboratories, Medical College of Virginia Hospitals, Richmond, Virginia).

Referral

After diagnostic testing, the primary care provider should strongly consider referring the patient to a cardiologist. The cardiologist, using information provided by the primary care physician, can decide whether to proceed with cardiac catheterization, which would identify a potentially surgically reversible lesion. Cardiac catheterization can answer several questions:

- Is coronary artery obstruction producing hibernating myocardium?
- Are the murmurs of mitral or tricuspid regurgitation primary or secondary?
- Is there a significant element of diastolic dysfunction?

Furthermore, the cardiologist will be able to distinguish the rare case of a restrictive cardiomyopathy from the more common congestive cardiomyopathy. On the basis of this consultation with the patient, the primary care physician and the cardiologist can decide whether a surgically correctable lesion is present and whether the patient is an acceptable candidate for cardiac surgery.

Radionuclide Studies

Radionuclide ventriculography and left ventricular angiography, like echocardiography, can demonstrate ventricular dilatation, impaired diastolic function, and other options that can be used to follow the course of the disease in response to therapy.

Invasive Studies

Cardiac catheterization is desirable in all patients in whom coronary artery disease is the underlying cause of congestive heart failure that is associated with concomitant coronary atherosclerosis. Reduced left ventricular function due to hibernating myocardium in coronary artery disease is potentially reversible by revascularization. **Hemodynamic studies** often demonstrate elevation in pulmonary capillary wedge pressure and left ventricular end-diastolic pressure. Elevations of right ventricular end-diastolic pressure, right atrial pressure, and central venous pressure may signify concomitant right ventricular dysfunction and a poor prognosis.

The therapeutic usefulness of myocardial biopsy in dilated congestive cardiomyopathies is controversial. The most common histologic findings are of myocyte hypertrophy and interstitial fibrosis. These findings, along with the electron microscopic findings of mitochondrial swelling, loss of myofibrils, and vacuolization of the sarcoplasmic reticulum, are not specific and do not seem to affect overall patient management. Myocardial biopsy is a useful research tool, but the anticipation that tissue diagnosis in dilated cardiomyopathies would help the primary care physician manage the patient with congestive heart failure has not come to fruition. Indeed, myocardial biopsy is not recommended except in carefully selected cases, which should be discussed in detail with the referring cardiologist.

Summary of Diagnosis

- Causes include
  - Coronary artery disease
  - Cardiomyopathy
  - Valvular heart disease
  - Hypertension
- Male preponderance with coronary artery disease and cardiomyopathy
- History
  - Shortness of breath
  - Orthopnea
  - Paroxysmal nocturnal dyspnea
  - Peripheral edema
  - Fatigue
- Physical examination
  - Bilateral rales
  - S_3 gallop
  - Murmur of mitral regurgitation
  - Jugular venous distention
  - Pulsatile liver
  - Ascites
  - Peripheral edema
- Laboratory testing
  - Electrocardiographic findings vary.
  - Echocardiography reveals left ventricular ejection fraction less than 40%.
  - Chest radiography indicates cardiomegaly and pulmonary venous hypertension.

MANAGEMENT

Nonpharmacologic

The management of congestive heart failure, especially by nonpharmacologic means, is important (Table 19.2). The physician must maintain a positive attitude. At the authors' institution, physicians tell all of their patients that the "ultimate goal is to return you (the patient) to a lifestyle that you and your family define—not a lifestyle defined by a gray-haired doctor in a long white coat."

TABLE 19.2. Lifestyle Modifications in Patients with Congestive Heart Failure

Encourage isotonic exercise
- Walking, hiking, golf, etc.

Forbid isometric exercise
- Pushing cars, weight lifting, moving heavy furniture, etc.

Eliminate the salt shaker
- Extreme strict salt restriction difficult to achieve

Eliminate cigarette smoking

Minimize alcohol consumption
- Only in moderation and then discourage

Maintain good basic nutrition

Encourage attainment of ideal body weight

Encourage a normal, healthy lifestyle

Encourage a positive attitude

Nonpharmacologic management requires a great deal of physician time and patient education. Initial bedrest during the symptomatic period should be encouraged but should be followed rapidly by a progressive exercise program. This program helps to alleviate the signs and symptoms of heart failure; conditioning improves skeletal muscle function and contributes to the patient's overall well-being and quality of life (see Appendix B).

Salt restriction, together with an adequately balanced diet ensuring good caloric intake, is important. Because patients with symptomatic heart failure are in a negative nitrogen balance, the maintenance of nutrition becomes extremely important. An extremely important part of dietary control is maintenance of an ideal body weight. The obese patient should be encouraged to lose weight because excess weight represents an increased load to the heart. A carefully constructed exercise program can aid in achieving this goal.

Administration of low-flow oxygen continues to be part of the standard of care in the initial decompensated period, especially in patients with pulmonary hypertension. It is now well-documented that patients with symptomatic heart failure have significant sleep abnormalities and that nocturnal oxygen can improve the sleep difficulties. Moderate alcohol consumption and cessation of cigarette smoking are also mandatory. These important nonpharmacologic principles of heart failure management should not be underemphasized in favor of pharmacologic therapy.

Pharmacology

Pharmacologic therapy for symptomatic congestive heart failure has significantly changed and improved in the past 10 years. For many years, digoxin and diuretics alone or in combination were used to treat patients with heart failure, and they continue to be part of the mainstay of pharmacologic therapy.

Digoxin

Digoxin is the oldest drug used to treat congestive heart failure, especially in patients with superimposed supraventricular arrhythmias (Table 19.3). Digoxin alone has not been shown to improve survival, but it has clearly been shown to improve quality of life. Because medical professionals have been using digoxin for a long time, much is known about this drug. It can be given as monotherapy, and it can be loaded orally with the loading dose independent of the renal function. A simple guideline for the loading dose is the following:

0.25 mg every 6 hours in four doses,
for a total of 1 mg

The maintenance dose is then titrated to the patient's age, lean body mass, and renal function. As a general guideline, octogenarians, patients with a lower-than-average body mass, and patients with a serum creatinine level greater than 3.0 mg/dL should be maintained on 0.125 mg/day. Patients with normal renal function and younger patients can be maintained on 0.25 mg/day. The half-life of digoxin is in the range of 33 hours; 85% is renally excreted and only 15% is excreted via the enterohepatic circulation. Electrocardiography is very sensitive to the effects of digoxin (should the primary care physician desire a serum level, the radioimmunoassay of serum digoxin is readily available). There is absolutely no need to balance the serum digoxin level in the therapeutic range between 0.1 and 0.2 ng/mL. A major value of the serum digoxin level is to answer the question, "Is the patient ingesting and absorbing the digoxin, or do they have a great deal of excessive digoxin on board?" Furthermore, it must be kept in mind that the control of atrial fibrillation requires higher than normal serum digoxin level, in the range of 2 to 3 ng/dL.

Loop Diuretics

Loop diuretics are the cornerstone of diuretic therapy in the United States (Table 19.4); the loop diuretic furosemide remains the gold standard, having been used for 30 years. Furosemide is available in generic form in the United States, and its cost is therefore low compared with the proprietary version. Proprietary diuretics tend to be somewhat more predictable and somewhat shorter acting but are more expensive. Furthermore, furosemide has been used in all the trials that have demonstrated an

Pharmacologic Management of the Patient with Congestive Heart Failure by Using Digoxin **TABLE 19.3.**

Improves quality of life but does not increase survival
Once per day—monotherapy
Loading dose is independent of the renal function: e.g., 0.25 mg orally every 6 hours for four doses to a total dose of 1.0 mg
Titrate maintenance dose to age, lean body mass, and renal function
Radioimmunoassay is readily available
Electrocardiography is very sensitive to "digoxin toxicity"
Monitor for hypokalemia

Pharmacologic Management of the Patient with Congestive Failure by Using Furosemide **TABLE 19.4.**

30-year experience; now generic in the United States
Wide and safe dosing range
Available for both intravenous and oral use
Hypokalemia is a direct effect of the drug
May cause hyperuricemia or may cause clinical gout
Ototoxicity at high doses
Additive effect with metolazone (2.5–5.0 mg/d); watch for significant hypokalemia

increase in survival with combination therapy in congestive heart failure.

Hypokalemia is a direct result of furosemide therapy; when the drug is used in combination with digoxin, the patient's serum potassium level must be monitored carefully. If the serum potassium level begins to decrease to less than 4.0 mEq/L (to the range of 3.5 to 4.0 mEq/L), the patient's drug regimen should be supplemented with oral potassium. The dose range of furosemide is extremely wide (between 20 mg/d and 320 to 640 mg/d). Above these levels, ototoxicity may appear. The primary care physician must become adept at diagnosing and treating gout because high-dose furosemide therapy in combination with the congestive heart failure syndrome increases serum uric acid levels and sometimes leads to clinical gout.

Vasodilator Therapy

Vasodilator therapy, especially with angiotensin-converting enzyme (ACE) inhibitors, has revolutionized the treatment of heart failure (Table 19.5). The concept of vasodilator therapy with ACE inhibitors was first demonstrated in 1987 from Scandinavia in patients with functional New York Heart Association class III and class IV heart failure. The combination of digoxin, furosemide, and a long-acting ACE inhibitor (enalapril) significantly improved survival in these patients.

The superiority of triple drug therapy—digoxin, furosemide, and a long-acting ACE inhibitor—was further demonstrated in two hallmark studies performed in the United States. In 1991, the first of these studies showed that this therapy was efficacious in improving survival compared with the combination of digoxin, lasix, hydralazine, and isordil in patients with New York Heart Association class II and class III heart failure. In the second study, performed with a cross-sectional representation of the U.S. population, the comparison group was digoxin, furosemide, and any vasodilator combination the physician wished to put together. Eighty- five percent of these patients were receiving oral nitrate preparations. The study treatment was digoxin, furosemide, and enalapril. After 4 years, survival significantly increased in patients receiving digoxin, furosemide, and enalapril. Little doubt remains that the standard of care in congestive heart failure is digoxin, furosemide, and a long-acting ACE inhibitor (Table 19.6). Recently, the angiotensin-I receptor blocker losartan has been found to be beneficial in patients with New York Heart Association class II and class III heart failure. Patients who cannot tolerate ACE inhibitors can be switched safely to losartan (50 mg/d).

TABLE 19.5. **Pharmacologic Management of the Patients with Congestive Heart Failure Using Angiotensin-Converting Enzyme Inhibitors**

Enalapril increases survival in patients with NYHA class II, III, and IV heart failure
Hyperkalemia in the absence of renal dysfunction is usually not a problem and may decrease potassium chloride requirements
Before instituting therapy, ensure an arterial pressure of 90 mm Hg or greater and a serum sodium level greater than 134 mEq/L
Angioneurotic edema is class specific
Incidence of bothersome cough, 4–8% of patients
First-line therapy in NYHA class I, II, III, and IV heart failure

NYHA, New York Heart Association.

TABLE 19.6. **Standard of Care for Patients with Congestive Heart Failure in the United States**

New York Heart Association Heart Disease Class	Pharmacologic Treatment
Class I	Long-acting ACE inhibitor
Class II, III, and IV	Digoxin
	Loop diuretics (furosemide)
	ACE diuretics (survival benefit demonstrated with enalapril)

ACE, angiotensin-converting enzyme inhibitor.

A growing literature indicates that β-blockers may increase survival in patients with congestive heart failure. If the primary care physician is considering β-blocker therapy with carvedilol, the patient should be referred to the cardiologist for institution and upward titration of the drug. Carvedilol is not meant to be used in the decompensated patient.

Asymptomatic Patients

Class I heart failure is now defined as ejection fraction of less than 40% without symptoms. In a landmark study, asymptomatic patients were randomly assigned to receive placebo or enalapril. At the end of 4 years, the survival statistics clearly demonstrated a prolongation to the time of the onset of heart failure, a marked decrease in morbid events, and a marked decrease in hospital admissions in patients treated with enalapril and demonstrated the cost-effectiveness of this form of therapy.

A second major study in asymptomatic patients was performed in patients after myocardial infarction. The ejection fraction was measured 7 to 13 days after infarction; if it was less than 40%, the patients were randomly assigned to receive captopril (50 mg three times daily) or placebo plus their post–myocardial infarction drugs. Beginning 6 months after myocardial infarction and continuing for the 4 years of the study, there was a significant improvement in survival additive to the effects of thrombolytic therapy and β-blockers.

In summary, all major classes of heart failure should include long-acting ACE inhibitors as front-line therapy (Table 19.6).

Anticoagulation

The role of long-term anticoagulation is controversial. The current recommendation is that patients with normal sinus rhythm and congestive heart failure should not be submitted to the rigors of long-term warfarin therapy. The risks seem to outweigh the benefits in this patient population. However, the patient with heart failure and atrial fibrillation is a candidate for long-term anticoagulation; thus, a fourth or fifth drug—warfarin—must be added to their medical program. This necessitates careful monitoring of the prothrombin time and frequent adjustment of doses.

Other Considerations

Decompensated Heart Failure on an Adequate Oral Program

Decompensated congestive heart failure in symptomatic patients taking digoxin, furosemide, and an ACE inhibitor continues to carry unacceptable mortality and

Summary of Treatment

Nonpharmacologic treatment includes the following lifestyle modifications:

- Weight reduction
- Cessation of cigarette smoking
- Limitation of salt intake
- Regular exercise (forbid isometric exercise)
- Balanced diet
- Adequate rest

Pharmacologic treatment includes:
Class I heart failure:

- Left ventricular ejection failure less than 40% in the asymptomatic patient: long-acting ACE inhibitors

Class II, III, and IV (ambulatory) heart failure:

- Digoxin, furosemide, and long-acting ACE inhibitors
  - Digoxin, loading dose 0.75 to 1.25 mg
  - Maintenance dose adjusted to age, lean body mass, and renal function.
  - Furosemide, 20 to 1.20 mg; watch for hypokalemia and clinical gout
  - Long-acting ACE inhibitors, (e.g., enalapril, 5 to 10 mg twice daily)
- Potassium chloride supplementation to maintain serum potassium level at greater than 4.0 mEq/L
- Consider adding metolazone, 5 to 10 mg every other day, when furosemide dose exceeds 160 to 320 mg/d

morbidity rates. The Scandinavian trial reported a 45% mortality rate at 1 year in patients with class III and class IV congestive heart failure. When drug treatment proves inadequate, the primary care physician should seek cardiology consultation, which may lead to use of intravenous inotropic therapy.

Obviously, cardiac transplantation is an option, and the primary care physician should consider referring the candidate patient early in the course of their disease process. The cardiac transplantation procedure is donor-limited; only 3000 transplantations are performed per year. This is a small number of patients with heart failure. Intravenous inotropic therapy is the most common treatment currently used in patients with decompensated congestive heart failure. The two major drugs used include dobutamine (a sympathomimetic amine) and milrinone (a phosphodiesterase inhibitor). Patients with congestive heart failure are generally admitted to the hospital in the decompensated state and receive pharmacologic therapy for 3 to 5 days. Numerous programs of intermittent inotropic therapy in the outpatient and home environment have been devised for certain patients; these programs represent the forefront of clinical investigation. The primary care physician is urged to seek cardiology consultation when considering inotropic therapy. Evidence is promising that long-term intermittent therapy with either dobutamine or milrinone can significantly improve the patient's quality of life and reduce the number of hospitalizations. However, no data are available on long-term survival.

Sudden Death in Patients with Congestive Heart Failure

Data show that between 20% and 40% of patients with symptomatic heart failure die suddenly. Most sudden deaths are results of the fatal ventricular rhythms—ventricular tachycardia and ventricular fibrillation. Patients in class III heart failure are more predisposed to sudden death than patients in class IV failure. Electrocardiography with long rhythm strips, Holter monitoring, and telemetry performed in patients in class III heart failure often show nonsustained ventricular tachycardia. The problem in the patient with congestive heart failure is that all type I antiarrhythmics have been found to be "proarrhythmic"; that is, these drugs increase the incidence of ventricular tachycardia and ventricular fibrillation, thus increasing the incidence of sudden death. The newer antiarrhythmic agent, amiodarone, although showing some promise, has not been proven to decrease incidence of sudden death. Patients at risk for sudden death should be treated aggressively for their underlying heart failure; antiarrhythmic agents should not be administered. Indeed, some evidence shows that the aggressive therapy for heart failure decreases the incidence of sudden death. Patients who experience an episode of near–sudden death and survive should be referred for the placement of an automatic internal cardiac defibrillator. Evidence of long-term benefit to patients is currently under investigation.

Diastolic Dysfunction

Diastolic dysfunction is seen in patients with thick, noncompliant left ventricles, as is common with aortic stenosis and chronic hypertension. The function of hearts with diastolic dysfunction is characterized by small changes in volume that create large changes in pressure. Thus, the patient with diastolic dysfunction who is in a state of fluid overload develops pulmonary edema and may have an echocardiogram demonstrating an ejection fraction of 50%. (This is also commonly seen in hypertrophic obstructive cardiomyopathies.) Diastolic dysfunction is a difficult problem to manage because pharmacologic management is extremely limited. All efforts are aimed at maintaining an adequate intravascular volume while not causing overdiuresis. The next goal is to add calcium-channel blockers or β-blockers as negative inotropic agents in an effort to improve the compliance of the still, inelastic ventricle.

Currently recommended drugs include the β-blockers metoprolol, in the range of 50 to 100 mg twice daily, and sustained-release verapamil, 240 mg/d. Most of these data have been gathered from the literature on hypertrophic obstructive myopathy; by analogy, they are extended to the treatment of the hypertensive patient with diastolic dysfunction. This problem is extremely difficult to manage, and referral to a cardiologist for long-term care is suggested.

Acute Decompensated Heart Failure

Acute decompensated heart failure presenting with pulmonary edema, hypotension, and tachycardia, with or without tachyarrhythmias, should be treated as a life-threatening medical emergency. The patient should be transported to the emergency department with nasal oxygen and telemetry, and the following actions should be taken:

- The patient should be managed in the sitting position as much as possible.
- The airway should be patent, and, if necessary, the patient should be intubated and ventilated.
- A large peripheral intravenous line is inserted and malignant tachyarrhythmias treated immediately; if necessary, direct-current cardioversion is used.
- Rotating tourniquets are useful for treating acute pulmonary edema.
- Intravenous morphine, 2 to 4 mg, acts as a venodilator and relieves central nervous system anxiety.
- Sublingual nitroglycerin can be given immediately.
- Intravenous furosemide at 80 to 240 mg can be given to initiate diuresis and increase venous capacitance.
- Initiation of peripherally administered dobutamine or milrinone is the method for the most rapid cardiovascular stabilization.
- Hypertension that is not responding to oxygen, nitroglycerin, and morphine should be aggressively treated.
- Upon stabilization, the patient should be transferred to an intensive care unit, preferably a coronary care unit.
- Patients in the intensive care unit or coronary care unit should be evaluated for acute ischemia or myocardial infarction; arrhythmias should be controlled.

After 24 hours of inotropic therapy, treatment with digoxin, furosemide, and a long-acting ACE inhibitor can be initiated. These patients require a careful search for the cause of their decompensation.

Restrictive Cardiomyopathy

Restrictive cardiomyopathy is an uncommon form of primary "cardiac muscle disease" that is physiologically characterized by a marked decrease in compliance of both ventricles caused by an infiltration process. Thus, this form of heart disease is a unique subset of diastolic dysfunction—a failure to adequately fill the ventricle. Pathophysiologically, this form of heart disease behaves like constrictive pericardial disease. This distinction between constrictive pericardial disease and restrictive myocardial disease is one of the most difficult in clinical cardiology, and patients suspected of having either disease should be referred to a cardiologist.

The classic example of restrictive cardiomyopathy is amyloid heart disease. Other causes are iron overload states, sarcoidosis, and acute cardiac allograft rejection. In these processes, the heart is infiltrated with noncontractile material, including amyloid, protein, iron, and immunoretroactive cells. This infiltrate causes a stiff, noncompliant ventricle with resistance to filling and a subsequent decrease in end-diastolic volume. This, in turn, produces a decrease in stroke volume, a reflex resting tachycardia, and a decrease in cardiac output. The patients then develop the signs and symptoms of "forward failure": fatigue, dyspnea on exertion, and shortness of breath.

Because this is a problem of compliance, the reduced end-diastolic volume increases end-diastolic pressure, resulting in biatrial enlargement. On the left side, left atrial pressure and pulmonary venous pressure increase. These patients frequently develop bilateral pleural effusions. On the right side of the system, both pulmonary artery and systemic venous hypertension develop. The patient then develops jugular venous distention, ascites, and peripheral edema.

The patient will then present to the primary care team with the signs and symptoms of congestive heart failure with several perplexing findings:

- Electrocardiography generally demonstrates low voltage as a result of the infiltrative process.

- Chest radiography does not show cardiomegaly but rather a normal silhouette.
- Echocardiography demonstrates small ventricular chambers, a normal to slightly reduced ejection fraction, and biatrial enlargement.

With such findings, the cardiologist may wish to proceed with endomyocardial biopsy to diagnose an infiltrative process. Biopsy can be performed safely in these patients because of their thickened, infiltrated ventricles.

The distinction between restrictive and congestive cardiomyopathy is important because therapy for these conditions is diametrically opposed. Digoxin, diuretics, and ACE inhibitors are of little benefit to patients with restrictive cardiomyopathy. In fact, overdiuresis can lead to profound low-output syndromes and even shock because these patients entirely depend on an adequate preload to maintain cardiac output. This is an opportune time to recall the physician's oath: "First, do no harm." The patients must be told that they will maintain some peripheral edema; the usefulness of diuretic becomes a balancing act in order to make the patient comfortable. Because of the paucity of therapy (phlebotomy may be of benefit in iron-overload states) these patients require patience and perseverance from the primary care provider.

SUMMARY

Enormous progress has been made in the treatment of the congestive heart failure syndrome. Health professionals can improve the quality of life and improve survival with a better quality of life in all four classes of heart failure. Even in the best of circumstances, however, congestive heart failure still carries a high rate of morbidity and mortality; for example, the annual mortality rate for patients with class III and class IV heart failure is 40 to 50%. Herein lies the challenge. With increasing progress in pharmacologic, surgical, and nonpharmacologic management of congestive heart failure, physicians are at a threshold of new and innovative advances in therapeutics based on the understanding of the molecular pathology involved in the heart failure syndrome. These new concepts of therapeutics and management require careful dedication and hard work. Eventually, these seemingly insolvable problems can be solved with the discipline and imagination of the investigator.

KEY POINTS

- Look for the correctable lesion (e.g., valvular aortic stenosis, valvular or mitral insufficiency, or mitral stenosis.
- Ensure that coronary artery anatomy is noncorrectable. Cardiac catheterization indicates intracardiac pressures and coronary anatomy.
- Perform coronary bypass surgery or percutaneous transluminal coronary angioplasty if indicated
- Symptoms of ventricular tachycardia include
  - Syncope
  - Near-syncope
  - Near–sudden death (survivable)

Refer for electrophysiology study and possible intracardiac converter-defibrillator.

- Younger patients with class III or class IV heart failure: consider immediate referral to a transplant center.
- Patients with decompensated heart failure receiving an adequate oral program: consider referral to cardiologist for inotropic therapy.
- Continued patient education for lifestyle modifications and complex medical therapy.
- Newer forms of therapy include β-blockers and AT_2 receptor blockers.

SUGGESTED READINGS

Cohn JH, Archibald DG, Ziesche S, et al. Effect of vasodilator therapy on mortality in chronic congestive heart failure: results of a Veterans Administration Cooperative Study. N Engl J Med 1986;314:1547–1552.

Cohn JN, Johnson G, Ziesche S, et al. A comparison of enalapril with hydralazine-isosorbide dinitrate in the treatment of chronic congestive heart failure. N Engl J Med 1991;325:303–310.

CONSENSUS Trial Study Group. Effects of enalapril on mortality in severe congestive heart failure: Results of the Cooperative North Scandinavian Enalapril Survival Study (CONSENSUS). N Engl J Med 1987;316:1429–1435.

Hess ML, Pathak S. Dilated cardiomyopathies. In: O'Rourke RA, ed. Hurst's the heart. Update I.. New York: McGraw-Hill; 1996:124–145.

Kavinsky CJ, Parillo JE. Severe heart failure in cardiomyopathy: pathogenesis and treatment. In: Ayres SM, Grenvik A, Holbrook PR, et al, eds. Textbook of critical care. Philadelphia: W.B. Saunders; 1995:583–595.

McCall D. Advances in the treatment of congestive heart failure. In: O'Rourke RA, ed. Hurst's the heart. Update I. New York: McGraw-Hill; 1996:144–164.

Packer M, Lee WH, Kestler PD. Role of neurohumoral mechanisms in determining survival in patients with severe chronic heart failure. Circulation 1987;75(Suppl IV):80–92.

Parmley WW. Congestive heart failure. In: Messerli FH, ed. Cardiovascular drug therapy. Philadelphia: W.B. Saunders; 1996:10–13.

The SOLVD Investigators. Effect of enalapril on mortality and the development of heart failure in asymptomatic patients with reduced left ventricular ejection fractions. N Engl J Med 1992;327:685–691.

The SOLVD Investigators. Effect of enalapril on survival in patients with reduced left ventricular ejection fractions and congestive heart failure. N Engl J Med 1991;325:293–302.

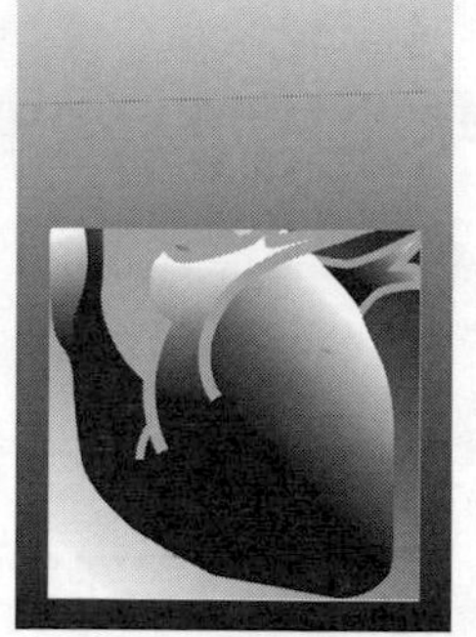

CHAPTER 20

Noncardiac Surgery

David W. Richardson

Philosopher Albert Camus
Says our knowledge is all askew.
Our beliefs all absurd
Was his final word.
About noncardiac surg'ry his view is too true
DWR

INTRODUCTION

Physicians often face requests to evaluate the risk for catastrophe in a person with known or suspected heart disease who is facing noncardiac surgery. Cardiologists extend the evaluation to consider whether intervention can reduce the risks, especially risk for death and myocardial infarction (the common, irrevocable complications of surgery). Our knowledge of the risks of noncardiac surgery can be stated only in terms of probabilities based on rather small numbers; this is not much guidance for a patient in whom the risk for coronary thrombosis after surgery is unknown. Coronary stenoses of 40 to 50% by angiography are more likely to progress to complete occlusion within months than are stenoses of 90%. Angiography cannot detect which of the former category of stenoses will rupture and obstruct the artery or when this would happen. It is simply not known whether the technologic cascade of diagnosis and treatment reduces the risks associated with noncardiac surgery.

PREVALENCE OF NONCARDIAC SURGERY

Data from the National Center for Health Statistics estimate the following:

- Three million major operations are performed annually in the United States.
- One million of these patients have coronary disease or more than two risk factors.
- Seventy-five thousand die or have myocardial infarction.
- Eighty thousand develop serious cardiac arrhythmia, congestive heart failure, or unstable angina.

Physicians have frequent opportunities to reduce physical, emotional, and financial distress by avoiding complex preoperative evaluation. Physicians are reluctant to depend on history and physical examination because of the insensitivity of these tests, especially for coronary disease.

TYPES OF HEART TROUBLE

Coronary artery disease is the most severe problem because of its prevalence and especially its unpredictability. One cannot foresee when or in whom myocardial infarction or sudden death will strike, but it is certain that myocardial infarction commonly complicates noncardiac surgery and is attended by high mortality rates after surgery. Myocardial ischemia without infarction occurs frequently during the first few days after surgery and is often a precursor of myocardial infarction. No data are available on whether intervention with drugs or revascularization benefits patients with myocardial ischemia. Congestive heart failure may delay surgery until the patient can lie flat without breathlessness; however, management of this condition with current drug therapy, although requiring attentiveness, does not necessarily suggest that surgery is contraindicated. Cardiac arrhythmia, recognized early by the ever-present monitors, is usually manageable but is cause for concern. Valvular disease presents little problem in planning for surgery if the patient can perform ordinary activities of daily life. Even aortic stenosis, with the accompanying threat of sudden death and the recognition that it is a big risk (according to the seminal study by Goldman and colleagues), can be managed safely. In 49 patients seen at the Mayo Clinic (mean age $>$ 70 years and mean transaortic pressure gradient $>$ 70 mm Hg), noncardiac surgery resulted in no deaths.

GOALS OF PREOPERATIVE CONSULTATION

In evaluating a candidate for noncardiac surgery, the physician's major goals are to

- Prevent death
- Prevent myocardial infarction
- Reduce suffering
- Limit cost

Although health professionals still cannot prevent perioperative myocardial infarction or death attributable to this event, the physician can recognize myocardial infarction after surgery. Myocardial infarction most often occurs several (3 to 6) days after surgery; thus, it may be overlooked if the most recent electrocardiogram was obtained 1 day after surgery. Preoperative attention to congestive failure, bronchitis, hypertension, and chronic renal failure will smooth the course. Minimization of suffering, pain, and anxiety from investigative procedures requires careful attention to each patient's understanding and fears, as well as physical limitations and the presence of noncardiac disease. The monetary cost of diagnostic procedures is important and easily estimated, but the cost in terms of patient fear and complications should also be considered. Cost becomes a problem as the number of consultants used increases. Should the generalist manage asthmatic bronchitis that leads to postoperative pneumonia, modest renal failure, or preoperatively obvious coronary disease? At the authors' institution, primary care physicians typically request consultation with a pulmonologist, nephrologist, and cardiologist, believing that no expense is too great to ensure the greatest safety for the patient. Subspecialists are likely to prefer procedures to interviews, and the generalist may prove best when several body systems are failing.

CORONARY REVASCULARIZATION BEFORE NONCARDIAC SURGERY

The cardiologist's first thought is not estimation of the risk of noncardiac surgery but rather what can be done to lessen the risk. Interventions to improve blood flow through narrowed coronary arteries or through a diseased valve are readily available.

However, no evidence suggests that preoperative cardiac intervention decreases the rate of perioperative death or myocardial infarction. The Coronary Artery Surgery Study (CASS) observed 1600 patients who underwent annual coronary angiography for suspected coronary arterial disease for 4 years and then had noncardiac surgery within 1 year. The rate of death from noncardiac surgery was 2.4% in patients who did not have coronary artery bypass grafting (CABG) and 0.9% in those who did have CABG. However, the mortality rate within 30 days of the procedure was 1.4% (Fig. 20.1). Myocardial infarction occurred after noncardiac surgery in about 1% of those who had previously undergone CABG and those who had not. The CASS investigation is a good study of coronary intervention before noncardiac surgery; it suggests that previous coronary revascularization provides no benefit.

Angioplasty, with its negligible procedure-related mortality rate, seems an attractive means to relieve myocardial ischemia before noncardiac surgery. No large or randomized study has examined its efficacy in reducing complications of noncardiac surgery. In 1992, Huber and colleagues at the Mayo Clinic reported on 50 patients (31 of whom had class III or class IV angina and a positive stress test result) who had noncardiac surgery an average of 9 days after angioplasty. Angioplasty itself induced one non–Q-wave myocardial infarction and five emergency coronary bypass graft operations. Noncardiac surgery after successful angioplasty led to death in one patient and myocardial infarction in two patients. These results do not inspire enthusiasm.

In summary, no current knowledge suggests that intervention on coronary arteries lessens the risk for death or myocardial infarction (or, of course, for heart failure or cardiac arrhythmia) after noncardiac surgery. Need for noncardiac surgery provides an opportunity to recognize patients with coronary disease so that surgical treatment can allow them to live longer and better lives.

GUIDANCE FROM THE NATURAL HISTORY OF CORONARY DISEASE

The Veterans Administration Cooperative Study observed nearly 700 men with angiographically proven coronary disease who were randomly assigned to CABG or medical treatment. Only patients with stenoses of all three major coronary arteries and left ventricular ejection fractions less than 50% showed benefit from CABG (Fig. 20.2). Similarly, in CASS, 780 women and men with mild or no symptoms but angiographically proven coronary disease were randomly assigned to CABG or medical treatment. Mortality rates decreased only in patients with ejection fractions less than 50% and at least 70% stenosis of all three major coronary arteries (Fig. 20.3). Both the Veterans Administration study and CASS excluded patients with severe angina and those with more than 50% stenosis of the left main coronary artery because CABG was already known to relieve angina and prolong life in patients with stenosis of the left main coronary artery. Both studies reported that among patients with angiographically proven coronary

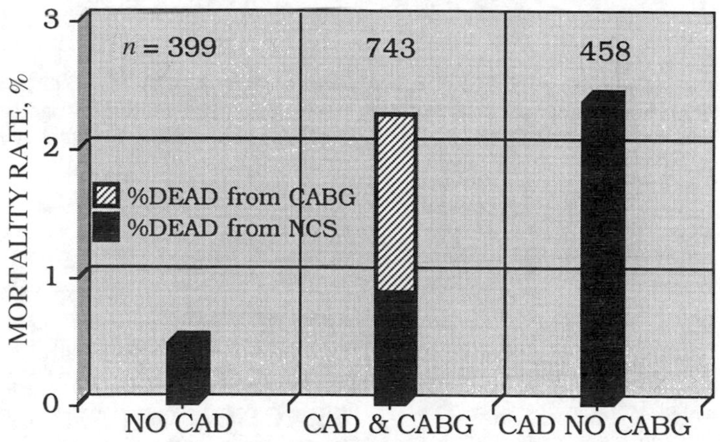

FIGURE 20.1.

Mortality from noncardiac surgery in Coronary Artery Surgery Study (CASS). A total of 1600 patients had coronary angiography for suspected coronary disease between 1971 and 1975 and underwent noncardiac surgery within 1 year. The "CAD + CABG" group had bypass surgery before noncardiac surgery. The mortality rate from noncardiac surgery was lower in patients who had CABG first (*middle column*), but the mortality from CABG itself almost canceled this benefit. *CABG,* coronary artery bypass grafting; *CAD,* coronary artery disease.

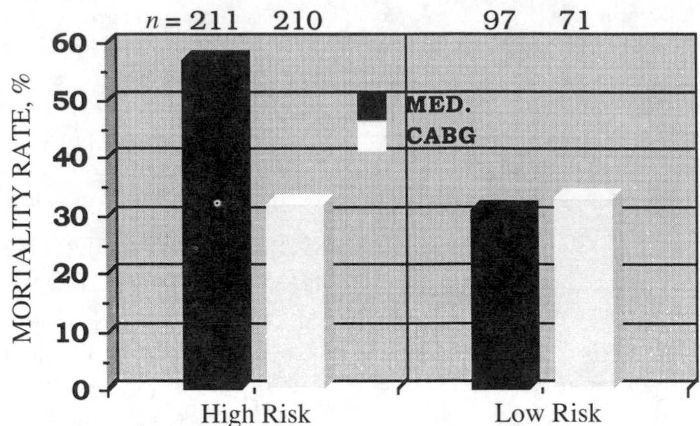

FIGURE 20.2.

Deaths occurring over a 7-year period in the Veterans Administration Cooperative Study. A total of 686 men with coronary artery disease shown by angiography were randomly assigned to medical treatment (*MED*) or coronary artery bypass grafting (*CABG*). High risk means that patients had stenoses in all three major coronary arteries plus a left ventricular ejection fraction less than 50%. Low risk means one or two vessel diseases and normal ejection fractions. Patients at low risk did not benefit from CABG.

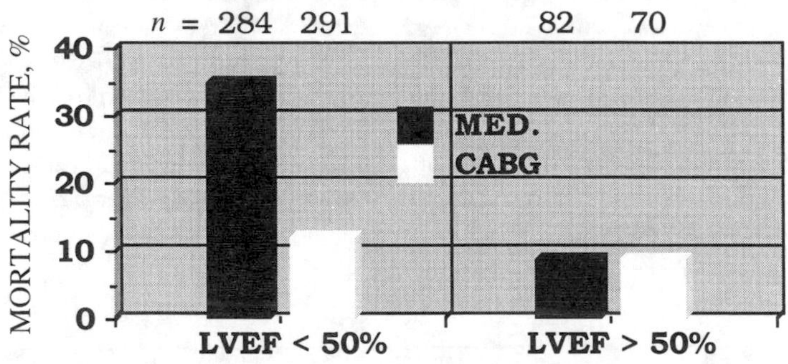

FIGURE 20.3.

Mortality rates at 7 years in the Coronary Artery Surgery Study (CASS). A total of 780 patients with stenosis of all three major coronary arteries shown by arteriography were randomly assigned to medical treatment (*MED*) or coronary artery bypass grafting (*CABG*). Only patients with three-vessel disease plus a left ventricular ejection fraction (*LVEF*) less than 50% benefited from CABG.

stenoses but mild or no angina, bypass surgery prolonged life only in those with stenoses in all three major coronary arteries plus ejection fraction less than 50%. The primary care physician whose patient will undergo noncardiac surgery should remember that no presurgical intervention is known to prevent perioperative cardiac death or myocardial infarction. However, opening or bypassing coronary stenoses in patients with severe angina, stenosis of the left main coronary artery, or three-vessel disease plus reduced left ventricular ejection fraction permits the patient to lead a longer, healthier life.

No one has suggested that any drug treatment before noncardiac surgery reduces the likelihood of myocardial infarction or death. Because of the long-term benefit from β-adrenergic blocking drugs after myocardial infarction, these drugs can be recommended for use before and after noncardiac operations.

SELECTION OF PATIENTS AT HIGH RISK FOR NONCARDIAC SURGERY

Peripheral Vascular Disease

Coronary and peripheral vascular disease are closely intertwined. For example, within 5 years after successful repair of abdominal aortic aneurysm, 35% of patients without overt coronary disease and 57% with uncorrected coronary disease die; 80% of these deaths are caused by coronary artery disease.

Coronary Artery Surgery Study

The CASS investigators examined the 8-year outcome of patients with peripheral vascular disease evident on angiography done at study entry. Of the 557 patients who had three-vessel coronary stenoses, more than 70% underwent CABG soon after entry and 284 did not. In the CABG group, 4% died and 6% had myocardial infarction within 30 days of CABG. Within 3 years, however, the group that did not have surgery surpassed the CABG group in number of deaths and myocardial infarction. At 8 years, death or myocardial infarction occurred in 50% of the patients in the no-surgery group and 35% of the patients in the CABG group (Fig. 20.4). Again, benefit from CABG occurred only in patients with left ventricular ejection fractions less than 50%. This study of peripheral vascular disease emphasizes the likelihood that severe coronary artery disease, even when minimally symptomatic, will develop in patients with peripheral arterial disease.

Veterans Administration Cooperative Study

The Veterans Administration investigators did almost as well in selecting patients who benefited from CABG by using simple clinical criteria as in selecting patients by using the angiographic criteria of three-vessel disease and ejection fraction less than 50%. The clinical criteria were hypertension, previous myocardial infarction, and ST-segment depression on resting electrocardiography. Coronary artery bypass grafting reduced mortality rates in patients who met at least two of the three clinical criteria and did not reduce mortality rates in patients who met one criterion or none, even though the patients had three-vessel disease and low ejection fraction.

Noninvasive Testing

As noted in CASS and the Veterans Administration Cooperative Study, left ventricular ejection fraction greater than 50% makes prognosis for life so good that intervention could hardly decrease mortality rates, even in patients with stenoses in all three coronary arteries. Two subsequent studies of patients with recent myocardial infarction emphasize the excellent prognosis with ejection fractions exceeding 50%. In the Thrombolysis in Myocardial Infarction Phase II Study, for example, the mortality rate during the first year after myocardial infarction was 1% in patients with a resting left ventricular ejection fraction exceeding 49% and 10% in patients with an ejection fraction less than 30%. A normal ejection fraction also indicates that few complications will occur after noncardiac surgery and that no further study is needed in a patient facing noncardiac surgery. However, a subnormal ejection fraction does not predict which patients will have cardiac problems after noncardiac surgery. Similar statements apply to other noninvasive tests.

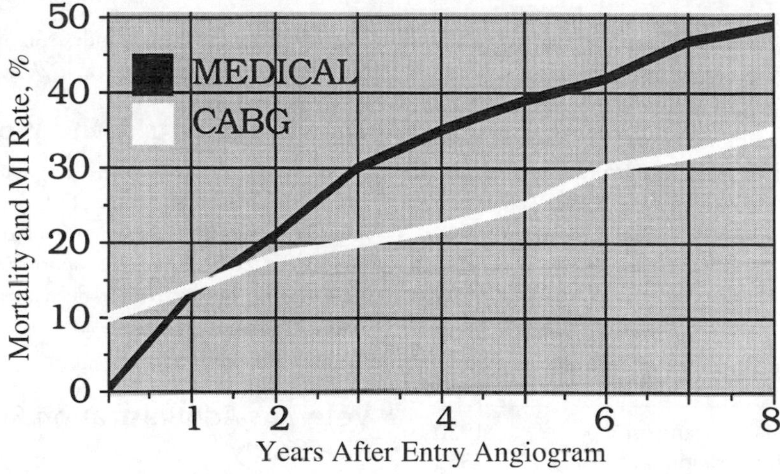

FIGURE 20.4.

Peripheral vascular disease in the Coronary Artery Surgery Study (CASS): death plus myocardial infarction (*MI*) in the 8 years after coronary angiography in patients who had stenoses in all three major coronary arteries and peripheral vascular disease. A total of 557 patients underwent coronary bypass grafting (*CABG*); 284 patients continued medical treatment. Although the immediate mortality rate from CABG was 10%, mortality was lower in survivors of CABG once 2 years had passed.

TABLE 20.1.

Test	Death or Myocardial Infarction after Noncardiac Surgery, %	
	Negative Result	Positive Result
Dipyridamole thallium scanning	1	17
Dipyridamole echocardiography	2	7–0
Dobutamine echocardiography	3	7–3
24-Hour electrocardiography	1	13–8
Treadmill alone (without thallium scanning)	14	27
Coronary angiography	0.5	4

Other Noninvasive Tests

The popular tests indicate that no complications will follow noncardiac surgery if test results are normal; however, many patients with abnormal test results experience little trouble with noncardiac surgery.

Treadmill testing alone (without thallium) is nonspecific as well as insensitive. The positive coronary angiogram includes single-, double-, and triple-vessel disease and any ejection fraction as a positive test and is therefore very sensitive and very specific.

All of the noninvasive tests seem to perform about equally. Except for the treadmill-only test, a normal result on any of these tests predicts a low rate of death or myocardial infarction after noncardiac surgery. An abnormal result predicts a higher rate of complications after noncardiac surgery but does not identify which patients will have complications. Coronary angiograms showing three-vessel disease and reduced ejection fraction suggest that an intervention should be done to prolong life; this could be performed before elective noncardiac surgery. The startling financial cost of these tests, obtained from 1998 charges at the Medical College of Virginia, follows (Table 20.2).

TABLE 20.2.

Test	Cost, $
Dipyridamole thallium scanning	1950
Dipyridamole echocardiography	1350
Dobutamine echocardiography	1350
24-hour electrocardiography	700
Treadmill alone (without thallium scanning)	625
Coronary angiography with left ventriculography	6475

ESTIMATING THE RISK OF NONCARDIAC SURGERY

Patients facing noncardiac surgery and their physicians need an estimate of risk for death and myocardial infarction. The latter leads to death within 30 days in about half its victims and irreversibly damages the heart in its survivors. Several plans have evolved.

The Goldman Criteria

In a basic paper, Goldman and colleagues found nine **predictors of fatal and life-threatening cardiac complications of noncardiac surgery.** These predictors, with their relative weights expressed as points, are listed in Table 20.3.

The following cardiac risk index summarizes the points for an individual patient in Table 20.4.

The Plan of Detsky and Wong

Detsky and colleagues added **angina** and **diabetes** as risk factors, and the results of dipyridamole thallium tests to derive the schema presented by Detsky and Wong (Fig. 20.5). This plan is popular with physicians, but care must be taken not to delay consideration of the diagnosis while awaiting results of the dipyridamole thallium stress test.

Veterans Administration Surgical Risk Study

The Veterans Administration Surgical Risk Study has reported on 16,000 men older than 40 years of age who underwent nonvascular surgery. Eighty percent of the operations were for gastrointestinal disorders and 26% were for cancer. The end point was **postoperative myocardial infarction diagnosed by new Q waves on the**

TABLE 20.3.

Predictor	Points
S_3 or jugular venous distention	11
Myocardial infarction in preceding 6 months	10
Dysrhythmias other than sinus or premature atrial contractions on preoperative electrocardiography	7
More than 5 premature ventricular contractions/min at any time before surgery	7
Age > 60 years	5
Emergency operation	4
Intraperitoneal, intrathoracic, or aortic operation	3
Significant aortic stenosis	3
General status	3
$Po_2 < 60$ mm Hg or $Pco_2 > 50$ mm Hg	
Potassium < 3.0 mEq/L or $HCO_3 < 20$ mEq/L	
Blood urea nitrogen > 50 mg/dL or creatinine > 3.0 mg/dL	
Signs of chronic liver disease	
Bedridden from noncardiac causes	

TABLE 20.4. Summing the points for an individual led to a cardiac risk index as follows:

Class	Total Points	Life-threatening Complications (n=39), %[a]	Cardiac Death, % (n=19)
I (n=537)	0–5	0.7	0.2
II (n=316)	6–12	5.0	2.0
III (n =130)	13–25	11.0	2.0
IV (n=18)	>25	22.0	56.0

[a] Myocardial infarction, pulmonary edema, ventricular tachycardia, each associated with 25% mortality rate.

electrocardiogram. Forty-three percent of patients with infarction died compared with 5% of those without infarction. Significant predictors of myocardial infarction in a randomly selected training set of 8000 patients were as follows (Table 20.5):

The investigators performed multivariate analysis to determine the odds ratios and point scores. Adding the point scores for each patient strongly predicted the occurrence of myocardial infarction in the other half (the validation set). The sum of points also predicted total mortality after noncardiac surgery (Fig. 20.6).

Patients with none or one of these predictors seem unlikely to need further study before noncardiac surgery. Even in the second risk group, almost 95% survived. These simple data provide a well-validated guide, derived from a very large group, of

TABLE 20.5.

Predictor	Odds Ratio	Points
Creatinine > 4.5 mg/dL	5.2	4
Angina in past month	3.3	3
Age > 60 years	3.1	3
Cerebrovascular accident with residual	3.1	3
Myocardial infarction in past 6 months	2.6	2
Preoperative glucose > 250 mg/dL	2.3	2
Emergency operation	2.2	2
Previous vascular surgery	2.1	2

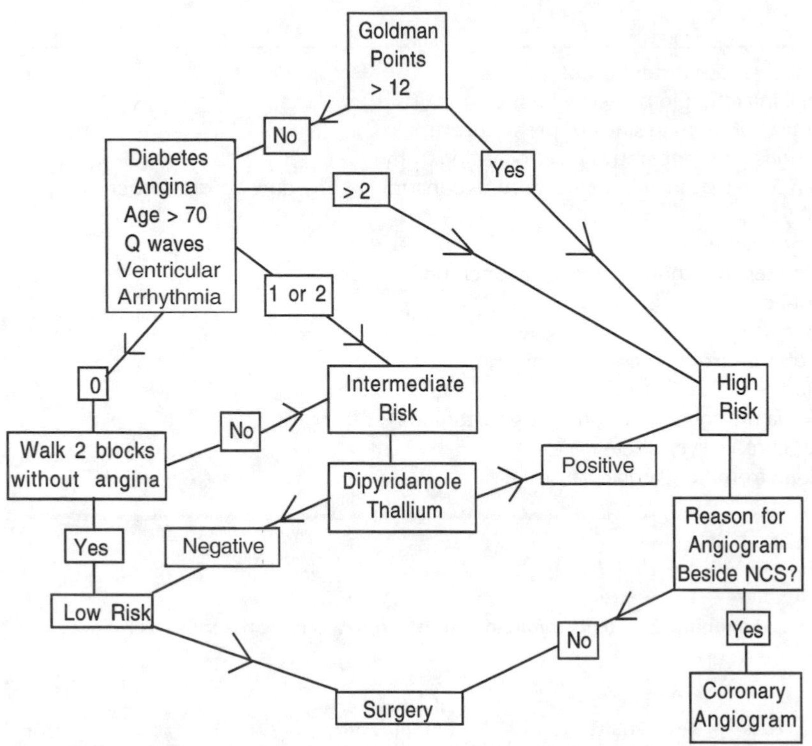

FIGURE 20.5.
The plan of Detsky and Wong. *NCS,* noncardiac surgery.

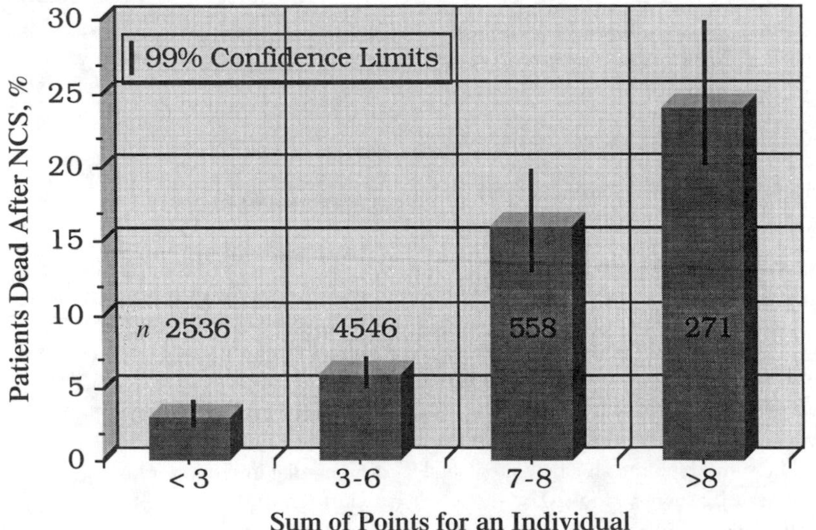

FIGURE 20.6.
Veterans Administration Surgical Risk Study. Simple measurements (see text) predicted death after noncardiac surgery (*NCS*) among 16,000 men. Vertical bars represent 99% confidence limits.

the risk of noncardiac surgery for men older than 40 years of age.

Braunwald's Textbook

In the 1997 edition of Braunwald's textbook of cardiology, Goldman states that patients can undergo **most operations with acceptable risk** if they can carry two grocery bags or a small child up a flight of steps without stopping, have normal findings on ambulatory electrocardiography for ischemia, or have a normal dipyridamole thallium scan. Goldman suggests that inability to perform the carrying task or an abnormal test result should lead to intensification of medical treatment if possible; if the abnormality persists, coronary angiography should be done to determine the feasibility of coronary revascularization. Braunwald's textbook presents the standard of practice for the cardiology community.

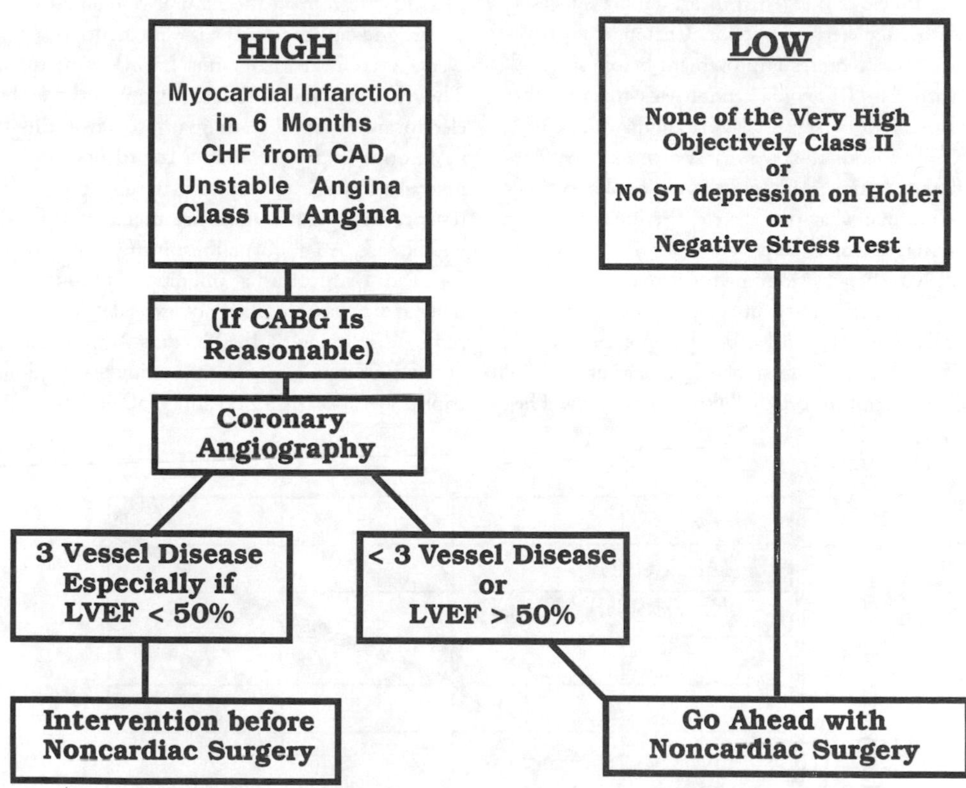

FIGURE 20.7.
Suggested plan for the primary care provider. *CABG,* coronary artery bypass grafting; *CAD,* coronary artery disease; *CHF,* congestive heart failure; *LVEF,* left ventricular ejection fraction.

Suggested Plan for the Primary Care Provider

The following plan was developed from the author's belief that

- One cannot predict which patient or even which group of patients will do better after noncardiac surgery if they first have an intervention to restore flow through narrow or blocked coronary arteries.
- Patients with severe disease of all three major coronaries plus a subnormal left ventricular ejection fraction will live longer if CABG is done.

Most of the information required in this plan (Fig. 20.7) can be quickly obtained from patient and hospital records. Previous congestive heart failure suggests low left ventricular ejection fraction. Current congestive failure, of course, requires improvement before surgery. Patients with class III angina cannot walk three blocks or climb one flight of steps. Class II angina can be objectively established if the physician watches the patient climb a flight of steps, perhaps carrying books to simulate Dr. Goldman's bag of groceries. Peripheral vascular disease suggests more severe coronary disease, which is more likely to benefit from intervention.

Among noninvasive tests, ambulatory electrocardiography is relatively inexpensive but has not been used much because health professionals have succumbed to the flood of literature on thallium scintigraphy. The electrocardiography laboratory must be told in advance that ST segments are the data of interest so that the portable recorders can be calibrated correctly.

The Asymptomatic Cardiac Ischemia Pilot Trial studied 558 patients who had coronary anatomy suitable for revascularization and had ischemia displayed during 48 hours of ambulatory electrocardiography. They were randomly assigned to revascularization (angioplasty or bypass surgery, depending on coronary anatomy) or medical treatment. After 1 year, 3% of patients in the revascularization group had died or had sustained an acute myocardial infarction compared with 7% of patients in the medical treatment group (P = 0.03) (Fig. 20.8). This trial supports the usefulness of ambulatory electrocardiography to predict the effect of revascularization on the natural outcome of coronary disease and emphasizes the low incidence of irreversible events even in patients not having revascularization. These findings and the relatively low cost of ambulatory electrocardiography leads many to favor this type of monitoring as the noninvasive test of first choice before noncardiac surgery. A normal result on a noninvasive test provides great reassurance that noncardiac surgery will be safe. An abnormal result indicates a higher risk for death or myocardial infarction, although the mortality rate probably does not exceed 5% (see the preceding discussion of the Veterans Administration Surgical Risk Study). Even if that estimate were doubled or tripled because of uncertainty about test outcomes,

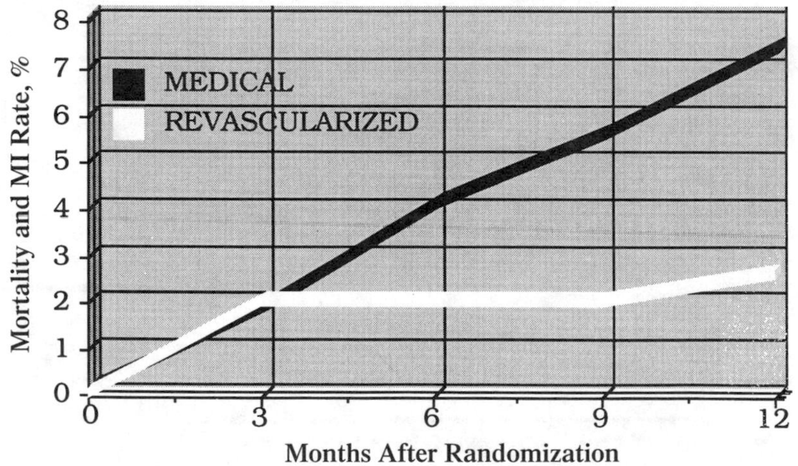

FIGURE 20.8.
Asymptomatic cardiac ischemia pilot study. A total of 558 patients had coronary anatomy suitable for revascularization and ischemia, as shown by 48-hour ambulatory electrocardiography. Patients were randomly assigned to continue medical treatment or to receive revascularization by angioplasty or coronary artery bypass grafting. In patients with electrocardiographic evidence of ischemia, revascularization appears beneficial.

many clinicians would prefer that risk to the discomfort, risk, and uncertainty associated with catheterization, angioplasty, and CABG.

SUMMARY

No intervention before noncardiac surgery is known to alter the risk of the surgery for patients with coronary artery disease or other heart disease. Revascularization by CABG reduces morbidity and mortality in the subsequent 7 to 10 years in patients with major narrowing of all three coronaries and subnormal left ventricular ejection fraction. Intervention before noncardiac surgery may prove beneficial for this group. Peripheral vascular disease and ischemia during ambulatory electrocardiography mark patients who are likely to derive long-term benefit from intervention with CABG or angioplasty. Several alternate plans are presented to estimate the cardiac risk in patients with coronary disease who face noncardiac surgery.

ACKNOWLEDGMENT

The author would like to thank Dr. Gottlieb Friesinger of the Verterans Administration Surgical Risk Study for Table 20.5.

KEY POINTS

When to worry about the risk for a cardiac event with noncardiac surgery:

- Known presence of coronary artery disease or active ischemia
- Valvular heart disease
- Congestive heart failure

For patients with one of these conditions, consider a cardiology consultation.

Coronary revascularization before noncardiac surgery: Case-by-case evaluation

- No strong evidence suggests that the preoperative intervention lessens morbidity (from myocardial infarction) or mortality rates.
- Guidelines: Triple-vessel disease with left ventricular ejection fraction less than 50% benefit from CABG.

Identification of patients at high risk for cardiac events undergoing noncardiac surgery: history and physical examination

- Presence of peripheral vascular disease.
- Left ventricular ejection fraction less than 50% with coronary artery disease.

A negative result on noninvasive evaluation is generally associated with a decrease in morbidity (from myocardial infarction) and mortality rates.

Estimating the cardiac risk in noncardiac surgery:

- Goldman criteria (in descending order):
  - S_3 gallop
  - Myocardial infarction within 6 months
  - Dysrhythmia (except premature atrial contractions on preoperative electrocardiogram)
  - More than five premature ventricular contractions/min
  - Age older than 60 years
- Emergency procedures, aortic stenosis, intraperitoneal, thoracic or aortic procedures, general status (chronic obstructive pulmonary disease, hypokalemia, renal insufficiency). The greater the point scale score, the greater the morbidity and mortality rates.
- Additional information: Angina, diabetes, and dipyridamole thallium study.
- Common-sense guidelines: Carry two bags of groceries or a child up a flight of stairs, normal results on ambulatory electrocardiography for ischemia, normal dipyridamole thallium scan.

SUGGESTED READING

Eagle KA, Brundage BH, Chaitman BR, et al. Guidelines for preoperative cardiac for noncardiac surgery. Report of the American College of Cardiology American Heart Association Task Force on Practice Guidelines. J Am Coll Cardiol 1996;27:910–948.

Goldman L. General anesthesia and noncardiac surgery in patients with heart disease. In: Braunwald E, ed. Heart disease. 5th ed. Philadelphia: W.B. Saunders, 1997:1756–1766.

Rogers WR, Bourassa MG, Andrews TC, et al. Asymptomatic Cardiac Ischemia Pilot study: outcome at 1 year with asymptomatic cardiac ischemia randomized to medical therapy or revascularization. J Am Coll Cardiol 1995;26: 594–605.

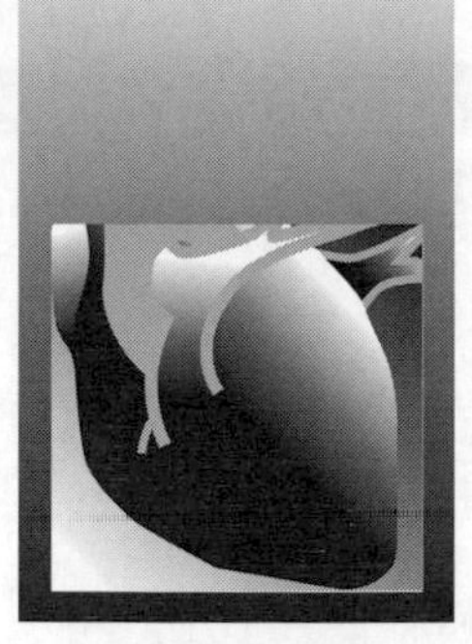

CHAPTER 21

Follow-up and Prevention

Michael L. Hess
Andrea Hastillo
William B. Moskowitz

BACKGROUND

The establishment of a firm and correct diagnosis is the first step in a logical approach to patient care. Next comes the formulation of an intelligent and meaningful treatment plan, whether medical, surgical, or a combination of the two. The next step, in some aspects more difficult than the first two, is appropriate follow-up and prevention. It is in this arena that the entire primary care team can participate fully and dynamically.

For the patient, appropriate follow-up and secondary prevention are essential to ensuring a full and complete life. For the long-term management of the patient, understanding of primary prevention is necessary for the patient's family and friends. The entire primary care team must fully support this concept.

PEDIATRIC AND ADOLESCENT CARDIOVASCULAR DISEASE

Complex congenital heart disease, corrected or uncorrected, should be managed by the primary care provider along with the pediatric cardiologist. Heart failure in a child requires modification of the drug dose over the course of treatment, a process necessitating careful communication between the primary care physician and the pediatric cardiologist. The primary care team has significant input.

Exercise and diet modifications (see Appendix B) can be reinforced on a routine, scheduled basis. Patient and family education about prophylaxis against subacute bacterial endocarditis should continue. Early education about the hazards of cigarettes and alcohol can be initiated. Consistent review of the medical program is absolutely required—keep it simple, with monotherapy if possible. Preach compliance; without compliance, success is impossible.

Corrected Atrial Septal Defects and Ligated Patent Ductus Arteriosus

Appropriate follow-up by the primary care team and awareness of when to refer to a specialist are essential. Corrected atrial septal defects and ligated patent ductus arteriosus with normal pulmonary artery pressures are among the rare cardiovascular conditions that can be cured. Patients who have undergone successful surgery for these two defects can lead a full and normal life (see Appendix B), do not require prophylaxis against subacute bacterial endocarditis, and, after the initial postoperative visit to the cardiac surgeon and pediatric cardiologist, can be followed by the primary care team.

Corrected Ventricular Septal Defects

Patients with corrected ventricular septal defects and normal pulmonary artery pressures can also lead a full and normal life (see Appendix B) but require careful prophylaxis against subacute bacterial endocarditis (see Appendix A). The presence of residual pulmonary hypertension should be managed by the primary care physician and the pediatric cardiologist, with referrals made at least once annually.

Marfan's Syndrome with Aortic Dilatation

The adolescent with newly diagnosed Marfan's syndrome plus aortic dilatation and the adolescent with hypertrophic cardiomyopathy present challenging problems. Not only must the appropriate medical program be followed and prophylaxis against subacute bacterial endocarditis be maintained, but profound lifestyle changes must be enforced. Contact sports and exercise done in "bursts" (e.g., sprinting) must be eliminated because of the predilection for sudden death from aortic dissection. This recommendation can be devastating to the adolescent and requires careful, compassionate counseling from the entire primary care team.

Valvular Heart Disease

Management of valvular heart disease, corrected or uncorrected, requires careful communication between the primary care team and the pediatric cardiologist. With uncorrected valvular heart disease (e.g., asymptomatic aortic stenosis or aortic insufficiency or mitral regurgitation), reinforcement of the medical program (such as long-acting angiotensin-converting enzyme [ACE] inhibitors) and education about subacute bacterial endocarditis are part of the regular routine. Mechanical valve replacement in the child or adolescent is a unique challenge when warfarin therapy is being used. Homograft valves are recommended in this population because of the risk for bleeding associated with warfarin therapy used to maintain the international normalized ratio to a value between 3 and 4 with mechanical valves. However, homograft valves in the young patient have a predilection for rapid and early malfunction. Homograft valve replacement dictates changes in exercise recommendations, diet modifications, and strict adherence to prophylaxis against subacute bacterial endocarditis. As a general rule, all patients with valvular heart disease should be seen by a pediatric cardiologist at least annually. The cardiologist typically examines the patient and performs echocardiography.

Hypertension

The major problem with the long-term management of the pediatric patient with hypertension is compliance. After a careful search for correctable causes of hypertension, the appropriate medical program must be simplified and continually reinforced. Appropriate diet and exercise modifications (see Appendix B) established in collaboration with the pediatric cardiologist must be continually reinforced.

Peer Pressure

The extra burden of peer pressure among children and adolescents must be constantly reviewed by the primary care team. Cigarettes, alcohol, and street drugs are problems ubiquitous in society. It is not enough to merely mention to the patient that these items are forbidden; the physician must reinforce this constantly. Cigarette smoke is an independent cause of type I vascular injury (along with sheer stress and hypercholesterolemia). Alcohol directly depresses myocardial function, and patients with primary cardiomyopathy, volume overload, or pressure overload who start to consume alcohol are creating a difficult and foreshortened life.

Finally, street drugs kill. Cocaine and amphetamines induce malignant ventricular rhythms that are magnified in the compromised heart. Needles, whether used intravenously, intramuscularly, or subcutaneously, lead to death; infections, whether caused by bacteria, HIV, or a hepatitis virus, are introduced; and endocarditis remains a fatal disease.

ADULT CARDIOVASCULAR DISEASE

Postintervention Care

Follow-up must be individualized for each adult patient with cardiovascular disease. In general, the primary care physician should be able to provide adequate follow-up of patients who do not have complications associated with the disease. Coronary artery disease and congestive heart failure occur so frequently that the primary care physician manages most patients with either disease. After a myocardial infarction, patients either undergo an intervention or do not. For those who undergo intervention, the usual procedure is cardiac catheterization followed by coronary artery bypass surgery, some form of angioplasty (with or without atherectomy, laser, or stent placement), or no further surgery.

Other patients may undergo risk stratification with some form of stress-testing after myocardial infarction and not undergo an invasive workup or procedure. In most institutions, the majority of patients who sustain a myocardial infarction undergo coronary angiography. This process probably excludes high-risk patients, such as patients who have postinfarction angina, patients who have had cardiogenic shock, and patients with a positive result on a submaximal stress test after myocardial infarction.

Angioplasty

Patients who have angioplasty have approximately a one-third chance of restenosis of the infarct-related coronary artery. Because of that possibility, it is prudent to obtain a "baseline" stress-nuclear test after percutaneous transluminal angioplasty. Recurrence of angina or the anginal equivalent should lead to immediate, repeated referral to the interventional cardiologist.

Post–Stent Placement

Post–stent placement therapy is in a state of flux. Anticoagulation with warfarin is used less frequently, and antiplatelet therapy is evolving as the key treatment to prevent occlusion of the stent. The use of short-term (30-day) ticlopidine therapy after stent placement requires careful follow-up (two to four times during the month) of the leukocyte and platelet count. It is hoped that the introduction of clopidogrel, with its decreased adverse effect profile, will replace ticlopidine. A postprocedure stress-nuclear test to define coronary flow should be obtained as a baseline, and any recurrence of angina or anginal equivalent should signal the need for emergency consultation with the cardiologist.

Bypass Grafts

Surgeons routinely discharge patients 1 week after bypass graft surgery. Postoperative problems specific to the surgery usually include wound infection, postoperative pericarditis, dysrhythmia (e.g., atrial fibrillation), and deconditioning. All but the last are usually resolved by the first postoperative visit to the surgeon. Most patients, provided they do not experience complications, can return to full-time work 6 weeks after surgery. A postoperative stress-nuclear test should be considered because patients with bypass grafts are likely to redevelop coronary disease and may require cardiovascular clearance for other than coronary grafting. Long-term, postbypass medical therapy should include aspirin (325 mg/d) and a coenzyme-A reductase inhibitor (a "statin" drug; e.g., pravastatin or simvastatin, 20 mg/d).

Post-Myocardial Infarction

Patients who have had myocardial infarction should be seen approximately 2 weeks, 6 weeks, 3 months, and 6 months after infarction. Once the patient's routine activity has been successfully reestablished, semiannual visits may suffice. Risk factors for coronary artery disease should be addressed repeatedly at each visit. Commonly administered postinfarction medications (ACE inhibitors, β-blockers [e.g., metaprolol 25–50 mg bid], cholesterol-lowering agents [Pravastatin or Simvastatin, 20 mg/d]) necessitate surveillance laboratory studies. Yearly electrocardiography is indicated.

Patients with complications, heart failure, residual unrevascularized coronary disease, persistent angina, or a multitude of risk factors require follow-up for electrocardiography more frequently than semiannually or annually. Patients with silent ischemia are problematic; annual electrocardiography and even stress-nuclear testing should be considered for these patients.

Congenital and Valvular Heart Disease

Patients with congenital and valvular heart disease are more difficult to manage and often require consultation with a cardiologist. Mechanical valve replacement requires long-term anticoagulation to prevent thrombosis. Warfarin therapy requires determinations of the international normalized ratio at least once per month, more frequently if the ratio is difficult to control. Echocardiography should be done after surgery to serve as a baseline in any patient undergoing valve replacement or valve repair. Valve surgery may leave abnormalities that mimic vegetations or other abnormalities; thus, a baseline for these abnormalities and chamber size and function is important. Any new symptoms or signs suggestive of endocarditis, valve leak, valve stenosis, or myocardial dysfunction should lead to consultation with a cardiologist and echocardiography. As long as the patient is asymptomatic, only semiannual visits may be needed in addition to determination of the international normalized ratio.

Porcine valves usually do not require anticoagulation. At about 10 years, however, they begin to deteriorate. At this time, annual echocardiography should begin. As with mechanical valves, certain signs and symptoms, especially the appearance of a new regurgitant murmur, should lead to immediate evaluation for valve dysfunction. Annual visits may be sufficient for the medically well-informed, compliant, asymptomatic patient.

Valve repair also requires postoperative echocardiography and electrocardiography; the frequency of follow-up visits depends on the patient's cardiac functional status and residual disease. Any patient who has valvular disease with residual and significant regurgitation should be followed carefully, with attention to the possibility of insidious myocardial dysfunction. Therefore, in patients with marked valvular insufficiency, concomitant cardiology consultation should be considered or, at least, echocardiography every 6 to 12 months with referral to a cardiologist if the ejection fraction declines. As noted in Chapter 9, normalization of the ejection fraction from a previously "supranormal" level in patients with aortic or mitral insufficiency means that significant myocardial functional loss has occurred and that the time for surgical intervention has probably arrived.

Congenital heart disease in adults often requires input from the cardiologist because so many of these patients are not cured. Congenital heart disease may

- Increase the potential for dysrhythmias
- Involve surgical procedures that involve implants that could deteriorate
- Be complicated by abnormal and irreversible hemodynamics
- Involve only temporizing therapies

Successful closure of a simple atrial septal defect, patent ductus arteriosus, ventricular septal defect, or coarctation of the aorta may require no special follow-up. Most other patients with congenital heart disease require cardiology consultation. Specific guidelines should be discussed with the cardiologist and information gathered from patient visits shared promptly.

Women with valve disease, coronary artery disease, and congenital disease may be at increased risk when they become pregnant. Consultation with the cardiologist followed by early counseling of the woman considering childbearing is important to the patient's care.

LONG-TERM OFFICE FOLLOW-UP OF THE ADULT PATIENT

Medical Management

Long-term follow-up of the adult patient with cardiovascular disease presents a unique challenge to the primary care term. Lifestyle modifications include

- Exercise recommendations (see Appendix B)
- Diet modifications (see Appendix B)
- Cigarette smoking cessation
- Decrease in or elimination of alcohol consumption

Lifestyle modifications must be constantly reinforced. In addition, many adverse drug effects, drug-drug interactions, and adverse drug reactions must be screened for and monitored carefully.

Coronary Artery Disease

The patient with coronary artery disease, whether surgically corrected or not, may receive four to five drugs per day. Typically, these patients receive 325 mg of enteric coated aspirin per day along with a β-blocker or oral nitrates, and a statin drug, with or without a long-acting ACE inhibitor. Compliance and cost becomes a major problem (see Appendix C). A history that includes

- Sexual history for **loss of libido** or **impotence** may incriminate the β-blocker.
- **Muscle aches and pains** many incriminate the myositis of the statin drugs.
- **Severe headaches** may incriminate the oral nitrates.
- **Chronic, nonproductive cough** may incriminate ACE inhibitors.

Nitroglycerin given as prophylaxis and therapy is a key drug for treatment of patients with coronary artery disease. Patients should be instructed to carry their nitroglycerin as far away from body heat as possible (in a purse or an outer pocket), carry only a small supply at any time, keep the "stock" supply in the refrigerator, and resupply from the "stock supply" every 4 to 8 weeks, thus ensuring an adequate supply of fresh nitroglycerin.

The use of the combination of aspirin and warfarin, which is increasing in patients with coronary artery disease or arterial fibrillation, requires careful monitoring. This combination is also used in most adult patients with mechanical valve replacements. Use of amiodarone plus warfarin requires careful monitoring of the international normalized ratio.

Prophylaxis against subacute bacterial endocarditis is mandatory in patients with adult congenital disease, corrected and uncorrected valvular disease, and hypertrophic cardiomyopathy (see Appendix A). Exercise modification in this patient population is also necessary.

Marfan's Syndrome

Like the adolescent, the young, asymptomatic adult with Marfan's syndrome and aortic dilatation or hypertrophic cardiomyopathy must be instructed to withdraw from contact sports. The patient with Marfan's syndrome requires extensive education and counseling. In the young adult, as with the adolescent, peer pressure for the use of cigarette smoking, alcohol consumption, and use of street drugs must be addressed. Street drugs kill young adults with cardiovascular disease, whether from the malignant rhythms of amphetamines, cocaine-induced acute myocardial infarction, or induction of severe hypertension with hallucinogens.

Congestive Heart Failure

Patients with congestive heart failure already receive a complex medical regimen with at least three to four drugs per day: digoxin, loop diuretics, long-acting ACE inhibitors, and aspirin. Warfarin is *not* recommended in patients with a reduced ejection fraction who maintain normal sinus rhythm.

Loop diuretics induce hypokalemia and hypocalcemia. Serum potassium and magnesium levels must be carefully monitored and, if low, supplemented. This supplementation adds another drug to the regimen. An added benefit of ACE inhibitors is protection against hypokalemia, thus benefiting the patient from both an economic and medical viewpoint. Patients receiving high-dose loop diuretics should be encouraged to take calcium supplements for their calcium loss. This is especially true when metolazone has been added to the medical program.

Most patients with New York Heart Association class III and class IV heart failure demonstrate ventricular ectopy or nonsustained ventricular tachycardia. Patients treated with type I antiarrhythmic drugs have been shown to be proarrhythmic. Even amiodarone has been shown *not* to be of benefit in these patients. Therefore, it is recommended that these asymptomatic rhythms not be treated with antiarrhythmic agents; rather, the underlying heart failure should be aggressively treated. If the patient develops the symptoms of syncope, near-syncope, or near–sudden death, that patient should be immediately referred to the electrophysiologist for evaluation for implantation of an automatic internal cardiac defibrillator.

Hypertension

The hypertensive patient truly presents a study of drug-drug interaction and a challenge for compliance. Every effort should be made for monotherapy or, if necessary, several drugs that can be taken only once per day. The physician can then instruct the patient to "put your drugs by the toothpaste and take them each morning." The recent development of long-acting preparations of ACE inhibitors, angiotensin-receptor blocking agents, β-blockers, and calcium-channel blockers makes this aim of once-daily therapy a viable goal. Short-acting calcium-channel blockers have become extremely controversial and probably should be completely avoided, but extended-release preparations continue to show benefit.

Lifestyle Modifications

Lifestyle modifications are just as important as pharmacology in the management and follow-up of the adult patient with cardiovascular disease. Obese patients with hypertension, coronary artery disease, or heart failure must be encouraged to lose weight and restrict salt and fat intake (see Appendix B). Regular, programmed exercise should become a part of the daily routine. Every effort to eliminate cigarette use and minimize or eliminate alcohol intake should be attempted. Every member of the care-provider office team should discuss and encourage these lifestyle modifications, not only with the patients but with their family, friends, and neighbors. Drugs do not help patients unless patients take responsibility for their care and become active participants with the entire primary care team.

KEY POINTS

Medical Management

- Nonpharmacologic lifestyle modifications are extremely important, including exercise, diet, cessation of cigarette smoking, decreased intake of alcohol, and obesity.
- Drug treatment after coronary artery disease (including treatment after percutaneous transluminal coronary angioplasty and coronary artery bypass grafting) should include 325 mg of aspirin per day and a statin drug.
- For patients receiving statin drugs, check liver function; decrease dosage for patients with muscle aches and pains (myositis).
- Ensure adequate dosing of oral nitrates.
- Check renal function and serum potassium levels in patients receiving ACE inhibitors.
- Ensure patient education and "drug freshness" of nitroglycerin.
- Administer prophylaxis against subacute bacterial endocarditis when indicated.
- Drug treatment for congestive heart failure includes

  DIgoxin (titrate dose to age 80 years, lean body mass, and renal function)

  Loop diuretics (monitor potassium, magnesium, uric acid levels)

  ACE inhibitors or angiotensin-I receptor blockers (monitor renal function and serum potassium levels)
- At signs or symptoms of malignant ventricular rhythms, refer to the cardiologist.
- Most patients receive their best and most accurate patient education in the office.
- Assign areas of expertise to each key member of the office team.
- Ensure that the office schedule allows sufficient time for patient education and risk factor modification.

PREVENTION

Pediatric Cardiovascular Disease

Cardiovascular diseases of all types may be genetic. This is certainly true for coronary artery disease, the risk factors of which cluster within families, but also for congenital heart disease. Genes and environment contribute to the cause of anatomic congenital heart disease. In approximately 10% of patients, the cause of congenital heart disease is solely attributable to genetic factors, with little contribution from the environment. Conversely, a small percentage of cases are purely environmental. Most cases (approximately 90%) are best explained by a gene-environment interaction known as the multifactorial inheritance.

Genetic Counseling

In families with a child with a congenital heart defect and a chromosomal abnormality, counseling is optimally performed by a clinical geneticist. The recurrence risk for heart lesions in subsequent offspring is related to the recurrence risk for the chromosomal anomaly. If the cardiac defect is part of a syndrome due to a single gene mutation, the gene will be transmitted in 50% of the offspring in cases of autosomal dominant genes and in 25% of the offspring in autosomal recessive genes. Other forms of inheritance produce a much lower risk for recurrence. If the first child has a congenital heart defect, the type of defect that may present itself in subsequent siblings is usually similar to that of the first sibling. The risk to the fetus if the mother or father has congenital heart disease ranges from 5 to 10%. Amniocentesis may be recommended during subsequent pregnancies to provide optimal information on recurrence risks. Fetal ultrasonography, which can detect significant heart defects during the early part of gestation, may also provide reassurance, as well as early detection of significant anatomic and functional heart disease.

Environmental Precautions

The importance of environmental contribution to the production of congenital heart disease is limited to specific situations. Known teratogens taken by women during gestation include lithium salts, which are associated with a higher incidence of Ebstein's disease. Diabetic women and women taking progesterone during pregnancy may have an increased risk for having offspring with congenital heart defects. The prevalence and severity of congenital heart disease in offspring with fetal alcohol syndrome depend on the amount of alcohol ingested by the parent. Specific infections, such as rubella (which is associated with peripheral pulmonary artery stenosis, patent ductus arteriosus, and, sometimes, pulmonary valve stenosis) are well-described. Other viruses may cause vasculitis and myocarditis. Intrauterine exposure to cigarette smoke is associated with high carboxyhemoglobin levels with a 2:1 fetus-to-mother gradient; this may result in significant fetal hypoxemia because of the lower birthweight, higher hemoglobin levels, and morbidity associated with premature delivery. Therefore, avoidance of known teratogens during pregnancy, as well as adequate prenatal care and adequate immunizations of women before pregnancy, can prevent many congenital heart defects.

Adult Cardiovascular Disease

Prevention in adult cardiovascular disease can be divided into primary and secondary prevention. In primary prevention, the goal is to have the asymptomatic patient assume a healthier lifestyle in order to prevent the disease from even occurring. With secondary prevention, a patient with a preexisting cardiovascular problem is encouraged to assume a healthier lifestyle in addition to learning about their disease in order to prevent a subsequent event. Both primary and secondary prevention can be focused on risk factor modifications (lifestyle modifications).

The concept of risk factor modifications involves extensive patient education, in which the entire primary care team can be included. The major risk factors to be addressed include

- Family history
- Obesity
- Hypertension
- Hypercholesterolemia
- Cigarette smoking
- Sedentary lifestyle

Family History

All too often, a pessimistic view of a family history of disease is accepted as a genetic predisposition to the disease process. To a certain extent this is true, but other environmental risk factors can cluster in the family environment and affect the patient. For example, a father and grandfather who died of myocardial infarction at a young age may have smoked two packs of cigarettes per day and had untreated hypertension. A definite family and cultural trend toward obesity is common. Finally, a predilection to a sedentary lifestyle can be "learned" from parents and siblings. Thus, once a positive family history is obtained, it behooves the physician to delve into this history to ascertain what is truly "genetic" and what is environmental and, therefore, what can be modified for both primary and secondary prevention.

Cigarette Smoking

Cigarette smoking represents a major modifiable risk factor for adult cardiovascular disease. Cigarette smoking has

- Strong correlation to peripheral vascular disease
- Moderate correlation to coronary artery disease in both sexes
- Weak correlation to cerebrovascular disease

Cigarette smoke is one of the three major causes of type I and type II endothelial injury and thus can adversely affect both the atherosclerotic process and hypertension. Primary prevention is imperative: if individuals do not smoke as adolescents, the chances are good that they will not smoke as adults. The primary care team can participate in local school campaigns and educational programs of the American Heart Association, American Lung Association, and American Cancer Society; they can also become proactive in government campaigns to further tax cigarettes and prohibit cigarette smoking in public areas.

Cigarette smoking adversely affects adults with hypertension, coronary artery disease, peripheral vascular disease, and heart failure. One must not simply tell the patient to "quit smoking" but rather must become involved in a program of cigarette smoking cessation. Numerous hospitals have evening classes aimed at this goal. A program using nicotine chewing gum and nicotine patches can be incorporated into the responsibility of the office nurse and nurse practitioner staff. Adolescents must be educated and committed not to start smoking. If patients already smoke, they must quit, and family and friends of the patient should be urged and educated to cease smoking as well.

Legal prohibition of cigarettes will not happen. It is the responsibility of the entire medical community to aid in education, legislation, and patient counseling to decrease the size of the problem.

Cholesterol

Hypercholesterolemia has been implicated as the single strongest risk factor for the development of accelerated coronary artery disease. An attack on this problem represents an attack on the entire atherosclerotic process. During the past 15 to 20 years, the incidence of coronary heart disease in the United States has significantly declined. This has been attributed to a diet lower in fat and a decrease in cigarette smoking. Simple, diet modifications for the family can be taught (see Appendix B): for example, switching from whole milk to skim milk and from butter to polyunsaturated margarines, decreasing red meat consumption, and consuming no-fat or low-fat dairy products. Weight loss is imperative because, in most patients, hypercholesterolemia is directly linked to obesity. Weight loss can normalize or decrease cholesterol levels in a large proportion of patients. For every 1 mg/dL decrease in serum cholesterol levels, there is a 1% decrease in the rate of death from coronary artery disease. Target cholesterol levels include a total cholesterol level less than 200 mg/dL, a low-density lipoprotein cholesterol level less than 140 mg/dL (preferably less than 100 mg/dL) and a high-density lipoprotein cholesterol level greater than 50 mg/dL. Exercise and weight loss remain the cornerstone of decreasing total cholesterol and low-density lipoprotein cholesterol levels while increasing high-density lipoprotein cholesterol levels. In women, estrogen therapy, when indicated, further increases high-density lipoprotein cholesterol levels. A natural example of this positive lifestyle change can be seen in a recent report that female marathon runners have significantly elevated high-density lipoprotein cholesterol levels.

The statin drugs have revolutionized the control of cholesterol levels. In the landmark 4S (Scandinavian Simvastatin Survival Study), the outcome of 4 years of therapy with simvastatin in patients with a coronary event (angina or myocardial infarction) was a 33% decrease in total mortality, myocardial infarction, the need for intervention (percutaneous transluminal coronary angioplasty or coronary artery bypass grafting), and hospitalization for unstable angina. However, these beneficial effects are not seen until plaque stabilization occurs, usually in approximately 6 months. Therefore, the earlier therapy with these drugs is started, the better. The target total cholesterol level in 4S was less than 180 mg/dL.

Recent, significant progress using Pravastatin has also been made in primary prevention. The impressive West of Scotland study reported decreased cardiovascular mortality and incidence of myocardial infarction in a high-risk population: asymptomatic men older than 45 years of age with at least one major risk factor. In elderly persons and in women, however, clinical judgment must dictate the use of the statin" drugs. Although these drugs can be expensive for daily use (see Appendix C), the overall decrease in morbidity and mortality and the cost-effectiveness more than offset the cost, which is truly less than a pack of cigarettes per day.

Obesity

The percentage of obese persons in the United States continues to increase. Obesity contributes to the morbidity of coronary atherosclerosis, hypertension, congestive heart failure, and diabetes. Recently, the former Surgeon General of the United States stated that obesity is the second largest killer in the United States. Thus, the entire primary care team must deal with this problem on a daily basis. Comprehensive office education on exercise and diet modification (see Appendix B) is essential.

Referral to weight reduction programs and programs such as Overeaters Anonymous should be encouraged. Carefully selected morbidly obese patients may benefit from surgical referral for gastric procedures. Finally, the recent introduction of centrally acting appetite suppressions may be of benefit. Careful avoidance of extreme diets should be encouraged. For example, some high-protein liquid diets have been associated with sudden death (ventricular tachycardia and fibrillation). Thus, the attack on the obesity problem should include diet, behavioral modification, exercise, referral if appropriate, and careful medical management.

Sedentary Lifestyle

A sedentary lifestyle is the risk factor most recently associated with heart disease. Physical education in schools should be supported, and a vigorous lifestyle encouraged, especially in children and adolescents. Activity learned as a child is likely to be translated into a more vigorous, active adult lifestyle.

Hypertension

The cardiovascular risk factor of hypertension is of such critical importance that a separate chapter has been devoted to the subject. Here we emphasize only nonpharmacologic lifestyle modifications.

Weight reduction with attainment and maintenance of ideal body weight appears to be the most difficult lifestyle change for many hypertensive patients. Furthermore, because the hypertensive syndrome includes hypercholesteremia, weight reduction assumes an even greater emphasis.

Cigarette smoking must cease. The combination of hypertension and cigarette smoking increases cardiovascular mortality in the hypercholesterolemic patient by more than fourfold (400%). Thus, there is a tight interplay between successful treatment of the hypertensive patient and risk factor modification.

Salt restriction continues to play an important component of hypertension management. The authors suggest a no-added-salt diet. Rather than suggesting prepared low-salt foods, the physician should emphasize to the patient the relative ease of simply not adding salt to foods and not eating heavily salted foods (see Appendix B).

Stress management and even biofeedback techniques have been implicated in the successful management of hypertension. The contribution of the chronic stress of family life, occupation, or environmental factors to the development of the atherosclerotic process of the hypertensive syndrome has not withstood critical analysis. Stress management techniques may be beyond the scope of the primary care team, but careful attention in the history to stressors in the patients life may indeed prove beneficial in the overall care of the patient.

Diabetes

The successful management of patients with type I and type II diabetes is obviously beyond the scope of this chapter. Suffice it to say that careful management of the glucose level, independent therapy for hypercholesterolemia with the statin drugs, and meticulous attention to the details of risk factor modifications have all been shown to decrease cardiovascular morbidity. The diabetic patient requires additional educational attention from the entire team.

Stress

The contributions of stress to death are controversial. There is no doubt that acute stress can precipitate angina and myocardial infarction. Obviously, identification of stressors in the patient's lifestyle is important for the overall management of the patient and deserves an in-depth analysis.

SUMMARY

In summary, lifestyle modifications and risk factor modification must play an important role in the management of the cardiovascular patient and the prevention of future cardiovascular events. This physician picks one major risk factor at a time and works on the problem. For example, the hypertensive, hypercholesterolemic patient with angina is first treated medically for the two treatable risk factors (hypertension and cholesterol); education and time are then devoted to cigarette smoking cessation. This is an opportunity for the entire primary care team to "subspecialize" in both primary and secondary prevention. The ultimate goal can be expressed in Robert Browning's famous quotation from Rabbi Ben Ezra: "Grow old along with me! The best is yet to be."

KEY POINTS

Pediatric and Adolescent Cardiovascular Disease

- Prophylaxis against subacute bacterial endocarditis: All corrected and uncorrected valves and shunts *except* corrected atrial septal defects and ligated patent ductus arteriosus.
- Complex, congenital heart disease and heart failure managed in consultation with the pediatric cardiologist.
- Reinforce lifestyle modifications and continuing education about limitations and exercise.
- Prevention of and education about cigarettes, alcohol, street drugs, and obesity.

Adult Cardiovascular Disease

- Individual patient care and education.
- After percutaneous transluminal coronary angioplasty and coronary artery bypass grafting, obtain baseline stress-nuclear study; 30% chance of restenosis.
- Monitor drug therapy: Ticlopidine, monitor neutrophil and platelet count; warfarin, maintain international normalized ratio at 2 to 3.
- After myocardial infarction: Monitor drug therapy, encourage lifestyle modifications, and minimize risk factors.
- After valve replacement: Monitor warfarin therapy (with mechanical valves, the international normalized ratio should be 3 to 4); prophylaxis against subacute bacterial endocarditis; yearly echocardiography and semiannual physical examination.
- Porcine valves may begin to degenerate at 10 years. Follow physical examination carefully. If changes are noted (reappearance of mitral or aortic insufficiency), perform echocardiography and refer back to the cardiologist.
- Valve repair: Postoperative echocardiography and prophylaxis against subacute bacterial endocarditis.
- Congenital disease in adults: Follow with the cardiologist; prophylaxis against subacute bacterial endocarditis.
- Women: Consider possibility of pregnancy in consultation with the cardiologist.

Medical Management in the Office

- Nonpharmacologic, lifestyle modifications extremely important: Exercise, diet, cigarette smoking, alcohol, obesity.
- Drug treatment for coronary artery disease (including after percutaneous transluminal coronary angioplasty and coronary artery bypass grafting): Aspirin, 325 mg/d.
- Statin drugs: Check liver function; decrease dosage for muscle aches and pains (myositis).
- Oral nitrates: Ensure adequate dosing.
- ACE inhibitors: Check renal function and potassium levels.
- Nitroglycerin: Ensure patient education and "drug freshness."
- Prophylaxis against subacute bacterial endocarditis when indicated.
- Drug treatment for congestive heart failure:

  Digoxin: Titrate dose to age, lean body mass, and renal function.

  Loop diuretics: Monitor potassium, magnesium, and uric acid levels.

  ACE inhibitors and angiotensin-1 receptor blockers: Monitor renal function and serum potassium levels.
- Signs or symptoms of malignant ventricular rhythms, refer back to the cardiologist.
- The role of the primary care physician and the entire "team" in prevention cannot be overemphasized.
- Assign areas of expertise to each key member of the office team.
- Ensure that the office schedule allows sufficient time for patient education and risk factor modification.

SUGGESTED READINGS

Modest GA. Cardiovascular risk factors: social determinants of cardiovascular disease. In: Noble JS, ed. Primary care medicine. St. Louis: Mosby–Year Book; 1996:148–178.

Multiple Risk Factors Intervention Group. Mortality after 10 years for hypertensive participants in the Multiple Risk Factor Intervention Trial. Circulation 1990;82: 1616–1628.

Rosscavio JE, Lewis B, Rifkind BM. The value of lowering cholesterol after myocardial infarction N Engl J Med 1990;323:1112–1119.

Scandinavian Simvastatin Survival Study Group. Randomized Trial of Cholesterol lowering in 4444 patients with coronary heart disease. The Scandinavian Simvastatin Survival Study (4S). Lancet 1994;344:1383–1389.

Shepherd JT, Weiss SM, eds. Conference on behavioral medicine and cardiovascular disease. Circulation. 1987;76(Suppl I):1–227.

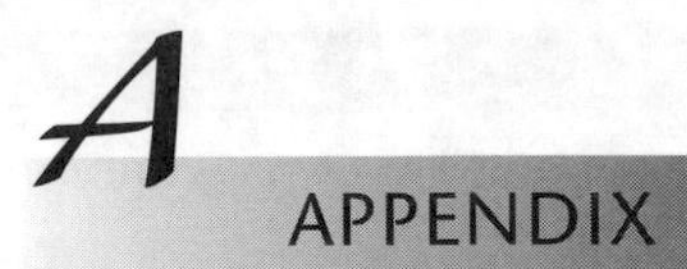

Subacute Endocarditis Prophylaxis: Antibiotic and Patient Selection

Michael L. Hess
William Moskowitz

A-1 For Dental, Oral, Upper Respiratory Tract, or Esophageal Procedures*

Situation	Agent	Regimen: Adult	Regimen: Child
Standard general prophylaxis	Amoxicillin	2.0 g	50 mg/kg†
		Orally 1 hour before procedure	
Unable to take oral medications	Ampicillin	2.0 g	50 mg/kg
		IM or IV within 30 minutes before procedure	
Allergic to penicillin	Clindamycin or Cephalexin	600 mg	20 mg/kg
	or Cefadroxil	2.0 g	50 mg/kg
	or Azithromycin or clarithromycin	500 mg	15 mg/kg
		Orally 1 hour before procedure	
Allergic to penicillin and unable to take oral medications	Clindamycin	600 mg	20 mg/kg
	or Cefazolin	1.0 g	25 mg/kg
		Clindamycin, IV 30 minutes before procedure; Cefazolin, IV or IM 50 minutes before procedure	

IM, intramuscular; *IV*, intravenous

*Adapted from Datani AS, et al. Prevention of bacterial endocarditis: recommendations by the American Heart Association. Circulation 1997;96:358–366.

†The following weight ranges may also be used for the initial pediatric dose of amoxicillin: <15 kg (33 lbs) = 750 mg; 15–30 kg (33–66 lbs) = 1500 mg; > 30 kg (66 lbs) = 3000 mg (full adult dose).

Kilogram to Pound Conversion: A-2
1 kilogram = 2.2 pounds

Kilogram	Pound
5	11.0
10	22.0
20	44.0
30	66.0
40	88.0
50	110.0

A-3 **For Genitourinary or Gastrointestinal Procedures***

Situation	Agents		Regimen
High-risk patients	Ampicillin plus gentamicin	Adult	*Within 30 minutes of starting procedure:* Ampicillin, 2.0 g IM or IV plus Gentamicin, 1.5 mg/kg (not to exceed 120 mg) *6 hours later:* Ampicillin 1 g IM or IV or Amoxicillin 1 g orally
		Child	*Within 30 minutes of starting procedure:* Ampicillin, 50 mg/kg IM or IV (not to exceed 2.0 g) plus Gentamicin, 1.5 mg/kg *6 hours later:* Ampicillin, 25 mg/kg IM or IV or Amoxicillin, 25 mg/kg orally
High-risk patients allergic to ampicillin or amoxicillin	Vancomycin plus gentamicin	Adult	*Within 30 minutes of starting procedure, complete injection or infusion administration of:* Vancomycin, 1.0 g IV over 1–2 hours, plus Gentamicin, 1.5 mg/kg IV or IM (not to exceed 120 mg)
		Child	*Within 30 minutes of starting procedure, complete injection or infusion administration of:* Vancomycin, 20 mg/kg IV over 1–2 hours plus Gentamicin, 1.5 mg/kg IV or IM
Moderate-risk patients	Amoxicillin or ampicillin	Adult	*1 hour before starting procedure:* Amoxicillin, 2.0 g orally or *Within 30 minutes of starting procedure:* Ampicillin, 2.0 g IM or IV
		Child	*1 hour before starting procedure:* Amoxicillin, 50 mg/kg orally or *Within 30 minutes of starting procedure:* Ampicillin, 50 mg/kg IM or IV
Moderate-risk patients allergic to ampicillin or amoxicillin	Vancomycin	Adult	*Within 30 minutes of starting procedure, complete infusion administration of:* Vancomycin, 1.0g IV over 1–2 hours
		Child	*Within 30 minutes of starting procedure, complete infusion administration of:* Vancomycin, 20 mg/kg IV over 1–2 hours

*Adapted from Datani AS, et al: Prevention of bacterial endocarditis: recommendations by the American Heart Association. Circulation 1997;96:358–366.

A-4 General Guidelines: Patients in Whom Prophylaxis Against Subacute Bacterial Endocarditis Is and Is Not Required*

SBE Prophylaxis Required	SBE Prophylaxis Not Required
Prosthetic heart valves—both tissue homografts and mechanical valves	Coronary artery bypass or percutaneous transluminal coronary angioplasty
Previous episodes of endocarditis, even in the absence of heart disease	Previous **Kawasaki's** disease or **rheumatic fever** without valve defects
Proven valvular heart disease—both stenotic and regurgitant valves (i.e., aortic, mitral, tricuspid, pulmonic stenosis or insufficiency)	Cardiac catheterization
Unrepaired **patent ductus arteriosis**	Repaired **patent ductus arteriosus,** 6 months after surgery
Mitral valve prolapse with regurgitation	**Mitral valve prolapse** in the absence of regurgitation
Hypertrophic cardiomyopathy with obstruction	**Primary cardiomyopathy**
Atrial septal defect and **ventricular septal defect** repairs within 6 months of surgery	**Repaired atrial septal defect** or **ventricular septal defect,** 6 months after surgery
Unrepaired **ventricular septal defects**	**Atrial septal defects** before surgery
Vaginal delivery in a patient with valvular heart disease in the presence of infection	**Vaginal delivery** in the absence of infection; delivery by cesarean section

SBE, subacute bacterial endocarditis.

A-5 Dental Procedures and Prophylaxis Against Subacute Bacterial Endocarditis*

Prophylaxis Recommended
- Dental extraction
- Periodontal procedures including surgery, scaling, root planing, probing, recall maintenance
- Dental implant placement and reimplanation of avulsed teeth
- Endodontic (root canal) instrumentation or surgery only beyond the apex
- Subgingival placement of antibiotic fibers or strips
- Initial placement of orthodontic bands, but not brackets
- Intraligamentary local anesthetic injections
- Prophylactic cleaning of teeth or implants where bleeding is anticipated

Prophylaxis not Recommended
- Restorative dentistry (operative and prosthodontic) with or without retraction cord
- Local anesthetic injections (nonintraligamentary)
- Intracanal endodontic treatment; post–placement and buildup
- Placement of rubber dams
- Postoperative suture removal
- Placement of removable prosthodontic or orthodontic appliances
- Taking of oral impressions
- Fluoride treatments
- Taking of oral radiographs
- Orthodontic appliance adjustment
- Shedding of primary teeth

*Recommended reading: Datani AD, et al: Prevention of bacterial endocarditis: recommendations by the American Heart Association. Circulation 1997;96:358–366.

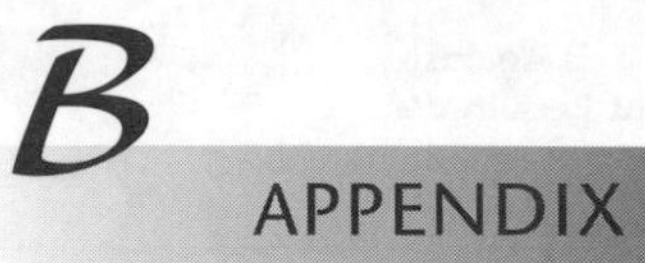

Exercise and Diet Recommendations in Heart Disease

Michael L. Hess

B-1 Isotonic and Isometric Exercise

Type of Exercise	Examples of Exercise
Isotonic exercise	Walking
	Hiking
	Golf
	Swimming
	Jogging
	Tennis (noncompetitive)
	Adult softball
Isometric exercise	Weight lifting
	Racquetball
	Football
	Hockey
	Basketball (competitive)
Sudden acceleration	Pushing cars
	Shoveling snow
	Moving heavy furniture
	Tennis (competitive)

Exercise in Pediatric and Adolescent Heart Disease B-2

Type of Disease	Situation	Exercise Recommendations
Unrepaired shunts	Left-to-right shunts that are deemed small (e.g., for atrial septal defects)	No restrictions
	Left-to-right shunts, moderate in size, with or without pulmonary hypertension	Preexercise evaluation by a pediatric cardiologist Low-intensity exercise
	Marked pulmonary hypertension	Low-intensity exercise only
	Repaired defects with no residual and normal pulmonary artery pressures	Unrestricted activity
Valvular disease	Unrepaired mild stenosis (e.g., aortic and pulmonic stenosis)	No restrictions
	Moderate stenosis	Preexercise, presport evaluation with a stress test by a pediatric cardiologist Typically, participation in noncontact sports allowable with a normal electrocardiogram and exercise test result
	Homografts (grafts and pacemakers)	No contact sports No isometric exercise
	Repaired coarctations	No contact sports for 1 year after repair Isometric exercise forbidden Normal activity allowed with resting gradient less than 20 mm Hg and normal exercise test result
	Kawasaki's disease	No restriction for patients with normal coronary artery anatomy as demonstrated by angiography With abnormal coronary arteries, annual exercise test following annual stress thallium study should be performed by a pediatric cardiologist
	Marfan's syndrome	With normal aorta, no restrictions; serial echocardiography must be performed With dilated aorta, no competitive sports; only low-intensity exercise
	Hypertrophic cardiomyopathy	No isometric exercise Low-intensity exercise only after examination by pediatric cardiologist

In the pediatric and adolescent population, all information should be shared with the family.

B-3 **Exercise in Adult Cardiovascular Disease**

Situation	Exercise Recommendations
General rule for cardiovascular disease	Increase isotonic exercise, especially walking
Coronary artery disease (unrepaired)	Exercise treadmill test to evaluate heart rate response to the onset of symptoms Exercise limited to isotonic exercise to the precalculated rate; heart rate in asymptomatic patient should be limited to 70–75% of maximal predicted heart rate Maximal predicted heart rate in adults is generally taken as 220 minus the age; 75% of this number is the calculated maximal predicted heart rate
Post–myocardial infarction Percutaneous transluminal coronary angioplasty Post coronary artery bypass grafting	After initial recovery period at home: Walking 5–7 days per week, 20–30 minutes per walk Increase frequency and duration to the point of symptoms Isometric exercise for tone are encouraged, but not for development of muscle mass; isometric exercise discouraged if patients need to hold their breath
Congestive heart failure	Isotonic exercise encouraged Standard walking program (5–7 days per week, 20–30 minutes per walk) Patients with symptoms: walk in a shopping mall to reap benefits of flat surface, air conditioning, and availability of benches
Hypertension	Isotonic exercise encouraged Avoid strenuous isometric exercise
Hypertrophic cardiomyopathy (documented by echocardiography)	Forbid contact sports, competitive exercise, and isometric exercise

B-4 **Meat and Seafood Recommendations for Patients with Heart Disease**

Choose only lean means and certain seafoods.
Limit portions to a 3-ounce serving (about the size of a deck of cards) no more than twice per day.
Limit the following meats to no more than three servings per week:
Beef: round, sirloin, chuck, loin
Pork: tenderloin, ham, leg (fresh)
Lamb: roast, loin, leg, arm
Veal: all trimmed cuts

Choose	Avoid
Skinless chicken breast	Liver, chitterlings, gizzards
Skinless turkey breast	Canned or potted meats
Smoked turkey breast	Red lunch meats
Ground turkey breast	Breaded and fried meats and fish
Fish and shellfish	Bologna and hot dogs (all types)
Wild game	Bacon and sausage (all types)
Canned salmon and tuna (packed in water)	Chicken and turkey wings
	Cheese

Cooking and Serving Suggestions for Patients with Heart Disease **B-5**

Type of Food	Cooking and Serving Suggestions
Meats	Buy meat, fish, and chicken without added salt, breading, or sauces Trim all visible fat from meat, chicken, and turkey Do not pan-fry or deep-fry Remove all skin from chicken and turkey before eating Bake, broil, roast, stew, grill, or pan-fry with a nonstick cooking spray Throw away all fat that cooks out of the meat
Soups and stews	Cool soups, stews, and sauces, and skim fat before serving
Eggs	Use egg whites and egg substitutes as desired Limit egg yolks to no more than three per week, including egg yolks used in cooking and baking
Dairy	Use skim milk or 1% milk instead of 2% milk or whole milk Avoid anything with the word "cream" in it: ice cream, sour cream, cream cheese, cream soup, coffee creamer (unless it is "light" or "fat free")
Vegetables	Eat unlimited quantities of vegetables Cook vegetables without fat or use only a small amount of oil or margarine Do not season with meat, bacon grease, fatback, or salt pork Avoid vegetables in cheese sauce or butter sauce.
Fruits and juices	Eat plenty of fruits and fruit juices; these are low in fat and are healthy choices
Breads	Eat rice, potatoes, pasta, breads, cereals. Substitute whole-grain (wheat) foods for refined (white) foods Best choices Brown rice Whole-wheat breads, bagels Bran cereals Whole-wheat pasta Limit intake or avoid Cornbread Spoonbread Biscuits Croissants Muffins Doughnuts and pastries
Fats	Oils and margarine are high in fat and calories; limit their use to 2 tablespoons per day Do not use shortening, butter, or bacon grease Use fat-free or "light" mayonnaise and salad dressings Use low-fat condiments Fresh, dried, powdered herbs and spices Liquid hickory smoke Catsup, mustard, barbecue sauce, steak sauce, vinegar, tabasco Jelly, jam, honey, syrup, chocolate syrup, sugar, and sugar substitute Extracts: e.g., vanilla, lemon, almond
Snacks (*For patients with high blood sugar or diabetes, use sugar-free food and sugar substitutes*)	Good choices Fruit, fruit juices, fruit juice bars Raw vegetable sticks Low-fat or fat-free yogurt Pretzels and fat-free popcorn

continued

B-5 Cooking and Serving Suggestions for Patients with Heart Disease

Type of Food	Cooking and Serving Suggestions
	Avoid
	Potato chips and dip
	Tortilla and corn chips
	Cheese puffs
	Regular popcorn
	Nuts and party mix
	Cakes, pies, cookies, candy bars, ice cream
	Eat in moderation
	Italian ice, sherbet, ice milk
	Graham crackers, vanilla wafers, gingersnaps, fig bars
	Angel food cake
Low-salt diets	Avoid
	Salt and salty seasonings (e.g., garlic salt)
	Olives, pickles, sauerkraut
	Canned vegetables
	Cured or smoked luncheon meats
	Canned meats
	Frozen dinners
	Salted snacks
	Stuffing, macaroni, rice mixes
	Instant soups
	Meat tenderizers
	Soy sauce and Accent®

Modified and used with permission from Martha Massie, Colleen Tansey, and John N. Clore from the General Clinical Research Center and Clinical Nutrition Services of the Virginia Commonwealth University, Medical College of Virginia campus, Richmond, Virginia.

APPENDIX C

Retail Price of Cardiovascular Drugs

Johnny Moore
Michael L. Hess

INTRODUCTION

The cost of drugs to patients is an extremely important concern to the primary care team. This concern takes on added responsibility when one considers that an extremely large percentage of patients with cardiovascular disease are either retired or on disability programs with fixed incomes and limited insurance coverage. In addition, patients with cardiovascular diseases tend to be receiving multiple-drug therapy. For example, the post–myocardial infarction patient can be taking aspirin, β-blockers, an angiotension-converting enzyme inhibitor, and a coenzyme A reductase inhibitor; the symptomatic patient with heart failure can be taking digoxin, a loop diuretic, and a long-acting angiotensin-converting enzyme inhibitor; and the hypertensive patient may be receiving several drugs plus a coenzyme A reductase inhibitor.

What follows is the retail cost to the patient, in units of 100 tablets, derived from a large retail pharmacy chain in Richmond, Virginia, as of mid-1998. Patients at our institution are urged to shop around and compare prices. The following now allows the person writing the prescription to do the same.

Drug	Dose (mg)	Cost/100 Tablets ($)
β-Blockers		
I. Betapase	80	206.97
Betapase	120	274.97
Betapase	160	342.97
Betapase	240	445.97
II. Corgard	20	122.97
Corgard	40	115.59
Corgard	80	194.97
Corgard	120	252.97
III. Nadolol	20	65.99
Nadolol	40	69.99
Nadolol	80	104.99
Nadolol	120	119.99
IV. Inderal	10	38.99
Inderal	20	49.69
Inderal	40	63.97
Inderal	80	95.79
V. Propranolol	10	12.99
Propranolol	20	13.59
Propranolol	40	13.59
Propranolol	80	15.99
VI. Lopressor	50	59.49
Lopressor	100	102.49
VII. Metoprolol	50	20.49
Metoprolol	100	23.99
VIII. Normodyne	100	67.99
Normodyne	200	92.97
Normodyne	300	114.97
IX. Sectral	200	123.97
Sectral	400	160.97
X. Acebutolol	200	76.99
Acebutolol	400	94.99
XI. Tenormin	25	100.69
Tenormin	50	91.99
Tenormin	100	149.99
XII. Atenolol	25	15.99
Atenolol	50	15.99
Atenolol	100	23.99
XIII. Toprol XL	50	67.97
Toprol XL	100	94.97
Toprol XL	200	173.97
XIV. Trandate	100	67.97
Trandate	200	90.97
Trandate	300	114.97
XV. Visken	5	99.59
Visken	10	137.97
α-Blockers		
I. Cardura	1	110.97
Cardura	2	110.97
Cardura	4	115.97
Cardura	8	119.97
II. Hytrin	1	134.99
Hytrin	2	134.99
Hytrin	5	134.99
Hytrin	10	134.99
III. Minipress	1	58.97
Minipress	2	75.97
Minipress	5	75.97
ACE Inhibitors		
I. Accupril	5	108.97
Accupril	10	108.97
Accupril	20	108.97
Accupril	40	108.97
II. Altace	1.25	89.97
Altace	2.5	89.97
Altace	5.0	95.97
Altace	10.0	107.97
III. Capoten	12.5	75.99
Capoten	25	75.29
Capoten	50	121.99
Capoten	100	201.97
IV. Captopril	12.5	28.79
Captopril	25	29.79
Captopril	50	44.99
Captopril	100	75.99
V. Lotensin	10	90.97
Lotensin	20	90.97
Lotensin	40	90.97
VI. Monopril	10	89.97
Monopril	20	89.97
Monopril	40	89.97
VII. Prinivil	2.5	64.29
Prinivil	5	84.99
Prinivil	10	85.99
Prinivil	20	90.99
Prinivil	40	133.97
VIII. Univase	7.5	58.79
Univasc	15	58.79
IX. Vasotec	2.5	94.97
Vasotec	5	84.97
Vasotec	10	88.64
Vasotec	20	129.99
X. Zestril	5	80.99
Zestril	10	80.99
Zestril	20	85.99
Zestril	40	128.99
Calcium-Channel Blockers		
I. Adalat	10	54.97
Adalat	20	90.97
Adalat	30	97.99
Adalat	40	167.99
II. Nifedipine	10	17.97
Nifedipine	20	24.97
III. Calan	40	51.97
Calan	80	68.97
Calan SR	120	114.97
Calan SR	180	117.99
Calan SR	240	133.99

Drug		Dose (mg)	Cost/100 Tablets ($)
IV.	Verapamil	40	23.99
	Verapamil	80	18.99
	Verapamil	120	19.99
	Verapamil SR	180	47.99
	Verapamil SR	240	49.99
V.	Cardene	20	57.97
	Cardene	30	83.97
	Cardene SR	30	84.97
	Cardene SR	45	123.97
	Cardene SR	60	145.97
VI.	Cardizem	30	46.99
	Cardizem	60	64.99
	Cardizem	90	81.89
	Cardizem SR	90	93.99
	Cardizem CD	120	102.99
	Cardizem CD	180	114.79
	Cardizem CD	240	166.99
	Cardizem CD	300	213.99
VII.	Diltiazem	30	16.79
	Diltiazem	60	23.99
	Diltiazem	90	29.99
VIII.	Dilacor XR	120	114.97
	Dilacor XR	180	130.97
	Dilacor XR	240	139.97
IX.	Dynacirc	2.5	81.97
	Dynacirc	5	112.97
X.	Norvasc	2.5	123.99
	Norvasc	5	120.99
	Norvasc	10	208.99
XI.	Plendil	2.5	107.97
	Plendil	5	112.97
	Plendil	10	191.97
XII.	Procardia XL	30	120.99
	Procardia XL	60	197.99
	Procardia XL	90	288.97
XIII.	Tiazac	120	100.97
	Tiazac	180	109.97
	Tiazac	240	148.97
	Tiazac	360	190.97
Coenzyme A Reductase Inhibitors			
I.	Zocor	5	158.99
	Zocor	10	180.49
	Zocor	20	320.99
	Zocor	40	320.99
II.	Pravachol	10	191.99
	Pravachol	20	193.99
	Pravachol	40	292.99
III.	Mevacor	10	144.97
	Mevacor	20	196.99
	Mevacor	40	357.99

Drug		Dose (mg)	Cost/100 Tablets ($)
IV.	Lescol	20	125.59
	Lescol	40	152.97
Diuretics			
I.	Lasix	20	22.99
	Lasix	40	22.99
	Lasix	80	43.99
II.	Bumex	0.5	45.98
	Bumex	1.0	58.97
	Bumex	2.0	90.97
III.	Demadex	5	64.97
	Demadex	10	70.97
	Demadex	20	79.97
	Demadex	100	258.97
IV.	Generic furosemide	20	9.99
	Generic furosemide	40	10.29
	Generic furosemide	80	13.99
V.	Generic bumetanide	0.5	25.99
	Generic bumetanide	1.0	30.99
	Generic bumetanide	2.0	35.99
Miscellaneous but Important			
I.	Cordarone	200	277.99
II.	Lanoxin	0.125	14.79
	Lanoxin	0.25	14.90
III.	Coumadin	1	55.99
	Warfarin	1	47.99
	Coumadin	2	56.99
	Warfarin	2	50.99
	Coumadin	2.5	58.99
	Warfarin	2.5	51.49
	Coumadin	4.0	60.19
	Warfarin	4.0	51.49
	Coumadin	5.0	55.99
	Warfarin	5.0	49.99
	Coumadin	7.5	89.19
	Warfarin	7.5	75.99
	Coumadin	10.0	92.39
	Warfarin	10.0	78.99
	Diovan	80	128.97
	Diovan	160	128.97
	Cozaar	2.5	117.99
	Cozaar	50	117.99
	Avapro	75	126.97
	Avapro	150	132.97
	Avapro	300	227.97

Index

Page numbers in *italics* denote figures; those followed by a "t" denote tables.